VITAMINS AND HORMONES

VOLUME 28

VITAMINS AND HORMONES
ADVANCES IN RESEARCH AND APPLICATIONS

Edited by

ROBERT S. HARRIS
University of Minnesota
Minneapolis, Minnesota

PAUL L. MUNSON
University of North Carolina
Chapel Hill, North Carolina

EGON DICZFALUSY
Karolinska Sjukhuset
Stockholm, Sweden

Consulting Editors

KENNETH V. THIMANN
University of California, Santa Cruz
Santa Cruz, California

IRA G. WOOL
University of Chicago
Chicago, Illinois

JOHN A. LORAINE
Medical Research Council
Edinburgh, Scotland

Volume 28
1970

ACADEMIC PRESS, New York and London

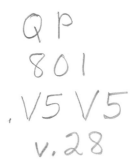

ACADEMIC PRESS, INC.
111 Fifth Avenue, New York, New York 10003

United Kingdom Edition published by
ACADEMIC PRESS, INC. (LONDON) LTD.
Berkeley Square House, London W1X 6BA

LIBRARY OF CONGRESS CATALOG CARD NUMBER: 43-10535

PRINTED IN THE UNITED STATES OF AMERICA

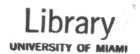

Contents

The Progressive Increase in Estrogen Production in Human Pregnancy: An Appraisal of the Factors Responsible

R. E. OAKEY

Insulin and the Pancreas

GEROLD M. GRODSKY

Regulation of Calcium Transport in Bone by Parathyroid Hormone

ROY V. TALMAGE, CARY W. COOPER, AND HAN Z. PARK

International Symposium on the Structures and Functions of Vitamin-Dependent Enzymes in Honor of Professor Hugo Theorell

Introductory Remarks

ROBERT S. HARRIS

Tribute to Professor Theorell

E. C. SLATER

Historical Survey and Introductory Remarks

HUGO THEORELL

Structure and Catalytic Role of the Functional Groups of Aspartate Aminotransferase

PAOLO FASELLA AND CARLO TURANO

Isoenzymes of NAD and NADP Dependent Dehydrogenases

G. PFLEIDERER

Role of Acetyl Coenzyme A Carboxylase in the Control of Fatty Acid Synthesis

S. NUMA, S. NAKANISHI, T. HASHIMOTO, N. IRITANI, AND T. OKAZAKI

Binding of Pyridoxal Phosphate to Apoenzymes as Studied by Optical Rotatory Dispersion and Circular Dichroism

OSAMU HAYAISHI AND YUTAKA SHIZUTA

Analogs of Pyridoxal or Pyridoxal Phosphate: Relation of Structure to Binding with Apoenzymes and to Catalytic Activity

ESMOND E. SNELL

Influences of Pyridoxine Derivatives on the Biosynthesis and Stability of Pyridoxal Phosphate Enzymes

FERNANDE CHATAGNER

Effect of Conformation on the Binding of Flavins to Flavoenzymes

K. V. RAJAGOPALAN, F. O. BRADY, AND M. KANDA

The Binding of NAD⁺ and NADH to Glyceraldehydephosphate Dehydrogenase

E. C. SLATER, J. J. M. DE VIJLDER, AND W. BOERS

The Role of Phosphopantetheine in the Yeast Fatty Acid Synthetase Complex

E. SCHWEIZER, K. WILLECKE, W. WINNEWISSER, AND F. LYNEN

Tricarboxylic Acid Activator-Induced Changes at the Active Site of Acetyl-CoA Carboxylase

M. DANIEL LANE, JOHN EDWARDS, ERWIN STOLL, AND JOEL MOSS

Thiamine Pyrophosphate-Catalyzed Enzymatic Decarboxylation of α-Oxo Acids

JOHANNES ULLRICH, YURI M. OSTROVSKY, JAIME EYZAGUIRRE, AND HELMUT HOLZER

Mechanism and Stereochemistry of Transamination

HARMON C. DUNATHAN

Roles of Vitamin B_{12} and Folic Acid in Methionine Synthesis

HERBERT WEISSBACH AND ROBERT T. TAYLOR

Chemical Properties of Flavins in Relation to Flavoprotein Catalysis

G. R. Penzer, G. K. Radda, J. A. Taylor, and M. B. Taylor

Model Studies on Flavin-Dependent Oxidoreduction

Peter Hemmerich

Flavin-Radical-Metal Chelates

Anders Ehrenberg

The Existence of Nonfunctional Active Sites in Milk Xanthine Oxidase; Reaction with Functional Active Site Inhibitors

Vincent Massey, Hirochika Komai, Graham Palmer, and Gertrude B. Elion

Quinones and Nicotinamide Nucleotides Associated with Electron Transfer

A. Kröger and M. Klingenberg

Au Revoir

Hugo Theorell

Contributors to Volume 28

Numbers in parentheses indicate the pages on which the authors' contributions begin.

W. Boers, *Laboratory of Biochemistry, B.C.P. Jansen Institute, University of Amsterdam, Amsterdam, The Netherlands* (315)

F. O. Brady,* *Department of Biochemistry, Duke University Medical Center, Durham, North Carolina* (303)

Fernande Chatagner, *Laboratoire de Chimie Biologique, Faculté des Sciences, Paris, France* (291)

Cary W. Cooper, *Department of Pharmacology, School of Medicine, University of North Carolina, Chapel Hill, North Carolina* (103)

J. J. M. De Vijlder, *Laboratory of Biochemistry, B.C.P. Jansen Institute, University of Amsterdam, Amsterdam, The Netherlands* (315)

Harmon C. Dunathan, *Haverford College, Haverford, Pennsylvania* (399)

John Edwards, *Department of Biochemistry, New York University School of Medicine, New York, New York* (345)

Anders Ehrenberg, *Department of Biophysics, Stockholm University, Karolinska Institutet, Stockholm 60, Sweden* (489)

Gertrude B. Elion, *The Wellcome Laboratories, Research Triangle Park, North Carolina* (505)

Jaime Eyzaguirre,† *Biochemisches Institut der Universität, Freiburg im Breisgau, Germany* (365)

---

* Present address: Institute for Cancer Research, Columbia University Medical Center, New York, New York.

† Present address: Department of Biochemistry, Catholic University, Santiago, Chile.

PAOLO FASELLA,* *Institute of Biochemistry, University of Parma, and Institute of Biological Chemistry, University of Perugia, and Center of Molecular Biology, C.N.R., Rome, Italy* (157)

GEROLD M. GRODSKY, *Metabolic Research Unit and Department of Biochemistry and Biophysics, University of California, San Francisco, California* (37)

ROBERT S. HARRIS,† *Massachusetts Institute of Technology, Cambridge, Massachusetts* (143)

T. HASHIMOTO, *Department of Medical Chemistry, Kyoto University Faculty of Medicine, Kyoto, Japan* (213)

OSAMU HAYAISHI, *Department of Medical Chemistry, Kyoto University Faculty of Medicine, Kyoto, Japan* (245)

PETER HEMMERICH, *Fachbereich Biologie, Universität Konstanz, Germany* (467)

HELMUT HOLZER, *Biochemisches Institut der Universität, Freiburg im Breisgau, Germany* (365)

N. IRITANI, *Department of Medical Chemistry, Kyoto University Faculty of Medicine, Kyoto, Japan* (213)

M. KANDA, *Department of Biochemistry, Duke University Medical Center, Durham, North Carolina* (303)

M. KLINGENBERG, *Institut für Physiologische Chemie und Physikalische Biochemie, University of Munich, Munich, Germany* (533)

HIROCHIKA KOMAI, *Department of Biological Chemistry and Biophysics Research Division, The University of Michigan, Ann Arbor, Michigan* (505)

A. KRÖGER, *Institut für Physiologische Chemie und Physikalische Biochemie, University of Munich, Munich, Germany* (533)

---

* Present address: Instituto di Biochimica, Università di Parma, Borgo Carissimi 10, Parma, Italy.
† Present address: University of Minnesota, Minneapolis, Minnesota.

M. DANIEL LANE, *Department of Physiological Chemistry, The Johns Hopkins University School of Medicine, Baltimore, Maryland and Department of Biochemistry, New York University School of Medicine, New York, New York* (345)

F. LYNEN, *Max-Planck-Institut für Zellchemie und Chemisches Laboratorium der Universität, Institut für Biochemie, Munich, Germany* (329)

VINCENT MASSEY, *Department of Biological Chemistry and Biophysics Research Division, The University of Michigan, Ann Arbor, Michigan* (505)

JOEL MOSS, *Department of Physiological Chemistry, The Johns Hopkins University School of Medicine, Baltimore, Maryland and Department of Biochemistry, New York University School of Medicine, New York, New York* (345)

S. NAKANISHI, *Department of Medical Chemistry, Kyoto University Faculty of Medicine, Kyoto, Japan* (213)

S. NUMA, *Department of Medical Chemistry, Kyoto University Faculty of Medicine, Kyoto, Japan* (213)

R. E. OAKEY, *Division of Steroid Endocrinology, Department of Chemical Pathology, School of Medicine, University of Leeds, Leeds, England* (1)

T. OKAZAKI, *Department of Medical Chemistry, Kyoto University Faculty of Medicine, Kyoto, Japan* (213)

YURI M. OSTROVSKY,[*] *Biochemisches Institut der Universität, Freiburg im Breisgau, Germany* (365)

GRAHAM PALMER, *Department of Biological Chemistry and Biophysics Research Division, The University of Michigan, Ann Arbor, Michigan* (505)

HAN Z. PARK, *Department of Anatomy, School of Medicine, University of Utah, Salt Lake City, Utah* (103)

[*] Present address: Department of Biochemistry, State Medical Institute, Grodno, Bielorussian SSR, USSR.

G. R. PENZER,* *Department of Biochemistry, University of Oxford, Oxford, England* (441)

G. PFLEIDERER, *Ruhr Universität Bochum, Bochum, Germany* (195)

G. K. RADDA, *Department of Biochemistry, University of Oxford, Oxford, England* (441)

K. V. RAJAGOPALAN, *Department of Biochemistry, Duke University Medical Center, Durham, North Carolina* (303)

E. SCHWEIZER,† *Max-Planck-Institut für Zellchemie und Chemisches Laboratorium der Universität, Institut für Biochemie, Munich, Germany* (329)

YUTAKA SHIZUTA, *Department of Medical Chemistry, Kyoto University Faculty of Medicine, Kyoto, Japan* (245)

E. C. SLATER, *Laboratory of Biochemistry, B.C.P. Jansen Institute, University of Amsterdam, Amsterdam, The Netherlands* (147, 315)

ESMOND E. SNELL, *Department of Biochemistry, University of California, Berkeley, California* (265)

ERWIN STOLL, *Department of Biochemistry, New York University School of Medicine, New York, New York* (345)

ROY V. TALMAGE,‡ *Division of Biology and Medicine, Atomic Energy Commission, Washington, D. C.* (103)

J. A. TAYLOR, *Department of Biochemistry, University of Oxford, Oxford, England* (441)

M. B. TAYLOR, *Department of Biochemistry, University of Oxford, Oxford, England* (441)

ROBERT T. TAYLOR, *Bio-Medical Division, Lawrence Radiation Laboratory, University of California, Livermore, California* (415)

---

* Present address: Department of Chemistry, University of York, England.

† Present address: Institut für Biochemie der Universitat Würzburg, 87 Würzburg, Germany.

‡ Present address: Orthopaedic Research Laboratory, Department of Surgery, School of Medicine, University of North Carolina, Chapel Hill, North Carolina.

Hugo Theorell, *Medicinska Nobelinstitutet, Stockholm, Sweden* (151, 575)

Carlo Turano,* *Institute of Biochemistry, University of Parma, and Institute of Biological Chemistry, University of Perugia, and Center of Molecular Biology, C.N.R., Rome, Italy* (157)

Johannes Ullrich, *Biochemisches Institut der Universität, Freiburg im Breisgau, Germany* (365)

Herbert Weissbach, *Roche Institute of Molecular Biology, Nutley, New Jersey* (415)

K. Willecke, *Max-Planck-Institut für Zellchemie und Chemisches Laboratorium der Universität, Institut für Biochemie, Munich, Germany* (329)

W. Winnewisser, *Max-Planck-Institut für Zellchemie und Chemisches Laboratorium der Universität, Institut für Biochemie, Munich, Germany* (329)

* Present address: Instituto di Chimica Biologica, Università, Perugia.

Preface

The Editors are pleased to present Volume 28 of *Vitamins and Hormones*.

This volume is composed of two parts. The first section contains three chapters reviewing estrogen production in human pregnancy (Oakey), insulin and the pancreas (Grodsky), and regulation of calcium transport in bone by parathyroid hormone (Talmage, Cooper, and Park).

The second section of this volume contains the twenty-one papers presented at the *International Symposium on the Structures and Functions of Vitamin-Dependent Enzymes* that was held at Lausanne-Ouchy, Switzerland on July 16 and 17, 1970. This symposium was dedicated to Professor Hugo Theorell, who, in addition to many other scientific achievements, was the first to demonstrate conclusively that an enzyme, the "yellow enzyme," was dependent for its activity on the presence of a nonprotein prosthetic group, the phosphate ester of the vitamin riboflavin. The papers of the symposium record and put into perspective the substantial additions to knowledge about the vitamin-dependent enzymes that have accumulated in the thirty-five years since Professor Theorell's pioneering discovery.

During the past twelve years, vitamin symposia have been published in six alternate volumes of *Vitamins and Hormones:* Vitamin A (Volume 18); Vitamin E (Volume 20); Vitamin B_6 (Volume 22); Vitamin K and Related Quinones (Volume 24); Vitamin-Related Anemias (Volume 26); and Vitamin-Dependent Enzymes (Volume 28). We are indebted to Hoffman-LaRoche, Inc., of Basel, Switzerland and Nutley, New Jersey for generously supporting these symposia and for underwriting the extra costs of publication of these proceedings.

With this volume we are obliged to announce that after seven years of energetic and dedicated service as an Editor of Volumes 21 through 27, Dr. John A. Loraine has resigned. We are happy that he will remain as a Consulting Editor, in which role we shall have the opportunity to benefit from his assistance and wise counsel.

We are happy to announce that Dr. John Glover, Professor of Biochemistry, University of Liverpool, England, will join the editorial board of *Vitamins and Hormones* beginning with Volume 29. As previously announced, Dr. Egon Diczfalusy, Professor of Reproductive Endocrinology and Director of the Reproductive Endocrinology Research Unit,

Swedish Medical Research Council, Karolinska Sjukhuset, Stockholm, became a co-editor of *Vitamins and Hormones* with the present volume.

ROBERT S. HARRIS
PAUL L. MUNSON
EGON DICZFALUSY

VITAMINS AND HORMONES

VOLUME 28

The Progressive Increase in Estrogen Production in Human Pregnancy: An Appraisal of the Factors Responsible

R. E. OAKEY

Division of Steroid Endocrinology, Department of Chemical Pathology, School of Medicine, University of Leeds, Leeds, England

I. Summary

From a brief review of the pathways of estrogen biosynthesis in late pregnancy, it is concluded that estrogens are synthesized in the placenta largely from androgen sulfates secreted by the fetal zone of the fetal adrenal. It is argued that the level of supply of these precursors determines the quantity of estrogen produced. Evidence is reviewed from which it is concluded that adrenocorticotropic hormone (ACTH) secreted by the fetal pituitary is the factor which stimulates androgen production by the fetal adrenal. In turn, the concentration of cortisol in the fetus is seen as regulating the secretion of ACTH.

Consideration is given to factors which modify the concentration of cortisol in the fetal circulation. These are discussed in terms of synthesis, metabolism, transport from the maternal system, and transport to the maternal system. It is concluded that in late pregnancy cortisol is largely synthesized by the fetal zone of the fetal adrenal from progesterone derived from the placenta. Cortisol is lost from the circulation by metab-

1

olism in the liver and by transport to the mother. A major factor in facilitating this cortisol transport is the smaller number of available binding sites for cortisol in the fetal plasma than in maternal plasma.

It is suggested that the imposition of this means of cortisol loss on the normal apparatus for cortisol homeostasis (i.e., hypothalamus-pituitary-adrenal axis and liver), in effect, increases the metabolic clearance rate of cortisol and provokes an increased secretion of ACTH from the fetal pituitary. In consequence, adrenal growth and steroid secretion are enhanced. However, due to deficiencies of certain enzymes required for cortisol biosynthesis from cholesterol, notably a lack of 3β-hydroxy-steroid dehydrogenase, the effect of increased ACTH secretion is to increase the production of pregnenolone sulfate and dehydroepiandrosterone sulfate and, therefore, to increase the supply of estrogen precursors to the placenta.

These conclusions are discussed in relation to other theories regarding the control of estrogen synthesis in pregnancy, the effect of corticosteroid treatment of the mother on adrenal function after birth and the degeneration of the fetal zone.

It is considered that the hypothesis presented reconciles many available data regarding estrogen production during the last half of human pregnancy. It is hoped that stimulation of interest in this subject will enable our understanding of these processes to be improved.

II. INTRODUCTION

A characteristic feature of human pregnancy is the progressive increase in the production of estrogens, in particular of estriol, as gestation advances. Significant increases in estrogen synthesis during pregnancy have been noted in other species, for example, in the cow (Mellin and Erb, 1965), the horse (Savard, 1961), the pig (Raeside, 1963), and the rhesus monkey (Hopper and Tullner, 1967), but the excretion of large quantities of estriol appears to be confined to human pregnancy. The presence of estrogens in pregnancy urine was recognized by Aschheim and Zondek (1927) on the basis of bioassays. Almost 30 years later, J. B. Brown (1956) made reliable quantitative measurements by a chemical method and substantiated the original observations.

Since 1956 knowledge of steroid biosynthesis and metabolism in pregnancy has advanced, stimulated by the techniques and investigations pioneered by Ryan and by Diczfalusy. From earlier ideas (Halban, 1905), it seemed that the placenta was responsible for the hormonal changes in pregnancy. It has since been recognized that the fetus plays an important role in many aspects of pregnancy and especially in estrogen production (Diczfalusy, 1964, 1969). Nevertheless, our present understanding is based, to a large extent, on the results of perfusion experiments carried out early in pregnancy or at midterm and on experiments *in vitro* with tissue obtained early in pregnancy or after delivery. Except in rare instances, information regarding steroid production by the fetus *in utero* has been, of necessity, indirect. While examination of cord blood provides valuable information (Eberlein, 1965), the influence of the stress of delivery or surgical intervention on the steroid content of such samples (Migeon *et al.*, 1956) must not be overlooked. Reservations such as these have rightly led to caution in the acceptance of the results as reflecting completely the physiological situation. Seen in the context of estrogen production in normal and pathological pregnancies, however, the pathways of estrogen biosynthesis in pregnancy appear to be firmly established.

While our understanding of the means by which estrogen is synthesized in pregnancy has improved, the factors responsible for stimulating the progressive increase in estrogen production have not yet been clearly defined. Fetal death or complications such as maternal hypertension or toxemia often reduce estrogen excretion and it is implied, reduce estrogen production. The extent of the reduction from the level in normal pregnancy often reflects the severity of the complications (e.g., Heys *et al.*, 1968, 1969). However, low estriol excretion in such situations is usually considered to be associated with poor function of the fetus, placenta or maternal kidney in general terms, rather than with a reversal of the specific mechanism(s) responsible for the increased production noted in uncomplicated pregnancies.

The production of a particular hormone by an endocrine gland has often been rationalized as satisfying a precise purpose, for example, in the case of insulin production by the pancreas or aldosterone production by the adrenal cortex. Such rationalizations have aided the exploration and identification of factors which stimulate or inhibit production of the hormone. No clear need has yet been recognized for the large quantities of estrogens produced in late pregnancy. This lack of understanding could perhaps have hindered the recognition of factors controlling estrogen production. Paradoxically, diversion of effort into a search for a requirement for estrogens in late pregnancy may have delayed the definition of the controlling factors.

The purpose of this article is to review current information relating to the control of estrogen production during the last half of pregnancies free from complications and to draw attention to factors responsible for the increased estrogen production which is observed. Deliberately, it was decided to confine information for the basis of this review almost entirely to that relating to human subjects. Many features of estrogen production appear, at present, to be peculiar to human pregnancy. Transposition of data obtained from other species to the human may be less justified than usual. As our understanding of other species improves it may be possible to consider their particular problems in the light of information drawn together in the present article.

III. Nomenclature

Most steroids are referred to by their trivial names; the systematic names are listed below.

Trivial name	Systematic name
Aldosterone	18,11-Hemiacetal of 11β,21-dihydroxy-3,20-dioxo-4-pregnen-18-al
Androstenedione	4-Androstene-3,17-dione
Cholesterol	5-Cholesten-3β-ol
Corticosterone	11β,21-Dihydroxy-4-pregnene-3,20-dione
Cortisol	11β,17α,21-Trihydroxy-4-pregnene-3,20-dione
Cortisone	17α,21-Dihydroxy-4-pregnene-3,11,20-trione
Dehydroepiandrosterone	3β-Hydroxy-5-androsten-17-one
Dehydroepiandrosterone sulfate	5-Androsten-3β-yl-sulfate-17-one
16α-Hydroxydehydro-epiandrosterone	3β,16α-Dihydroxy-5-androsten-17-one
16α-Hydroxydehydroepian-drosterone sulfate	16α-Hydroxy-5-androsten-3β-yl-sulfate-17-one
11-Deoxycortisol	17α,21-Dihydroxy-4-pregnene-3,20-dione
Dexamethasone	9α-Fluoro-16α-methyl-11β,17α,21-trihydroxy-1,4-pregnadiene-3,20-dione
16α-Hydroxyestrone	3,16α-Dihydroxy-1,3,5(10)-estratrien-17-one
Estradiol-17β	3,17β-Dihydroxy-1,3,5(10)-estratriene
Estriol	3,16α,17β-Trihydroxy-1,3,5(10)-estratriene
Estrone	3-Hydroxy-1,3,5(10)-estratrien-17-one
Prednisone	17α,21-Dihydroxy-1,4-pregnadiene-3,11,20-trione
Pregnanediol	3α,20α-Dihydroxy-5β-pregnane
Pregnenolone	3β-Hydroxy-5-pregnen-20-one
Pregnenolone sulfate	5-Pregnen-3β-yl-sulfate-20-one
17α-Hydroxypregnenolone	3β,17α-Dihydroxy-5-pregnen-20-one
Progesterone	4-Pregnene-3,20-dione
17α-Hydroxyprogesterone	17α-Hydroxy-4-pregnene-3,20-dione

IV. Quantitative Aspects

One week before menstruation a nonpregnant woman excretes approximately 20 μg of estriol, 10 μg of estrone, and 4 μg of estradiol-17β daily (J. B. Brown, 1959). The exact quantities vary widely in different individuals, but the total excretion rarely exceeds 100 μg (J. B. Brown et al., 1959). If pregnancy occurs, the quantity of estrogen excreted increases at once and progressively so that at term the daily excretion may be 40 mg of estriol, 2 mg of estrone, and 1 mg of estradiol-17β (J. B. Brown, 1956). Many other estrogens can also be found in late pregnancy urine in quantities greater than those in urine from nonpregnant women (for review, see Breuer, 1962), but estriol accounts for 85–90% of the estrogens which can be measured in late pregnancy urine (J. B. Brown, 1956; Hobkirk and Nilsen, 1962).

Some idea of the quantity of estrogen produced, as distinguished from that determined in maternal urine, can be obtained from a knowledge of the umbilical blood flow rate and the difference in concentration of recognized estrogen precursors in the umbilical artery and vein. Dawes (1968) reviewed published measurements of umbilical blood flow and concluded that the flow rate was likely to be 100–150 ml/kg/min and probably approached the higher value. Simmer et al. (1964) and Easterling et al. (1966) found mean arteriovenous differences of 32 μg per 100 ml of plasma for dehydroepiandrosterone sulfate and 70 μg per 100 ml of plasma for 16α-hydroxydehydroepiandrosterone sulfate. These compounds are now recognized as the major precursors of estrogen in late pregnancy (see Section V). It can be calculated from these data that approximately 330 mg of estrogen is produced daily near term by a fetus weighing 3 kg. Estimation of urinary estrogens can account for only a small portion of this calculated production rate. This discrepancy may arise because differences in the concentration of estrogen precursors in the umbilical artery and vein plasma, measured after delivery, fail to reflect accurately the utilization of the precursors by the placenta before delivery. Furthermore, the relative recovery of different estrogens from urine may also contribute to the inconsistency. For example, J. B. Brown (1960) found that the greater part of estradiol-17β administered to a nonpregnant woman could not be recovered as recognizable estrogens. Goebelsmann et al. (1965) infused women in mid-pregnancy with radioactive estriol conjugates and recovered 66–87% of this material as estrogen conjugates in the urine. The difficulties in the determination of estrogen secretion rates in pregnant women have been discussed by Gurpide et al. (1962). Firm conclusions cannot be reached at present as to the quantity of estrogen secreted daily, but the evidence discussed above suggests it is likely to be in excess of 100 mg.

V. ESTROGEN BIOSYNTHESIS IN PREGNANCY

In the first two months of pregnancy the maternal ovary and, in particular, the corpus luteum is responsible for estrogen production. Initially, estrogen and progesterone are necessary for the proper development and maintenance of the uterine endometrium for successful implantation of the fertilized egg. By the ninth week of pregnancy steroid production by the ovary wanes (Mikhail and Allen, 1967; Yoshimi *et al.*, 1969). After this time ovariectomy can be carried out with much less risk of interruption of the pregnancy (Ask-Upmark, 1926; Tulsky and Koff, 1957; Diczfalusy and Borell, 1961; Rebbe and Møller, 1966) than before (K. M. Wilson, 1937). Nevertheless, estrogen and progesterone production continue to increase. From this time onward the growing fetus and placenta, operating in concert, are responsible for the production of most of the estrogen and the placenta is responsible for the production of the progesterone.

The broad outline of the major pathways of estrogen biosynthesis during the latter half of pregnancy, when the so-called fetoplacental unit has assumed a dominant role in estrogen production, is shown in Fig. 1. The major route appears to be secretion of dehydroepiandrosterone sulfate by the fetal adrenal and, in particular, by the "fetal" zone (Colás and Heinrichs, 1965; Easterling *et al.*, 1966), hydroxylation at C-16α by the fetal liver (Slaunwhite *et al.*, 1965; Heinrichs *et al.*, 1966; Bolté *et al.*, 1966), and conversion of 16α-hydroxydehydroepiandrosterone sulfate to estriol by the placenta (Ryan, 1959; Kirschner *et al.*, 1966; Dell'Acqua *et al.*, 1967). A portion of the dehydroepiandrosterone sulfate secreted

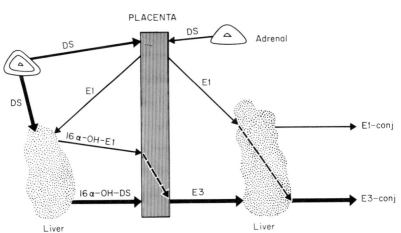

FIG. 1. Major pathways of estrogen biosynthesis in the fetoplacental unit in late pregnancy. Note secretion of dehydroepiandrosterone sulfate from the fetal and maternal adrenals, with major pathway (broad arrow) producing estriol. Abbreviations: *DS*, dehydroepiandrosterone sulfate; *16α-OH-DS*, 16α-hydroxydehydroepiandrosterone sulfate; *E1*, estrone; *E3*, estriol; *16α-OH-E1*, 16α-hydroxyestrone; *E1-conj*, estrone conjugates; *E3-conj*, estriol conjugates.

by the fetal adrenal is converted to estrone before hydroxylation at C-16α (Kirschner *et al.*, 1966). Metabolism of the estrone so formed ultimately yields some estriol; both the maternal and the fetal liver can effect this transformation (Bolte *et al.*, 1964b; Schwers *et al.*, 1965). Approximately 10% of the estrogen excreted in late pregnancy is produced from dehydroepiandrosterone sulfate secreted by the maternal adrenal (Frandsen and Stakemann, 1961; MacDonald and Siiteri, 1965). Little hydroxylation of this precursor at C-16α occurs in the maternal compartment before conversion to estrone (Kirschner *et al.*, 1966). Other minor pathways involving 16α-hydroxy C_{21} steroids have been suggested (Kirschner *et al.*, 1966; Shahwan *et al.*, 1969a).

More detailed aspects of the biosynthesis appear to depend on oxidation and reduction of C_{19} and C_{18} intermediates at C-17 and C-16 and the formation of estrogen conjugates by the fetal and maternal liver and intestinal tract. These pathways will not be described, since they do not significantly modify the generalized pathways described above.

From this evidence, estriol production in pregnancy can be recognized as essentially a feature of the participation of the fetus in estrogen biosynthesis and as a consequence of active 16α-steroid hydroxylase activities in fetal liver (Engel *et al.*, 1962; Slaunwhite *et al.*, 1965; Jungmann and Schweppe, 1967). The biosynthetic pathway described enables an understanding of the disproportionate increase in estriol production which is largely independent of estrone and estradiol-17β (Baulieu and Dray, 1963; Siiteri and MacDonald, 1963) and also an understanding of the necessity for a living fetus for continued estriol production (Cassmer, 1959).

A continuing and increasing level of estrogen production after the ninth week of pregnancy, therefore, depends primarily on an adequate and increasing supply of androgen sulfates, in particular of dehydroepiandrosterone sulfate and 16α-hydroxydehydroepiandrosterone sulfate, reaching the placenta from the fetus. That the "fetal" zone of the fetal adrenal is the most important source of these steroids or their precursors, at least at term, is demonstrated by the greatly reduced concentrations of these precursors in cord blood from anencephalic infants (Colás and Heinrichs, 1965; Easterling *et al.*, 1966). Contributions from the gonads are minimal in late pregnancy and may be neglected for the purpose of the present discussion. The ability of the healthy placenta to convert these precursors to estrogen appears to be unrestricted, since urinary estrogen values far in excess of the appropriate normal values have been recorded on occasions (Beischer *et al.*, 1968; Cathro *et al.*, 1969; Oakey, 1969). Scommegna *et al.* (1968) however incline to the view that the activity of the placental enzymes concerned with estrogen biosynthesis is the limiting factor in estrogen production. Their view is based on the low conversion (less than 1%) to urinary estriol of dehydroepiandrosterone or its sulfate introduced into the amniotic cavity (Frandsen and Stakemann, 1964; Michie, 1966). Some account must be taken of the transport of the precursor, introduced in this way, from the amniotic fluid to the fetal plasma. A much higher conversion (10%) of ^{14}C-labeled dehydroepiandrosterone sulfate to urinary estriol was found when the precursor was injected directly into the umbilical circulation (Bolté et al., 1964b). A slow transfer of steroid rather than saturated placental enzymes is probably the reason for the low conversions noted. More recently, Hausknecht and Mandelman (1969) recorded that in 4 normal pregnancies and in 2 pregnancies where retarded fetal growth was suspected, estriol excretion increased by 40–110% following intra-amniotic injection of 200 mg of dehydroepiandrosterone sulfate. These findings add weight to the belief that the efficiency of placental enzymes is not, in general, the limiting factor in sustaining the level of estrogen biosynthesis. In contrast, Laumas et al. (1968) found that less C_{19} precursor was converted to estrogen in vitro by extracts of placentas from pregnancies complicated by toxemia than was converted by placentas from normal pregnancies. This evidence, suggestive of deficiencies of placental enzymes in toxemic pregnancies warrants further investigation. Talbert and Easterling (1967) and Cleary et al. (1970), however, measured estrogen precursors in cord plasma in pregnancies complicated by hypertension and with low estriol excretion and found reduced values compared to normal pregnancies. This evidence points to a deficient supply of precursors in the complicated pregnancies.

Since the production of dehydroepiandrosterone sulfate by the fetal adrenal is clearly an important feature of estrogen biosynthesis in late pregnancy, some comment on the biosynthesis of this androgen is pertinent. Investigations have been carried out by perfusion of fetuses, obtained at midterm abortion, with radioactive substrates and by incubation of similar substrates with adrenal tissue from midterm fetuses and from newborn hydrocephalic and anencephalic infants. By means of these different experimental approaches, dehydroepiandrosterone, either free or conjugated, has been shown to be formed from acetate (Bloch and Benirschke, 1959; Jaffe et al., 1968; Telegdy et al., 1970), from cholesterol (Telegdy et al., 1970), from pregnenolone (C. A. Villee and Loring, 1965; Solomon et al., 1967; Cooke, 1968; Shahwan et al., 1969a,c), from pregnenolone sulfate (Pérez-Palacios et al., 1968), and from 17α-hydroxypregnenolone (Pion et al., 1967; Reynolds et al., 1969). The biosynthetic pathway acetate → cholesterol → pregnenolone → 17α-hydroxypregnenolone → dehydroepiandrosterone is in accord with these experimental results. Elucidation of the detailed pathway for the bio-synthesis of dehydroepiandrosterone sulfate awaits further experiments, although some evidence for a separate route from acetate has been pro-vided (Telegdy *et al.,* 1970).

For some years it has been widely considered that pregnenolone or pregnenolone sulfate secreted by the placenta is utilized by the fetal adrenal for androgen synthesis. This view appeared tenable since preg-nenolone but not cholesterol, could serve as precursor during fetal per-fusion (Solomon *et al.,* 1967; Coutts and Macnaughton, 1969). More recent evidence has pointed to the need for a modification of this view. Conrad *et al.* (1967) demonstrated that the fetus was secreting preg-nenolone sulfate to the placenta, rather than vice versa. Moreover, after modification of earlier techniques, the formation of free and conjugated dehydroepiandrosterone from acetate and cholesterol by the perfused midterm fetus has been demonstrated convincingly (Telegdy *et al.,* 1970). It would appear therefore that acetate and cholesterol in fetal plasma are important precursors of dehydroepiandrosterone and dehydro-epiandrosterone sulfate. (See also Section VIII.)

In the light of evidence presented in this section, the factors which limit estrogen production in normal pregnancy should be sought among those which modify androgen production by the fetal adrenal. These factors will be discussed next.

VI. Factors Influencing Androgen Production by the Fetal Adrenal

Ingestion of corticosteroids by the mother reduces the concentration of dehydroepiandrosterone sulfate and of 16α-hydroxydehydroepiandros-terone sulfate in cord blood (Simmer *et al.,* 1966). Urinary estrogen excretion is also suppressed by this treatment (Wray and Russell, 1964; Wallace and Michie, 1966; Oakey *et al.,* 1967; Oakey and Stitch, 1967; Warren and Cheatum, 1967; Scommegna *et al.,* 1968; J. B. Brown *et al.,* 1968; Driscoll, 1969; Morrison and Kilpatrick, 1969). This effect is inter-preted as a consequence of inhibition of adrenocorticotropic hormone (ACTH) secretion by the maternal and fetal pituitaries and, therefore, of a diminution of androgen secretion from the fetal and maternal adrenals. An effect of corticosteroids on the activity of the placental en-zymes involved in estrogen biosynthesis cannot entirely be ruled out, although pregnanediol excretion (a measure of progesterone synthesis by the placenta) remains within the normal range during treatment (Oakey and Stitch, 1967; Driscoll, 1969). Inhibition of placental enzymes would not easily explain the reduction in the production of androgens by the fetus, which is a clear response to the treatment (Simmer *et al.,* 1966).

ACTH injected into the mother increases the excretion of estriol
(Dässler, 1966; Scommegna *et al.*, 1968) and to a lesser extent the excretion of estrone and estradiol-17β also (Maeyama *et al.*, 1969). Since
estriol is predominantly of fetal origin, these findings imply that ACTH
crosses the placenta and stimulates the fetal adrenal. This suggestion is
borne out by a failure to detect a change in estriol excretion following
ACTH after intrauterine death of the fetus (Dässler, 1966; Maeyama
et al., 1969) or in pregnancies with an anencephalic fetus (Maeyama
et al., 1969). This evidence implicates ACTH as a factor which increases
androgen secretion by the fetal adrenal and raises the question whether
ACTH from the maternal compartment is a physiological factor controlling the fetal adrenal gland. In discussion of this point, it must be
noted that the rates of ACTH infusion used by these workers (3–5
IU/hour or 40 IU in a single injection) are at least 100 times greater
than the rate of ACTH infusion required to maintain a detectable stimulation of adrenal tissue in adults (Liddle *et al.*, 1962). It has also been
noted that the adrenals of fetuses born to adrenalectomized rodents are
heavier than normal (Ingle and Fisher, 1938) and that this response to
adrenalectomy is abolished by hypophysectomy of the mother (Knobil
and Briggs, 1955). From these observations, it is clear that ACTH can
cross the placenta when the concentration of this hormone in the maternal
circulation is excessive, for example, under conditions of infusion of large
quantities of ACTH, or after adrenalectomy. However, under physiological conditions, ACTH secreted by the maternal pituitary does not
cross to the fetus. This is illustrated by the atrophy of the fetal adrenal
in rats and rabbits after decapitation *in utero* (Wells, 1947; Jost, 1948),
in the fetal lamb after electrocoagulation of the hypophysis (Liggins and
Kennedy, 1968), and in the human anencephalic fetus (Angevine, 1938).
The balance of the evidence is, therefore, against a role for ACTH
secreted by the maternal pituitary gland in the regulation of the fetal
adrenal.

Metyrapone, a drug which stimulates ACTH secretion by interference
with cortisol biosynthesis (Liddle *et al.*, 1959) has been used to examine
the influence of ACTH on estrogen production. Scommegna *et al.* (1968)
and Dickey and Thompson (1969) found estriol excretion was increased
significantly in pregnant women treated with metyrapone. Oakey and
Heys (1969, 1970) confirmed these findings in 2 pregnancies with a hydrocephalic fetus and in 4 normal pregnancies. Significantly, no response was
detected in 3 pregnancies with an anencephalic fetus. Therefore, an intact hypothalamic-pituitary-adrenal axis in the fetus was necessary to
obtain a response. Androgens from the maternal adrenal make little or
no contribution to that response, since no increase in estrogen excretion
was observed in pregnancies with an anencephalic fetus.

Other conclusions, which have important implications, may also be drawn, especially when the mechanism by which metyrapone exerts its effect is considered (Oakey and Heys, 1970). Three alternatives are possible. Metyrapone may stimulate increased ACTH secretion by the maternal pituitary. Part of the increased amount of ACTH generated may cross the placenta and stimulate the fetal adrenal. However, metyrapone only increases plasma ACTH concentration by a factor of 2 (Liddle *et al.*, 1962; Strott *et al.*, 1969). It is unlikely, therefore, that transfer of ACTH to the fetus is responsible for the effect. Alternatively, the transient lowering of the cortisol concentration in maternal plasma may provoke transport of cortisol from the fetus to the maternal plasma. The consequent fall in concentration of cortisol in the fetal plasma would be expected to stimulate ACTH secretion by the fetal pituitary. The third possibility is that metyrapone (molecular weight 220) crosses the placenta and stimulates the fetal pituitary by interference with cortisol synthesis in the fetus. Such an inhibition of 11β-hydroxylation by metyrapone has been demonstrated during fetal perfusion experiments (Shimao *et al.*, 1968). Either or both of the last two suggested mechanisms may operate. In any event the secretion of ACTH by the fetal pituitary, and hence the production of androgens by the fetal adrenal, can be regulated by the concentration of cortisol in the fetal circulation. This conclusion is in keeping with the suppressive effects of corticosteroids on the concentration of androgen sulfate in cord plasma (Simmer *et al.*, 1966). Regulation of androgen production in the adult operates in a similar manner: ACTH increases androgen secretion (Migeon, 1955; Wieland *et al.*, 1965), treatment with active corticosteroids such as prednisone and dexamethasone suppresses it (Lamb *et al.*, 1964; Kirschner *et al.*, 1965).

To understand the control of androgen production by the fetus more thoroughly, it is necessary to examine the parameters which modify the concentration of cortisol and, more particularly, of biologically active (i.e., nonprotein bound) cortisol in the fetal plasma. It is this fraction of the total plasma cortisol which is accepted as regulating ACTH secretion.

VII. Factors Affecting the Concentration of Cortisol in the Fetal Plasma

Measurements of plasma cortisol concentrations in the fetus during intrauterine life have not been made. The concentration of cortisol in the fetal circulation must be regulated by the rates of secretion into and removal from the fetal plasma. Cortisol can be expected to enter the fetal plasma (a) by secretion from the fetal adrenal, (b) from the maternal circulation. Cortisol may be removed from the fetal plasma (c) by metabolism in peripheral tissues, (d) by transfer to the maternal circulation. These factors will be discussed separately.

A. SECRETION BY THE FETAL ADRENAL

It has not been practicable to demonstrate cortisol secretion by the fetal adrenal *in vivo*. Cortisol production by the fetus is implied by the report that an adrenalectomized pregnant woman, maintained on dexamethasone while measurements were made, had a cortisol production rate of 8.1 mg/day at 39 weeks gestation (Harkness *et al.*, 1966). Studies of the same patient in subsequent pregnancies gave cortisol production rates of 1.5 and 3.8 mg/day for the mother in late pregnancy (Charles *et al.*, 1970). Some allowance should perhaps be made for cortisol given therapeutically up to 51 hours before the determination. Nevertheless, the production rates recorded are close to the value of 3.7 ± 0.8 mg/day found in normal newborn infants (Kenny *et al.*, 1966a) and in the infants after birth (5.0 mg/day, Harkness *et al.*, 1966; 3.0 mg/day, Charles *et al.* 1970). James (1966) detected cortisol and cortisone in cord plasma at delivery of a pregnant woman with adrenal insufficiency who was maintained on prednisone (5 mg/day). These steroids could not be detected in maternal peripheral plasma at this time. Consequently, this evidence also suggests that the fetal adrenal secretes cortisol. Less specific information on this point has been provided by Abramovich and Wade (1969b), who found normal concentrations of 17-hydroxycorticosteroids in the amniotic fluid of a pregnant adrenalectomized woman. These steroids presumably originated in the fetal adrenal. Although the patient was maintained on prednisone (15 mg daily), this is unlikely to account for all the hydroxycorticosteroids found in the fluid. Other evidence that the fetal adrenal and, in particular, the "fetal" zone may secrete corticosteroids is derived from the observation (Oakey and Heys, 1970) that women pregnant with an anencephalic fetus excrete less 17-oxogenic steroids than do women with a normal or a hydrocephalic fetus. In 3 anencephalic pregnancies the excretion of 17-oxogenic steroids was 6.4–8.4 mg/24 hours (mean 7.3 mg/24 hours), and in 2 hydrocephalic and 4 normal pregnancies the values were 10.0–16.4 mg/24 hour (mean 13.5 mg/24 hour). These data, which require substantiation in a larger series, are contrary to accepted ideas, which are based, to a large extent, on the data of Frandsen and Stakemann (1964). These authors reported normal levels of urinary 17-oxogenic steroid excretion in women with an anencephalic fetus, but used nonpregnant women to define the normal range.

Indirect evidence must also be assessed. Newborn infants, whether normal or anencephalic, whether born at term or prematurely, whether delivered by cesarean section or *per vaginam*, or born to diabetic mothers or to mothers who received corticosteroids during pregnancy, have cortisol production rates similar to adults, when related to body area (Aarskog, 1965; Kenny et al., 1966a,b). About 0.5 mg of the production rate measured within 48 hours after birth is due to cortisol received from the mother during delivery (Kenny et al., 1966b). Nevertheless, the similarity of the production rates recorded in newborn infants implies an effective means of cortisol synthesis in utero or one which operates efficiently immediately after birth.

Experiments in vitro with fetal adrenal tissue demonstrate a potential for cortisol biosynthesis from precursors in the fetal plasma such as pregnenolone, present as pregnenolone sulfate (150–200 μg/100 ml plasma, Conrad et al., 1967) and progesterone (22–187 μg/100 ml plasma, Greig et al., 1962; 43–72 μg/100 ml, Harbert et al., 1964; 14–37 μg/100 ml, Zander, 1961). Cholesterol, although present in cord blood (114 mg per 100 ml of blood, Sabata and Novák, 1967) has not been examined as a precursor in vitro.

In any discussion of steroid biosynthesis by the fetal adrenal, the existence of the "fetal" and "definitive" zones must be recognized. The "fetal" zone, which forms 80% of the volume of the gland at term, is considered from indirect evidence to have a lower ability than the "definitive" zone to convert Δ^5-3β-hydroxysteroids to Δ^4-3-oxosteroids. The enzymes involved—3β-hydroxysteroid dehydrogenase, of which there may be several substrate-specific enzymes, and $\Delta^5 \rightarrow \Delta^4$-isomerase—are essential for the conversion of cholesterol and pregnenolone, but not of progesterone, to cortisol. In the absence of this enzyme complex, neither cholesterol nor pregnenolone can serve as substrates for cortisol synthesis. Bloch and Benirschke (1962) found that the ratio of dehydroepiandrosterone to androstenedione synthesized from radioactive acetate by the "fetal" zone was twice as great as that synthesized by the "definitive" zone. The problem is difficult to resolve exactly, since the "definitive" zone tissue used has usually been contaminated with "fetal" zone tissue (Bloch and Benirschke, 1959; Hillman et al., 1962; Solomon et al., 1958). Histochemical techniques, which enable exact characterization of the tissue under examination have been applied largely to the reaction dehydroepiandrosterone $\rightarrow$ androstenedione (Goldman et al., 1966). These authors found no 3β-hydroxysteroid dehydrogenase in the "fetal" zone throughout gestation, but a consistently high activity of this enzyme was detected in all samples of the "definitive" zone after 12 weeks' gestation. Niemi and Baillie (1965), however, found traces of a 3β-hydroxysteroid dehydrogenase for dehydroepiandrosterone and for pregnenolone throughout the entire "fetal" zone in adrenals from a fetus of 22 weeks' gestation. The nature of the steroids in cord plasma (Eberlein, 1965) supports the idea of a deficiency of the 3β-hydroxysteroid dehydrogenase activity. Fetal adrenals obtained after 16 or 22 weeks' gestation converted pregnenolone to cortisol *in vitro* (Klein and Giroud, 1967; Whitehouse and Vinson, 1968), but pregnenolone sulfate was not converted to cortisol when incubated under conditions to minimize cleavage of the sulfate group (Pérez-Palacios *et al.*, 1968). Incubations of pregnenolone with adrenals from a newborn hydrocephalic infant yielded cortisol (C. A. Villee and Loring, 1965). The "definitive" zone of the adrenal cortex is implicated in this conversion which can be demonstrated in adrenal tissue from newborn anencephalic infants (Cooke, 1968; Shahwan *et al.*, 1969b). Progesterone, which accumulates preferentially in the fetal adrenal on perfusion (Bengtsson *et al.*, 1964), can be converted to cortisol by adrenals from the newborn infant or the immature fetus (Lanman and Silverman, 1957; D. B. Villee *et al.*, 1959, 1961; C. A. Villee and Loring, 1965; Klein and Giroud, 1967; Whitehouse and Vinson, 1968). Incubation of acetate with slices of adrenal tissue from a fetus of 22 weeks' gestation yielded cortisol (Bloch and Benirschke, 1959). During tissue culture cortisol-like material was found to be secreted by slices of fetal adrenal obtained early in gestation. The effect was enhanced if ACTH was added to the incubation medium (Stark *et al.*, 1965).

In general, radioactive progesterone was found to be converted more efficiently to cortisol than was radioactive pregnenolone. This finding may be explicable in two ways. The pool of pregnenolone in the tissue may be larger than the pool of progesterone, thereby producing a substrate of lower specific activity within the cell and consequently a lower conversion to product of radioactive substrate, but not necessarily of mass of substrate.

Alternatively, some part of the pathway between pregnenolone and cortisol may be inhibited in this tissue, as discussed earlier. Kinetic studies by Whitehouse and Vinson (1968) strongly indicate a relative inactivity of at least one 3β-hydroxysteroid dehydrogenase in early fetal adrenal tissue.

Perfusion experiments, although necessarily performed before about 20 weeks of gestation, demonstrate a potential for cortisol synthesis, at least from progesterone. Solomon *et al.* (1967) failed to detect cortisol-^{14}C after injection of the fetus *in utero* with pregnenolone-[14]C. However, when progesterone-^{14}C was perfused, the adrenal tissue was found to contain cortisol-[14]C (Bird *et al.*, 1966). On perfusion of an adrenalectomized fetus (R. Wilson *et al.*, 1966) or an anencephalic infant (Zander *et al.*, 1965) with progesterone-^{14}C, cortisol-^{14}C could not be detected among the metabolites, emphasizing the importance of the adrenal and, in particular, the "fetal" zone in cortisol biosynthesis.

When ^{3}H-labeled $3\beta,17\alpha,21$-trihydroxy-5-pregnen-20-one was perfused through a fetus at mid-pregnancy cortisol-^{3}H was isolated from adrenal tissue (Pasqualini *et al.*, 1968). Similarly, when 17α-hydroxypregnenolone-^{3}H was injected into the umbilical circulation prior to midterm abortion cortisol-^{3}H was isolated from the fetal adrenal (Reynolds *et al.*, 1969). Jackanicz *et al.* (1969) also noted the formation of cortisol from 17α-hydroxypregnenolone and from 17α-hydroxyprogesterone during perfusion studies. Since the Δ^5-3β-hydroxysteroids mentioned can be isolated from cord blood (Eberlein, 1965), these experiments suggest other routes of cortisol biosynthesis. It is possible that cortisol synthesis could occur in the placenta from $3\beta,11\beta,17\alpha,21$-tetrahydroxy-5-pregnen-20-one, another constituent of the sulfate fraction from cord blood (Eberlein, 1965). Cholesterol-^{3}H perfused through previable fetuses did not yield corticosteroids (Solomon *et al.*, 1967; Coutts and Macnaughton, 1969). This is not unexpected in view of the relative quantities of cholesterol-^{3}H perfused and the plasma concentration of cholesterol, approximately 100 mg per 100 ml of blood (Sabata and Novák, 1967).

There appears to be good evidence that the fetus has a supply of precursors and enzymes necessary for the production of cortisol. Incubation studies with fetal and newborn adrenals demonstrate a potential for cortisol biosynthesis in the whole adrenal from progesterone and in the "definitive" zone from pregnenolone. Perfusion experiments imply that progesterone is the preferred precursor. Neither of these pathways of biosynthesis would be stimulated directly by ACTH (Stone and Hechter, 1954; Karaboyas and Koritz, 1965).

The measurement of cortisol production rates *in utero* and after birth also support the contention that the fetus synthesizes cortisol. The definitive experiment, in order to remove any doubts, would be to measure plasma cortisol concentrations in the adrenal artery and vein of the fetus *in utero* with the minimum of stress to mother and fetus. There would, of course, be considerable ethical and technical difficulties to this experiment.

B. Secretion from the Maternal Circulation

Injection of radioactive cortisol into the mother is followed by a transient appearance of up to 2% of the injected radioactivity in the cord blood (Migeon *et al.*, 1957). Abramovich and Wade (1969a) found less than 0.04% of injected radioactivity in amniotic fluid samples after infusion of the mother at mid-pregnancy with cortisol-^{3}H immediately prior to hysterectomy. Twenty minutes' delay between the end of the infusion and hysterectomy resulted in failure to detect tritium in the amniotic fluid. Transfer of corticosteroids from mother to fetus is il-

lustrated also by the finding that the quantities of 17-hydroxycortico-
steroids in maternal and cord blood are greater after delivery by vaginal
route than after cesarean section (Migeon et al., 1956), presumably
because of the greater stress of vaginal delivery. The ratio of the concentrations in maternal and cord plasma were similar whether delivery
followed normal labor or cesarean section, suggesting that the levels in
the cord merely reflected the concentration in the maternal circulation
(Migeon et al., 1962). It must be noted, however, that this ready transfer
of corticosteroids was demonstrated when the concentration in maternal
plasma was acutely raised to levels which exceed the binding capacity
of cortisol-binding globulin. Aarskog (1965) confirmed these findings
using a more specific assay for cortisol. After delivery, the concentration
of nonprotein bound cortisol was identical in maternal and cord plasma.
Corticosteroids given in large doses to the mother also appear to cross
the placenta (Section VI), but these findings are not evidence of physiological transfer during pregnancy.

Other considerations suggest that there is little net transfer of cortisol
from mother to fetus. For example, if a net gain of cortisol by the fetus
could occur under physiological conditions then the excessive production
of ACTH which occurs in fetuses affected by certain forms of congenital
adrenal hyperplasia should not take place. Consideration of the effect
of the binding of cortisol to plasma proteins (see below) also suggests
that there is little or no net transfer of cortisol from the maternal to the
fetal circulations under physiological conditions.

C. Removal by Metabolism in Peripheral Tissues

The means by which the fetus metabolizes cortisol have not been
investigated in vivo by dynamic studies. Migeon et al. (1961) found
that cortisol-^{14}C introduced into the amniotic fluid was transferred to the
maternal plasma. The behavior of cortisol introduced in this way cannot be equated with that of cortisol secreted by the adrenal.

Cortisol metabolism by the liver of the fetus is implied by the finding
of Leyssac (1961) that the cortisol concentration in plasma from the
fetal heart (82 μg/100 ml) was less than that in the umbilical vein (130
μg/100 ml) during experiments in which cortisol was infused into the
maternal circulation prior to abortion. Other evidence is available from
studies of infants and of amniotic fluid which may be pertinent.

6β-Hydroxycortisol and 6β,11β,17α,20β,21-pentahydroxy-4-pregnen-
3-one have been isolated from amniotic fluid (Lambert and Pennington,
1963, 1964). These compounds are presumably derived from cortisol
metabolism in the fetus. The capacity of the fetal liver to hydroxylate
cortisol at C-6 persists in infancy (Ulstrom et al., 1960; Birchall et al.,

1961). The half-life of cortisol is greater in infancy than in adult life (Migeon, 1959) while the ability of the liver to form glucuronosides and to reduce ring A is diminished (Reynolds et al., 1962). On the other hand, sulfate formation is greater in infancy than in the adult (Drayer and Giroud, 1965). Thus, the liver in infancy and presumably in the fetus inactivates cortisol, but probably by reactions rather different from those which operate in the adult.

Cortisol can also be removed from the plasma by oxidation to cortisone in the chorionic membrane (Osinski, 1960). This route appears to be an important means of biological inactivation, since the concentration of cortisone in cord plasma (14 μg/100 ml) exceeds that of cortisol (8 μg/100 ml) (Hillman and Giroud, 1965).

D. Transfer to the Maternal Circulation

Cortisol may also be removed from the fetus by transfer across the placenta to the maternal circulation. This process will be confined initially to that fraction of cortisol in fetal plasma which is not bound to cortisol binding globulin. However, since the pools of free and protein bound cortisol are in equilibrium, cortisol could be slowly removed from the binding protein and transferred. Extraction of a hormone, such as cortisol, from plasma is more efficient if there is little binding of the hormone to plasma proteins.

Sandberg and Slaunwhite (1962) demonstrated that cortisol metabolism by liver slices, in vitro, was reduced in the presence of cortisol binding globulin. Presumably, the transfer of cortisol into the cells was reduced by interaction with the large globulin molecule. Hepatic extraction of progesterone and aldosterone, which have little affinity for plasma proteins, is 90% (Little et al., 1962). In contrast, cortisol, of which 90% is bound to cortisol binding globulin, has a hepatic extraction of only 7–15% (Plager et al., 1957; Engell et al., 1961). Moreover, cortisol binding to plasma proteins is lower and hepatic extraction is higher in the dog than in man (Daughaday, 1958; Slaunwhite and Sandberg, 1959; Steenburg et al., 1960).

Fetal plasma has a lower capacity for cortisol binding than maternal plasma. This has been substantiated in several laboratories by different techniques. Sandberg and Slaunwhite (1959) dialyzed diluted plasma against saline containing cortisol-^{14}C. They found that 88% of the cortisol was bound to maternal plasma proteins, but only 64% to proteins in cord blood samples. Moreover, addition of nonradioactive cortisol (1 μg) to the system reduced the cortisol binding to maternal plasma by 10%, whereas a similar addition to the dialysis of cord plasma reduced cortisol binding by 17%. Sandberg and Slaunwhite (1959) concluded that less cortisol was bound to proteins in cord plasma than in maternal plasma and, more important, there were fewer binding sites available in cord plasma. De Moor *et al.* (1962) confirmed these conclusions. These authors separated protein-bound and free cortisol in plasma by gel filtration. Cord plasma bound 10.9 μg of cortisol per 100 ml whereas maternal plasma bound 52.4 μg of cortisol per 100 ml. Ultrafiltration studies on cord plasma after addition of radioactive cortisol also indicated that a smaller proportion of cortisol was bound than in samples of maternal plasma (Mills *et al.*, 1959). Daughaday *et al.* (1959) found the proportion of nonbound cortisol in cord plasma (16.2%) was greater than that in adult plasma (1.1%).

These results are often interpreted to indicate that there is less cortisol-binding globulin in cord plasma than in maternal plasma. This need not necessarily be the case. It must be recognized that the techniques used do not measure the quantity of cortisol-binding globulin in absolute terms. Furthermore, valid comparisons between samples can be made only if cortisol is the sole steroid in the samples which is significantly bound to the globulin. For many samples the assumption is justified. Corticosterone, 11-deoxycortisol, and progesterone, all of which bind to cortisol-binding globulin (De Moor *et al.*, 1962; Murphy, 1967; Nugent and Mayes, 1966; Rosenthal *et al.*, 1969; Strott *et al.*, 1969), are minor steroid constituents of adult plasma in comparison to cortisol (Fraser and James, 1968; Strott *et al.*, 1969; van der Molen and Groen, 1965). In pregnancy, both cord and maternal plasma contain relatively high concentrations of progesterone. For example, concentrations of up to 187 μg/100 ml have been recorded in umbilical vein plasma and up to 27 μg/100 ml in maternal peripheral plasma (Greig *et al.*, 1962). Progesterone competes with cortisol for cortisol binding globulin, and this effect is more marked at 37°C than at 4°C (Murphy, 1967; Rosenthal *et al.*, 1969). The high proportion of unbound cortisol in cord blood may reflect the competition from progesterone for the binding sites rather than a low quantity of cortisol binding globulin. So far these two alternatives have not been resolved, and the problem requires further investigation. Whichever explanation is correct, the net result will be the same—the number of binding sites available for cortisol is diminished.

Booth *et al.* (1961) found that 60% of the possible binding sites on cortisol-binding globulin in maternal plasma, obtained in late pregnancy, not at delivery, are vacant. Rosenthal *et al.* (1969) confirmed this result, calculating that 55% of the sites were free. The maternal and fetal circulations may be envisaged as two pools separated by a semipermeable membrane, the placenta. The fetal plasma contains relatively few sites available for cortisol binding, either because of a low concentration of cortisol-binding globulin or because of the high concentration of progesterone. Maternal plasma which contains much less progesterone, in contrast, has much higher numbers of available sites (Sandberg and Slaunwhite, 1959; De Moor *et al.*, 1962) and most of the sites are vacant. In consequence, the cortisol in fetal plasma, which is not bound to the binding globulin, will tend to pass to the maternal plasma. A net flow of cortisol in the reverse direction would require some form of pump against the gradient established by the different numbers of binding sites available in the two compartments. Passage of radioactive cortisol from mother to fetus, as observed by Migeon *et al.* (1957) and by Abramovich and Wade (1969a), will occur during equilibrium and exchange, in the placenta, of nonprotein bound cortisol from the maternal and fetal populations. De Moor *et al.* (1962) and Doe *et al.* (1964) demonstrated that the capacity of maternal plasma for cortisol binding doubles during the first 6 months of gestation and then remains fairly constant. Rosenthal *et al.* (1969) extended these observations using a refined technique. They found that the quantity of transcortin and the concentration of binding sites free from both cortisol and progesterone increased processively during pregnancy. This effect is generally accepted as a response to the increased concentrations of estrogen associated with pregnancy (Sandberg and Slaunwhite, 1959; De Moor *et al.*, 1962). Thus the attractive force for cortisol in the fetal plasma progressively increases during gestation. Zander (1961) calculated that half the progesterone synthesized by the placenta, at term, was secreted to the fetus. The placenta secretes increasing quantities of progesterone during pregnancy, as illustrated by the rising concentration of this hormone in maternal plasma (Short and Eton, 1959; Yannone *et al.*, 1968). It seems likely that the concentration of progesterone in fetal plasma increases in parallel. Thus, even if the quantity of cortisol binding globulin in the fetus increases, the competition from progesterone for binding sites will increase also. Therefore, the driving force for cortisol transfer to maternal plasma will also increase progessively during gestation. The net rate of cortisol transfer, therefore, appears to be related to the progressively increasing numbers of cortisol binding sites in maternal plasma and the increasing competition for binding sites in fetal plasma.

Cortisol transfer from the fetal to maternal plasma might be indicated by an increased cortisol production rate in pregnancy. Cope and Black (1959) found cortisol secretion rates of 15–40 mg (mean 25 mg) per day in late pregnancy, much greater than the values they recorded in nonpregnant women (6–24 mg/day). Migeon *et al.* (1968) could not confirm these findings and reported that cortisol production rates were lower in pregnancy than in nonpregnant women. These authors consider that this decreased secretion is due to increased cortisol binding related to an increased estrogen production in pregnancy. This effect obscures any contribution from the fetus and vitiates any attempt to measure the transfer of cortisol from the fetus, by this approach.

Progressive transfer to the mother of radioactive cortisol injected into the amniotic sac has been demonstrated (Migeon et al., 1961), although the physiological significance of this finding is doubtful. Three-quarters of this cortisol appears in the maternal urine, mainly as metabolites, within 22 hours. These experiments contrast strongly with the transient appearance in the fetus of cortisol injected into the mother which has already been mentioned (Migeon et al., 1957; Abramovich and Wade, 1969a). The gradient appears to be from fetus to mother.

From the evidence presented in this section it is suggested that the fetus produces cortisol using progesterone and, to a smaller extent, pregnenolone as precursors. The corticosteroid is lost from the fetal plasma through inactivation by the fetal liver and by transfer across the placenta to the mother. Both these processes are facilitated by the relatively low concentration of sites available for cortisol binding in fetal plasma. In the adult, cortisol homeostasis is achieved by a balance between inactivation of cortisol by the liver and stimulation of cortisol production by ACTH (Yates and Urquhart, 1962). The imposition on this system in the fetus of the loss of cortisol across the placenta essentially increases the metabolic clearance rate of cortisol. As Tait and Burstein (1964) pointed out, the consequence of an increased cortisol clearance rate is an increased secretion of ACTH. Such a consequence is well illustrated by reference to hyperthyroidism. Here, the metabolic clearance rate of cortisol is raised (Peterson et al., 1955; Levin and Daughaday, 1955; H. Brown et al., 1958); there is an increased secretion of ACTH (Hilton et al., 1962) while the cortisol concentration in plasma remains normal (Peterson, 1958).

It must be concluded that an increase in the metabolic clearance rate of cortisol leads to stimulation of ACTH secretion by the fetal pituitary. Although the secretion of ACTH has not been measured during gestation, Taylor et al. (1953) detected this hormone in pituitary glands of 16-week-old fetuses. Berson and Yalow (1968) reported that the mean concentration of ACTH in cord plasma was 161 pg/ml, three times greater than the value recorded for maternal plasma (56 pg/ml). This value for ACTH in cord plasma probably reflects the stress of delivery on the infant and demonstrates the capacity of the fetal pituitary for ACTH secretion.

The secretion of ACTH at an increased rate during gestation has important consequences for the growth of the adrenal tissues and for the level of steroid production by the gland. In the adult excessive ACTH secretion induces adrenal growth and increased steroid production (e.g., see Landon *et al.*, 1967). An analogous response would be expected from the adrenal of the fetus also. This will be discussed in the next section. Since cortisol is considered to be synthesized in the fetus largely from progesterone (see above) rather than from cholesterol, as in the adult (Borkowski *et al.* 1967), no direct stimulation of cortisol production by ACTH would be expected. Stone and Hechter (1954) demonstrated that ACTH stimulates corticosteroid biosynthesis from cholesterol, but not from progesterone.

VIII. The Adrenal Cortex of the Fetus

The development and growth of the fetal adrenal have been reviewed on numerous occasions (e.g., Lanman, 1953). It is proposed, therefore, only to summarize here the main and relevant conclusions. The fetal adrenal is composed of two distinct zones of tissue, an inner "fetal" zone and an outer "definitive" zone. Cells of the "fetal" zone are relatively large and contain abundant cytoplasm. Cells in the "definitive" zone, in contrast, are smaller, have prominent nuclei and contain little cytoplasm. The "fetal" zone is laid down during the third week of gestation while the "definitive" zone appears some 3 weeks later (Uotila, 1940). Information on the growth of these zones has been provided by Swinyard (1943) from fetuses examined after abortion. The conclusions are drawn from only five specimens, but the overall picture is clear. Between the 14th and 28th week of pregnancy the size of the "fetal" zone increases 7-fold, whereas the "definitive" zone grows more slowly from about 100 mm^3 to 400 mm^3. From the 28th week of pregnancy the "fetal" zone continues to grow rapidly. The volume of this zone increases from 1200 mm^3 to about 4000 mm^3. In contrast, the rate of growth of the "definitive" zone is much slower after 28 weeks of gestation than before. During this time the volume increases to 500 mm^3. Consequently, at term, the "fetal" zone occupies some 80% of the adrenal cortex. Furthermore, the weight of the adrenal glands, 7–9 gm per pair at birth (Keene and Hewer, 1927; Scammon, 1926), is 10–20 times greater than that of the adult adrenal relative to body weight. Growth of the fetal adrenal in intact or decapitated rodents and in the hypophysectomized fetal lamb is stimulated by ACTH (Wells, 1948; Kitchell and Wells, 1952; Liggins, 1968). In man, where experimental hypophysectomy is out of the question, the anencephalic fetus provides a demonstration of the role of the hypothalamus and pituitary in the development of the fetal adrenal. In the anencephalic fetus the hypothalamus is invariably absent, although the anterior lobe of the pituitary is present (Angevine, 1938). The adrenal cortex, at term, weighs 0.2–0.6 g and the small size is due mainly to a virtual absence of the "fetal" zone (Keene and Hewer, 1927; Angevine, 1938; Benirschke, 1956). The adrenal atrophy is usually considered to be related to the lack of some pituitary factor. Adrenocorticotropin (ACTH) has been implicated as the factor responsible for growth of the "fetal" zone (Lanman, 1962) since enlarged adrenals, with prominent "fetal" zones, were found in surviving anencephalic infants given ACTH. Johannisson (1968) found a decrease in lipophilic droplets in adrenals of anencephalic infants treated with ACTH at term and in normal fetuses of 16–18 weeks' gestation given ACTH at the time of therapeutic abortion. This response to ACTH is characteristic of the adult adrenal also (Symington, 1962). Human chorionic gonadotropin (HCG) has also been suggested as a

TABLE I

STEROIDS IN PLASMA FROM THE FETUS AND FROM PERIPHERAL PLASMA OF NONPREGNANT ADULTS[a]

Steroid	Source[b]	Concentration (μg/100ml)	Reference
Pregnenolone sulfate	U.A.	200	Conrad et al. (1967)
	U.V.	140	Conrad et al. (1967)
	P.C.	17–27	Eberlein (1965)
	Adult	5	Bègue (1965)
Dehydroepiandrosterone sulfate	U.A.	81	Colás et al. (1964)
	U.V.	68	Colás et al. (1964)
	U.A.	162	Simmer et al. (1964)
	U.V.	130	Simmer et al. (1964)
	Adult	41–137	Eberlein et al. (1967)
16α-Hydroxydehydroepi-androsterone	U.A.	147	Colás et al. (1964)
	U.V.	114	Colás et al. (1964)
	U.A.	110	Easterling et al. (1966)
	U.V.	87	Easterling et al. (1966)
	Adult*	<10	Easterling et al. (1966)
Cortisol	P.C.	8	Hillman and Giroud (1965)
	P.C.	17	Aarskog (1965)
	Adult	12	Fraser and James (1968)
Progesterone	U.A.	14	Zander (1961)
	U.V.	37	Zander (1961)
	U.A.	57	Greig et al. (1962)
	U.V.	102	Greig et al. (1962)
	U.A.	43	Harbert et al. (1964)
	U.V.	72	Harbert et al. (1964)
	Adult	<3	van der Molen and Groen (1965)

[a] All values are means of authors' results.
[b] U.A. = umbilical artery; U.V. = umbilical vein; P.C. = pooled umbilical cord sample; Adult* = pregnant adult subjects; Adult = nonpregnant adult subjects.

factor required for development of the "fetal" zone. Meyer (1912), Kiyono (1925), and Benirschke (1956) noted that the fetal adrenal developed normally in anencephaly up to 20 weeks of gestation, which implies some extrapituitary factor is involved in maintaining adrenal growth during early gestation. Depletion of lipid particles was noted in the "fetal" zone of the adrenals of fetuses given HCG between 14 and 17 weeks gestation (Johannisson, 1968). Furthermore, in perfusion of fetuses of similar gestation with blood containing an anti-HCG serum, the transition zone between the "adult" and "fetal" zones of the fetal adrenals showed a distinct increase in the numbers of dark cells present. These cells contained numerous osmiophilic droplets, and the observations are consistent with a low secretory activity (Johannisson, 1968). In contrast, the fetal adrenal showed no growth response to HCG at term (Lanman, 1962). It must be concluded that ACTH secreted by the fetal pituitary is a factor required for continued growth and development of the "fetal" zone at least during the last 20 weeks of gestation.

The fetal adrenal secretes sulfates of Δ^5-3β-hydroxysteroid exemplified by dehydroepiandrosterone sulfate and pregnenolone sulfate. Examination of the concentration of steroids in plasma from the umbilical cord and from adults (Table I) demonstrates the relatively high concentrations of these steroids in the cord artery at term. The fetal adrenal is an active

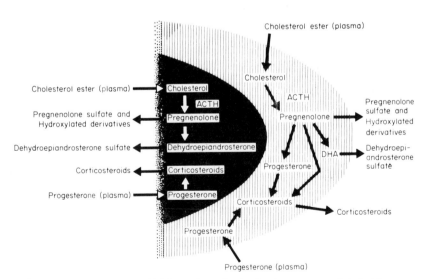

FIG. 2. Pathways of steroid biosynthesis in the fetal zone ▦, and definitive zone ▥ of the human fetal adrenal. Note that ACTH stimulation of steroid biosynthesis in the fetal zone leads to increased formation of dehydroepiandrosterone sulfate. Corticosteroid formation in this zone is derived from progesterone.

gland of steroid secretion in relation to its size. This activity must reflect the influence of ACTH on the growth of the gland and also in stimulating steroid biosynthesis directly. The lack of 3β-hydroxysteroid dehydrogenase activity in the "fetal" zone (Goldman *et al.*, 1966) leads to the formation of pregnenolone, dehydroepiandrosterone, and their sulfates rather than of cortisol from acetate, cholesterol, and pregnenolone sulfate (Telegdy *et al.*, 1969, 1970; Pérez-Palacios *et al.*, 1968).

A schematic illustration of steroid biosynthesis in the fetal adrenal is shown in Fig. 2. A direct action of ACTH on the formation of pregnenolone from cholesterol (Stone and Hechter, 1954; Karaboyas and Koritz, 1965) would reinforce the production of dehydroepiandrosterone and pregnenolone sulfates. Increasing concentrations of ACTH would, therefore, provide the stimulus for an increasing production of dehydroepiandrosterone sulfate and of pregnenolone sulfate in late pregnancy. Cortisol production from progesterone might also be enhanced by an increased turnover of this precursor in the enlarged adrenal.

IX. Conclusion

The increasing production of estrogens in the second half of gestation arises from an increasing production of androgen sulfates by the fetal adrenal associated with progressive growth of and stimulation of steroid biosynthesis in this gland which, in turn, are provoked by an elevated secretion of ACTH from the fetal pituitary. The secretion of ACTH in increased quantities is a response to an increased metabolic clearance rate of cortisol from the fetal plasma. A major factor concerned in the increased clearance of cortisol is the disparity in the number of available binding sites for cortisol in fetal and maternal plasma.

X. Discussion

Many factors, in addition to those concerned directly with the fetal adrenal, modify estrogen synthesis in pregnancy (Klopper, 1968). It is not proposed to discuss here these extra-adrenal factors, but to consider estrogen production in situations devoid of these complications. The evidence presented has been taken, almost entirely, from measurements in the human. While there is a vast body of information relating to the hypophyseal control of the function of the fetal adrenal in rodents (e.g., Jost, 1966), this has not been utilized for this discussion, since only in the human is the association between the enlarged fetal adrenal and estrogen excretion accepted.

The conclusions drawn in this review rest mainly on information obtained either by measurement of steroid biosynthesis and metabolism *in vitro* or during perfusion or from measurements of the steroid content of cord blood obtained after delivery. No data on the concentration of ACTH, androgen sulfates, cortisol, progesterone, or cortisol-binding globulin in fetal plasma during gestation have been obtained so far. Bearing in mind the ethical problems posed by such measurements, this lack of information is understandable. It seemed pertinent, therefore, to review the data available in order to stimulate consideration of the problems involved and to invite attempts at their solution.

Since the basis for the conclusions drawn about events during gestation is often, of necessity, indirect, the conclusions must be considered in relation to information that is well founded. The increasing quantities of androgen secreted by the fetal adrenal are well established, provided estriol excretion during pregnancy is accepted as an index of androgen production. Suppression of androgen production in the fetus through treatment of the mother with corticosteroids (Simmer *et al.*, 1966) relates androgen production to the activity of the hypothalamic-pituitary-adrenal axis of the fetus. The experiments with metyrapone (Oakey and Heys, 1970) indicate the reverse effect, that is, stimulation of androgen production by the fetus in response to a reduced cortisol concentration in the fetus. That different numbers of available cortisol binding sites exist in maternal and fetal plasma is demonstrated by data from at least four laboratories. Four important proposals are made, however, which have not been fully substantiated. These are that the fetus secretes cortisol *in utero;* that a substantial portion of this cortisol is transferred to the maternal circulation; that this transfer increases the metabolic clearance rate of cortisol; and that ACTH secretion by the fetus increases to compensate for this increased cortisol clearance rate.

Certain features of the conclusions reached have been suggested previously. Lanman (1961) recognized that the fetal adrenal was enlarged and argued that this was due to stimulation by ACTH rather than by other tropic factors, for example, HGG, estrogens, or growth hormone. Although a response of atropic "fetal" zone tissue to ACTH could be demonstrated (Lanman, 1961, 1962), the proposal did not meet with wide acceptance, since the stimulus suggested for ACTH secretion was not altogether convincing. Lanman (1961) considered that a major reason for this stimulus was the inability of the fetus to produce cortisol. This theory, however, did not distinguish between a normal fetus and one afflicted with congenital adrenal hyperplasia associated with an inability for cortisol biosynthesis, where in any case adrenal enlargement was much greater than normal.

Mills (1964) and Cope (1965) both suggested that cortisol secreted by the fetus might pass to the mother, in view of the lower capacity for cortisol binding in the fetal plasma. A transfer of cortisol in the reverse direction had been recognized (Migeon *et al.*, 1956; Aarskog, 1965) but occurs at delivery when, under stress, the maternal cortisol production rate increases (Migeon *et al.*, 1968) and large quantities of nonprotein bound cortisol are available for diffusion from mother to fetus.

It is argued here that the fetus has a degree of adrenal hyperplasia resulting from an increased secretion of ACTH. The situation in the normal fetus must differ from that in a fetus affected by congenital adrenal hyperplasia associated with an incomplete complement of steroid hydroxylase activities necessary for cortisol biosynthesis. In such a situation less cortisol will be available and ACTH secretion is higher than normal (Sydnor, *et al.*, 1953). Affected infants have larger adrenals than normal (Blackman, 1946). Moreover, adrenal androgen production is greater than normal in this condition (Eberlein, 1965) and is reflected by an increased maternal estriol excretion (Cathro *et al.*, 1969).

It has been noticed that infants born to women treated with corticosteroids during pregnancy rarely suffer from adrenal insufficiency after birth. Bongiovanni and McPadden (1960) reviewed the literature and found only one case of adrenal insufficiency after birth in 260 treated pregnancies. Yackel *et al.* (1966) noted that none of the 26 infants born to 21 women treated with corticosteroids during their pregnancies showed signs of adrenal insufficiency. While it is apparent that corticosteroids given therapeutically will cross the placenta and suppress ACTH production (Section VI), this will not of necessity suppress the production of cortisol after birth. From the data presented in this review, it has been concluded that the fetus synthesizes cortisol largely from progesterone in the "fetal" zone, which is the zone responsive to ACTH. After birth, cortisol production must proceed mainly in the "definitive" zone from cholesterol as in the adult (Borkowski *et al.*, 1967), since the supply of progesterone from the placenta is withdrawn and the "fetal" zone degenerates. The "definitive" zone *in utero* appears to be relatively independent of ACTH. Therefore, inhibition of ACTH secretion in the fetus should leave cortisol production by the fetus (from progesterone) and by the infant (from cholesterol) virtually undisturbed. Hypoplasia of adrenals in infants born to women treated with corticosteroids has been recognized. In a case presenting at Leeds Maternity Hospital, the mother received 7.5 mg of prednisone daily and the hypoplasia was confined to the "fetal" zone, but other congenital abnormalities were observed (Cowen and Kohler, 1968). Oppenheimer (1964) recorded a case in which the mother received at least 40 mg of prednisone daily and where the infant had atrophic adrenals with histological changes in the "definitive" zone also. Two infants born to women given 10–15 mg prednisone daily showed no adrenal atrophy at autopsy (Simmer *et al.*, 1966). It is likely that the degree of adrenal atrophy is related to the dose of steroid given. The key feature of the relationship is that cortisol production *in utero* is believed to occur without direct stimulation by ACTH in a tissue whose growth is sensitive to ACTH. The "definitive" zone of the fetal adrenal probably accounts for little cortisol production *in utero* and most of the cortisol production after birth.

The apparent paradox between the observation that corticosteroids given therapeutically will cross the placenta to the fetus while there is little net transfer of cortisol formed by the mother, can be readily resolved. In order to demonstrate suppression of estriol production in late pregnancy more than 75 mg of cortisol needs to be given daily, either as cortisol or as one of the synthetic analogs (Oakey, 1970). Thus, the capacity of the binding globulin in maternal plasma will be exceeded, as happens at delivery, and free corticosteroid will be available to cross the placenta. If synthetic corticosteroids are given a similar effect is seen, since these steroids have little or no affinity for cortisol binding globulin (Murphy, 1967).

The hyperplastic "fetal" zone degenerates after birth and involutes within about 3 months (Tahka, 1951). Steroid production by the "fetal" zone also declines during this period, if the concentration of Δ^5-3β-hydroxysteroid sulfates in infant plasma (Eberlein, 1965) and urine (Reynolds, 1965) during this period is taken to indicate the function of the "fetal" zone. The infant adrenal, composed of "definitive" zone tissue and degenerating "fetal" zone responds to ACTH by increases of 17-hydroxycorticosteroids and cortisol production (Bertrand *et al.*, 1962; Hillman and Giroud, 1965; Ducharme *et al.*, 1970) and, to a much lesser degree, of Δ^5-3β-hydroxysteroids (Lauritzen *et al.*, 1968). Gradually the latter activity wanes and returns only after puberty (Mills *et al.*, 1962). The reason for the involution of the "fetal" zone is not known. Possibly, as ACTH secretion falls after birth in response to a reduction in cortisol clearance rate, the hyperplastic structure cannot be maintained and, therefore, degenerates. However, in the newborn infant affected by congenital adrenal hyperplasia, where plasma ACTH secretion is considered to be high and remains high without treatment (Sydnor *et al.*, 1953) the "fetal" zone degenerates (Blackman, 1946). A reduction in plasma ACTH cannot, therefore, be the only factor responsible for initiation of the degeneration of the"fetal" zone.

The role of human chorionic gonadotropin in control of androgen production should also be explored. The influence of this hormone is removed at birth. Pauerstein and Solomon (1966) have demonstrated a role for HCG in the control of adrenal androgen production in the adult. Despite the finding of Lanman (1962) that human chorionic gonadotropin did not stimulate adrenal growth in anencephalic infants, a function in the regulation of androgen production deserves consideration, especially in the period prior to the 20th week of pregnancy.

While the increased estrogen production in late pregnancy can be understood on the basis of ideas put forward here, the means by which the process is initiated is not clear. Several possibilities can be envisaged. The rise in estrogen production in early pregnancy, derived from the corpus luteum, is sufficient to provoke an increase in the concentration of cortisol binding globulin in maternal plasma (Doe *et al.*, 1964). This may, in turn, provide the stimulus for transfer of cortisol from fetus to mother. It is doubtful, however, whether the fetus is sufficiently integrated, at this early stage of gestation, to respond in the manner which has been described essentially for the second half of pregnancy. The competitive role of progesterone, described above, may be a more important factor in initiating a net transfer of cortisol from fetus to mother. It must be recognized also that the production of increased quantities of estrogen, including estrone and estradiol-17β, will enhance the production of cortisol binding globulin. To some extent, therefore, the process outlined, once initiated, may be self-generating.

Many attempts have been made to explain the increased estrogen excretion in pregnancy. Investigators have sought a requirement for estrogens, either to maintain the pregnancy or as a factor in the induction of parturition. While estrogens are essential in early pregnancy for implantation of the fertilized egg, no clear necessity for large quantities of estrogens in late pregnancy has been demonstrated (Hytten and Leitch, 1964; Benirschke and Driscoll, 1967; Klopper, 1968). Infants born to mothers excreting very low quantities of estrogens (e.g., in anencephaly, congenital adrenal hypoplasia, or congenital sulfatase deficiency) often survive to term and are of almost normal body weight (Milic and Adamsons, 1969; Uttley, 1968; O'Donohoe and Holland, 1968; France and Liggins, 1969). A requirement for large quantities of estrogen for nutrition and development of the fetus must, therefore, be questioned. Since expulsion of the fetus often occurs only after a long delay following death *in utero,* estrogens do not appear to be involved directly in the initiation of labor (reviewed by Csapo and Wood, 1968). A similar conclusion was drawn by Klopper *et al.* (1969), who injected estriol sulfate into the amniotic cavity near term, without hastening delivery. This treatment, however, modified uterine contractile activity. The adrenal of the fetal lamb (Liggins, 1968) and possibly of the human fetus (Anderson *et al.*, 1969) is involved in the initiation of parturition.

This appears to be a manifestation of corticosteroid production (Liggins, 1968, 1969). The competition between cortisol and progesterone for binding sites in the fetal plasma and the suggested increase in ACTH secretion by the fetal pituitary may possibly play some role in this process. The present hypothesis recalls an earlier proposal of Bolté *et al.* (1964a) that estrogen production is a means of disposing of androgens. It must be concluded from the present review and in the limited state of our knowledge that estrogens are a by-product of an unusual pattern of steroid secretion in the fetus and that estrogen biosynthesis by the placenta is an efficient means of removing androgenic steroids.

The conclusions drawn and the hypothesis put forward in this review leave many questions unanswered. The drive for the high production of androgen sulfates from the fetal adrenal can be traced ultimately, to an inequality in the number of sites available for cortisol binding in the fetal and maternal plasma. As discussed earlier, whether this is due to absolute differences in the concentration of the binding globulin in the two circulations, or to the competitive effect of progesterone, requires further study. The failure of 3β-hydroxysteroid dehydrogenase enzymes in the fetal adrenal to be active in gestation also needs investigation. D. B. Villee (1966) claims to have demonstrated an inhibitory effect of progesterone on these enzymes *in vitro* and this effect should be explored *in vivo*. Similarly, the effect of ACTH on steroid biosynthesis in both "fetal" and "definitive" zone tissue has been largely neglected, although this problem is being studied in our laboratory. Perhaps a more detailed understanding of the problems will be difficult to obtain from studies during human pregnancy, and a more rewarding approach may be made with animals amenable to surgical interference in mid-gestation.

It is considered that the hypothesis proposed reconciles much apparently conflicting evidence, especially that relating to the effects of corticosteroid treatment in pregnancy and the failure of corticosteroids in the maternal circulation to suppress excessive ACTH secretion by the fetal pituitary. It enables a clear distinction to be drawn between the adrenal hyperplasia seen in the normal fetus and the more gross form evident in fetuses with little ability for cortisol biosynthesis.

It is hoped that other workers interested in this field, and those at present outside it, will be encouraged to take up some of the problems outstanding. If this results in an improved and more complete understanding of the complex relationship between mother, placenta, and fetus, the real purpose of this review will have been achieved.

Acknowledgments

Encouragement and constructive comments from Professor G. H. Lathe, Drs. M. J. Levell, M. M. Shahwan, S. R. Stitch, and A. D. Tait and financial support from the Medical Research Council and the Wellcome Trust are gratefully acknowledged.

REFERENCES

Aarskog, D. (1965). *Acta Paediat. Scand.* Suppl. 158.

Abramovich, D. R., and Wade, A. P. (1969a). *J. Obstet. Gynaecol. Brit. Commonw.* **76**, 610.

Abramovich, D. R., and Wade, A. P. (1969b). *J. Obstet. Gynaecol. Brit. Commonw.* **76**, 893.

Anderson, A. B. M., Laurence, K. M., and Turnbull, A. C. (1969). *J. Obstet. Gynaecol. Brit. Commonw.* **76**, 196.

Angevine, D. M. (1938). *Arch. Pathol.* **26**, 507.

Aschheim, S., and Zondek, B. (1927). *Klin. Wochenschr.* **6**, 1322.

Ask-Upmark, M. E. (1926). *Acta Obstet. Gynecol. Scand.* **5**, 211.

Baulieu, E. E., and Dray. M. F. (1963). *J. Clin. Endocrinol. Metab.* **23**, 1298.

Bègue, J. A. (1965). *C. R. Acad. Sci.* **260**, 3777.

Beischer, N. A., Brown, J. B., and Smith, M. A. (1968). *J. Obstet. Gynaecol. Brit. Commonw.* **75**, 622.

Bengtsson, G., Ullberg, S., Wiqvist, N., and Diczfalusy, E. (1964). *Acta Endocrinol. (Copenhagen)* **46**, 544.

Benirschke, K. (1956). *Obstet. Gynecol.* **8**, 412.

Benirschke, K., and Driscoll, S. G. (1967). *In* "The Pathology of the Human Placenta," p. 446. Springer, Berlin.

Berson, S. A., and Yalow, R. S. (1968). *J. Clin. Invest.* **47**, 2725.

Bertrand, J., Gilly, R., and Loras, B. (1962). *In* "The Human Adrenal Cortex" (A. R. Currie, T. Symington, and J. K. Grant, eds.), p. 608. Livingstone, Edinburgh and London.

Birchall, K., Cathro, D. M., Forsyth, C. C., and Mitchell, F. L. (1961). *Lancet* **1**, 26.

Bird, C. E., Wiqvist, N., Diczfalusy, E., and Solomon, S. (1966). *J. Clin. Endocrinol. Metab.* **26**, 1144.

Blackman, S. S. (1946). *Bull. Johns Hopkins Hosp.* **78**, 180.

Bloch, E., and Benirschke, K. (1959). *J. Biol. Chem.* **234**, 1085.

Bloch, E., and Benirschke, K. (1962). *In* "The Human Adrenal Cortex" (A. R. Currie, T. Symington, and J. K. Grant, eds.), p. 589. Livingstone, Edinburgh and London.

Bolté, E., Mancuso, S., Eriksson, G., Wiqvist, N., and Diczfalusy, E. (1964a). *Acta Endocrinol. (Copenhagen)* **45**, 535.

Bolté. E., Mancuso, S., Eriksson, G., Wiqvist, N., and Diczfalusy, E. (1964b). *Acta Endocrinol. (Copenhagen)* **45**, 576.

Bolté, E., Wiqvist, N., and Diczfalusy, E. (1966). *Acta Endocrinol. (Copenhagen)* **52**, 583.

Bongiovanni, A. M., and McPadden, A. J. (1960). *Fert. Steril.* **11**, 181.

Booth, M., Dixon, P. F., Gray, C. H., Greenaway, J. M., and Holness, N. J. (1961). *J. Endocrinol.* **23**, 25.

Borkowski, A. J., Levin, S., Delcroix, C., Mahler, A., and Verhas, V. (1967). *J. Clin. Invest.* **46**, 797.

Breuer, H. (1962). *Vitam. Horm. (New York)* **20**, 285.

Brown, H., Englert, E., and Wallach, S. (1958). *J. Clin. Endocrinol. Metab.* **18**, 167.

Brown, J. B. (1956). *Lancet* **1**, 704.

Brown, J. B. (1959). *J. Obstet. Gynaecol. Brit. Emp.* **66**, 795.

Brown, J. B. (1960). *Advan. Clin. Chem.* **3,** 157.
Brown, J. B., Kellar, R., and Matthew, G. D. (1959). *J. Obstet. Gynaecol. Brit. Emp.* **66,** 177.
Brown, J. B., Beischer, N. A., and Smith. M. A. (1968). *J. Obstet. Gynaecol. Brit. Commonw.* **75,** 819.
Cassmer, O. (1959). *Acta Endocrinol. (Copenhagen)* Suppl. 45.
Cathro, D. M., Bertrand, J., and Coyle, M. G. (1969). *Lancet* **1,** 732.
Charles, D., Harkness, R. A., Kenny, F. M., Menini, E., Ismail, A. A. A., Durkin, J. W., and Loraine, J. A. (1970). *Amer. J. Obstet. Gynecol.* **106,** 66.
Cleary, R. E., Depp, R., and Pion, R. (1970). *Amer. J. Obstet. Gynecol.* **106,** 534.
Colás, A., and Heinrichs, W. L. (1965). *Steroids* **5,** 753.
Colás, A., Heinrichs, W. L., and Tatum, H. J. (1964). *Steroids* **3,** 417.
Conrad, S. H., Pion, R. J., and Kitchin, J. D. (1967). *J. Clin. Endocrinol. Metab.* **27,** 114.
Cooke, B. A. (1968). *J. Endocrinol.* **41,** xxiii.
Cope, C. L. (1965). *In* "Adrenal Steroids in Health and Disease," p. 68. Pitman Medical, London.
Cope, C. L., and Black, E. (1959). *J. Obstet. Gynaecol. Brit. Emp.* **66,** 404.
Coutts, J. R. T., and Macnaughton, M. C. (1969). *J. Endocrinol.* **44,** 481.
Cowen, P. N., and Kohler, H. G. (1968). Personal communication.
Csapo, A. I., and Wood, C. (1968). *In* "Recent Advances in Endocrinology" (V. H. T. James, ed.), p. 207. Churchill. London.
Dässler, C. G. (1966). *Acta Endocrinol. (Copenhagen)* **53,** 401.
Daughaday, W. H. (1958). *Arch. Intern. Med.* **101,** 286.
Daughaday, W. H., Kozak, I., and Biederman, O. (1959). *J. Clin. Invest.* **38,** 998.
Dawes, G. S. (1968). *In* "Foetal and Neonatal Physiology," p. 76. Year Book Publ., Chicago, Illinois.
Dell'Acqua, S., Mancuso, S., Eriksson, G., Ruse, J. L., Solomon, S., and Diczfalusy, E. (1967). *Acta Endocrinol. (Copenhagen)* **55,** 401.
De Moor, P., Heirwegh, K., Heremans, J. F., and Declerck-Raskin, M. (1962). *J. Clin. Invest.* **41,** 816.
Dickey, R. P., and Thompson, J. P. (1969). *J. Clin. Endocrinol. Metab.* **29,** 701.
Diczfalusy, E. (1964). *Fed. Proc., Fed. Amer. Soc. Exp. Biol.* **23,** 791.
Diczfalusy, E. (1969). *In* "The Foeto-Placental Unit" (A. Pecile and C. Finzi, eds.), p. 65. Excerpta Med. Found., Amsterdam.
Diczfalusy, E., and Borell, U. (1961). *J. Clin. Endocrinol. Metab.* **21,** 1119.
Doe, R. P., Fernandez, R., and Seal, U. S. (1964). *J. Clin. Endocrinol. Metab.* **24,** 1029.
Drayer, N. M., and Giroud, C. J. P. (1965). *Steroids* **5,** 289.
Driscoll, A. M. (1969). *Brit. Med. J.* **1,** 556.
Ducharme, J. R., Leboeuf, G., and Sandor, T. (1970). *J. Clin. Endocrinol. Metab.* **30,** 96.
Easterling, W. E., Simmer, H. H., Dignam. W. J., Frankland, M. V., and Naftolin, F. (1966). *Steroids* **8,** 157.
Eberlein, W. R. (1965). *J. Clin. Endocrinol. Metab.* **25,** 1101.
Eberlein, W. R., Winter, J., and Rosenfield, R. L. (1967). *In* "Hormones in Blood" (C. H. Gray and A. L. Bacharach, eds.), 2nd rev. ed., Vol. 2, p. 187. Academic Press, New York.
Engel, L. L., Baggett, B., and Halla, M. (1962). *Endocrinology* **70,** 907.
Engell, H. C., Winkler, K., Tygstrup, N., and Buus, O. (1961). *Ann. Surg.* **154,** 269.

France, J. T., and Liggins, G. C. (1969). *J. Clin. Endocrinol. Metab.* **29**, 138.

Frandsen, V. A., and Stakemann, G. (1961). *Acta Endocrinol. (Copenhagen)* **38**, 383.

Frandsen, V. A., and Stakemann, G. (1964). *Acta Endocrinol. (Copenhagen)* **47**, 265.

Fraser, R., and James, V. H. T. (1968). *J. Endocrinol.* **40**, 59.

Goebelsmann, U., Eriksson, G., Wiqvist, N., and Diczfalusy, E. (1965). *Acta Endocrinol. (Copenhagen)* **50**, 273.

Goldman, A. S., Yakovac, W. C., and Bongiovanni, A. M. (1966). *J. Clin. Endocrinol. Metab.* **26**, 14.

Greig, M., Coyle, M. G., Cooper, W., and Walker, J. (1962). *J. Obstet. Gynaecol. Brit. Commonw.* **69**, 772.

Gurpide, E., Angers, M., Vande Wiele, R. L., and Lieberman, S. (1962). *J. Clin. Endocrinol. Metab.* **22**, 935.

Halban, J. (1905). *Arch. Gynaekol.* **75**, 353.

Harbert, G. M., McGaughey, H. S., Scoggin, W. A., and Thornton, W. N. (1964). *Obstet. Gynecol.* **23**, 413.

Harkness, R. A., Menini, E., Charles, D., Kenny, F. M., and Rombaut, R. (1966). *Acta Endocrinol. (Copenhagen)* **52**, 409.

Hausknecht, R. U., and Mandelman, N. (1969). *Amer. J. Obstet. Gynecol.* **104**, 433.

Heinrichs, W. L., Feder, H. H., and Colás, A. (1966). *Steroids* **7**, 91.

Heys, R. F., Scott, J. S., Oakey, R. E., and Stitch, S. R. (1968). *Lancet* **1**, 328.

Heys, R. F., Scott, J. S., Oakey, R. E., and Stitch, S. R. (1969). *Obstet. Gynecol.* **33**, 390.

Hillman, D. A., and Giroud, C. J. P. (1965). *J. Clin. Endocrinol. Metab.* **25**, 243.

Hillman, D. A., Stachenko, J., and Giroud, C. J. P. (1962). *In* "The Human Adrenal Cortex" (A. R. Currie, T. Symington, and J. K. Grant, eds.), p. 596. Livingstone, Edinburgh and London.

Hilton, J. G., Black, W. C., Athos, W., McHugh, B., and Westermann, C. D. (1962). *J. Clin. Endocrinol. Metab.* **22**, 900.

Hobkirk, R., and Nilsen, M. (1962). *J. Clin. Endocrinol. Metab.* **22**, 134.

Hopper, B. R., and Tullner, W. W. (1967). *Steroids* **9**, 517.

Hytten, F. E., and Leitch, I. (1964). *In* "Physiology of Human Pregnancy," p. 155. Blackwell, Oxford.

Ingle, D. J., and Fisher, G. T. (1938). *Proc. Soc. Exp. Biol. Med.* **39**, 149.

Jackanicz, T. M., Wiqvist, N., and Diczfalusy, E. (1969). *Biochim. Biophys. Acta* **176**, 883.

Jaffé, R. B., Pérez-Palacios, G., Lamont, K. G., and Givner, M. L. (1968). *J. Clin. Endocrinol. Metab.* **28**, 1671.

James, V. H. T. (1966). *J. Eur. Steroides* **1**, 5.

Johannisson, E. (1968). *Acta Endocrinol. (Copenhagen)* Suppl. 130.

Jost, A. (1948). *C. R. Soc. Biol.* **142**, 273.

Jost, A. (1966). *Recent Progr. Horm. Res.* **22**, 541.

Jungmann, R. A., and Schweppe, J. S. (1967). *J. Clin. Endocrinol. Metab.* **27**, 1151.

Karaboyas, G. C., and Koritz, S. B. (1965). *Biochemistry* **4**, 462.

Keene, M. F. L., and Hewer, E. E. (1927). *J. Anat.* **61**, 302.

Kenny, F. M., Preeyasombat, S. C., and Migeon, C. J. (1966a). *Pediatrics* **37**, 34.

Kenny, F. M., Preeyasombat, S. C., Spaulding, J. S., and Migeon, C. J. (1966b). *Pediatrics* **37**, 960.

Kirschner, M. A., Lipsett, M. B., and Collins, D. R. (1965). *J. Clin. Invest.* **44**, 657.

Kirschner, M. A., Wiqvist, N., and Diczfalusy, E. (1966). *Acta Endocrinol. (Copenhagen)* **53**, 584.

Kitchell, R. L., and Wells, L. J. (1952). *Anat. Rec.* **112**, 561.

Kiyono, H. (1925). *Virchow's Arch. Pathol. Anat. Physiol.* **257**, 441.

Klein, G. P., and Giroud, C. J. P. (1967). *Steroids* **9**, 113.

Klopper, A. I. (1968). *Obstet. Gynecol. Surv.* **23**, 813.

Klopper, A. I., Dennis, K. J., and Farr, V. (1969). *Brit. Med. J.* **2**, 786.

Knobil, E., and Briggs, F. N. (1955). *Endocrinology* **57**, 147.

Lamb, E. J., Dignam, W. J., Pion, R. J., and Simmer, H. H. (1964). *Acta Endocrinol. (Copenhagen)* **45**, 243.

Lambert, M., and Pennington, G. W. (1963). *Nature (London)* **197**, 391.

Lambert, M., and Pennington, G. W. (1964). *Nature (London)* **203**, 656.

Landon, J., James, V. H. T., and Peart, W. S. (1967). *Acta Endocrinol. (Copenhagen)* **56**, 321.

Lanman, J. T. (1953). *Medicine (Baltimore)* **32**, 389.

Lanman, J. T. (1961). *Pediatrics* **27**, 140.

Lanman, J. T. (1962). *In* "The Human Adrenal Cortex" (A. R. Currie, T. Symington, and J. K. Grant, eds.), p. 547. Livingstone, Edinburgh and London.

Lanman, J. T., and Silverman, L. M. (1957). *Endocrinology* **60**, 433.

Laumas, K. R., Malkini, P. K., Koshti, G. S., and Hingorani, V. (1968). *Amer. J. Obstet. Gynecol.* **101**, 1062.

Lauritzen, C., Shackleton, C. H. L., and Mitchell, F. L. (1968). *Acta Endocrinol. (Copenhagen)* **58**, 655.

Levin, M. E., and Daughaday, W. H. (1955). *J. Clin. Endocrinol. Metab.* **15**, 1499.

Leyssac, P. (1961). *Acta Obstet. Gynecol. Scand.* **40**, 181.

Liddle, G. W., Estep, H. L., Kendall, J. W., Williams, W. C., and Townes, A. W. (1959). *J. Clin. Endocrinol. Metab.* **19**, 875.

Liddle, G. W., Island, D., and Meador, C. K. (1962). *Recent Progr. Horm. Res.* **18**, 125.

Liggins, G. C. (1968). *J. Endocrinol.* **42**, 323.

Liggins, G. C. (1969). *In* "Foetal Autonomy" (G. E. W. Wolstenholme and M. O'Connor, eds.), p. 218. Churchill, London.

Liggins, G. C., and Kennedy, P. C. (1968). *J. Endocrinol.* **40**, 371.

Little, B., Bougas, J., Tait, J. F., and Tait, S. A. S. (1962). *Proc. Endocrine Soc.* p. 17.

MacDonald, P. C., and Siiteri, P. K. (1965). *J. Clin. Invest.* **44**, 465.

Maeyama, M., Nakagawa, T., Tuchida, Y., and Matuoka, H. (1969). *Steroids* **13**, 59.

Mellin, T. N., and Erb, R. E. (1965). *J. Dairy Sci.* **48**, 687.

Meyer, R. (1912). *Virchow's Arch. Pathol. Anat. Physiol.* **210**, 158.

Michie, E. A. (1966). *Acta Endocrinol. (Copenhagen)* **51**, 535.

Migeon, C. J. (1955). *Ciba Found. Colloq. Endocrinol.* **8**, 141.

Migeon, C. J. (1959). *J. Pediat.* **55**, 280.

Migeon, C. J., Prystowsky, H., Grumbach, M. M., and Byron, M. C. (1956). *J. Clin. Invest.* **35**, 488.

Migeon, C. J., Bertrand, J., and Wall, P. E. (1957). *J. Clin. Invest.* **36**, 1350.

Migeon, C. J., Bertrand, J., and Gemzell, C. A. (1961). *Recent Progr. Horm. Res.* **17**, 207.

Migeon, C. J., Bertrand, J., and Gemzell, C. A. (1962). *In* "The Human Adrenal Cortex" (A. R. Currie, T. Symington, and J. K. Grant, eds.), p. 580. Livingstone, Edinburgh and London.

Migeon, C. J., Kenny, F. M., and Taylor, F. H. (1968). *J. Clin. Endocrinol. Metab.* **28**, 661.

Mikhail, G., and Allen, W. M. (1967). *Amer. J. Obstet. Gynecol.* **99**, 308.

Milic, A. B., and Adamsons, K. (1969). *J. Obstet. Gynaecol.* **76**, 102.

Mills, I. H. (1964). *In* "Clinical Aspects of Adrenal Function," p. 101. Blackwell, Oxford.

Mills, I. H., Chen, P. S., and Bartter, F. C. (1959). *J. Endocrinol.* **18**, xxx.

Mills, I. H., Brooks, R. V., and Prunty, F. T. G. (1962). *In* "The Human Adrenal Cortex" (A. R. Currie, T. Symington, and J. K. Grant, eds.), p. 204. Livingstone, Edinburgh and London.

Morrison, J., and Kilpatrick, N. (1969). *J. Obstet. Gynaecol. Brit. Commonw.* **76**, 719.

Murphy, B. E. P. (1967). *J. Clin. Endocrinol. Metab.* **27**, 973.

Niemi, M., and Baillie, A. H. (1965). *Acta Endocrinol. (Copenhagen)* **48**, 423.

Nugent, C. A., and Mayes, D. M. (1966). *J. Clin. Endocrinol. Metab.* **26**, 1116.

Oakey, R. E. (1969). *Lancet* **1**, 886.

Oakey, R. E. (1970). *J. Obstet. Gynaecol. Brit. Commonw.* **76**, 922.

Oakey, R. E., and Heys, R. F. (1969). *J. Endocrinol.* **45**, xxiii.

Oakey, R. E., and Heys, R. F. (1970). *Acta Endocrinol.* **65**, 502.

Oakey, R. E., and Stitch, S. R. (1967). *J. Endocrinol.* **38**, xxiii.

Oakey, R. E., Bradshaw, L. R. A., Eccles, S. S., Stitch, S. R., and Heys, R. F. (1967). *Clin. Chim. Acta* **15**, 35.

O'Donohoe, N. V., and Holland, P. D. J. (1968). *Arch. Dis. Childhood* **43**, 717.

Oppenheimer, E. H. (1964). *Bull. Johns Hopkins Hosp.* **114**, 146.

Osinski, P. A. (1960). *Nature (London)* **187**, 777.

Pasqualini, J. R., Lowy, J., Wiqvist, N., and Diczfalusy, E. (1968). *Biochim. Biophys. Acta* **152**, 648.

Pauerstein, C. J., and Solomon, D. (1966). *Obstet. Gynecol.* **28**, 692.

Pérez-Palacios, G., Pérez, A. E., and Jaffé, R. B. (1968). *J. Clin. Endocrinol. Metab.* **28**, 19.

Peterson, R. E. (1958). *J. Clin. Invest.* **37**, 736.

Peterson, R. E., Wyngaarden, J. B., Guerra, S. L., Brodie, B. B., and Bunim, J. J. (1955). *J. Clin. Invest.* **34**, 1779.

Pion, R. J., Jaffé, R. B., Wiqvist, N., and Diczfalusy, E. (1967). *Biochim. Biophys. Acta* **137**, 584.

Plager, J. E., Samuels, L. T., Ballard, A., Tyler, F. H., and Hecht, H. H. (1957). *J. Clin. Endocrinol. Metab.* **17**, 1.

Raeside, J. I. (1963). *J. Reprod. Fert.* **6**, 427.

Rebbe, H., and Møller, K. J. A. (1966). *Acta Obstet. Gynecol. Scand.* **45**, 261.

Reynolds, J. W. (1965). *J. Clin. Endocrinol. Metab.* **25**, 416.

Reynolds, J. W., Colle, E., and Ulstrom, R. A. (1962). *J. Clin. Endocrinol. Metab.* **22**, 245.

Reynolds, J. W., Wiqvist, N., and Diczfalusy, E. (1969). *Acta Endocrinol. (Copenhagen)* **61**, 533.

Rosenthal, H. E., Slaunwhite, W. R., and Sandberg, A. A. (1969). *J. Clin. Endocrinol. Metab.* **29**, 352.

Ryan, K. J. (1959). *J. Biol. Chem.* **234**, 2006.

Sabata, V., and Novák, M. (1967). *Gynaecologia* **163**, 179.

Sandberg, A. A., and Slaunwhite, W. R. (1959). *J. Clin. Invest.* **38**, 1290.

Sandberg, A. A., and Slaunwhite, W. R. (1962). *J. Clin. Invest.* **41**, 1396.

Savard, K. (1961). *Endocrinology* **68**, 411.

Scammon, R. E. (1926). *Proc. Soc. Exp. Biol. Med.* **23**, 809.

Schwers, J., Eriksson, G., and Diczfalusy, E. (1965). *Acta Endocrinol. (Copenhagen)* 49, 65.

Scommegna, A., Nedoss, B. R., and Chattoraj, S. C. (1968). *Obstet. Gynecol.* 31, 526.

Shahwan, M. M., Oakey, R. E., and Stitch, S. R. (1969a). *Acta Endocrinol. (Copenhagen)* 60, 491.

Shahwan, M. M., Oakey, R. E., and Stitch, S. R. (1969b). *J. Endocrinol.* 44, 557.

Shahwan, M. M., Oakey, R. E., and Stitch, S. R. (1969c). *J. Endocrinol.* 45, xxiv.

Shimao, S., Wiqvist, N., Diczfalusy, E., and Solomon, S. (1968). *Can. J. Biochem.* 46, 663.

Short, R. V., and Eton, B. (1959). *J. Endocrinol.* 18, 418.

Siiteri, P. K., and MacDonald, P. C. (1963). *Steroids* 2, 713.

Simmer, H. H., Easterling, W. E., Pion, R. J., and Dignam, W. J. (1964). *Steroids* 4, 125.

Simmer, H. H., Dignam, W. J., Easterling, W. E., Frankland, M. V., and Naftolin, F. (1966). *Steroids* 8, 179.

Slaunwhite, W. R., and Sandberg, A. A. (1959). *J. Clin. Invest.* 38, 384.

Slaunwhite, W. R., Karsay, M. A., Hollmer, A., Sandberg, A. A., and Niswander, K. (1965). *Steroids* Suppl. 2, 211.

Solomon, S., Lanman, J. T., Lind, J., and Lieberman, S. (1958). *J. Biol. Chem.* 233, 1084.

Solomon, S., Bird, C. E., Ling, W., Iwamiya, M., and Young, P. C. M. (1967). *Recent Progr. Horm. Res.* 23, 297.

Stark, E., Gyévai, A., Szalay, K., and Acs, Z. (1965). *Can. J. Physiol. Pharmacol.* 43, 1.

Steenburg, R. W., Smith, L. L., Shoemaker, W. C., and Moore, F. D. (1960). *Surg., Gynecol. Obstet.* 111, 697.

Stone, D., and Hechter, O. (1954). *Arch. Biochem. Biophys.* 51, 457.

Strott, C. A., West, C. D., Nakagawa, K., Kondo, T., and Tyler, F. H. (1969). *J. Clin. Endocrinol. Metab.* 29, 6.

Swinyard, C. A. (1943). *Anat. Rec.* 87, 141.

Symington, T. (1962). *In* "The Human Adrenal Cortex" (A. R. Currie, T. Symington, and J. K. Grant, eds.), p. 9. Livingstone, Edinburgh and London.

Sydnor, K. L., Kelley, V. C., Raile, R. B., Ely, R. S., and Sayers, G. (1953). *Proc. Soc. Exp. Biol. Med.* 82, 695.

Tahka, H. (1951). *Acta Paediat. Scand.* 40, Suppl. 81.

Tait, J. F., and Burstein, S. (1964). *In* "The Hormones" (G. Pincus, K. V. Thimann, and E. B. Astwood, eds.), Vol. 5, p. 441. Academic Press, New York.

Talbert, L. M., and Easterling, W. E. (1967). *Amer. J. Obstet. Gynecol.* 99, 923.

Taylor, N. R. W., Loraine, J. A., and Robertson, H. A. (1953). *J. Endocrinol.* 9, 334.

Telegdy, G., Weeks, J. W., Wiqvist, N., and Diczfalusy, E. (1969). *Acta Endocrinol. (Copenhagen)* Suppl. 138, 54.

Telegdy, G., Weeks, J. W., Archer, D. F., Wiqvist, N., and Diczfalusy, E. (1970). *Acta Endocrinol (Copenhagen)* 63, 119.

Tulsky, A. S., and Koff, A. K. (1957). *Fert. Steril.* 8, 118.

Ulstrom, R. A., Colle, E., Burley, J., and Gunville, R. (1960). *J. Clin. Endocrinol. Metab.* 20, 1080.

Uotila, U. (1940). *Anat. Rec.* 76, 183.

Uttley, W. S. (1968). *Arch. Dis. Childhood* 43, 724.

van der Molen, H. J., and Groen, D. (1965). *J. Clin. Endocrinol. Metab.* **25**, 1625.

Villee, C. A., and Loring, J. (1965). *J. Clin. Endocrinol. Metab.* **25**, 307.

Villee, D. B. (1966). *Advan. Enzyme Regul.* **4**, 269.

Villee, D. B., Engel, L. L., and Villee, C. A. (1959). *Endocrinology* **65**, 465.

Villee, D. B., Engel, L. L., Loring, J. M., and Villee, C. A. (1961). *Endocrinology* **69**, 354.

Wallace, S. J., and Michie, E. A. (1966). *Lancet* **2**, 560.

Warren, J. C., and Cheatum, S. G. (1967). *J. Clin. Endocrinol. Metab.* **27**, 433.

Wells, L. J. (1947). *Anat. Rec.* **97**, 409.

Wells, L. J. (1948). *Proc. Soc. Exp. Biol. Med.* **68**, 487.

Whitehouse, B. J., and Vinson, G. P. (1968). *Steroids* **11**, 245.

Wieland, R. G., de Courcy, C., Levy, R. P., Zala, A. P., and Hirschmann, H. (1965). *J. Clin. Invest.* **44**, 159.

Wilson, K. M. (1937). *Amer. J. Obstet. Gynecol.* **34**, 977.

Wilson, R., Bird, C. E., Wiqvist, N., Solomon, S., and Diczfalusy, E. (1966). *J. Clin. Endocrinol. Metab.* **26**, 1155.

Wray, P. M., and Russell, C. S. (1964). *J. Obstet. Gynaecol. Brit. Commonw.* **71**, 97.

Yackel, D. B., Kempers, R. D., and McConahey, W. M. (1966). *Amer. J. Obstet. Gynecol.* **96**, 985.

Yannone, M. E., McCurdy, J. R., and Goldfien, A. (1968). *Amer. J. Obstet. Gynecol.* **101**, 1058.

Yates, F. E., and Urquhart, J. (1962). *Physiol. Rev.* **42**, 359.

Yoshimi, T., Strott, C. A., Marshall, J. R., and Lipsett, M. B. (1969). *J. Clin. Endocrinol. Metab.* **29**, 225.

Zander, J. (1961). *Ciba Found. Study Group* No. 9, 32.

Zander, J., Holzmann, K., and Bengtsson, L. P. (1965). *Acta Obstet. Gynecol. Scand.* **44**, 204.

Insulin and the Pancreas

GEROLD M. GRODSKY

Metabolic Research Unit and Department of Biochemistry and Biophysics, University of California, San Francisco, California

I. Foreword

Since our earlier review (Grodsky and Forsham, 1966) numerous studies have established that many hormones, lipids, amino acids, and drugs affect the release of insulin (see reviews by Frohman, 1969; Mayhew *et al.*, 1969[*]). Currently, areas of widespread interest include: the nature of the basic multiple phenomena leading to release, how these phenomena are controlled, and on which ones the various agents act. Indeed, this may be a poor time for a review since established methods permit clarification, within the next year or two, of areas which at the moment are almost undecipherable. In the hope that this manuscript will have some extended usefulness, I have attempted to review the field in depth,[†] including pertinent material discussed in my original review (Grodsky and Forsham, 1966).

[*] The latter review was brought to our attention after final completion of this manuscript.

[†] To January 1970.

In addition, considerable speculative considerations (not always my own conceptions) were introduced which may serve to stimulate further investigations by others.

A complete review of an area of such extensive interest is impossible; I am therefore deeply grateful to the many investigators who kindly sent preprints of their current work and apologize to those whom I may have inadvertently overlooked.

II. CHEMICAL STRUCTURE AND ACTIVITY OF INSULIN

A. THE PRIMARY STRUCTURE OF INSULIN

The primary structure of insulin from a variety of species has been determined (Sanger, 1956, 1960; L. F. Smith, 1966). All insulins so far studied consist of an acidic (A) and a basic (B) chain usually containing 21 and 30 amino acids, respectively. The two chains are interconnected by two disulfide bridges. On the A chain an additional intradisulfide bond connects the half-cystines at positions 6 and 11. Many mammalian insulins, including those from the horse, sheep, pig, sperm whale, and cow, differ from each other only at amino acids 8, 9, and 10 beneath the internal disulfide bridge of the A chain (Harris et al., 1956); structures of porcine, sperm whale, and canine insulins are identical. Insulins from the cow and goat also have the same structure (F. G. Young, 1961). Human, porcine, and leporine insulins are identical, with the single exception of amino acid 30 on the carboxyl end of the B chain (threonine, alanine, or serine, respectively) (Nicol and Smith, 1960). Because of its structural similarity to human insulin, porcine insulin has been used for treating normal and insulin-resistant diabetic subjects (Akre et al., 1964; Boshell et al., 1964a; R. Feldman et al., 1963; Berson and Yalow. 1963). Porcine insulin is usually less antigenic and occasionally more effective, particularly in those subjects with high levels of circulating antibody to commercial mixtures of bovine and porcine insulins.

Large structural variations in mammalian insulins can occur; insulins from the rat and guinea pig, for example, differ from that of the pig by more than 17 of their 51 amino acid residues. The extremely poor cross-reaction of insulin from the capybara and the coypu with antisera made against a variety of insulins suggests that these mammalian insulins also contain many amino acid variations (Davidson et al., 1969). Mammalian insulins may also vary among subspecies since structural differences exist between insulin of the sei whale (finned) and the sperm whale (toothed) (Ishihara et al., 1958).

Nonmammalian insulins of the chicken or a variety of fish consistently vary broadly from insulin of higher mammals. A comparison of the sequences of cod and bovine insulins shows nine differences on the A chains and eight on the B chains (Reid *et al.*, 1968). Additionally, fish insulins differ in the alignment of amino acids in the B chain, each having an additional N-terminal amino acid, but ending at the C-terminus with one less amino acid (L. F. Smith, 1966; Reid *et al.*, 1968; Humbel and Crestfield, 1965).

Despite the large structural variations between species, the biologic potency of the various insulins is still 10–100% of bovine or porcine insulin when tested in mammals (Wilson and Dixon, 1961). The potency of cod insulin, for example, has been variably reported as 11 to 20 U/mg compared to an average of 25 U/mg for bovine insulin (Falkmer and Wilson, 1967; Reid *et al.*, 1968). Since most variations between species with similar biologic activity occur at amino acids A 8-10 under the disulfide bridge, A_{12-15}, B_{1-3}, and B_{30}, these portions of the molecule may not be at the active site of the hormone. Possibly histidine and serine residues are important for insulin activity; cod, hagfish, and guinea pig insulins have fewer serine and histidines in both chains and, concomitantly, reduced biologic activity (Weitzel *et al.*, 1967; Bosshard *et al.*, 1969).

More than one insulin may exist in a single species. Rat insulin contains two different B chains (L. F. Smith, 1964a), and certain fish insulins have four different chains (two A's and two B's) (Humbel, 1963). Although these observations suggest that more than one gene for insulin can occur in the same animal they could also indicate the occurrence of an interchange of amino acids at the translational level of insulin synthesis.

Crystallized insulin from common mammalian species is heterogeneous, consisting of many minor fractions with varying biologic and immunologic potencies (Mirsky and Kawamura, 1966). Although several of these components are precursors involved in the biosynthesis of insulin (Steiner *et al.*, 1967) or insulins with different levels of amidation (Harferist and Craig, 1952), the possibility that some may represent insulins with different primary amino acid structure should not be excluded. No abnormal insulin has yet been observed from normal human pancreas (L. F. Smith, 1964b) or islet cell tumors (Taylor and Sheldon, 1964; Brunfeldt *et al.*, 1969a), though a single amino acid substitution in insulin from one of eight diabetic subjects is reported (Kimmel and Pollock, 1967).

B. SECONDARY AND TERTIARY STRUCTURES OF INSULIN

The secondary and tertiary structures of porcine insulin crystals were recently analyzed by X-ray diffraction (Adams *et al.*, 1969). In the dimer configuration (Fig. 1), the A chain in each molecule is a compact unit

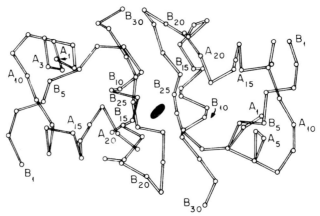

Fig. 1. Structure of the dimer of insulin. A chain, black: B chain, open. From Adams *et al.* (1969).

around which the terminal parts of the B chain are wrapped. The intra-disulfide loop of the A chain is directed away from the surface of the molecule, which is of particular interest since the opening of this loop may be involved in the action of insulin at the molecular level (Fong *et al.*, 1962; Whitney *et al.*, 1963). The highly folded structure of the A chain is maintained in part by hydrogen bonding at specific tyrosines. The center of the B chain supplies rigid structure to the molecule and contains more helices than the A chain. It also provides at B_{23-28} the sole contacts for the two molecules of insulin in the dimer. The adjacent B chains are arranged in antiparallel fashion, as pleated sheets. The hexamer of insulin is an oblate spheroid formed by the coordination of three insulin dimers around two zinc ions. Each zinc ion is in contact with three B_{10} histidine residues in each dimer. Additional reactions of the zinc ions with the oxygen of water and with additional tyrosines and histidines are probable. Hydrogen bonding between the dimers, particularly at glutamic acid residues, also contributes to the structure of the hexamer.

The secondary structure of a crystallized protein may not always be identical with the structure in solution; however, the X-ray studies are supported by other observations. Thus, a pleated sheet configuration (Hodgkin and Oughton, 1956) and in addition a right-handed helix consisting of about 20% of the molecule (Markus, 1964) were proposed on the basis of absorption spectra. Helical structure of insulin requires juxtaposition of the two chains, since the separated chains exist as random coils (Markus, 1964). The helical nature of the B chain as well as its involvement in dimer formation in the unexposed portion of the molecule may explain why tyrosines in this chain are often less reactive with iodine (Semeijns de Vries van Doesburgh and Havinga, 1964; Springell, 1962; De Zoeten *et al.*, 1961a,b) or detergents (Cowgill, 1964) than those in the A chain. Tyrosines on the separated A and B chains are equally susceptible to iodination (Semeijns de Vries van Doesburgh and Havinga, 1964). Numerous studies confirm that binding of zinc to insulin in solution involves the histidine residues (for review, see Brunfeldt *et al.*, 1969b; Brill and Venable, 1968; Covelli and Wolff, 1967). Arquilla *et al.* (1969) compared the immunologic cross-reactivity of modified insulins with antibody developed in pure strains of guina pigs, and independently suggested a structure for insulin similar to that proposed by the X-ray diffraction analysis.

The minimum chemical molecular weight of insulin must be 6000 (Sanger and Thompson, 1953); however, the degree of polymerization in solution will vary with the temperature, concentration, and pH (Fredericq, 1956; Marcker, 1960a; Harferist and Craig, 1952). Insulin exists as the dimer in mild acid and as the monomer in 30% acetic acid (Sluyterman, 1955). For this reason acetic acid is often used during the chemical separation of insulin from its larger precursors (proinsulins) since it minimizes dimer formation and misinterpretation of results. Most estimates of molecular weight of insulin in solution by physicochemical techniques vary from 12,000 to 48,000 (Gutfreund, 1952; Tietze and Neurath, 1952; Fredericq, 1957). Based on sedimentation rates, normal insulin in solution corresponded to a hexamer of 36,000 mol. wt. (Arquilla *et al.*, 1969), but with progressive addition of large molecules of fluorescein onto the amino side chains it dissociates to the monomer. Molecular weights are also dependent on zinc concentration (Fredericq, 1956) and can increase to 300,00 with increments of zinc, as large aggregates form. Insulin bound to antibody is not in monomeric form but has a molecular weight reported as 13,000 to 30,000 (Jones and Cunliffe, 1961; Birkinshaw, 1962). Studies to date refer to molecular weights of insulin in various artificial buffers; the physiologic molecular weight of insulin, and whether it changes with physiologic conditions, is not established.

C. STRUCTURE-ACTIVITY RELATIONSHIPS

The sites on the insulin molecule responsible for biologic activity are investigated both by comparing activity with structure of insulins from different species and by measuring changes in activity after controlled modification of side chains and end groups. These latter studies are complicated, since chemical changes on a single side chain may grossly modify the total secondary and tertiary structures, which in turn may alter a binding site far removed from the original modification.

Masking of amino groups at the terminal amino acids or on the lysine side chains, in itself, does not interfere with biologic activity (Fraenkel-Conrat and Fraenkel-Conrat, 1950); however, reaction with molecules large enough to produce steric hindrance may cause inactivation. Thus, tagging of amino side chains with acetylhomocysteine thiolactone (Virupaksha and Tarver, 1964), or more than one molecule of fluorescein isothiocyanate, decreases biologic activity. However, this loss of activity is associated with gross structural changes, indicated by conversion to the monomer, decrease in helices, and decreased combination with antibody (Brandenburg, 1969; Arquilla et al., 1969; Tietze et al., 1962; Haliken and Arquilla, 1961; Seidler et al., 1964).

Two-thirds of the available carboxyl groups can be esterified with small molecular-weight alcohols without loss of function (Mommaerts and Neurath, 1950). Further esterification causes a decrease in activity; however, this is accompanied with gross changes in the secondary structure (Grodsky et al., 1959) that may cause nonspecific inactivation. Limited sulfation of the hydroxyl groups of serine and threonine does not affect biologic activity (Reitz et al., 1946; Moloney et al., 1964). Since mild sulfation of these side chains causes a preferential decrease in combining power to antibody, sulfated insulin has been used in the treatment of insulin-treated diabetic subjects whose circulating antibody normally binds and inactivates unmodified insulin. Unfortunately, oversulfation progressively decreases biologic activity, and sulfated insulin with sufficient biologic activity, but little or no immunologic activity, is difficult to prepare reproducibly; thus clinical results have been inconsistent (Goldschmied and Laurian, 1968; Little and Arnott, 1966).

The A_{19} tyrosine in the C-terminal portion of the A chain of insulin may be particularly involved in the active site. Iodine at less than 1 molar equivalent is primarily directed to this particular tyrosine group (Rosa et al., 1967); Arquilla et al. (1968) prepared insulin-^{125}I with as little as 0.1 atom of iodine per molecule, chemically separated the monoiodoinsulin from the unlabeled hormone, and found it to have no significant biologic activity and attenuated immunologic activity. These studies question the usefulness of ^{131}I or ^{125}I tagged insulins as biologic tracers. However, the biologic integrity of the radioactive iodoinsulin may vary among laboratories (Yalow and Berson, 1966), since tagging insulin with ^{131}I or ^{125}I may produce nonspecific changes due to varying contamination in the labeled iodine preparations used. Iodoinsulin retains some immunologic activity and can be effectively used in radioimmunoassays where identical cross-reactivity of the labeled tracer with the unknown or standard insulins is not required.

In addition to the A_{19} tyrosine, the C-terminal amino acid of the A chain, asparagine, is required for the biologic function of insulin (Harris et al., 1956) though the amide group on this amino acid is not necessary. The importance of this asparagine (or aspartic acid) is further indicated by the observation that it is a constituent of all insulins thus far isolated. Removal of the C-terminal amino acid on the B chain (alanine in the case of bovine or porcine insulins) is rapidly achieved by carboxypeptidase digestion, without loss of biologic activity (Harris and Li, 1952; Nicol, 1961). The resulting dealaninated porcine insulin has an amino acid structure almost identical with human insulin, except that it is shorter by one amino acid. It is used as a substitute for bovine or porcine insulin in resistant diabetic subjects (Akre et al., 1964; Boshell et al., 1964a; Burt, 1965), particularly those with high circulating insulin antibodies. In most cases, however, the clinical and immunologic characteristics of dealaninated porcine insulin is identical with and often offers no advantage over intact porcine insulin. If the C-terminal octapeptide from the B-chain is removed by tryptic digestion, biologic inactivation results. This portion of the insulin molecule is important for maintaining secondary structure, since its loss results in gross changes in the physical chemical characteristics of the molecule (Arquilla et al., 1969). Some amino acids in the N-terminal portion of insulin are not required and can be removed by digestion with leucine aminopeptidase without diminution of biologic activity (E. L. Smith et al., 1958). As noted previously (page 41), histidines are particularly involved in maintaining the tertiary structure of insulin; their reduction in insulin from certain species or their destruction by photo-oxidation or cyanoethylation correlates with decreased biologic activity (see discussion in Reid et al., 1968).

Disruption of the disulfide bonds connecting the A and B chains of insulin results in the immediate loss of activity (Fraenkel-Conrat and Fraenkel-Conrat, 1950; Miller and Anderson, 1942; Lens and Neutelings, 1950). Since inactivation may occur after reduction of only 10% of these bonds, it is possible that disruption of a single inner connecting link may cause inactivation (or labilization) of a polymeric form of the hormone. Evidence is not conclusive (Fong et al., 1962; Whitney et al., 1963) that cleavage of the A chain intradisulfide bridge is involved in the hormone's biologic action but, if so, it suggests that it is the interchain disulfide bridges that must remain intact to maintain biologic activity.

Isolated A and B chains of insulin were originally reported to have small amounts of residual activity (Fisher and Zachariah, 1960; Langdon, 1960; Nicol, 1959). However, these chains were prepared originally from insulin and probably contained some of the intact hormone as an impurity. Completely synthetic A chain, either in the thiol form or with its disulfide bridge intact, or highly purified B chain, had no detectable biologic activity (Marglin and Cushman, 1967; Surmaczynska and Metz, 1969). Completely synthetic insulins with deliberate variance of amino acid structure in both the A and B chains have been prepared (Hörnle *et al.*, 1968). In time, these and other synthetic insulins will permit less equivocal evaluation of structure-activity relationships by eliminating conditions in which contaminating proteins or heterologous forms of insulin interfere.

D. PROINSULIN

In recent experiments measuring the rate of incorporation of radioactive amino acids into insulin in human islet cell adenomas, Steiner and associates (Steiner and Oyer, 1967) observed that the isotope was first incorporated into a protein of higher molecular weight (approximately 9000). This precursor or proinsulin reacted with anti-insulin antibodies and was thus related in structure to insulin. Similar proinsulins have been isolated from islet tissue of the rat (Clark and Steiner, 1969; Steiner *et al.*, 1967), codfish (Grant and Reid, 1968), angler fish (Bauer, 1968), Chinese hamster (Chang, 1970), and fetal calf (Tung and Yip, 1968). Commercial insulins contain about 1% proinsulin as an impurity and serve as a convenient source for its isolation in sufficient quantity to permit structural determination. Proinsulin is a single polypeptide chain which begins with the N-terminus of the B-chain sequence of insulin and terminates with the A-chain sequence; the two chains are connected by a polypeptide of approximately 3000 molecular weight consisting of 30 (bovine) or 33 (porcine) amino acids (Rubenstein and Steiner, 1970a; Chance *et al.*, 1968; Schmidt and Arens, 1968). The structure for porcine proinsulin is shown in Fig. 2. Although the primary structure of porcine and bovine insulins differs by only two amino acids, the connecting peptides differ in 17 of 33 positions (Chance *et al.*, 1968). Gross differences are also seen among connecting peptides in proinsulin from the rat, codfish, and human (Grant and Reid, 1968; Clark *et al.*, 1969). Two different proinsulins are found in rat islets, corresponding to the two insulins produced by this animal (Clark and Steiner, 1969). Large variation in the connecting peptide suggests that many amino acids in the connecting link are not vital in maintaining the shape of the molecule; each of the proinsulins thus far studied, however, contains arginine as both the initiating and terminating portions of the segment, making the connecting link particularly sensitive to tryptic digestion at these points. Hydrolysis of proinsulin with trypsin causes the conversion of the biologically inactive proinsulin to a fully active insulin derivative (Fig. 2). During this process the two arginines at the C- and N-terminals are released, result-

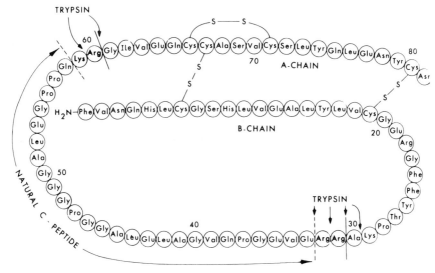

FIG. 2. Structure of bovine proinsulin.

ing in separation of the C peptide, which is one amino acid longer (lysine) than that resulting from natural cleavage. Trypsin hydrolysis also results in the nonbiologic removal of alanine from the C-30 position of the B chain. Therefore, trypsin does not exactly duplicate biologic conversion. Intermediates in the conversion of proinsulin to insulin have been isolated, in which one of the linkages at the carboxyl terminus of the connecting segment is hydrolyzed, resulting in a double-chain peptide that still retains most of the connecting peptide and has a molecular weight approximately that of proinsulin (Steiner *et al.*, 1968; Tung and Yip, 1969). Since varying amounts of proinsulin may be released from the pancreas (Goldsmith *et al.*, 1969; Roth *et al.*, 1968; Rubenstein *et al.*, 1968a; Gorden and Roth, 1969), its biologic activity in peripheral tissues is of interest. Purified proinsulin has 2–5% of the activity of insulin on carbohydrate and lipid metabolism in the isolated fat cell (Challoner, 1969) and frog muscle (Narahara, 1968) *in vitro*. When incubated with adipose tissue or diaphragm muscle, however, proinsulin is 20–35% as active as insulin on various parameters of glucose, glycogen, and triglyceride metabolism (Roth *et al.*, 1968; Rubenstein *et al.*, 1969, 1970a; Ryan and Robbins, 1969; Schmidt and Arens, 1968; Shaw and Chance, 1968a). These effects are completely blocked by the addition of Kunitz pancreatic trypsin inhibitor. Shaw and Chance (1968a) concluded that proinsulin has little intrinsic biologic activity, but that enzyme systems in adipose and muscle tissues can hydrolyze it to active insulin. In the intact animal, proinsulin can cause hypoglycemia; however, its biologic activity is about 10–15% that of insulin (Chance and Ellis, 1969; Chance et al., 1968). This low activity is consistent with the observations that little proinsulin-^{131}I is converted to insulin-^{131}I when injected into the intact animal (Rubenstein and Steiner, 1970a).

The double-chain intermediate has a biologic activity greater than that of proinsulin but less than of insulin (Steiner et al., 1968). Biologic activity of the C-peptide, secreted from the pancreas in equimolar concentrations with insulin (Rubenstein and Steiner, 1970a), has not been adequately explored; because its structure has little in common with insulin, extensive insulinlike activity is unlikely.

Proinsulin cross-reacts variably with anti-insulin antibodies, depending on the species of proinsulin and the species of both the insulin and the animal used to make the antibodies (Rubenstein and Steiner, 1970a). Thus, it can interfere in estimations of plasma insulin (Lawrence and Kirsteins, 1969). Improved sensitivity and specificity for assay of proinsulin is usually obtained when antiserum is prepared using proinsulin as the antigen. After adsorption of the antiserum with insulin, it can be used for radioimmunologic measurement of proinsulin without interference by insulin (Yip and Logothetopoulos, 1969; Rubenstein et al., 1969). Antibody against bovine or porcine proinsulin cross-reacts poorly with human proinsulin (Rubenstein and Steiner, 1970a); a specific radioimmunoassay for the human precursor, therefore, must await the availability of antihuman proinsulin sera. Since the C-peptide may cross-react in such a system, discriminating assay of proinsulin, insulin, and the C-peptide in plasma, may require their prior separation by gel filtration or by thin-layer gel chromatography (Ryan and Robbins, 1969). (See Section III for biosynthesis and secretion of insulin precursors and the C-peptide.)

Some unidentified proteins with molecular weights greater than insulin, but with some insulin activity, have been found in commercial insulin. These are not convertible to insulin by trypsin digestion, have a molecular weight comparable to insulin dimers, and may or may not be precursors of insulin (Steiner et al., 1968). Removal of high molecular weight contamination results in a "mono-component insulin" of clinical interest because of its reduced antigenicity (Schlichtkrull, 1970).

E. Chemical Synthesis of Insulin

Simultaneously, Katsoyannis (1963, 1964; Katsoyannis et al., 1963) and Meienhofer et al., (1963) chemically synthesized both the A and B chains of insulin and effected their combination to produce a wholly synthesized insulin molecule with biologic, immunologic, and chemical characteristics identical with the natural hormone. When the A and B chains were mixed under mildly oxidative conditions that permitted their highly reactive thiol groups to form disulfide linkages, low yields of insulin resulted, varying from 0.5 to 10% (Wilson et al., 1962; Chen-lu et al., 1961). Under optimal conditions a maximum resynthesis of 50% was obtained (Yu-cang et al., 1965; Rong-qing et al., 1963). It is apparent that A and B chains do not naturally align to form insulin but react to form nonspecific polymers. The discovery that insulin is biologically synthesized from a precursor (proinsulin) in which the two chains are connected and maintained in specific alignment by an additional peptide segment shows that the total peptide chain is first synthesized, the proper disulfide bridges and tertiary structure are formed, and the connecting peptide is removed by subsequent proteolytic activity. After the disulfide bridges of proinsulin are cleaved by reduction in $8 M$ urea, subsequent oxidation results in the reappearance of 60–70% of the original immunologic reactivity (Bromer and Patterson, 1969; Steiner and Clark, 1968). Therefore it can be anticipated that high yields of chemically synthesized insulin may be achieved by starting with a synthesized single chain proinsulin.

III. Biosynthesis, Storage, and Secretion of Insulin

A. Insulin and the Islets of Langerhans

The pancreatic islets of Langerhans, the primary sources of insulin, are histologically discrete cell groups which represent, in man, 1% of the pancreas by weight and number 1 to 2 million. The pancreatic islets may not be the sole source of insulin, since insulinlike activity has also been found in some nonpancreatic tumors (Perkoff and Simons, 1963; Boshell et al., 1964b; Whitney and Massey, 1961; August and Hiatt, 1958; Oleesky et al., 1962). Usually, however, immunologically active insulin is undetectable in these tumors (Genuth and Lebowitz, 1964; Love et al., 1965) or, when present, could be trapped insulin from the circulation (Unger et al., 1964). Extrapancreatic tissue capable of producing insulin may also be present in the duck, which cannot be made diabetic by surgical pancreatectomy though it becomes hyperglycemic after administration of anti-insulin antibody (Mirskey et al., 1964). However, in the normal animal, the pancreas, because of its size and insulin concentration, is the major and probably only significant source of insulin.

Primitive islet cells with immunologically active insulinlike material are found in orders as low as the tunicates and are usually associated with the hepatopancreas or gut in snails, starfish, and the earliest vertebrates. [For a summary of the ontogenetic and phylogenetic differentiation of endocrine pancreatic tissue, see Renold (1970).] Development of islets begins in the rat at day 13 of gestation (Hard, 1944) and insulinogenic function begins around day 17 or 18. Insulin granules are usually detectable by electron microscopy around this time. In man and rat (Ogilvie, 1937; Hellman, 1959a,b) the number and size of islets, beta cell granulation, and total weight of islet tissue increase until maturity. In man, this increase is faster than body growth for the first two years, falls behind during the growth period at 3–12 years and parallels growth from 13 to 21 years. It is at age 3 to 12 years that islet development lags, corresponding to the period of greatest incidence of juvenile diabetes. Changes in the islets of diabetic and prediabetic subjects and newborn infants of diabetic mothers have been reviewed (Ogilvie, 1964) and discussed by us previously (Grodsky and Forsham, 1966). In chronic juvenile diabetes, both size and number of islets and the ratio of beta to alpha cells are sharply decreased. In the mild maturity-onset diabetic, indication of hyperactivity is often observed though this may be a function of the obesity frequently found in these subjects (Steinke et al., 1961; Yalow and Berson, 1961). Recently Gepts et al. (1970) noted that islets from overt maturity-onset diabetics have about half the insulin of islets from normal subjects, though the number of beta cells is not changed; part of this decreased content may be due to concomitant fasting hyperglycemia. In obese nondiabetic humans, rats, and mice, islet mass and pancreatic insulin content are abnormally increased (Ogilvie, 1964), corresponding to the hyperinsulinemia observed in this state (Karam et al., 1963; Rabinowitz and Zierler, 1962; Bagdade et al., 1967; Benedetti et al., 1967; Kreisberg et al., 1967; Malaisse et al., 1968a; Genuth, 1969).

Though some controversy still exists, it is generally recognized that obesity in the mild diabetic increases the tendency for hyperinsulin response to a variety of stimulants but that this response is attenuated in subjects with increased severity of their diabetes. Progressive disease occurs in some animals with genetic propensity toward diabetes; this is characterized by enlarged islets with high insulin levels in the early stages followed in time with a state of pancreatic deficiency and hypofunction (Malaisse et al., 1968b).

Neoformation of islets and β cells is seen in special circumstances. Thus, ligation of the pancreatic duct, prolonged administration of anti-insulin antibody or alloxan, cause increased mitosis as measured by thymidine-^{3}H incorporation into nuclear DNA, as well as neoformation of β cells (Logothetopoulos and Bell, 1966; Logothetopoulos et al., 1970). In the alloxanized animals, proliferation of differentiated beta cells and the increase in mitosis occurred for only 1 week was not quantitatively sufficient to repair total damage.

B. Biosynthesis and Release of Insulin

1. *Proinsulin*

The rough endoplasmic reticulum (RER) of the β cell has a lamellar appearance with ribosomes attached on the outer surfaces (Fig. 3). During stimulation of insulin synthesis (e.g., the recovery period following depletion of the pancreas by tolbutamide) a pale gray amorphous material is observed in this organelle (Lacy, 1964; Volk and Lazarus, 1964). Presumably this contains the proinsulin polypeptide chain synthesized by the ribosomes, consisting of the B chain, connecting segment, and A chain (Fig. 2). The mechanism for folding of the chain to form appropriate disulfide linkages is unknown; this may be spontaneous, since proper alignment and production of proinsulin occurs with high yield *in vitro* under mild oxidative conditions (Rubenstein and Steiner, 1970a). Only proinsulin or its precursors is made in the endoplasmic reticulum since (1) proinsulin is found in the isolated microsomes but insulin is not (Tung and Yip, 1969; Grant *et al.*, 1970); and (2) localization of labeled amino acid in the RER corresponds in time to the period of maximum incorporation into proinsulin (Clark *et al.*, 1970).

Normally, proinsulin represents 2–5% of total pancreatic insulin (Clark and Steiner, 1968) though this estimate may be much higher in some islet cell tumors or in the newborn (Tung and Yip, 1969; N. R. Lazarus *et al.*, 1969; Goldsmith *et al.*, 1969).

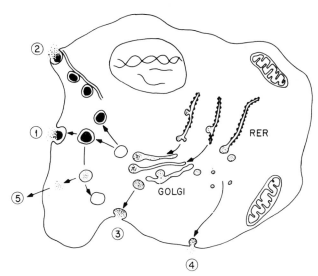

Fig. 3. Schematic representation of possible mechanisms of insulin secretion. RER, rough endoplasmic reticulum.

Paradoxically, after pulse labeling, when the specific activities of a recurring amino acid are measured at each of its sites in the insulin molecule, results are inconsistent with the single-chain hypothesis for insulin synthesis; specific activities do not progressively increase with distance from the N-terminal portion of the B chain as would be expected (Humbel, 1965; Konikova et al., 1969; Vaughan and Anfinsen, 1954). Possibly the atypical labeling results from the existence of anticodons for a given amino acid along the messenger-RNA coding the insulin molecule. Since the major pathway for the synthesis of insulin involves the prior production of single-chain proinsulin, appearance of A and B chains in plasma may reflect pancreatic or peripheral catabolism of insulin. Radioimmunoassays specific for each chain have been described (Meek et al., 1968; Varandani, 1968). Surprisingly, fasting plasma levels for both chains were 4 and 25 times insulin levels, the B chain increasing after glucose stimulation. Both chains prepared from insulin have variably been reported to be inactive, to have minor insulinlike activity, or, particularly in the case of the B chain, to be inhibitors of insulin action. Since these chains are usually prepared from insulin, part of their "effects" may have been due to contamination by intact hormone; synthesized A chain is biologically inert (see Surmaczynska and Metz, 1969, for general review). In these studies, the unfortunate investigator must choose between using the isolated A and B chains with chemically masked thiol groups as stable but nonphysiologic chemical derivatives or using the chains in their free thiol form which rapidly interreact to produce nonspecific polymers.

2. Packaging and Conversion of Proinsulin to Insulin

Previously it was held that the synthesized peptides were "packaged" as a result of vesicular modification of the membranes in the RER (Lacey, 1961). There is now ample evidence that the proinsulin in the RER is transferred to the smooth cisternae of the Golgi complex where most of the "packaging" occurs (Fig. 3). Hyperactivity, coated microvesicles, and new granules have been visualized in the Golgi when insulin synthesis was stimulated (Batts, 1959; Bencosme and Martinez-Palomo, 1968; Grodsky and Lee, 1970; Orci et al., 1969; Logothetopoulos, 1966; Lacy and Howell, 1970). Orci et al. (1969) suggested from electron microscopic studies that the smooth endoplasmic reticulum forms buds, and subsequently microvesicles, which are an obligatory step for packaging in the Golgi. Electron radioautography during pulse-labeling experiments show that newly synthesized protein is concentrated in the Golgi before appearing in cytoplasmic granules (Lacy, 1970).

Transformation of proinsulin to insulin probably occurs within the granule, either while it is still in the Golgi complex or shortly after. The half-life of conversion was estimated as about 60 minutes, a value that was not influenced by glucose (Clark et al., 1970). Conversion requires the initial cleavage of the connecting segment at either its N- or C-terminal to produce the two-chain intermediate with the molecular weight approximating that of proinsulin (Tung and Yip, 1969; Steiner et al., 1968) (see Fig. 2). With time, the other terminus is cleaved and the C-peptide is released. Though tryptic digestion can duplicate the removal of the arginines and the release of the connecting segment, lysine adjacent to the carboxyl terminus of the segment is also removed during natural production of the C-peptide (Clark et al., 1969). Thus, if trypsin is involved, a second enzymatic activity similar to that of carboxypeptidase-B would be required. Since conversion takes place within the membrane-enclosed granule, the C-peptide formed is retained. During stimulation, the C-peptide was shown to be released from the granules into the circulation in equimolar ratio with insulin (Rubenstein and Steiner, 1970a).

3. Storage, Compartmentalization, and Secretion

a. The Beta Granule and Emeiocytosis. The beta granule is the primary storage site of the finished insulin. A direct correlation between the degree of granulation of beta cells and insulin content has been documented, using aldehyde fuchsin stains (Hartroft and Wrenshall, 1955; Logothetopoulos et al., 1965; Morgan et al., 1965). The granule is surrounded by a smooth membranous sac which is probably lipo- and glycoprotein in nature since it can be solubilized with saponin and deoxycholate (Lazarow et al., 1964a). Two types of granules—pale and dense—are observed by electron microscopy (S. S. Lazarus et al., 1967; Bencosme and Martinez-Palomo, 1968). Both types are membrane-enclosed; however, the more predominant, dense granule contains material of a higher electron density, which does not fill the sac. The pale granule contains less dense, amorphous, material, distributed more evenly. The latter also contains insulin, since it reacts with insulin antibody. Furthermore, insulin is recovered from the pancreases of newborn rabbits which consist almost exclusively of pale granules (Wellman et al., 1969). The origin of the pale granule is in dispute; it may arise from the endoplasmic reticulum, or it can be an immature granule normally packaged in the Golgi apparatus (see Bencosme and Martinez-Palomo, 1968, for discussion). Regardless of its immediate source, the pale granule probably represents an early form of storage granule.

The shape of the granular material in the more prominent dense granules varies among species, suggesting a significant difference in crystalline structure (Lacy, 1957; Falkmer and Olsson, 1962). They are round in the rat and rabbit, oval in the hagfish, rectangular in the dog, and composed of dense prismatic structures in the cat. Since all these structures can be found within a single β cell in man, it is unlikely the pattern of granulation reflects differences in the amino acid structure of the insulins among species. This conclusion is supported by recent observations that differences in crystalline structure are seen between porcine and canine granules though their insulins are chemically identical. (Coore et al., 1967). Williamson et al., (1961) described one process for insulin secretion that involves movement of the granules to the plasma membranes of the cell, fusing of the granule surface membrane with the cell membrane, rupture of the membranes, and liberation of the granular contents into the intracellular pericapillary space (emeiocytosis). The multiple concavities created at the surface of the cell by this disruptive process are presumably responsible for the microvilli extending from the surface of the beta cell into the intracellular and pericapsular spaces.

b. *Storage Compartments.* Though emeiocytosis may represent the final mechanism for the release of insulin, it may not always reflect identical processes (Fig. 3). Considerable evidence is accumulating that release of insulin is a discontinuous process in which more than one general compartment may coexist with varying sensitivity to stimulating agents. In addition to the pale and dense granules discussed above, the small vesicles produced in the Golgi and seen throughout the cytoplasm, including those in possible contact with the plasma membranes, may represent important storage compartments (Orci et al., 1969). Microtubules associated with certain granules have been observed in the cytoplasm of the islet cell, and may connect to the plasma membrane (Lacy et al., 1968). It was suggested that, during stimulation, this microtubular system contracts or, in some manner, imparts a motive force to the granules resulting in their displacement to the cell surface where release can occur by emeiocytosis. Though there is as yet little direct evidence for this theory, colchicine, which destroys microtubular elements, inhibits glucose-stimulated insulin release though general protein synthesis is unaffected (Lacy et al., 1968). Thus, those granules associated with the microtubular system could also represent a small compartment of rapidly available insulin. The relationship of compartments of stored insulin to patterns of insulin release is discussed on page 61.

Granules have been isolated from islets after homogenization and differential centrifugation (Howell et al., 1969; Coore et al., 1969; Sorenson et al., 1969; Lambert et al., 1970; Lindall et al., 1969). At least 14 different proteins and various lipids are found in granules from the goosefish. Isolated granules are extremely labile at pH 7.4 and could only be maintained around pH 6. At this acid pH, glucose, its metabolites such as glucose 6-phosphate and citrate, cyclic AMP, and the sulfonylureas had marginal, if any, direct effect on the solubilization of the granules and release of insulin. Only deoxycholate was consistently effective, presumably acting by dissolving the granular membrane. Although the failure of these agents to release insulin from the granules *in vitro* has been used as an argument that they do not act directly to solubilize insulin within the beta cell, the studies were performed at neutral pH, where an unusual stability may be artificially created, and in the absence of the metabolic machinery through which stimulating agents act to produce the ultimate release signal.

c. "Soluble" Insulin. That insulin may be stored or exist within the beta cell in a soluble nongranular "compartment" is controversial. The arguments favoring existence of soluble insulin are summarized by Creutzfeldt *et al.* (1970) and include:

1. Granular membranes are often thin and incomplete, thus making granule dissolution a possibility (Lever and Findlay, 1966; Creutzfeldt *et al.*, 1970).

2. Pancreatic tissue with depleted β granules often contains large amounts of extractable insulin and secrete insulin when stimulated. Examples include degranulated pancreas after prolonged tolbutamide (Creutzfeldt *et al.*, 1970), certain islet cell adenomas (Creutzfeldt *et al.*, 1970; Pollen *et al.*, 1961), and developing fetal tissue (Willes *et al.*, 1969; Dixit *et al.*, 1964).

3. During stimulation there is a pronounced increase in the number of cytoplasmic vesicles and structures resembling the beta granules, with intact membranes, but with increasingly smaller amounts of electron-dense content (Orci *et al.*, 1969).

Unfortunately, the significance of insulin content in microvesicles and pale granules and the poor quantitation associated with electron microscopic studies complicate interpretations. Evidence favoring granular secretion of insulin include: (a) visualization of emeiocytosis; (b) occasional observation of intact granular material in the extracellular capillary lumen where soluble insulin would be invisible (Théret and Tamboise, 1963; Lee *et al.*, 1970); (c) both insulin and the C-peptide, stored together in the granules, are secreted into extracellular fluid in equimolar concentration.

4. Turnover of Insulin in the Pancreas

Most current investigation has emphasized synthesis and secretion of insulin with no precise data on hormone turnover within the pancreas. However, a degradation system for insulin may exist and vary with the metabolic state. Thus, Creutzfeldt *et al.* (1969) found that when normal release was blocked by diazoxide, many beta cells displayed multigranular sacs and granule-containing dense bodies, suggesting intracellular digestion by lysosomes. Glutathione-insulin transhydrogenase, which degrades insulin to its respective A and B chains, is found in rat and fish islets (Lazarow *et al.*, 1964a; Kotoulas *et al.*, 1965) and may serve as a natural degradation system. Idahl and Täljedal (1968) found that islet cells are particularly rich in general peptidases.

IV. Metabolism of Islet Cells

A. General Considerations

Although histologic studies have been employed to establish the existence of specific enzymes in islets from various species (reviewed by Grodsky and Forsham, 1966) recent microchemical methods permit quantitative estimation of enzymes and intermediates and have provided considerable information on islet metabolic pathways (Fig. 4). Usually the isolated islet is used from the rat in which the beta cell makes up more than half the tissue, or from the obese hyperglycemic mouse con-

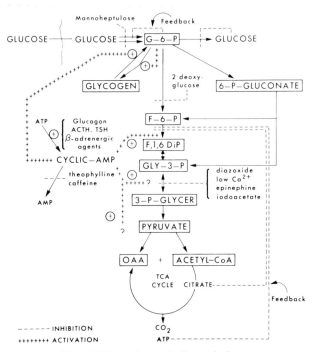

Fig. 4. Islet cell metabolism of glucose.

taining 90% beta cells. Unfortunately, most studies have been on the metabolism of carbohydrate, since interest is primarily directed to a better understanding of how glucose regulates insulin synthesis and release. Isolated islets, however, have been shown to respire for hours in glucose-free media, suggesting that the major source of basal fuel in this tissue is lipid or other noncarbohydrates (Hellerström, 1967; Stork et al., 1969). Consistent with this hypothesis is the observation that inhibition of glycolysis with iodoacetate only partially inhibits basal respiration. Presumably, as glucose is increased it progressively contributes to respiration. Islet respiration resembles that of liver in that rates are comparatively low (Hellerström, 1964).

B. GLUCOSE

1. *Glycolysis*

Glucose rapidly enters the beta cell of both the fish and mammals by a specific but unknown process, resulting in a rapid equilibrium of extra- and intracellular glucose (Field, 1964; Goetz and Cooperstein, 1962; Matschinsky and Ellerman, 1968; Idahl and Hellman, 1968). Entry is unaffected by phlorizin (Coore and Randle, 1964) or high concentration of nonmetabolizable sugars (Grodsky et al., 1963). Similar to the case in liver, glucose entrance into the islet is not insulin-sensitive, insulin having no direct effect on glucose uptake or its oxidation to CO_2 (Field, 1964; Jarrett, 1968). The islets, therefore, are ideally sensitive to changing levels of circulating glucose and at the same time are free to respond under conditions of insulin insufficiency, which could inhibit the metabolism of some other tissues.

Having entered the cell, glucose is rapidly phosphorylated to glucose 6-phosphate, an increase being detectable within 30 seconds after glucose administration. Glucose 6-phosphate levels parallel extracellular glucose; however, the glucose/glucose 6-phosphate levels are greater than one (Idahl and Hellman, 1970). Thus, phosphorylation is more rate-limiting than transport, though not necessarily the rate-limiting step for total glucose metabolism.

Two different phosphorylating enzymes have been detected, one a hexo-kinase with a low K_m, the other with a K_m of about 20 mM, which may prove similar to the glucokinase in liver (Randle and Ashcroft, 1969). The low K_m hexokinase is similar to hexokinases from other tissues, in that it is inhibited by glucose 6-phosphate (Matschinsky and Ellerman, 1968; Randle and Ashcroft, 1969), thereby providing a possible site for feedback regulation of glucose metabolism (see page 63) (Fig. 4). Mannoheptulose effectively blocks glycolysis by inhibiting glucose phosphorylation (Ashcroft *et al.*, 1968). Once glucose 6-phosphate is formed, enzyme pathways are available for glycolysis, the pentose pathway, glycogen synthesis, or conversion back to glucose. All enzymes of the glycolytic pathway, as well as lactic acid dehydrogenase, have been detected both histochemically and by microenzymatic assay in isolated islets (Lacy, 1962a; S. S. Lazarus and Bradshaw, 1959; Dixit and Lazarow, 1969). Glycerol phosphate dehydrogenase is low in the islets, suggesting that this tissue is poorly equipped to metabolize glycerol. Pyruvatekinase is high; however, both phosphofructokinase and glyceraldehyde-3-phosphate dehydrogenase are comparatively low, indicating that they may be important sites for the regulation of islet glycolysis. 2-Deoxyglucose is a potent inhibitor of glucose 6-phosphate isomerase. However, its effect on insulin release in the pancreas is variable (Devrim and Recant, 1966; Malaisse *et al.*, 1967a; Coore and Randle, 1964; Grodsky *et al.*, 1963; Lambert *et al.*, 1969a) so that its specific action is probably highly sensitive to concentration and method of administration. Matschinsky *et al.* (1968) found that citrate and ATP effectively inhibited islet phosphofructokinase, providing another site of possible feedback control (Fig. 4). Possibly fatty acids may also inhibit this enzyme. On the basis of the sensitivity of phosphofructokinase to ATP levels, agents such as tolbutamide which increase ADP/ATP ratios, could be expected to increase glycolysis at this step (Hellman *et al.*, 1969). As shown by Montague and Taylor (1969), citrate causes an increase in metabolism through the pentose pathway, presumably by blocking phosphofructokinase.

Important regulation of glycolysis may also occur at the glyceraldehyde-3-PO_4 dehydrogenase-phosphoglyceratekinase steps, catalyzing the conversion of glyceraldehyde 3-phosphate to 3-phosphoglycerate; elegant cross-over studies show that many agents inhibiting insulin release (e.g., diazoxide, calcium deprivation, and epinephrine), inhibit glycolysis at this step (Hellman, 1970). Iodoacetate may also block here (Webb, 1966). Hexoses other than glucose can be metabolized through the glycolytic pathway. Mannose metabolism is almost as rapid as glucose, while fructose is used at a much slower rate (Hellman and Larsson, 1961; Humbel and Renold, 1963) and galactose is comparatively inactive (Lazarow *et al.*, 1964b).

2. Citric Acid Cycle

Since islets can readily convert glucose to CO_2 (Humbel and Renold, 1963; Field and Lazarow, 1960) the citric acid cycle is operative. Evaluating the citric acid cycle by studying the effect of the intermediates is complicated by the possibility that some have limited permeability

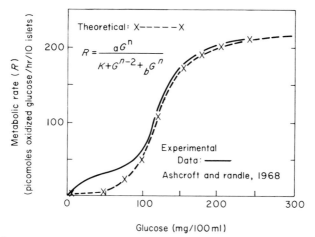

FIG. 5. Effect of glucose concentration on glucose metabolism in rat islets. Mathematical simulation by V. Licko and G. Grodsky. Experimental data from Ashcroft and Randle (1968a).

through the cellular and mitochondrial membranes. In adult tissue, pyruvate is poorly metabolized to CO_2, though it is not clear whether this is the result of poor permeability or a rapid conversion to lactic acid. The increased effectiveness of pyruvate in fetal tissue incubated in the presence of caffeine suggests islet metabolism of this intermediate may be controlled by cyclic AMP (Lambert et al., 1969a). Succinate, citrate, and oxaloacetate stimulate oxygen uptake by islets (Friz et al., 1960; Hellerström et al., 1970); thus these agents may facilitate maintenance of the pancreas by serving as an energy source (Coore and Randle, 1964); to date they have not been effective as direct signals for insulin release.

The overall metabolism of glucose to CO_2 follows a sigmoidal curve (Fig. 5) (Ashcroft and Randle, 1968a; Jarrett and Keen, 1966). In the rat, glucose is poorly metabolized up to a concentration of 5 mM (90 mg/100 ml). The K_m occurs at 7 mM (130 mg/100 ml), and the maximum effectiveness of glucose is 12 mM (around 220 mg/100 ml). The sigmoidal response is a power function of glucose concentration (Fig. 5) and is almost identical with the effect of glucose on insulin release (see p. 67).

3. Pentose Pathway

Experiments using specifically labeled glucose indicate that the pentose pathway may be an important route for the metabolism of glucose (Keen et al., 1965; Jarrett and Keen, 1966; Lazarow, 1963). All the enzymes in this pathway have been demonstrated (Field, 1964; Humbel and

Renold, 1963; Hellman and Hellerstöm, 1962a), though sometimes the levels are lower in the beta cells than in adjacent exocrine tissue. Xylitol and ribose may serve as substrates for the pentose pathway, and under certain circumstances may provide the necessary signals for insulin release (see page 69). Montague and Taylor (1969) found the pattern of increase of 6-phosphogluconate paralleled the sigmoidal curve for overall glucose metabolism. Additionally, tolbutamide, theophylline, and glucagon caused increased 6-phosphogluconate in a manner consistent with their ability to stimulate insulin release. The latter observations indicate that cyclic AMP causes increased activity of the pentose pathway, though it may not be a direct effect. The total significance of this pathway remains unclear since, in other laboratories, xylitol had no effect on glucose respiration (Hellerström *et al.*, 1970).

4. *Gluconeogenesis*

Glucose production from amino acids or lactate, or by reversal of glycolysis, may not occur since islets are very low in the enzyme, fructose-1,6-diphosphatase (Brolin *et al.*, 1968). Glucose 6-phosphatase, however, is found in a variety of species (S. S. Lazarus and Bradshaw, 1959; Hellman and Hellerström, 1962b; Schätzle, 1958; Täljedal, 1967, 1969; Ashcroft and Randle, 1968b; Petkov, 1966), levels being particularly high in the obese hyperglycemic mouse and in animals after cortisone treatment (Täljedal, 1969). The enzyme is microsomal and, similar to hepatic glucose 6-phosphatase, is inhibited by glucose (Täljedal, 1969). Thus a high concentration of glucose would facilitate its own effectiveness by inhibiting glucose 6-phosphatase. Conversely, at low glucose concentration the mobilization of glycogen by glucagon, for example, may be particularly ineffective since the glucose 6-phosphate produced may be converted back to glucose and lost to the cell (see Fig. 4). S. S. Lazarus and Bradshaw (1959) noted decreased glucose-6-phosphatase activity after administration of tolbutamide, and suggested this agent could stimulate insulin release by increasing the quantity of available glucose 6-phosphate in the beta cells. However, this effect of tolbutamide has not been confirmed (Ashcroft and Randle, 1968b). In some species, glucose-6-phosphatase may have only a limited effect on glucose metabolism; levels are very low, for example, in islets of the hamster and man (Wegman and Petkov, 1965).

5. *Glycogen*

Glycogen synthesis in the islet was demonstrated when the hydropic degeneration of diabetes was identified as this substance (Toreson, 1951).

The beta cell appears to store glycogen selectively in response to hyperglycemia, whereas acinar tissue and islet alpha cells do not (S. S. Lazarus and Volk, 1962). Glycogen synthetase activity is generally low (Lazarow, 1963; Brolin and Berne, 1970); however, the functional rate may increase with glucose concentration since the enzyme is activated by glucose 6-phosphate (Matschinsky and Ellerman, 1968). In normal mammals, glycogen levels are low, ranging from 3 to 10 mmoles/kg dry weight, though levels in the obese hyperglycemic mouse are about 3 times greater (Hellman and Idahl, 1970; Matschinsky and Ellerman, 1968). Malaisse et al. (1967a) showed that prolonged glucose administration can increase islet glycogen to levels that permit glucagon to stimulate insulin release in vitro without the added glucose normally required. However, even in the obese hyperglycemic mouse, glycogen is a limited source of substrate; Hellman and Idahl (1970) found ischemia to cause glycogen breakdown of 3 mmoles/kg dry weight in 5 minutes which, after correcting for wet weight, would have increased cellular glucose equivalents only 16 mg/100 ml. Total instant mobilization of all islet glycogen in these animals would provide about 150 mg/100 ml of glucose equivalents. Glucagon, cyclic AMP, theophylline, and tolbutamide mobilize glycogen; however, islet glycogen is often surprisingly insensitive to glucagon (Hellman and Idahl, 1970; Jarrett and Keen, 1968); sensitivity may prove a function of the levels of exogenous glucose or endogenous glycogen.

6. Amino Acids

Islets can synthesize amino acids from added glucose or fructose (Hellman and Larsson, 1961; Humbel and Renold, 1963), and synthesis of protein, including insulin from labeled amino acids, has been shown (Taylor et al., 1962; Vaughan and Anfinsen, 1954; Grodsky and Tarver, 1956; Steiner et al., 1967). Both amino acid dehydrogenases and transaminases have been detected (C. H. Smith and Lacy, 1962; Kissane and Brolin, 1963), and leucine-^{14}C can be decarboxylated and oxidized completely to $^{14}CO_2$ (Hellerström et al., 1970; Friz et al., 1960). Unfortunately, the metabolism of arginine and other amino acids that also stimulate insulin release has not been adequately studied.

ATP is high in islets (Wettermark et al., 1970; Matschinsky et al., 1968), levels of 10 mmoles/kg dry weight being found in those of the obese mouse. This may be the result of the high levels of ATP-generating dehydrogenases; characteristic of islet tissue (Brolin et al., 1967; Wegman and Petkov, 1965). Glucose increases ATP levels, and this may be useful as an energy source to permit the multiple effects of glucose on synthesis and release of insulin (see page 61). Since sulfonylureas decrease

ATP (Hellman *et al.*, 1969), the final signal for insulin release is probably not this nucleotide. ATPase has been found in some, but not all, beta cells from different species (Hellman and Hellerström, 1962b; S. S. Lazarus *et al.*, 1962; Gepts and Toussaint, 1964). When found, its concentration is highest in the membrane surrounding insulin granules. Though this enzyme may be affected by cation changes known to influence insulin secretion, its role in the production or secretion of insulin is not established.

7. *Nucleotides*

Both reduced and oxidized di- and triphosphorpyridine nucleotides are found in islets (Lazarow *et al.*, 1964a; Petkov *et al.*, 1968); in the fish, the ratio to oxidized to reduced forms is greater in islets than in other tissues investigated (Lazarow *et al.*, 1964a).

V. FACTORS INFLUENCING SECRETION OF INSULIN

A. GENERAL CONSIDERATIONS

A large number of *in vitro* preparations are now available for the study of insulin release including the perfused pancreas (Grodsky *et al.*, 1963; Sussman and Vaughan, 1967), isolated islets (Lacy and Kostianovsky, 1967; Keen *et al.*, 1965), and incubated pancreatic segments (Grodsky and Tarver, 1956; Coore and Randle, 1964; R-Candela, 1964; Frerichs *et al.*, 1965; Lambert *et al.*, 1967; Malaisse *et al.*, 1967b). Since our review (Grodsky and Forsham, 1966) it has been established by these methods that a variety of carbohydrates, amino acids, lipids, and nucleotides can directly affect insulin release from the pancreas.

These agents, however, may differ not only in their metabolic mode of action but also in the pancreatic phenomenon on which they act. Release of insulin can be the result of stimulation of synthesis of precursors, conversion of precursors to finished hormone, packaging, and the direct release from compartments of stored hormone (see Section V,A,1). Each mechanism differs in its time relationships; release of prestored insulin can occur in seconds after stimulation (Grodsky *et al.*, 1967a) but release of hormone as a result of increased synthesis or packaging can require minutes or hours (Howell and Taylor, 1967; Steiner *et al.*, 1967). Thus, insulin released during constant stimulation may not reflect the same pancreatic action at different times during the stimulatory period. Some agents such as glucose may act on more than one of these mechanisms. Better understanding of the time relations of these phenomena should prove useful in the analysis of insulin release patterns in subjects with impaired response to glucose.

1. *Multiphasic Aspects of Insulin Release*

a. Compartmentalization. The *in vitro* perfused pancreas, in which total perfusate is collected at short intervals after a single passage through the tissues, provides a dynamic system for measuring changes in the rates of insulin release during controlled, constant stimulation (Grodsky *et al.*, 1967a). In this system, glucose or tolbutamide produces a multiphasic response (Grodsky *et al.*, 1967a; Curry *et al.*, 1968a) (Fig. 6). Insulin release is immediate, occurring within 30–60 seconds after initiating either agent. However, in minutes, and although the stimulator concentration is maintained, secretion rates rapidly decrease. This phase is presumed to represent the release of preformed insulin, since it occurred rapidly and was not affected by inhibition of protein synthesis with puromycin. Insulin released is only 1–3% of total pancreatic content; thus this phase cannot represent total exhaustion of pancreatic stores. After several minutes of high levels of glucose, there is a secondary rise in insulin secretion rate (Curry *et al.*, 1968a). Since this third phase could be partially inhibited by puromycin, it reflects a phenomenon different from that involved in the initial release. The studies also illustrate that different agents may act similarly on one phase of release, but not on another: though tolbutamide stimulates the rapid release phase, in contrast to glucose, it has little positive effect on secondary release. Similar multiphasic patterns during constant stimulation have been observed in intact animals and man (Porte and Pupo, 1969; Waddell *et al.*, 1969). A two-

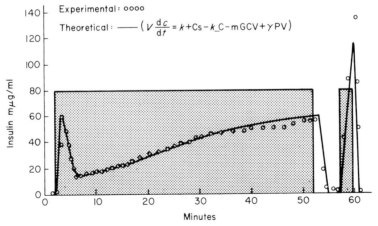

FIG. 6. Effect of prolonged perfusion of glucose on secretion of insulin. Perfusion was followed by a 5-minute rest period and subsequent readdition of glucose. From Grodsky *et al.* (1969), p. 554.

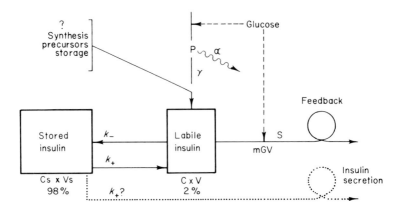

$$V\frac{dc}{dt} = k_+Cs - k_-C - mGCV + \gamma PV$$

$$S = mGCV$$

FIG. 7. Two-compartmental model for insulin secretion incorporating feedback inhibition.

compartmental model has been devised as a partial explanation for the multiphasic response (Grodsky *et al.*, 1969, 1970).

The model (Fig. 7) proposes a small compartment of insulin, which is particularly labile to stimulating agents. It is emphasized that no mathematical model can describe a highly complicated process such as pancreatic production and release of insulin. However, the model is described in some detail since it illustrates certain phenomena of insulin release that are often unsuspected but can be subject to further testing by more definitive means.

The initial release of insulin, shown in Fig. 6, reflects partial depletion of the small compartment which, in turn, can explain the refractory state to further stimulation that can occur in pancreas at this time (Grodsky *et al.*, 1967b).

Agents such as glucose, and probably mannose, can provide additional insulin to the small compartment, though this effect is comparatively slow and produces the second increasing phase of insulin release. In the model this is accomplished by a hypothetical potentiator, *P* (Fig. 7). Insulin secretion stops immediately after a stimulus is removed; however, after prolonged glucose stimulation, provision of insulin to the small compartment continues (until the residual potentiator is dissipated by independent processes). During this period, readily available insulin in the small compartment may exceed normal amounts; this may explain the hyperinsulin response that occurs both *in vivo* and *in vitro* when a prolonged stimulation with glucose is followed by a brief rest and subsequent restimulation (Grodsky *et al.*, 1969; Porte and Pupo, 1969) (Fig. 6). The model partially explains how glucose may produce a relatively insensitive or, conversely, a hypersensitive pancreatic state, depending on the period of glucose stimulation. The source of the insulin provided to the labile compartment is not known. It may be from *de novo* synthesis of amino acids, since glucose is known to stimulate this process (Howell and Taylor, 1967), though conversion of precursors or activation of the packaging process is equally probable. In any of these cases, the model suggests the novel hypothesis that newly synthesized insulin or its precursors may enter the more labile compartment and be preferentially secreted. Only if not immediately secreted is insulin shunted into the more stable, large, storage compartment. Observations in man (Roth *et al.*, 1968; Goldsmith *et al.*, 1969) and *in vitro* (Burr *et al.*, 1969) that significant amounts of "big" or proinsulin are released when the pancreas is strongly stimulated, support this hypothesis of preferential excretion of new, or even incompletely finished, insulin. Additionally, Clark and Steiner (1969) found in pulse-labeling experiments that glucose increased the relative proportion of labeled proinsulin secreted into the media. Similar results, indicating preferential release of newly formed hormone may be a general characteristic of endocrine systems, are described for release of vasopressin (Sachs and Haller, 1968) and thyroxine (Haibach and Kobayashi, 1970).

The small labile compartment may be that insulin stored in the pale immature granules or that associated with the microvesicles in the Golgi and cytoplasm (Fig. 3). There is as yet no evidence whether these granules are particularly sensitive to stimulating agents.

Finally, compartmentalization may still occur in a more conventional process, by which insulin in the major storage granules provides the source for the released insulin. In this case, the provisionary effect of glucose would occur by activating the stable granules. The small compartment could be those granules associated with the cytoplasmic tubules seen by Lacy *et al.* (1968).

The above considerations have used the term *compartmentalization* literally. It is also possible that the "compartment" may be a metabolic one and that the multiphasic insulin responses result from depletion and resynthesis of an intracellular substance controlling insulin release.

Regardless of the specific details, the dual action of glucose on release and subsequent provision, seems necessary to explain insulin-release patterns during stimulation.

b. Feedback Inhibition. Other studies suggest the initial diphasic insulin response to constant stimulation may in part result from stimulator-induced feedback inhibition (Grodsky *et al.*, 1967b; Bennett and Grodsky, 1969) (see Fig. 8). At constant, low, stimulating concentrations of glucose (100 mg/100 ml), the perfused pancreas still responds in a diphasic manner. The decreased rate of insulin release occurring after a few minutes during this stimulation can be almost 5-fold, which on the basis of a simple compartmental theory (Fig. 7) could only be explained by an almost-complete emptying of the source of available insulin. However, an additional increase in glucose concentration (150 mg/100 ml) elicits yet a larger diphasic response. This additional response can be explained if the labile compartment is assumed to contain a gaussian distribution of islets with different thresholds of sensitivity to the stimulator (Grodsky *et al.*, 1971). These results are also consistent with a feedback inhibition phenomenon in which each increase in the stimulator concentration results in temporary additional release until the new level of inhibition occurs. When glucose levels are raised to near maximum effectiveness, additional response in the face of the existing inhibition is marginal, and less insulin is released than at the lower glucose concentrations. Figure 8 illustrates that increasing concentrations of glucose may result in an apparent increased response (compare peaks at 100 and 150 mg/100 ml) or a refractory state (compare peaks at 150 and 300 mg/100 ml), yet all cases reflect a predicted response on the basis of feedback inhibition. Almost identical curves have been produced in man after stepwise stimulation with glucose (Karam *et al.*, 1970). The concept of feedback inhibition or gaussian distribution of islets can be incorporated into the compartmental model with no major modification in basic concepts.

Glucose-induced feedback could occur as inhibition of hexokinase by

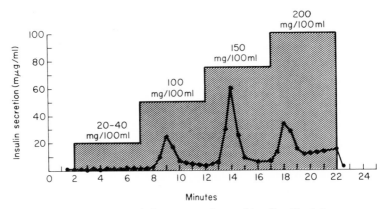

Fig. 8. Effect of increments of glucose on release of insulin. Shaded area represents period of glucose infusion.

glucose 6-phosphate, or as inhibition of phosphofructokinase by ATP (Fig. 4). It is of interest that glucagon, which increases cyclic AMP, may act to deinhibit insulin release (Bennett and Grodsky, 1969). In other tissues, cyclic AMP overcomes inhibition of phosphofructokinase by competing at allosteric sites with the inhibitor, ATP. It is likely that many other steps in glucose metabolism, particularly those involving kinases, could provide other sites for feedback control.

Insulin, itself, may contribute to a feedback inhibition. However evidence obtained both *in vivo* and *in vitro* is conflicting regarding the quantitative effect of exogenous insulin on secretion (see page 82). Extracts of the D cell in the pancreas, presumably a source of gastrin, can also inhibit insulin release, though it is not known whether this material increases during glucose stimulation (Hellman and Lernmark, 1969a).

A combination of all these factors may be responsible for the oscillating patterns for glucose and insulin occasionally reported *in vivo* (G. E. Anderson *et al.*, 1967; Iberall *et al.*, 1968; J. D. Young and Jenkinson, 1968).

Though the exact explanation for the multiphasic phenomenon of insulin release is not established, it is apparent that a constant linear relationship between glucose levels and insulin secretion over a prolonged period (such as during a glucose tolerance test) is not probable (Goodner *et al.*, 1969; Bierman *et al.*, 1968). In man, rapidly changing levels of growth hormone (Boden *et al.*, 1968; Yalow *et al.*, 1969) and glucagon (Ohneda *et al.*, 1969) add to the complication of interpreting patterns of insulin release. *In vivo*, mathematical models for the secretion and degradation of insulin, the production and utilization of glucose, and their multiple interrelationships have been discussed (Cerasi and Luft, 1967b; Izzo and Bartlett, 1969).

2. Enhancement or Potentiation

Many agents that "stimulate the secretion of insulin" actually are comparatively ineffective but act to potentiate or enhance the action of a primary stimulating agent, such as glucose. We therefore propose that stimulating agents be divided into two categories:

1. *Independent* agents that directly cause the release of insulin in the absence of a primary stimulating agent. Included are glucose, tolbutamide, leucine, and potassium ion.

2. *Dependent* agents requiring a substimulating concentration of an independent agent from category 1. Included in this group are glucagon, ACTH, TSH, certain amino acids (possibly arginine), cyclic AMP and cyclic AMP-generating substances (such as caffeine, theophylline, or beta adrenergic drugs).

Since glucose is necessarily present in all *in vivo* studies and is often used as an energy source in *in vitro* experiments, adequate data on the effectiveness of agents in the presence or absence of glucose is not always available. The distinction, however, can be useful in differentiating the basic action of different substances.

3. *Variable Roles of Stimulating Agents*

Five general mechanisms by which agents can act on the release of stored insulin have been suggested (Renold, 1970): (1) to provide the specific metabolic signal or signals which control insulin release; (2) to influence calcium and potassium availability which may affect the membrane-bound phase of insulin release; (3) to provide cyclic 3′,5′-AMP; (4) to influence beta and alpha autonomous-nervous system receptors, which in turn are probably involved in accumulating cyclic AMP; (5) to provide an energy source to permit the various islet cell processes, though not directly affecting the release mechanism.

Although these mechanisms are interrelated and overlap, they currently may be useful to distinguish the actions of dependent from independent stimulating agents.

B. SPECIFIC AGENTS AFFECTING INSULIN RELEASE

1. *Action of Carbohydrates*

As noted previously, glucose freely enters the pancreatic islet. However some metabolite or cofactor resulting from glucose metabolism rather than glucose itself probably provides the signal for insulin release.* Thus, a metabolizable sugar, such as mannose, stimulates insulin release while the nonmetabolizable sugar, galactose, does not (Grodsky *et al.*, 1963; Coore and Randle, 1964). *In vivo*, galactose can cause an increase in circulating insulin (Goetz *et al.*, 1964; Rommel *et al.*, 1969), but this may be an indirect effect on stimulation of intestinal factors that can enhance pancreatic response (see page 80). Fructose, which is metabolized about a third as well as glucose in islets (Hellman and Larsson, 1961; Humbel and Renold, 1963), is only partially (Grodsky *et al.*, 1963; Kilo *et al.*, 1962) or insignificantly (Coore and Randle, 1964; Frerichs *et al.*, 1965) effective in stimulating insulin release *in vitro*. Fructose *in vivo* stimulates some insulin secretion; this is probably not entirely due to the conversion of fructose to glucose since some stimulation occurs in patients with glucose-6-phosphatase deficiency (Hug and Schubert, 1967). Finally, glucose-induced secretion is blocked by inhibition of glucose metabolism

---

* Though most studies are consistent with this probability, Matschinsky (1970) did not obtain the expected increase in selected glycolytic intermediates in rat islets; the possibility that a membrane "glucoreceptor" triggers the intermediate intracellular events must still be considered.

with mannoheptulose (Coore et al., 1963), glucosamine (Martin and Bamber, 1964), and high concentrations of 2-deoxyglucose (Kilo et al., 1962; R-Candela et al., 1964; Martin and Bamber, 1964).

Glucose stimulates a variety of pancreatic mechanisms resulting in insulin release. Within seconds, it can cause secretion of some stored insulin, independent of any processes requiring synthesis of insulin or protein (Grodsky and Bennett, 1963; Curry et al., 1968a; Grodsky et al., 1967b).

In addition, it has a marked though slower effect on provision of additional insulin to the secretion system (see Fig. 7). Glucose stimulates islet synthetic machinery: (1) by increasing the synthesis of RNA, particularly transfer-RNA, (Jarrett et al., 1967, 1968) an (2) by increasing synthesis of proinsulin from labeled amino acids (Clark and Steiner, 1969), which results in increased synthesis of labeled insulin (Howell and Taylor, 1967; Wagle, 1965). An effect of glucose on insulinogenesis is further supported by evidence that the secondary or provisionary phase of insulin release (Fig. 6) is partially inhibited by puromycin. The action of glucose on insulin synthesis is also probably through one of its metabolites, since the metabolizable sugar, mannose, is effective (Jarrett et al., 1967; Howell and Taylor, 1967), but it is not known whether the same metabolic signals are required for both release and synthesis. Glucose may affect the packaging process since its action is usually associated with increased activity and size of the Golgi (Batts, 1959) and often with increased new granules in this organelle (see Section V,A,1). Preliminary studies indicate glucose does not affect conversion of proinsulin to insulin, the half-life for proinsulin remaining about 60 minutes (see discussion in Steiner, 1970). That glucose metabolites may convert the more stable granules to a more labile storage form is possible (see Fig. 7); however, such a mechanism has not been directly investigated.

Ashcroft and Randle (1968a) showed that the metabolism of glucose to CO_2 follows a sigmoidal curve (Fig. 5). Within experimental variation, a similar curve is obtained when glucose concentration is plotted against insulin release (Malaisse et al., 1967b; Grodsky et al., 1971). Several theoretical points have not been previously discussed but can be derived from this curve (though experimental confirmation is available, so far, in only a few instances):

1. As demonstrated by the superimposed curve in Fig. 5 provided in cooperation with Dr. V. Licko, a sigmoidal curve may reflect a cooperative effect in which the change in CO_2 production or insulin release is a *power function* of glucose concentration (G^n). The exact power of n must be determined from other experimental data. It seems obvious, however, that attempts to relate insulin to glucose concentrations as a linear function are adequate only for crude approximations and are particularly unsuitable at basal glucose levels or at concentrations over 180 mg/100 ml.

2. The sigmoidal response creates a natural threshold at or around basal glucose levels. In the case of the rat pancreas, increased insulin

secretion (Malaisse et al., 1967b; Grodsky et al., 1967b; Mariani, 1969) is first detectable at 70–90 mg/100 ml, the range of the fasting basal blood glucose in this animal. Rapid changes in rates of insulin secretion occur with small changes in blood glucose above basal levels. Referring to Fig. 5, a change in blood glucose of 25 mg/100 ml would cause a 3-fold change in the rate of insulin secretion. Often studies on the effect of in vivo agents on insulin release may be misinterpreted because only "minor changes" of blood sugar are noted and not considered significant.

3. At basal levels in the intact animal, glucose may be comparatively ineffective in the control of insulin release. Thus, lipids, amino acids and other hormones may play a proportionately greater role in this state than during hyperglycemia. Epinephrine, which inhibits glucose-stimulated insulin release, has little effect on basal secretion (Sussman et al., 1969), and a poor correlation of plasma basal insulin to glucose levels has been noted in man (Goodner et al., 1969; Bierman et al., 1968). On the same basis, it would appear that if homeostatic conditions are not changed, different levels of hypoglycemia have virtually no effect on insulin release; in these states insulin may affect glucose levels, but glucose would have little effect on insulin secretion.

4. Potentiation is usually defined as a condition occurring when the admixture of two agents produces a greater insulin release than the arithmetic sum of the effects of either agent alone. By this definition, glucose could appear as a potentiator of its own action. For example, glucose at 100 mg/100 ml is a mild stimulator, while at 50 mg/100 ml it is almost inactive. However, the concentration of 150 mg/100 ml is much more effective than the sum of either alone. Thus, "potentiation" can often reflect a simple additive effect in a nonlinear system. This should be distinguished from situations representing a different phenomenon in which agents increase the maximum effect of another. Malaisse found that mannose can "potentiate" glucose response but not when glucose is stimulating maximally (Malaisse and Malaisse-Lagae, 1970). Similar observations have been made with tolbutamide (Pfeiffer, 1969). Many agents, such as glucagon, ACTH, intestinal hormones, and cyclic AMP also act to enhance glucose action (Malaisse et al., 1967b; Grodsky et al., 1969; Buchanan et al., 1969; Vecchio et al., 1967), but the distinction between maximal and submaximal potentiation was either not made or resulted in conflicting conclusions.

Glucose produces the signals for insulin release; however, the nature of these signals in unknown. Clarification is complicated by experimental difficulties in distinguishing the different actions of glucose on synthesis, packaging, and secretion, which may differ in their controlling signals and energetic requirements. In addition, the same signal or source of energy can arise from different metabolic sites in glucose metabolism. Thus, TPNH can be generated not only in the pentose pathway but also during succinate or malate metabolism. ATP production also is not limited to a single metabolic step.

Though glucose may enter the glycolytic pathway and eventually produce these metabolic signals, it is unlikely that intermediates in the glycolytic pathway are directly involved. Insulin release is inhibited by anoxia (Coore and Randle, 1964; Grodsky and Tarver, 1956; Frerichs et al., 1965), DNP (Coore and Randle, 1964), oligomycin (Renold, 1970), and cyanide (Frerichs et al., 1965)—conditions that would be expected to increase glycolysis. Other observations further support the concept that the signal is at, or below, the level of the trioses. Iodoacetate, which blocks glycolysis at the level of glyceraldehyde-3-phosphate dehydrogenase (Webb, 1966), inhibits insulin release when stimulated with glucose or tolbutamide, but not by pyruvate (Renold, 1970). In elegant crossover studies, Hellman (1970) found that inhibition of insulin release by epinephrine or diazoxide, or deficiency of calcium ion was associated with a block between fructose 1,6-diphosphate and 3-phosphoglycerate. There was a striking accumulation of fructose 1,6-diphosphate as well as other intermediates of glucose above this metabolic step, though insulin release was inhibited. It is probable that the step involving the sequence catalyzed by phosphoglyceraldehyde dehydrogenase-phosphoglyceratekinase may be another important regulatory site for cyclic AMP and ADP activation, and ATP inhibition (see Fig. 4).

Pyruvate normally does not stimulate insulin release in adult tissue; however, in the presence of caffeine, cultures of fetal pancreas do respond (Lambert et al., 1969a). Since pyruvate probably cannot be reconverted to the higher glycolytic intermediates (at least above fructose 1,6-diphosphate) (Brolin et al., 1968), it has been concluded that the elusive signal for insulin release lies below pyruvate (Lambert et al., 1969a). The possible conversion of pyruvate to lactic acid in this special system was not measured; however, it is unlikely that lactate synthesis is advantageous for insulin release since it generates oxidized nucleotides, which do not favor secretion (Watkins et al., 1968).

Glucose stimulation is accompanied by an increase in CO_2 production via the pentose pathway (Keen et al., 1965). Xylitol, a pentitol that enters the pentose pathway, is reported to stimulate insulin release in vivo (Kuzuya and Kanazawa, 1969; Kuzuya et al., 1969; Hirata et al., 1966) and in vitro (Montague and Taylor, 1968a). Montague and Taylor have extended these studies in isolated islets to show that the increase in 6-phosphogluconate with increasing glucose concentration follows the sigmoidal pattern associated with insulin release (Fig. 5). A large number

of agents that stimulate insulin release, including tolbutamide, theophylline, and glucagon, caused a rapid increase in 6-phosphogluconate which
was more striking than the rise in glucose 6-phosphate (Montague and
Taylor, 1969). Citrate and octanoate increased insulin release and the
levels of 6-phosphogluconate [presumably by blocking glycolysis at phosphofructokinase (Matschinsky et al., 1968)], thereby shunting fructose
6-phosphate into the pentose pathway. Until more intermediates in the
pentose pathway are studied, it is difficult to establish whether a rise in
6-phosphogluconate reflects increased flux through this path or decreased
flux resulting from inhibition at a subsequent metabolic step. It is an
intriguing possibility that the primary effect of the pentose pathway is
to generate TPNH, which in turn—at least in the fish islet—can stimulate
insulin release (Watkins et al., 1968). Montague and Taylor (1968a)
argued that TPNH is not the signal in the pentose pathway since ribose
also stimulates insulin release but is not expected to generate TPNH
(though this could occur by recycling of ribose through fructose 6-phos-
phate and glucose 6-phosphate). However, ribose usually does not stimulate release in vivo in other laboratories (Grodsky et al., 1963; Coore
and Randle, 1964; Frerichs et al., 1965) and xylitol does not stimulate
in all species (Kuzuya et al., 1969). The experiments of Montague and
Taylor were all performed in the presence of low, but significant, concentrations of glucose; thus, xylitol may be a "dependent" stimulant
(page 65). This is supported by recent observations that xylitol works
only in the presence of glucose (Malaisse and Malaisse-Lagae, 1969a).
Finally, xylitol in contrast to glucose does not stimulate insulinogenesis (Taylor, 1968a). Therefore, although the pentose pathway may
provide signals contributing to insulin release, the total glucose effect in
the pancreas may not be limited to metabolism through this pathway.

A dependence of the secretory mechanism on the tricarboxylic acid
cycle is possible since insulin release requires oxygen, is inhibited by
cyanide, and release by glucose in vitro is facilitated when pyruvic,
fumaric, and glutamic acids are present (Coore and Randle, 1964). However, certain tricarboxylic acid (TCA) cycle intermediates do not stimulate release (Coore and Randle, 1964), though many are permeable to
islet mitochondria since they can stimulate respiration (Hellerström et al.,
1970).

Citrate, under specific circumstances, stimulates release (Montague and
Taylor, 1969; R-Candela et al., 1964), but this action may reflect the
inhibition of glycolytic or other kinases and shunting of glucose into the
pentose or other pathways. Furthermore, stimulation by citrate is not consistently observed (Frerichs et al., 1965). That malonate did not inhibit
insulin release (Coore and Randle, 1964), though it does inhibit respira-

tion (Hellerström *et al.*, 1970), would indicate the TCA pathway to be unimportant; however, the two observations were made in different types of pancreatic preparations and the doses of malonate may not have been equivalent. In summary, the dependence of insulin release on ATP (Renold, 1970; Coore and Randle, 1964) indicates that the TCA cycle contributes to insulin release by providing energy, but there is little proof that intermediates in this pathway act as release signals.

In the normal islets, glycogen levels are sufficient to enhance a glucose stimulation, but in the absence of glucose levels do not create sufficient intermediates to provide the necessary signals (see page 58). Thus, agents which deplete glycogen such as glucagon, ACTH, cyclic AMP, or those that increase intracellular cyclic AMP normally require glucose for insulin release (Malaisse *et al.*, 1967b). In animals chronically treated with glucose, glycogen stores can be increased to sufficient levels so that glucagon, for example, will stimulate in the absence of added glucose (Malaisse *et al.*, 1967b). Since glucose 6-phosphatase is found in the beta cell, it is possible that glycogen stores can be dissipated to glucose and diffused from the cell when extracellular glucose levels are low (Fig. 4). Glycogen mobilization for insulin release does not require an intermediate conversion to glucose; mannoheptulose inhibits glucose phosphorylation and stimulation of insulin release by glucose, but it had no effect on stimulation when glycogen breakdown was induced (Malaisse *et al.*, 1967b). Thus, although there may be some conditions where glycogen stores are not readily mobilized (Jarrett and Keen, 1968), glycogen serves as a ready, though limited, source of glucose intermediates. Part of tolbutamide's action may lie in its ability to deplete glycogen (Hellman and Idahl, 1970).

Some attention must be given to a current, completely unexplained phenomenon, namely, that many agents have increased effects on insulin release when glucose metabolism is inhibited. Thus, stimulation by citrate, pyruvate, and tolbutamide is greatly enhanced in the presence of mannoheptulose or 2-deoxyglucose (Renold, 1970; R-Candela *et al.*, 1964; Gagliardino and Martin, 1966). These observations may relate to those of Hellerström *et al.* (1970), who found that oxidation of endogenous noncarbohydrate substrates in the islet cells is inhibited when there is a rich supply of glucose. Apparently certain metabolic pathways that can provide signals for insulin release are normally suppressed in the presence of glucose but become active when glucose is unavailable.

2. Action of Nucleotides

Various nucleotides may be intimately involved in the control of insulin release. Of these, cyclic AMP has been the most extensively studied.

The beta cells contain the adenylcyclase-phosphodiesterase system for the synthesis and breakdown, respectively, of cyclic AMP (Turtle and Kipnis, 1967). Agents that increase the availability of cyclic AMP cause a prompt release in insulin; these include cyclic AMP or its dibutyl derivative (Sussman et al., 1966), theophylline (Grodsky et al., 1967a), stimulators of the beta adrenergic receptors such as isoproterenol (Porte, 1967; Malaisse et al., 1967c), and a variety of polypeptide hormones such as glucagon, ACTH, and TSH (Grodsky et al., 1967a; Lebovitz and Pooler, 1967; Malaisse et al., 1967a; Sussman et al., 1966). Cyclic AMP apparently does not serve as a primary signal for insulin release, but it enhances the stimulating action of glucose and other primary stimulators such as tolbutamide (Grodsky et al., 1969; Lambert et al., 1969b) and leucine (Malaisse and Malaisse-Lagae, 1970). In a glucose-stimulated system, inhibition of glucose metabolism by 2-deoxyglucose completely abolishes the action of cyclic AMP-generating agents. Further evidence that cyclic AMP acts to enhance the action of stimulators, rather than to serve as a final signal, was the observation that glucose still stimulates insulin release when cyclic AMP levels are depleted by imidazole activation of phosphodiesterase (Malaisse et al., 1968c). Cyclic AMP-generating agents are particularly effective when the beta cell contains large amounts of glycogen (Malaisse et al., 1967a). However, it is unlikely that activation of phosphophosphorylase (and glycogenolysis) is the sole, or even most important, site of action for these agents. Recent studies indicate that cyclic AMP activates or deinhibits a variety of kinase enzymes (Kuo and Greengard, 1969; Walsh et al., 1968). Although no evidence is yet available, activation is possible at the level of phosphofructokinase, phosphoglyceratekinase, and other kinases involved in the metabolism of carbohydrate, lipids, and proteins (Fig. 4). It is of interest that epinephrine, which depletes cyclic AMP in the islet (Turtle and Kipnis, 1967), produces as a major effect decreased activity around the enzyme, phosphoglycerokinase (see page 69).

Glucagon, presumably through cyclic AMP, can activate gluconeogenesis in the liver at the level of pyruvic carboxylase or phosphoenolpyruvate carboxykinase. It is not known whether these gluconeogenic enzymes exist in the beta cells; however, fructose-1,6-diphosphatase is low (Brolin et al., 1968), suggesting that this potentially inhibitory action of cyclic AMP-generating agents is minimal in this tissue. Cyclic AMP can activate special protein kinases (Walsh et al., 1968; Langan, 1968) capable of phosphorylating various proteins, including protamines and histones, suggesting that cyclic AMP eventually may be shown to play a major role in the induction or repression of islet protein synthesis.

Cyclic AMP-generating compounds may prove particularly important in the diagnosis and possible treatment of diabetes. Simpson *et al.* (1966) and Raptis *et al.* (1968) observed that the impaired early release of insulin in the maturity-onset diabetic patient is partially repaired with glucagon. Similar observations have been made using aminophyllene (Cerasi and Luft, 1968). The development of similar agents with a directed affinity to the beta cell may provide a new class of drugs for the treatment of maturity-onset diabetes. Cyclic AMP also increases permeability of calcium into membranes of other tissues (Rasmussen and Tenenhouse, 1968). Thus it may play an important role in maintaining membrane structures and regulating calcium ion known to be required for insulin release (Grodsky and Bennett, 1966; Milner and Hales, 1967).

In vitro, ATP can be a minor stimulator of insulin release (Sussman *et al.,* 1969; R-Candela *et al.,* 1963). In addition, the inhibition of respiration and ATP synthesis by oligomycin inhibits secretion (Renold, 1970). Dinitrophenol, however, which presumably uncouples oxidative phosphorylation and the synthesis of ATP, may or may not inhibit secretion (Grodsky *et al.,* 1963; Coore and Randle, 1964). Also, levels of ATP after glucose administration do not correlate with release (Matschinsky and Ellerman, 1968). Hellman *et al.* (1969) found that sulfonylureas decreased ATP levels, though these substances are potent stimulators of insulin release. He suggested that the increase in ADP/ATP ratios could serve to activate kinases in the glycolytic pathway and in oxidative phosphorylation. This would explain the increased oxygen uptake seen when microdissected islets are exposed to the sulfonylureas (Stork *et al.,* 1969). Thus, though ATP synthesis probably cannot be completely inhibited (some ATP would be required for the initial phosphorylation of glucose, and as an energy source for the secretion process), ATP may not be a direct release signal.

TPNH may prove to be one of the insulin-release signals, since it reportedly stimulates release in fish islets (Watkins *et al.,* 1968) ; however, this observation has not yet been confirmed in mammalian tissue. The suggested importance of the pentose pathway in providing a necessary signal (see page 69) is consistent with the possible significance of this nucleotide. The mammalian beta cell is particularly well equipped to maintain the reduced nucleotides, since it is a low oxygen tension tissue similar to liver (Hellman and Lernmark, 1969b).

Tolbutamide, glucose, and leucine (all class 1 agents that directly stimulate insulin release) produce action potentials in isolated islets (Dean and Matthews, 1968). These effects are almost instantaneous and consistent in time with the rapid release of insulin (Grodsky *et al.,* 1967a). Studies of membrane potentials may eventually clarify how metabolic signals are transformed into a physicochemical phenomenon resulting in activation of granular or cellular membranes and insulin release.

3. Action of the Sulfonylureas

The hypoglycemic action of the sulfonamide derivatives was first demonstrated by Loubatières (1946), who suggested that these agents directly stimulate the pancreas to secrete insulin. An increase in measurable insulin occurs in plasma after tolbutamide administration (Yalow et al., 1960; Pfeiffer et al., 1959; Recant and Fischer, 1957), and a direct effect by the sulfonylureas on the pancreas in vitro was shown in the perfused rat and dog pancreases (Grodsky et al., 1967b; Kilo et al., 1962; Mehnert et al., 1962; Mariani, 1969; Pfeiffer, 1969), incubated segments of pancreas (Coore and Randle, 1964; Bouman and Gaarenstroom, 1961), and isolated islets (Malaisse et al., 1967d).

The sulfonylureas belong to the class 1 type of stimulating agents since they effectively stimulate insulin secretion in vitro in the absence of added glucose and are still effective when glucose action is blocked with mannoheptulose (Coore et al., 1963). Sulfonylureas, therefore, may act on the pancreas when glucose regulation is made inoperative either by hypoglycemia or impairment of glucose metabolism. The efficacy of these agents in maturity-onset diabetic subjects or in patients with islet cell tumors whose pancreases do not respond to hyperglycemia is probably a reflection of this phenomenon.

Tolbutamide in vitro causes an immediate release of insulin. Contrary to glucose, there is little effect on the provisionary (Curry et al., 1968a) or insulinogenic phase (Taylor and Parry, 1967). Secretory patterns of insulin in the intact animal (Seltzer, 1962) and man (Cerasi and Luft, 1967a,c) support the suggestion that the primary effect of the sulfonylureas is on release of stored insulin. Emeiocytosis, closely resembling that after glucose, is seen when tolbutamide is administered in vivo (Lacy, 1964). With prolonged stimulation, the sulfonylureas cause more dramatic degranulation than glucose (Pfeiffer et al., 1957), presumably since they do not stimulate resynthesis of the hormone. Sulfonylureas, in high concentration, produce a refractory state in the pancreas to glucose or further sulfonylurea stimulation (Bennett and Grodsky, 1969), indicating they may create metabolic feedback inhibition or they may compete with glucose for available insulin in a labile compartment or both (Section V,A,1).* Since caffeine or glucagon enhance the tolbutamide effect in the absence of glucose, some of its independent processes may be stimulated by cyclic AMP (Grodsky et al., 1969; Lambert et al., 1969b). As with glucose, the final signal is probably not cyclic AMP since high concen-

---

* In addition, high concentrations of sulfonylureas with low glucose stimulate β cell lysosomes and cytosegresomes (Lee et al., 1970). Possibly, this suggestion of increased autodigestion may contribute to an inhibition of the provisionary phase in vitro.

trations of imidazole did not inhibit its effectiveness (Malaisse and Malaisse-Lagae, 1970).

Although the sulfonylureas can act independently of glucose, they also enhance a submaximal glucose stimulation; a maximum glucose effect, however, is not potentiated (Lambert et al., 1967; Pfeiffer, 1969; Mariani, 1969). These observations parallel the capacity of sulfonylureas to stimulate basal respiration, enhance glucose respiration, but not to have an effect on either respiration or CO_2 production at maximal glucose concentrations (Stork et al., 1970). Data are consistent with the possibility that both glucose and the sulfonylureas share a common metabolic effect which is maximized with high glucose alone. Tolbutamide may enhance a submaximal glucose stimulation by decreasing islet ADP/ATP ratios (Hellman et al., 1969). This would result in the stimulation of glycolysis, increased respiration, and glycogen mobilization. A direct effect by sulfonylureas to decrease glucose-6-phosphatase (S. S. Lazarus and Bradshaw, 1959) would theoretically enhance glucose metabolism, but such an action has not been confirmed (Ashcroft and Randle, 1968b). Thus in the intact animal where glucose is always present, sustained levels of sulfonylureas may enhance the action of glucose both on synthesis and release of insulin.

Sulfonylureas also enhance response of the pancreas to leucine (Floyd et al., 1963). Since leucine, rather than its metabolites, is reportedly the stimulating agent (page 77), the sulfonylureas may act in part by decreasing leucine catabolism. Tolbutamide decreases conversion of leucine to CO_2 in islets (Stork et al., 1970) and decreases leucine transamination, decarboxylation, and incorporation into protein in peripheral tissues (Penttilä, 1966; De Schepper, 1967).

The sulfonylureas complex heavy metals, including zinc (Yoshinaga and Yamamoto, 1966). Although availability of certain metal ions is important in insulin release (page 83), direct action of the sulfonylureas at the cation level of islet function is not established.

Sulfonylureas may influence other pancreatic functions besides insulin release; they decrease the monoamines, dopamine, and 5-hydroxytryptamine in islets (Cegrell et al., 1964), and stimulate secretion of catalytic enzymes from acinar tissue (Knick et al., 1964; Gulzow et al., 1963). Samols et al. (1969) suggested that part of the hypoglycemic effect of tolbutamide was to inhibit release of glucagon from the adjacent alpha cells. However, the direct inhibition of glucagon release by tolbutamide at the pancreatic level is not consistently observed (Buchanan et al., 1969; Chesney and Schoffield, 1969).

Prolonged treatment with sulfonylureas in man may improve pancreatic function by exerting a trophic effect on the pancreas, as indicated by increased volume and weight of islets and their ratio to total pancreas (Loubatières, 1960; Loubatières et al., 1963, 1969; Bander et al., 1957). In vivo, tolbutamide increases size and DNA content of nuclei with evidence of extrusion of RNA from the nucleoles, all suggesting an increased protein synthetic activity (Sandritter *et al.*, 1964). However, these experiments are necessarily performed in the presence of glucose and may represent an enhancement by sulfonylureas of a glucose effect. In addition, the findings could have been the result of compensation known to occur when insulin in the beta cell is chronically depleted (Logothetopoulos and Bell, 1966). *In vitro,* and in the absence of glucose, tolbutamide stimulates the Golgi apparatus even though new insulin is not available to be packaged (Lee *et al.*, 1970). Early studies showing improved carbohydrate tolerance in mild diabetic subjects or in animals treated with tolbutamide (Fajans and Conn, 1962) still have not been consistently supported (Sheldon *et al.*, 1966; Fox *et al.*, 1967; Reaven and Dray, 1967; Sussman *et al.*, 1967).

Although the sulfonylureas directly stimulate insulin release from the beta cells, this may not be the sole mechanism by which they affect blood sugar levels. Thus, action of exogenously administered insulin is enhanced by the sulfonylureas in pancreatectomized animals (Linke, 1961; Lacy, 1962b). A large number of extrapancreatic metabolic effects of tolbutamide on liver, adipose tissue, and muscle *in vitro* have been observed and are reviewed by J. M. Feldman and Lebovitz (1969a). These include decreased hepatic and muscle synthesis of protein, decreased hepatic glucose output, and decreased lipolysis in adipose tissue. In plasma, sulfonylureas can competitively displace substances such as thyroxine from serum proteins, thereby indirectly influencing many metabolic parameters (Hershman and Konerding, 1968). Recently, J. M. Feldman and Lebovitz (1969b) and Tagg *et al.* (1967) found that the tolbutamide derivatives, hydroxymethyltolbutamide and carboxytolbutamide, can effectively stimulate insulin release but cannot duplicate the total action of tolbutamide on blood glucose *in vivo.*

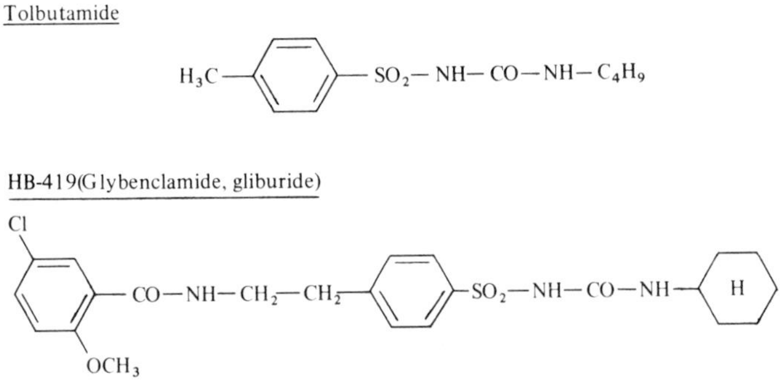

Tolbutamide

H_3C—⟨benzene ring⟩—SO_2—NH—CO—NH—C_4H_9

HB-419(Glybenclamide, gliburide)

Cl⟨benzene ring⟩—CO—NH—CH_2—CH_2—⟨benzene ring⟩—SO_2—NH—CO—NH—⟨cyclohexane ring H⟩

OCH_3

FIG. 9. Structural formulas of tolbutamide and glibenclamide.

A new sulfonylurea (glibenclamide, glyburide, HB-419) (Fig. 9) is 100–1000 times more potent than tolbutamide, both on blood glucose and insulin release *in vitro* and *in vivo* (Symposium, 1969). The pattern of insulin release that it stimulates in the perfused pancreas differs slightly from that of tolbutamide, though part of these effects may be due to dosage (Pfeiffer, 1969; Loubatières, 1969; Grodsky *et al.*, 1969).

4. *Action of Amino Acids*

Ingestion of protein or the intravenous administration of amino acids causes increased insulin levels (Floyd *et al.*, 1966a,b; Rabinowitz and Merimee, 1968; Dupré *et al.*, 1969). Among the amino acids, arginine is the most potent in man (Floyd *et al.*, 1966b), leucine, lysine, phenylalanine, and histidine being less active. *In vitro*, many amino acids directly stimulate insulin release, though the comparable effectiveness of each varies among investigators (Sussman *et al.*, 1967; Lambert *et al.*, 1969b; Edgar *et al.*, 1969; Milner, 1969a; Malaisse and Malaisse-Lagae, 1968a; Milner and Hales, 1967).

In vivo, leucine is distinguished from other amino acids, since its action is inhibited by diazoxide and is enhanced by prior treatment with sulfonylureas (Fajans *et al.*, 1966, 1967). Additionally, leucine induces severe hypoglycemia in some children with spontaneous hypoglycemia (Cochrane *et al.*, 1956) and in subjects with functioning islet cell tumors (Flanagan *et al.*, 1961); leucine may be the active agent, since its metabolic derivatives, isovalerate and acetoacetate, do not affect blood glucose in man (Knopf *et al.*, 1963). As previously discussed, the sulfonylureas may enhance leucine activity by decreasing its catabolism in liver, diaphragm, and pancreatic islets (page 75).

In vitro almost all amino acids tested in adult tissue require glucose or tolbutamide to be active (Edgar *et al.*, 1969); this is supported by observations in man that protein and glucose have a mutually enhancing effect on insulin secretion (Rabinowitz *et al.*, 1966). It is probable that the amino acids act primarily by altering the internal environment of the beta cell, making it more responsive to the action of a primary insulin-releasing stimulant. Leucine may prove unique among the amino acids in that under some circumstances it stimulates insulin release in the absence of glucose and can substitute for glucose in permitting the stimulatory action of arginine or cyclic AMP (Milner, 1969b). Therefore, it has tentatively been assigned to category 1. Possibly the use of new synthetic amino acids (Christensen and Cullen, 1969) that are not metabolized, but produce hypoglycemia in the intact animal and stimulate insulin from incubating fetal islets (Renold, 1970), may elucidate this action of the amino acids on insulin release.

5. *Action of Lipids and Ketones*

The ketones, β-hydroxybutyrate and acetoacetate, are reported to stimulate insulin release into the pancreatic vein of anesthetized dogs (Mebane and Madison, 1962). However, they are usually inactive when administered to man (Balasse and Ooms, 1968). Although the ketones enhance the effect of submaximal concentrations of glucose on insulin release in some studies (Malaisse and Malaisse-Lagae, 1968a) they are inactive in most *in vitro* pancreatic systems (Coore and Randle, 1964; R-Candela *et al.*, 1962; Rojas *et al.*, 1964; Montague and Taylor, 1968b; Lambert *et al.*, 1969b).

Short-chain fatty acids such as octanoate stimulate insulin release *in vivo* (Linscheer *et al.*, 1967) and *in vitro* (Sanbar and Martin, 1967; Lambert *et al.*, 1969b; R-Candela and Salinas, 1970) though this effect could be related to their ability to direct glucose metabolism toward the pentose shunt. Both octanoate and butyrate enhanced glucose stimulation *in vitro* (Montague and Taylor, 1968b) suggesting that these agents can serve to provide additional substrate to processes regulating release of insulin. Propionate and butyrate stimulate in ruminants, where they are important sources of metabolic energy, but do not in rats, rabbits, or pigs (Manns and Boda, 1967; Horino *et al.*, 1968). Long-chain fatty acids, such as oleate and palmitate, may increase insulin levels *in vivo* and *in vitro*, but the effects are usually small and sometimes undetectable (Greenough *et al.*, 1967; Madison *et al.*, 1968; Crespin *et al.*, 1969; Balasse and Ooms, 1968). Generally, situations associated with endogenous lipid mobilization, and high fat diets (Genuth, 1966; Malaisse *et al.*, 1967e) result in impaired insulin release in response to glucose stimulation (for discussion, see Malaisse *et al.*, 1969).

6. *Action of Hormones*

A variety of hormones have been shown to influence insulin release. Most of these effects, however, require pharmacologic concentrations; the significance of the results in terms of physiologic control is uncertain. Much confusion between *in vivo* and *in vitro* studies occurs, since most of the hormones studied are in category 2. Thus, their action is dependent on the presence of glucose or other sources of metabolic signals and energy.

Prolonged administration of *growth hormone* causes diabetes in dogs and in partially pancreatectomized cats (Fajans *et al.*, 1963), characterized by peripheral resistance to glucose and insulin. Evidence of overactivity and proliferation is found in the beta cell (Ogilvie, 1944). This peripheral resistance to glucose and islet proliferation are associated with hyperinsulinism after glucose stimulation in normal humans treated with growth hormone (Pavlatos *et al.*, 1964; Kipnis and Stein, 1964; Yalow and Berson, 1960) and in acromegalic subjects (Grodsky and Forsham, 1960; Yalow and Berson, 1960; Daughaday and Kipnis, 1966) or in animals with growth hormone-secreting tumors (Peake *et al.*, 1969). The hormone has no acute direct action at the pancreatic level since it does not stimulate insulin release *in vitro* (Grodsky *et al.*, 1962; E. Anderson and Long, 1948; Coore and Randle, 1964); at extremely high concentrations it can actually be inhibitory (Coore and Randle, 1964). A direct chronic effect on the pancreas by growth hormone is not excluded by the short *in vitro* experiments. *In vivo*, chronic treatment with growth hormone in the intact animal results in hyperglycemia, increased lipids, etc., which may stimulate the pancreas to increase its metabolic machinery for insulin release; pancreases taken from animals with growth hormone-producing tumors secrete a proportionately large amount of their pancreatic insulin when stimulated with glucose (Malaisse *et al.*, 1968d; Martin *et al.*, 1968). *Placental lactogen* probably acts similar to growth hormone since its administration *in vivo* results in a hyperinsulin response to glucose (Beck and Daughaday, 1967; Samaan *et al.*, 1968).

The *steroids*, notably cortisone, progesterone, and estrogen, also produce peripheral resistance to glucose and insulin, resulting in high insulin secretion in response to stimulation. Chronic cortisone administration produces islet changes similar to those after HGH (Volk and Lazarus, 1963; Hausberger, 1961); the steroids also have no effects on the pancreas *in vitro* (Coore and Randle, 1964), though these are necessarily short-term experiments. The similar action of the female hormones probably contributes to the hyperinsulinism in pregnancy (Beck, 1969; Lopez-Quijada *et al.*, 1967; Kitabchi *et al.*, 1968). By the same mechanism, combined estrogen and progesterone derivatives, administered as ovulatory suppressants, result in the hyperinsulin response (Spellacy *et al.*, 1967).

Glucagon and to a lesser extent *ACTH*, and *TSH*, act not only to stimulate the pancreas by indirectly increasing circulating glucose and peripheral resistance, but also can directly affect insulin release. *In vivo*, glucagon stimulates insulin release under conditions in which blood glucose levels are unchanged (Karam *et al.*, 1965; Samols *et al.*, 1965; Crockford *et al.*, 1966). *In vitro*, crystalline or synthetic glucagon directly stimulates insulin release (R-Candela *et al.*, 1965; Grodsky *et al.*, 1967a; Turner and McIntyre, 1966; Devrim and Recant, 1966; Weiniges *et al.*, 1969; Coll-Garcia and Gill, 1969; Vance *et al.*, 1968) though, as emphasized by Malaisse *et al.* (1967a), glucose or a large source of intracellular glycogen is required. Glucagon may also enhance a primary stimulation by tolbutamide (Grodsky *et al.*, 1969). Thus, these hormones belong to category 2. Since they raise islet cyclic AMP levels (Turtle and Kipnis, 1967), their primary action may be to activate adenylcyclase, thereby increasing glycogen breakdown and possibly activation of the various kinases that facilitate the metabolism of glucose and other agents (Fig. 4). Characteristic of agents increasing cyclic AMP, they can potentiate a maximal stimulus by glucose. Recent evidence that glucagon may deinhibit feedback inhibition induced by glucose (Bennett and Grodsky, 1969) could be another manifestation of these functions. Activation of the pentose pathway has been suggested since glucagon is known to increase 6-phosphogluconic acid (Montague and Taylor, 1969).

The acute effect of glucagon occurs within seconds (Grodsky *et al.*, 1967a) and is independent of protein synthesis since pancreatic response is not blocked by puromycin (Bennett and Grodsky, 1969). Glucagon is reported not to affect insulinogenesis (Taylor, 1968b) or RNA synthesis (McIntyre and Turner, 1970) in acute, *in vitro* experiments, but these phenomena have not been studied at high glucose concentration, where insulinogenesis may occur more rapidly. As all pancreatic effects by glucagon require high concentrations of the hormone, the role of physiologic levels on insulin release may be insignificant. Thus, Ohneda *et al.* (1969) and Malaisse *et al.* (1968c) found no effect on insulin secretion when endogenous glucagon levels were increased. Glucagon-like material from the intestine may not stimulate insulin release (Buchanan *et al.*, 1968).

That some *enteric* factor modifies the pancreatic secretion of insulin was suggested by the demonstration that oral glucose is cleared from plasma more rapidly than that administered intravenously (McIntyre *et al.*, 1964) and that the oral route for glucose and amino acids is associated with a greater rise in plasma insulin levels (Dupré, 1964; Ohneda *et al.*, 1968). In a combined intestinal and pancreatic *in vitro* preparation, glucose administered into the small intestine elicited a greater insulin response than glucose presented directly to the pancreas (Penhos *et al.*, 1969).

Intestinal hormones such as pancreozymin, secretin, gastrin, and intestinal glucagon may contribute to this insulin release. Presumably these agents, when active, operate by way of cyclic AMP and require the presence of basic stimulating agents, such as glucose or certain amino acids (Floyd *et al.*, 1966b; Dupré *et al.*, 1968; for review, see Unger and Eisentraut, 1969). Reports are remarkably inconsistent regarding the stimulating effect, either *in vivo* or *in vitro* of purified pancreozymin, secretin, or gastrin. Pancreozymin can sometimes cause the secretion of insulin *in vivo*, particularly in dogs, though this is not always observed; it appears completely inactive in the absence of glucose *in vitro* (Buchanan *et al.*, 1969; Turner, 1968). Secretin may cause increased insulin release *in vivo*, but the response is transient and not always detected (Unger and Eisentraut, 1969; Chisholm *et al.*, 1969); except for isolated reports (Pfeiffer *et al.*, 1965), purified secretin is inactive *in vitro*.*

The dog may be particularly sensitive to gastrin since a synthesized tetrapeptide of gastrin was active in this animal (Kaneto *et al.*, 1969). *In vitro*, it is a poor stimulator of insulin release (Buchanan *et al.*, 1969; Jarrett and Cohen, 1967), and at some concentration has actually been shown to inhibit stimulation by glucose (Lernmark *et al.*, 1969). Gastrin may be produced in the alpha cells within the islet (Gregory *et al.*, 1967; Lomský *et al.*, 1969); an extract of pigeon islets, which are rich in alpha cells, inhibited insulin release as does purified gastrin (Hellman and Lernmark, 1969a). It is not yet clear whether the intra-islet release of this hormone plays any role in the control of insulin secretion.

Despite the inconsistencies, there is ample evidence that crude extracts from the ileum and jejunum stimulate insulin release in the presence of glucose (Moody *et al.*, 1970). Turner (1968) concluded that none of the three purified hormones are effective and suggested that an undiscovered hormone ("Incretin") may be the major intestinal factor influencing insulin release. Possibly the active hormone or hormones are present to variable extent as impurities in available intestinal preparations.

Epinephrine inhibits insulin release *in vivo* (Porte *et al.*, 1966) or *in vitro* (Coore and Randle, 1964; Malaisse and Malaisse-Lagae, 1968b). This direct inhibition by epinephrine may explain why patients in shock have decreased insulin release (Allison *et al.*, 1968); shock, stress, or epinephrine in rats cause similar impaired insulin release from pancreas excised from the animals and stimulated *in vitro* with glucose (Wright and Malaisse, 1968). Epinephrine appears to act by stimulating both alpha and beta receptors, but in the beta cell the alpha receptor predominates (Porte *et al.*, 1966). Alpha adrenergic stimulation in the pancreatic islets results in decreased cyclic AMP (Turtle and Kipnis, 1967), thereby reducing insulin secretion. Phentolamine, an alpha blocker, in combination with epinephrine results in enhanced insulin secretion. Thus when the alpha-stimulating action of epinephrine is inhibited, its lesser, but significant, beta adrenergic action results in a rise of cyclic AMP and increase in insulin release. Isoproterenol, a beta adrenergic stimulating agent, causes a direct rise in insulin levels with no effect on blood glucose (Porte, 1967).

A block in glycolysis at the triosphosphate level by epinephrine was recently observed in cross-over studies (Hellman, 1970). Since a similar block occurs with calcium depletion, there may be an interrelationship

---

* Raptis *et al.* (1970) recently suggested that pancreozymin and secretin are active on the β cell only in the presence of exocrine pancreatic tissue. Thus, these agents may not work on pure islet preparations.

between epinephrine action and cation requirements in the islet. Epinephrine is a vasoconstrictor; thus part of its effect *in vivo* may be to decrease microcirculation in the islets (Bunnag *et al.*, 1963). However, the inhibitory characteristics of this hormone *in vitro* suggest that vasoconstriction is not necessary for the hormone's function on the beta cell.

Thyroxine in vitro does not affect insulin secretion (Malaisse *et al.*, 1967f). Paradoxically, both thyroidectomy and treatment with pharmacologic doses of thyroxine decrease insulin output *in vivo*. The depressed release with high concentrations of thyroxine may be a secondary result of stimulation of glucose uptake by peripheral tissues and reduced glucose-stimulated insulin secretion of the pancreas.

Both *oxytocin* and *vasopressin* can cause the release of insulin when infused into dogs (Kaneto *et al.*, 1967b). In contrast, *angiotensin-II* when administered *in vivo*, diminishes insulin response to glucose or to tolbutamide (Mintz *et al.*, 1967). No evidence is yet available whether these hormones directly act at the pancreatic level.

The role of *insulin* on secretion of insulin at the pancreatic level is unclear. Chronic administration of insulin *in vivo* at low levels insufficient to produce hypoglycemia has been reported to decrease insulin release (Kosaka *et al.*, 1964) and prevent degranulation (Erlandsen *et al.*, 1967). The concomitant decrease in pancreatic content of insulin has suggested that insulin *in vivo* may inhibit its own synthesis as well as release (Malaisse and Malaisse-Lagae, 1969b; Sodoyez *et al.*, 1969b). Usually, however, the small amounts of insulin necessarily used are ineffective (Chu and Goodner, 1968; Mintz *et al.*, 1968; Colwell and Colwell, 1966). The injection of anti-insulin serum effectively blocks the action of circulating insulin, and under conditions of artificially maintained normal glucose levels, antisera caused degranulation and other pancreatic evidence of increased insulin secretion (Logothetopoulos *et al.*, 1965). This may not be unequivocal evidence of a direct feedback, since insulin antisera added directly to pancreatic tissue *in vitro* did not affect insulin release (Malaisse *et al.*, 1967g).

In vitro, the measurement of small changes in endogenous hormone secretion in the presence of large amounts of added insulin are technically complicated and results have been inconsistent (Malaisse *et al.*, 1967h; Frerichs *et al.*, 1965). However, recent *in vitro* studies indicate that insulin can have a feedback effect on its own release (Sodoyez *et al.*, 1969a; Loubatières *et al.*, 1968; Boder *et al.*, 1969). Fish insulin has been used in feedback studies since its structural dissimilarity from mammalian insulin allows it to be added in large quantities without interfering in the immunologic assay of endogenous hormone. Both *in vitro* and *in vivo*, fish insulin does not inhibit insulin release in mammals, though it is fully active biologically (Grodsky *et al.*, 1968; Kanazawa, 1969). Possibly, therefore, feedback inhibition by insulin, if it occurs, may be due to its structural rather than hormonal characteristics. Hormonal inactivity of insulin in islets is suggested by the observation that metabolism of glucose to CO_2 is not affected by added insulin (Jarrett, 1968).

7. *Action of Metal Ions*

Since the original observations that calcium is absolutely required for insulin release and that release can be stimulated by either very high or very low potassium (Grodsky and Bennett, 1966; Milner and Hales, 1968), it has become apparent that cations, particularly potassium, sodium and calcium, are vitally involved in controlling the release of insulin during stimulation by a variety of agents (Milner and Hales, 1968, 1970; Lambert *et al.*, 1969b; Bennett *et al.*, 1969; Hales and Milner, 1968a; Howell and Taylor, 1968; Curry *et al.*, 1968b).

Insulin secretion is enhanced by phenomena that increase membrane depolarization and calcium uptake. Similar dependencies are seen in other secreting tissues (Douglas, 1968). Intracellular sodium levels probably play a major role in these phenomena; agents that raise intracellular sodium increase calcium uptake and insulin secretion. Thus, high extracellular potassium may stimulate release by increasing sodium permeability into cells, while low potassium or ouabain stimulate by inhibiting the sodium pump. Total potassium uptake into tissues is, in itself, not a necessary requirement for secretion, since ^{42}K uptake was not affected by tolbutamide (Howell and Taylor, 1968). Barium can often substitute for calcium in permitting release (Milner and Hales, 1968); in contrast, magnesium at high magnesium/calcium ratios effectively blocks secretion (Bennett *et al.*, 1969). The cations probably affect the late stages of insulin release at the membrane level since cation abnormalities can influence the action of glucagon, cyclic AMP, tolbutamide, amino acids, and glucose. Since the effects of ouabain or barium are blocked by 2,4-dinitrophenol, the action of cations may be energy-dependent (Milner and Hales, 1970); the adenylcyclase system and cyclic AMP have also been implicated (Lambert *et al.*, 1969b).

Diphenylhydantoin (DPH) causes hyperglycemia and decreased plasma insulin *in vivo* (Peters and Samaan, 1969) and directly inhibits insulin release *in vitro* (Levin *et al.*, 1970). The inhibitory action of this drug may relate to its effects on cation transfer previously shown in other tissues.

In cattle, normal hypocalcemia occurring with lactation or postparturition causes decreased insulin release in response to glucose stimulation (Littledike *et al.*, 1968). Insulin secretion is also depressed in subjects with low total body potassium, including anemia, and in animals on low potassium diets (Spergel *et al.*, 1967; Mondon *et al.*, 1968; Conn, 1965). In addition, the decreased total body potassium normally associated with different forms of diabetes may contribute to the impaired insulin release observed in this state (Telfer, 1966).

The role of zinc in storage and secretion of insulin remains uncertain. This ion is found directly associated with the granules in the beta cells (Boquist *et al.*, 1968; Yokoh *et al.*, 1969; Pihl, 1968). Zinc concentration in the beta cells decreases after glucose administration (Maske, 1957; Logothetopoulos *et al.*, 1964), and animals fed a low zinc diet have decreased content of pancreatic insulin. Zinc complexes with insulin primarily on the imidazole and terminal amino groups (Tangford and Epstein, 1954; Summerell *et al.*, 1965; Marcker, 1960b) (page 41); however, zinc is not required for biologic activity of insulin, zinc-free insulin being fully potent.

Other metals such as cobalt, copper, nickel, and iron will combine with insulin (Graig, 1962; Cunningham *et al.*, 1955), and cobalt can rapidly and specifically accumulate after its administration in the beta cells of certain fish (Falkmer *et al.*, 1964). However, there is currently no direct evidence that zinc or any of these metals are important factors influencing insulin synthesis or release.

8. *Action of the Central Nervous System*

This subject has been recently reviewed by Frohman (1969). Stimulation of the vagus nerve causes an immediate release of insulin (Frohman, 1969; Frohman *et al.*, 1967; Kaneto *et al.*, 1967a; Daniel and Henderson, 1967), which is inhibited by atropine (Frohman *et al.*, 1967). Similarly, stimulation of insulin release *in vivo* by derivatives of acetylcholine is blocked by atropine (Kajinuma *et al.*, 1968; Kaneto *et al.*, 1968). A direct stimulating effect of cholinergic drugs on the pancreas has been demonstrated *in vitro* (Mayhew *et al.*, 1968).

In the hypothalamus, destruction of the ventromedial nucleus results in increased adiposity and increased insulin. Though adiposity could produce the hyperinsulinism (Karam *et al.*, 1963; Parry and Taylor, 1966), it has been suggested that the increased hormone release was the result of a concomitant ventrolateral stimulation of the vagus nerve rather than a secondary effect of hyperphagia (Frohman *et al.*, 1969).

C. Variations of Pancreatic Sensitivity to Stimulating Agents

The previous discussions have primarily focused on regulation of insulin synthesis and secretion in the adult mammalian pancreas; however, differences in characteristics are observed among different species and vary with the stages of development in a given species. In the mature ruminant, where lipids provide the main source of energy, short-chain fatty acids, such as propionate and butyrate, are more effective than glucose in stimulating insulin release (Hertelendy et al., 1969; Manns et al., 1967; Manns and Boda, 1967). That the sensitivity to fatty acids in ruminants is also genetic, as well as an acquired characteristic, is supported by observations that fatty acids are still effective in the newborn lamb at a time when it functions as a monogastric animal. In fish, the amino acids are a major source of energy and prove more effective than glucose in stimulating pancreatic insulin release (Tashima and Cahill, 1968).

Fetal tissue from a variety of mammals, including the rat (Vecchio et al., 1967; Asplund et al., 1969), sheep (Willes and Boda, 1968), monkey (Mintz et al., 1969), and man (Grasso et al., 1968; Cornblath and Schwartz, 1966; Jorgensen et al., 1966; Adam et al., 1969), is comparatively insensitive to glucose. Most evidence suggests that the fetal pancreas contains adequate releasable insulin since it may still respond to tolbutamide, amino acids, or glucagon (Mintz et al., 1969; Grasso et al., 1968; Lambert et al., 1967). Lambert found that secretion is enhanced by caffeine, and suggested that fetal tissue is normally high in phosphodiesterase activity which rapidly destroys cyclic AMP, thereby reducing sensitivity to glucose. Tung and Yip (1968) observed that leucine-^{3}H is incorporated to a larger percentage into the proinsulin of incubating fetal pancreas and that synthesis of finished insulin is much slower than in adult tissue. Thus, in addition to impaired release of preformed hormone, fetal tissue may have impaired synthesis of insulin from amino acids or its precursors.

VI. Conclusion

A large variety of substances are now known to affect "release" of insulin, including carbohydrates, sulfonylureas, amino acids, hormones, β-adrenergic agents and possibly lipids. "Release," however, is not a single phenomenon, but is the resultant of many pancreatic processes. Sufficient evidence is available to show that some agents affecting release can differ in the pancreatic site on which they act. Thus, release should be considered, not only in terms of the effective concentration of stimulator, but also in terms of a stimulator's qualitative site of pancreatic action and the available insulin at that site.

The pancreatic processes involved in the production and storage of insulin have been partially elucidated; the biosynthesis of insulin and its precursors is well established, but the mechanisms controlling these processes are poorly understood. Even less is known of the storage mechanisms, though current studies indicate the existence of compartments with differing labilities.

Efforts to find a common metabolic signal for release are complicated by the probability that the signals controlling various pancreatic steps may differ. Furthermore some agents, such as glucose, sulfonylureas, and leucine can act independently while most other "releasing" substances (e.g., agents which increase islet cyclic AMP) actually require the presence of one of the independent stimulators. Nevertheless, it appears that intermediates of the glycolytic pathway do not act as signals, though cofactors arising from the pentose pathway or metabolites of acetyl-CoA may do so. The quantitative effect of most stimulators may be controlled by feedback inhibition induced by the stimulator and/or secreted insulin. A final common site of action is indicated at the membrane level where changes in electrical potential are associated with the availability of Na, K and Ca.

As the actions of individual agents are clarified, the mechanisms by which they act in concert may be established. Current observations indicate some combinations may mutually enhance submaximally in non-linear systems (such as glucose with the sulfonylureas); while others (glucose with glucagon or cyclic AMP) may potentiate maximal responses. In the latter case, concepts of deinhibition or newly available compartments should be considered.

Most forms of diabetes are characterized by defects of insulin release; however, the nature of these defects is unknown. It is expected that new testing procedures will be devised in which agents with known sites and mechanism of action will be administered singly or in conjunction with each other to establish not only the quantitative but also the qualitative nature of the defects. With time, new forms of treatment, in which agents are employed to specifically stimulate an impaired pancreatic function, are anticipated. Indeed, glucagon or drugs which increase cyclic AMP have already been employed to overcome the defect in "early release" occurring in certain mild diabetics. Though these latter agents may or may not prove clinically useful, a similar approach, based on a thorough understanding of the factors controlling pancreatic synthesis and secretion of insulin, should prove extremely important for novel treatment of the diabetic.

REFERENCES

Adam, P. A. J., Teramo, K., Raiha, N., Gitlin, D., and Schwartz, R. (1969). *Diabetes* **18**, 409.

Adams, M. J., Blundell, T. L., Dodson, E. J., Dodson, G. G., Vijayan, M. (1969). *Nature (London)* **224**, 491.

Akre, P. R., Kirtley, W. R., and Galloway, J. A. (1964). *Diabetes* **13**, 135.

Allison, S. P., Hinton, P., and Chamberlain, M. J. (1968). *Lancet* **2**, 1113.

Anderson, E., and Long, J. A. (1948). *Recent Progr. Horm. Res.* **2**, 209.

Anderson, G. E., Kologlu, Y., and Papadopoulos, C. (1967). *Metab., Clin. Exp.* **16**, 586.

Arquilla, E. R., Ooms, H., and Mercola, K. (1968). *J. Clin. Invest.* **47**, 474.

Arquilla, E. R., Bromer, W. W., and Mercola, D. (1969). *Diabetes* **18**, 193.

Ashcroft, S. J. H., and Randle, P. J. (1968a). *Lancet* **1**, 278.

Ashcroft, S. J. H., and Randle, P. J. (1968b). *Nature (London)* **219**, 857.

Ashcroft, S. J. H., Coll-Garcia, E., Gill, J. R., and Randle, P. J. (1968). *Diabetologia* **4**, 178.

Asplund, K., Westman, S., and Hellerström, C. (1969). *Diabetologia* **5**, 260.

August, J. T., and Hiatt, H. H. (1958). *N. Engl. J. Med.* **258**, 17.

Bagdade, J. D., Bierman, E. L., and Porte, D., Jr. (1967). *J. Clin. Invest.* **46**, 1549.

Balasse, E., and Ooms, H. A. (1968). *Diabetologia* **4**, 133.

Bander, A., Häussler, A., and Scholz, J. (1957). *Deut. Med. Wochenschr.* **82**, 1557.

Batts, A. (1959). *Ann. N. Y. Acad. Sci.* **82**, 302.

Bauer, G. E. (1968). Personal communication.

Beck, P. (1969). *Diabetes* **18**, 146.

Beck, P., and Daughaday, W. H. (1967). *J. Clin. Invest.* **46**, 103.

Bencosme, S. A., and Martinez-Palomo, A. (1968). *Lab. Invest.* **18**, 746.

Benedetti, A., Simpson, R. G., Grodsky, G. M., and Forsham, P. H. (1967). *Diabetes* **16**, 666.

Bennett, L. L., and Grodsky, G. M. (1969). *In* "Diabetes" (J. Östman and R. D. G. Milner, eds.), pp. 462–469. Excerpta Med. Found., Amsterdam.

Bennett, L. L., Curry, D. L., and Grodsky, G. M. (1969). *Endocrinology* **85**, 594.

Berson, S. A., and Yalow, R. S. (1963). *Science* **139**, 844.

Bierman, E. L., Bagdade, J. D., and Porte, D., Jr. (1968). *Amer. J. Clin. Nutr.* **21**, 1434.

Birkinshaw, V. J. (1962). *Nature (London)* **193**, 1089.

Boden, G., Soeldner, J. S., Gleason, R. E., and Marble, A. (1968). *J. Clin. Invest.* **47**, 729.

Boder, G. B., Root, M. A., Chance, R. E., and Johnson, I. S. (1969). *Proc. Soc. Exp. Biol. Med.* **131**, 507.

Boquist, L., Havu, N., Pihl, E., and Falkmer, S. (1968). *Diabetologia* **4**, 246.

Boshell, B. R., Barrett, J. C., Wilensky, A. S., and Patton, T. B. (1964a). *Diabetes* **13**, 144.

Boshell, B. R., Kirschenfeld, J. J., and Soteres, P. S. (1964b). *N. Engl. J. Med.* **270**, 338.

Bosshard, H. R., Jorgensen, K. H., and Humbel, R. E. (1969). *Eur. J. Biochem.* **9**, 353.

Bouman, P. R., and Gaarenstroom, J. H. (1961). *Metab., Clin. Exp.* **10**, 1095.

Brandenburg, D. (1969). *Hoppe-Seyler's Z. Physiol. Chem.* **350**, 741.

Brill, A. S., and Venable, J. H. (1968). *J. Mol. Biol.* **36**, 343.

Brolin, S. E., and Berne, C. (1970). In "The Structure and Metabolism of the Pancreatic Islets" (S. Falkmer, B. Hellman and I. B. Täljedal, eds.), p. 245. Pergamon Press, Oxford.

Brolin, S. E., Berne, C., and Linde, B. (1967). Diabetes 16, 21.

Brolin, S. E., Berne, C., Petersson, B., and Larsson, A. (1968). J. Histochem. Cytochem. 16, 654.

Bromer, W. W., and Patterson, J. M. (1969). Fed. Proc., Fed. Amer. Soc. Exp. Biol. 28, 343.

Brunfeldt, K., Deckert, T., and Thomsen, J. (1969a). Acta Endocrinol. 60, 543.

Brunfeldt, K., Hansen, B. A., and Nielsen, J. H. (1969b). Acta Endocrinol. 61, 561.

Buchanan, K. D., Vance, J. E., Morgan, A., and Williams, R. H. (1968). Diabetologia 4, 376.

Buchanan, K. D., Vance, J. E., and Williams, R. H. (1969). Diabetes 18, 381.

Bunnag, S. C., Bunnag, S., and Warner, N. E. (1963). Anat. Rec. 146, 117.

Burr, I. M., Stauffacher, W., Balant, L., Renold, A. E., and Grodsky, G. M. (1969). Lancet 2, 882.

Burt, R. L. (1965). Obstet. Gynecol. 25, 43.

Cegrell, L., Falck, B., and Hellman, B. (1964). In "The Structure and Metabolism of the Pancreatic Islets" (S. E. Brolin, B. Hellman, and Knutson, eds.), p. 429. Macmillan, New York.

Cerasi, E., and Luft, R. (1967a). Acta Endocrinol. 55, 278.

Cerasi, E., and Luft, R. (1967b). Acta Endocrinol. 55, 305.

Cerasi, E., and Luft, R. (1967c). Acta Endocrinol. 55, 330.

Cerasi, E., and Luft, R. (1968). Horm. Metab. Res. 1, 162.

Challoner, D. R. (1969). 61st Annu. Meet., Proc. Amer. Soc. Clin. Invest.

Chance, R. E., and Ellis, R. M. (1969). Arch. Intern. Med. 123, 229.

Chance, R. E., Ellis, R. M., and Bromer, W. W. (1968). Science 161, 165.

Chang, A. Y. (1970). In "The Structure and Metabolism of the Pancreatic Islets" (S. Falkmer, B. Hellman, and I. B. Täljedal, eds.), p. 515. Pergamon Press, Oxford.

Chen-lu, T., Yu-cang, D., and Geng-jun, S. (1961). Sci. Sinica 10, 332.

Chesney, T. McC., and Schoffield, J. G. (1969). Diabetes 18, 627.

Chisholm, D. J., Young, J. D., and Lazarus, L. (1969). J. Clin. Invest. 48, 1453.

Christensen, H. N., and Cullen, A. M. (1969). J. Biol. Chem. 244, 1521.

Chu, P. C., and Goodner, C. J. (1968). Endocrinology 82, 296.

Clark, J. L., and Steiner, D. F. (1968). Diabetes 17, 309.

Clark, J. L., and Steiner, D. F. (1969). Proc. Nat. Acad. Sci. U. S. [N.S.] 62, 278.

Clark, J. L., Cho, S., Rubenstein, A. H., and Steiner, D. F. (1969). Biochem. Biophys. Res. Commun. 35, 456.

Clark, J. L., Rubenstein, A. H., Oyer, P. E., MacKenzie, J. J., Cho, S., and Steiner, D. F. (1970). In "The Structure and Metabolism of the Pancreatic Islets" (S. Falkmer, B. Hellman, and I. B. Täljedal, eds.), p. 339. Pergamon Press, Oxford.

Cochrane, W. A., Payne, W. W., Simpkiss, M. J., and Woolf, L. L. (1956). J. Clin. Invest. 35, 411.

Coll-Garcia, E., and Gill, J. R. (1969). Diabetologia 5, 61.

Colwell, J. A., and Colwell, A. R., Jr. (1966). Diabetes 15, 123.

Conn, J. W. (1965). N. Engl. J. Med. 273, 1135.

Coore, H. G., and Randle, P. J. (1964). Biochem. J. 93, 66.

Coore, H. G., Randle, P. J., Simon, E., Kraicer, P. F., and Shelesnyak, M. C. (1963). Nature (London) 197, 1264.

Coore, H. G., Hellman, B., Idahl, L. Å., and Täljedal, I. B. (1967). *Opusc. Med.* **12,** 285.

Coore, H. G., Hellman, B., Pihl, E., and Täljedal, I. B. (1969). *Biochem. J.* **111,** 107.

Cornblath, M., and Schwartz, R. (1966). *In* "Major Problems in Clinical Pediatrics" (A. J. Schaffer, ed.), Vol. III, p. 48. Saunders, Philadelphia, Pennsylvania.

Covelli, I., and Wolff, J. (1967). *J. Biol. Chem.* **242,** 881.

Cowgill, R. W. (1964). *Arch. Biochem. Biophys.* **104,** 84.

Crespin, S. R., Greenough, W. B., III, and Steinberg, D. (1969). *J. Clin. Invest.* **48,** 1934.

Creutzfeldt, W., Frerichs, H., and Creutzfeldt, C. (1969). *In* "Diabetes" (J. Östman and R. D. G. Milner, eds.), p. 110. Excerpta Med. Found., Amsterdam.

Creutzfeldt, W., Creutzfeldt, C., and Frerichs, H. (1970). *In* "The Structure and Metabolism of the Pancreatic Islets" (S. Falkmer, B. Hellman, and I. B. Täljedal, eds.), p. 181. Pergamon Press, Oxford.

Crockford, P. M., Porte, D., Jr., Wood, F. C., Jr., and Williams, R. H. (1966). *Metab., Clin. Exp.* **15,** 114.

Cunningham, L. W., Fischer, R. L., and Vestling, C. S. (1955). *J. Amer. Chem. Soc.* **77,** 5703.

Curry, D. L., Bennett, L. L., and Grodsky, G. M. (1968a). *Endocrinology* **83,** 572.

Curry, D. L., Bennett, L. L., and Grodsky, G. M. (1968b). *Amer. J. Physiol.* **214,** 174.

Daniel, P. M., and Henderson, J. R. (1967). *J. Physiol. (London)* **192,** 317.

Daughaday, W. H., and Kipnis, D. M. (1966). *Recent Progr. Horm. Res.* **22,** 49.

Davidson, J. K., Zeigler, M., and Haist, R. E. (1969). *Diabetes* **18,** 212.

Dean, P. M., and Matthews, E. K. (1968). *Nature (London)* **219,** 389.

De Schepper, P. J. (1967). *Biochem. Pharmacol.* **16,** 2337.

Devrim, S., and Recant, L. (1966). *Lancet* **2,** 1227.

De Zoeten, L. W., De Bruin, O. A., and Everse, J. (1961a). *Rec. Trav. Chim. Pays-Bas* **80,** 907.

De Zoeten, L. W., Havinga, E., and Everse, J. (1961b). *Rec. Trav. Chim. Pays-Bas* **80,** 917.

Dixit, P. K., and Lazarow, A. (1969). *Diabetes* **18,** 589.

Dixit, P. K., Lowe, I. P., Heggestad, C. B., and Lazarow, A. (1964). *Diabetes* **13,** 71.

Douglas, W. W. (1968). *Pharmacology* **34,** 451.

Dupré, J. (1964). *J. Physiol. (London)* **175,** 58P.

Dupré, J., Curtis, J. D., Waddell, R. W., and Beck, J. C. (1968). *Lancet* **2,** 28.

Dupré, J., Curtis, J. D., Unger, R. H., Waddell, R. W., and Beck, J. C. (1969). *J. Clin. Invest.* **48,** 745.

Edgar, P., Rabinowitz, D., and Merimee, T. J. (1969). *Endocrinology* **84,** 835.

Erlandsen, S. L., Wells, L. J., and Lazarow, A. (1967). *Anat. Rec.* **157,** 415.

Fajans, S. S., and Conn, J. W. (1962). *Diabetes* **11,** Suppl., 123.

Fajans, S. S., Knopf, R. F., Floyd, J. C., Jr., Power, L., and Conn, J. W. (1963). *J. Clin. Invest.* **42,** 216.

Fajans, S. S., Floyd, J. C., Jr., Knopf, R. F., Rull, J., Guntsche, E. M., and Conn, J. W. (1966). *J. Clin. Invest.* **45,** 481.

Fajans, S. S., Floyd, J. C., Jr., Knopf, R. F., Guntsche, E. M., Rull, J. A., Thiffault, C. A., and Conn, J. W. (1967). *J. Clin. Endocrinol.* **27,** 1600.

Falkmer, S., and Olsson, R. (1962). *Acta Endocrinol.* **39,** 32.

Falkmer, S., and Wilson, S. (1967). *Diabetologica* **3,** 519.

Falkmer, S., Knutson, F., and Voigt, G. E. (1964). *Diabetes* **13,** 400.

Farquhar, J. W., Silvers, A., Reaven, G. M., and Shen, S.-W. (1968). *Diabetes* **17**, Suppl. 1, 323.

Feldman, J. M., and Lebovitz, H. E. (1969a). *Arch. Intern. Med.* **123**, 314.

Feldman, J. M., and Lebovitz, H. E. (1969b). *Diabetes* **18**, 529.

Feldman, R., Grodsky, G. M., Kohout, F. W., and McWilliams, N. B. (1963). *Amer. J. Med.* **35**, 411.

Field, J. B. (1964). *Amer. J. Med.* **36**, 867.

Field, J. B., and Lazarow, A. (1960). *Biol. Bull.* **119**, 313.

Fisher, R. B., and Zachariah, P. (1960). *Biochem. J.* **76**, 155.

Flanagan, G. C., Schwartz, T. B., and Ryan, W. G. (1961). *J. Clin. Endocrinol. Metab.* **21**, 401.

Floyd, J. C., Jr., Fajans, S. S., Knopf, R. F., and Conn, J. W. (1963). *J. Clin. Invest.* **42**, 1714.

Floyd, J. C., Jr., Fajans, S. S., Conn, J. W., Knopf, R. F., and Rull, J. (1966a). *J Clin. Invest.* **45**, 1479.

Floyd, J. C., Jr., Fajans, S. S., Conn, J. W., Knopf, R. F., and Rull, J. (1966b). *J. Clin. Invest.* **45**, 1487.

Fong, C. T. O., Silver, L., Popenoe, E. A., and Debons, A. F. (1962). *Biochim. Biophys. Acta* **56**, 190.

Fox, O. J., McAdams, G. L., and Boshell, B. R. (1967). *Clin. Res.* **15**, 43.

Fraenkel-Conrat, J., and Fraenkel-Conrat, H. (1950). *Biochim. Biophys. Acta* **5**, 89.

Fredericq, E. (1956). *Arch. Biochem. Biophys.* **65**, 218.

Fredericq, E. (1957). *J. Amer. Chem. Soc.* **79**, 599.

Frerichs, H., Reich, U., and Creutzfeldt, W. (1965). *Klin. Wochenschr.* **43**, 136.

Friz, C. T., Lazarow, A., and Cooperstein, S. J. (1960). *Biol. Bull.* **119**, 161.

Frohman, L. A., Ezdinli, E. Z., and Javid, R. (1967). *Diabetes* **16**, 443.

Frohman, L. A. (1969). *Annu. Rev. Physiol.* **31**, 353.

Frohman, L. A., Bernardis, L. L., Schnatz, J. D., and Burek, L. (1969). *Amer. J. Physiol.* **216**, 1496.

Gagliardino, J. J., and Martin, J. M. (1966). *Metab., Clin. Exp.* **15**, 1068.

Genuth, S. M. (1966). *Diabetes* **15**, 798.

Genuth, S. M. (1969). *Endocrinology* **84**, 386.

Genuth, S., and Lebovitz, H. E. (1964). *Clin. Res.* **12**, 267.

Gepts, W., and Toussaint, D. (1964). *In* "The Structure and Metabolism of the Pancreatic Islets" (S. E. Brolin, B. Hellman, and H. Knutson, eds.), p. 357. Macmillan, New York.

Gepts, W., Gregoire, F., Van Assche, A., and de Gasparo, M. (1970). *In* "The Structure and Metabolism of the Pancreatic Islets" (S. Falkmer, B. Hellman, and I. B. Täljedal, eds.), p. 283. Pergamon Press, Oxford.

Goetz, F. C., and Cooperstein, S. J. (1962). *Biol. Bull.* **123**, 496.

Goetz, F. C., Maney, J., and Greenberg, B. Z. (1964). *Excerpta Med.* **74**, 135.

Goldschmied, A., and Laurian, L. (1968). *Lancet* **2**, 405.

Goldsmith, S. J., Yalow, R. S., and Berson, S. A. (1969). *Diabetes* **18**, 834.

Goodner, C. J., Conway, M. J., and Werrbach, J. H. (1969). *J. Clin. Invest.* **48**, 1878.

Gorden, P., and Roth, J. (1969). *Arch. Intern. Med.* **123**, 237.

Graig, F. A. (1962). *N. Y. State J. Med.* **62**, 75.

Grant, P. T., and Reid, K. B. M. (1968). *Biochem. J.* **110**, 281.

Grant, P. T., Reid, K., Coombs, T., Youngen, A., and Thomas, A. (1970). *In* "The Structure and Metabolism of the Pancreatic Islets" (S. Falkmer, B. Hellman, and I. B. Täljedal, eds.), p. 349. Pergamon Press, Oxford.

Grasso, S., Messina, A., Saporito, N., and Reitano, G. (1968). *Lancet* **2**, 755.

Greenough, W. B., III, Crespin, S. R., and Steinberg, D. (1967). *Lancet* **2**, 1335.

Gregory, R. A., Grossman, M. I., Tracy, H. J., and Bentley, P. H. (1967). *Lancet* **2**, 543.

Grodsky, G. M., and Bennett, L. L. (1963). *Proc. Soc. Exp. Biol. Med.* **114**, 769.

Grodsky, G. M., and Bennett, L. L. (1966). *Diabetes* **15**, 910.

Grodsky, G. M., and Forsham, P. H. (1960). *J. Clin. Invest.* **39**, 1070.

Grodsky, G. M., and Forsham, P. H. (1966). *Annu. Rev. Physiol.* **28**, 347.

Grodsky, G. M., and Tarver, H. (1956). *Nature (London)* **223**, 4501.

Grodsky, G. M., Peng, C. T., and Forsham, P. H. (1959). *Arch. Biochem. Biophys.* **81**, 264.

Grodsky, G. M., Bennett, L. L., Batts, A., McWilliams, N., and Vcella, C. (1962). *Fed. Proc., Fed. Amer. Soc. Exp. Biol.* **21**, 202.

Grodsky, G. M., Batts, A. A., Bennett, L. L., Vcella, C., McWilliams, N. B., and Smith, D. F. (1963). *Amer. J. Physiol.* **205**, 638.

Grodsky, G. M., Bennett, L. L., Smith, D. F., and Schmid, F. G. (1967a). *Metab., Clin. Exp.* **16**, 222.

Grodsky, G. M., Bennett, L. L., Smith, D., and Nemechek, K. (1967b). *In* "Tolbut-amide—After Ten Years" (W. J. H. Butterfield and W. Van Westering, eds.), Int. Congr. Ser. No. 149, p. 11. Excerpta Med. Found., Amsterdam.

Grodsky, G. M., Curry, D. L., Bennett, L. L., and Rodrigo, J. J. (1968). *Acta Diabetol. Latina* **5**, Suppl. 1, 140.

Grodsky, G. M., Curry, D., Landahl, H., and Bennett, L. L. (1969). *Acta Diabetol. Latina* **6**, Suppl. 1, 554.

Grodsky, G., Landahl, H., Curry, D., and Bennett, L. L. (1970). *In* "Early Diabetes" (R. A. Camerini-Davalos and H. S. Cole, eds.), Suppl. 1, p. 45. Academic Press, New York.

Grodsky, G. M., Lee, J. C., Licko, V., and Landahl, H. (1971). *Excerpta Med.* (in press).

Gulzow, M., Diwok, K., and Trettin, H. J. (1963). *Deut. Z. Verdau.- Stoffwechselkr.* **23**, 7.

Gutfreund, H. (1952). *Biochem. J.* **50**, 564.

Haibach, H., and Kobayashi, I. (1970). *Clin. Res.* **18**, 121.

Haist, R. E. (1965). *In* "On the Nature and Treatment of Diabetes" (B. S. Leibal and G. A. Wrenshall, eds.), p. 12. Excerpta Med. Found., Amsterdam.

Hales, C. N., and Milner, R. D. G. (1968a). *J. Physiol. (London)* **194**, 725.

Hales, C. N., and Milner, R. D. G. (1968b). *J. Physiol. (London)* **199**, 177.

Haliken, D. N., and Arquilla, E. R. (1961). *Diabetes* **10**, 142.

Hard, W. L. (1944). *Amer. J. Anat.* **75**, 369.

Harferist, E. J., and Craig, L. C. (1952). *J. Amer. Chem. Soc.* **74**, 3083 and 3087.

Harris, J. I., and Li, C. H. (1952). *J. Amer. Chem. Soc.* **74**, 2945.

Harris, J. I., Sanger, F., and Naughton, N. A. (1956). *Arch. Biochem. Biophys.* **65**, 427.

Hartroft, W. S., and Wrenshall, G. A. (1955). *Diabetes* **4**, 1.

Hausberger, F. X. (1961). *Acta Endocrinol.* **37**, 336.

Hellerström, C. (1964). *Acta Endocrinol.* **45**, 122.

Hellerström, C. (1967). *Endocrinology* **81**, 105.

Hellerström, C., Westman, S., Marsden, N., and Turner, D. (1970). *In* "The Structure and Metabolism of the Pancreatic Islets" (S. Falkmer, B. Hellman, and I. B. Täljedal, eds.), p. 315. Pergamon Press, Oxford.

Hellman, B. (1959a). *Acta Endocrinol.* 31, 91.

Hellman, B. (1959b). *Acta Endocrinol.* 32, 63.

Hellman, B. (1970). *Minkowski Award-Lect.* (in press).

Hellman, B., and Hellerström, C. (1962a). *Z. Zellforsch. Mikrosk. Anat.* 56, 97.

Hellman, B., and Hellerström, C. (1962b). *Acta Endocrinol.* 39, 474.

Hellman, B., and Idahl, L. Å. (1970). *In* "The Structure and Metabolism of the Pancreatic Islets" (S. Falkmer, B. Hellman, and I. B. Täljedal, eds.), p. 253. Pergamon Press, Oxford.

Hellman, B., and Larsson, S. (1961). *Acta Endocrinol.* 38, 303.

Hellman, B., and Lernmark, Å. (1969a). *Endocrinology* 84, 1484.

Hellman, B., and Lernmark, Å. (1969b). *Diabetologia* 5, 22.

Hellman, B., Idahl, L. Å., and Danielsson, A. (1969). *Diabetes* 18, 509.

Hershman, J. M., and Konerding, K. (1968). *Endocrinology* 83, 74.

Hertelendy, F., Machlin, L., and Kipnis, D. M. (1969). *Endocrinology* 84, 192.

Hirata, Y., Fujisawa, M., Sato, H., Asano, T., and Katsuki, S. (1966). *Biochem. Biophys. Res. Commun.* 24, 471.

Hodgkin, D. C., and Oughton, B. (1956). *Ciba Found. Colloq. Endocrinol.* 9, 133.

Horino, M., Machlin, L. J., Hertelendy, F., and Kipnis, D. M. (1968). *Endocrinology* 83, 118.

Hörnle, V. S., Weber, U., and Weitzel, G. (1968). *Hoppe-Seyler's Z. Physiol. Chem.* 349, 1428 and 1431.

Howell, S. L., and Taylor, K. W. (1967). *Biochem. J.* 102, 922.

Howell, S. L., and Taylor, K. W. (1968). *Biochem. J.* 108, 17.

Howell, S. L., Young, D. A., and Lacy, P. E. (1969). *J. Cell Biol.* 41, 167.

Hug, G., and Schubert, W. K. (1967). *Diabetes* 16, 791.

Humbel, R. E. (1963). *Biochim. Biophys. Acta* 74, 96.

Humbel, R. E. (1965). *Proc. Nat. Acad. Sci. U. S.* 53, 853.

Humbel, R. E., and Crestfield, A. M. (1965). *Biochemistry* 4, 1044.

Humbel, R. E., and Renold, A. E. (1963). *Biochim. Biophys. Acta* 74, 84.

Iberall, A., Ehrenberg, M., Cardon, S., and Simenhoff, M. (1968). *Metab., Clin. Exp.* 17, 1119.

Idahl, L. Å., and Hellman, B. (1968). *Acta Endocrinol.* 59, 479.

Idahl, L. Å., and Hellman, B. (1970). *Acta Endocrinol.* (in press).

Idahl, L. Å., and Täljedal, I. B. (1968). *Biochem. J.* 106, 161.

Ishihara, Y., Saito, T., Ito, Y., and Fujino, M. (1958). *Nature (London)* 181, 1468.

Izzo, J. L., and Bartlett, J. W. (1969). *Arch. Intern. Med.* 123, 272.

Jarrett, R. J. (1968). *Diabetologia* 4, 178 (abstr.).

Jarrett, R. J., and Cohen, N. M. (1967). *Lancet* 2, 861.

Jarrett, R. J., and Keen, H. (1966). *Lancet* 1, 633.

Jarrett, R. J., and Keen, H. (1968). *Diabetologia* 4, 249.

Jarrett, R. J., Keen, H., and Track, N. (1967). *Nature (London)* 213, 634.

Jarrett, R. J., Keen, H., and Track, N. S. (1968). *Diabetologia* 4, 394.

Jones, V. E., and Cunliffe, A. C. (1961). *Nature (London)* 192, 136.

Jorgensen, K. R., Deckert, T., Pedersen, L. M., and Pedersen, J. (1966). *Acta Endocrinol.* 52, 154.

Kajinuma, H., Kaneto, A., Kuzuya, T., and Nakao, K. (1968). *J. Clin. Endocrinol.*

Metab. **28**, 1384.

Kanazawa, Y. (1969). Personal communication.

Kaneto, A., Kosaka, K., and Nakao, K. (1967a). *Endocrinology* **80**, 530.

Kaneto, A., Kosaka, K., and Nakao, K. (1967b). *Endocrinology* **81**, 783.

Kaneto, A., Kajinuma, H., Kosaka, K., and Nakao, K. (1968). *Endocrinology* **83**, 651.

Kaneto, A., Tasaka, Y., Kosaka, K., and Nakao, K. (1969). *Endocrinology* **84**, 1098.

Karam, J. H., Grodsky, G. M., and Forsham, P. H. (1963). *Diabetes* **12**, 197.

Karam, J. H., Grasso, S. G., Wegienka, L. C., Grodsky, G. M., and Forsham, P. H. (1965). *Diabetes* **14**, 444.

Karam, J. H., Grodsky, G. M., Burrill, K., and Ching, K. N. (1970). Unpublished observations.

Katsoyannis, P. G. (1963). *Chem. Eng. News* **41**, 42 and 45.

Katsoyannis, P. G. (1964). *Diabetes* **13**, 339.

Katsoyannis, P. G., Tometsko, A., and Fukuda, K. (1963). *J. Amer. Chem. Soc.* **85**, 2863.

Keen, H., Sells, R., and Jarrett, R. J. (1965). *Diabetologia* **1**, 28.

Kilo, C., Long, C. L., Jr., Bailey, R. M., Koch, M. B., and Recant, L. (1962). *J. Clin. Invest.* **41**, 1372.

Kimmel, J. R., and Pollock, H. G. (1967). *Diabetes* **16**, 687.

Kipnis, D. M., and Stein, M. F. (1964). *Ciba Found. Colloq. Endocrinol.* **15**, 156.

Kissane, J. M., and Brolin, S. E. (1963). *J. Histochem. Cytochem.* **11**, 197.

Kitabchi, A. E., Buchanan, K. D., Vance, J. E., and Williams, R. H. (1968). *J. Clin. Endocrinol. Metab.* **28**, 1479.

Knick, B., Lange, H. J., Baier, H., Jäger, H., Jöckel, H., and Haas-Scheuren, G. (1964). *Klin. Wochenschr.* **42**, 507.

Knopf, R. F., Fajans, S. S., Floyd, J. C., Jr., and Conn, J. W. (1963). *J. Clin. Endocrinol.* **23**, 519.

Konikova, A. S., Morenkova, S. A., and Kritzman, M. G. (1969). *Biochim. Biophys. Acta* **168**, 252.

Kosaka, K., Ide, T., Kuzuya, T., and Miki, E. (1964). *Excerpta Med.* **74**, 45.

Kotoulas, O. B., Morrison, G. R., and Recant, L. (1965). *Biochim. Biophys. Acta* **97**, 350.

Kreisberg, R. A., Boshell, B. R., Di Placido, J., and Roddam, R. F. (1967). *N. Engl. J. Med.* **276**, 314.

Kuo, J. F., and Greengard, P. (1969). *J. Biol. Chem.* **244**, 3417.

Kuzuya, T., and Kanazawa, Y. (1969). *Diabetologia* **5**, 248.

Kuzuya, T., Kanazawa, Y., and Kosaka, K. (1969). *Endocrinology* **84**, 200.

Lacy, P. E. (1957). *Diabetes* **6**, 489.

Lacy, P. E. (1961). *Amer. J. Med.* **31**, 851.

Lacey, P. E. (1962a). *Diabetes* **11**, 101.

Lacey, P. E. (1962b). *Diabetes* **11**, Suppl., 1.

Lacy, P. E. (1964). *Ciba Found. Colloq. Endocrinol.* **15**, 75.

Lacy, P. E. (1967). *N. Engl. J. Med.* **276**, 187.

Lacy, P. E. (1970). *In* "Thirteenth Nobel Symposium on the Pathogenesis of Diabetes Mellitus" (R. Luft and E. Cerasi, eds.), Stockholm (in press).

Lacy, P. E., and Howell, S. L. (1970). *In* "The Structure and Metabolism of the Pancreatic Islets" (S. Falkmer, B. Helman, and I. B. Täljedal, eds.), p. 171. Pergamon Press, Oxford.

Lacy, P. E., and Kostianovsky, M. (1967). *Diabetes* **16**, 35.

Lacy, P. E., Howell, S. L., Young, D. A., and Fink, C. J. (1968). *Nature (London)* **219**, 1177.

Lambert, A., Vecchio, D., Gonet, A., Jeanrenaud, B., and Renold, A. E. (1967). *In* "Tolbutamide—After Ten Years" (W. J. H. Butterfield and W. Van Westering, eds.), Int. Congr. Ser. No. 149, pp. 61–82. Excerpta Med. Found., Amsterdam.

Lambert, A. E., Junod, A., Stauffacher, W., Jeanrenaud, B., and Renold, A. E. (1969a). *Biochim. Biophys. Acta* **184**, 529.

Lambert, A. E., Jeanrenaud, B., Junod, A., and Renold, A. E. (1969b). *Biochim. Biophys. Acta* **184**, 540.

Lambert, A. E., Orci, L., Kanazawa, Y., and Renold, A. E. (1969c). *Acta Diabetol. Latina* **6**, Suppl. 1, 505.

Lambert, A. E., Kanazawa, Y., and Grodsky, G. M. (1970). *In* "The Structure and Metabolism of the Pancreatic Islets" (S. Falkmer, B. Hellman, and I. B. Täljedal, eds.), p. 397. Pergamon Press, Oxford.

Langan, T. A. (1968). *Science* **162**, 579.

Langdon, R. G. (1960). *J. Biol. Chem.* **235**, PC15–PC16.

Lawrence, A. M., and Kirsteins, L. (1969). *Proc. Soc. Exp. Biol. Med.* **131**, 1142.

Lazarow, A. (1963). *Recent Progr. Horm. Res.* **19**, 489.

Lazarow, A., Bauer, G. E., and Lindall, A. (1964a). *In* "The Structure and Metabolism of the Pancreatic Islets" (S. E. Brolin, B. Hellman, and H. Knutson, eds.), p. 203. Macmillan, New York.

Lazarow, A., Dixit, P. K., Lindall, A., Moran, J., Hostetler, K., and Cooperstein, S. J. (1964b). *In* "The Structure and Metabolism of the Pancreatic Islets" (S. E. Brolin, B. Hellman, and H. Knutson, eds.), p. 249. Macmillan, New York.

Lazarus, N. R., Tanese, T., and Recant, L. (1969). *Diabetes* **18**, 340.

Lazarus, S. S., and Bradshaw, M. (1959). *Proc. Soc. Exp. Biol. Med.* **102**, 463.

Lazarus, S. S., and Volk, B. (1962). *In* "The Pancreas in Human and Experimental Diabetes," p. 51. Grune & Stratton, New York.

Lazarus, S. S., Barden, H., and Bradshaw, M. (1962). *Arch. Pathol.* **73**, 210.

Lazarus, S. S., Shapiro, S. H., and Volk, B. W. (1967). *Lab. Invest.* **16**, 330.

Lebovitz, H. E., and Pooler, K. (1967). *Endocrinology* **80**, 656.

Lee, J. C., Grodsky, G. M., Bennett, L. L., Smith-Kyle, D. F., and Craw, L. (1970). *Diabetologia* (in press).

Lens, J., and Neutelings, J. (1950). *Biochim. Biophys. Acta* **4**, 501.

Lernmark, Å., Hellman, B., and Coore, H. G. (1969). *J. Endocrinology* **43**, 371.

Lever, J. D., and Findlay, J. A. (1966). *Z. Zellforsch. Mikrosk. Anat.* **74**, 317.

Levin, S. R., Booker, J., Jr., Smith, D. F., and Grodsky, G. M. (1970). *J. Clin. Endocrinol. Metab.* **30**, 400.

Lindall, A., Steffes, M., and Sorenson, R. (1969). *Endocrinology* **85**, 218.

Linke, A. (1961). *Ger. Med. Mon.* **6**, 177.

Linscheer, W. G., Slone, D., and Chalmers, T. C. (1967). *Lancet* **1**, 593.

Little, J. A., and Arnott, J. H. (1966). *Diabetes* **15**, 457.

Littledike, E. T., Witzel, D. A., and Whipp, S. C. (1968). *Proc. Soc. Exp. Biol. Med.* **129**, 136.

Logothetopoulos, J. (1966). *Diabetes* **15**, 823.

Logothetopoulos, J., and Bell, E. G. (1966). *Diabetes* **15**, 205.

Logothetopoulos, J., Kaneto, M., Wrenshall, G. A., and Best, C. H. (1964). *In* "The Structure and Metabolism of the Pancreatic Islets" (S. E. Brolin, B. Hellman, and H. Knutson, eds.), p. 333. Macmillan, New York.

Logothetopoulos, J., Davidson, J. K., Haist, R. E., and Best, C. H. (1965). *Diabetes* **14**, 493.

Logothetopoulos, J., Brosky, G., and Kern, H. (1970). *In* "The Structure and Metabolism of the Pancreatic Islets" (S. Falkmer, B. Hellman, and I. B. Täljedal, eds.), p. 15. Pergamon Press, Oxford.

Lomský, R., Langr, F., and Vortel, V. (1969). *Nature (London)* **223**, 618.

Lopez-Quijada, C., Gomez-Acebo, J., and R-Candela, J. L. (1967). *Diabetologia* **3**, 435.

Loubatières, A. (1946). *Arch. Int. Physiol.* **54**, 174.

Loubatières, A. (1960). *Presse Med.* **68**, 1421.

Loubatières, A. (1969). *Acta Diabetol. Latina* **6**, Suppl. 1, 216.

Loubatières, A., Fruteau de Laclos, C., Houareau, M. H., and Alric, R. (1963). *C. R. Soc. Biol.* **157**, 1652.

Loubatières, A., Mariani, M. M., and Chapel, J. (1968). *C. R. Acad. Sci., Ser. D* **266**, 2245.

Loubatières, A., Mariani, M. M., Alric, R., Ribes, G., de Malbosc, H., and Houareau, M. H. (1969). *Diabetologia* **5**, 219.

Love, T. A., Sussman, K. E., and Timmer, R. F. (1965). *Metab., Clin. Exp.* **14**, 632.

McIntyre, N., and Turner, D. S. (1970). Personal communication.

McIntyre, N., Holdsworth, C. D., and Turner, D. S. (1964). *Lancet* **2**, 20.

Madison, L. L., Seyffert, W. A., Jr., Unger, R. H., and Barker, B. (1968). *Metab., Clin. Exp.* **17**, 301.

Malaisse, W. J., and Malaisse-Lagae, F. (1968a). *J. Lab. Clin. Med.* **72**, 438.

Malaisse, W. J., and Malaisse-Lagae, F. (1968b). *Arch. Int. Pharmacodyn. Ther.* **171**, 235.

Malaisse, W. J., and Malaisse-Lagae, F. (1969a). *Arch. Int. Physiol. Biochim.* **77**, 366.

Malaisse, W. J., and Malaisse-Lagae, F. (1969b). *Diabetologia* **5**, 349.

Malaisse, W. J., and Malaisse-Lagae, F. (1970). *In* "The Structure and Metabolism of the Pancreatic Islets" (S. Falkmer, B. Hellman, and I. B. Täljedal, eds.), p. 435. Pergamon Press, Oxford.

Malaisse, W. J., Malaisse-Lagae, F., and Mayhew, D. (1967a). *J. Clin. Invest.* **46**, 1724.

Malaisse, W. J., Malaisse-Lagae, F., and Wright, P. H. (1967b). *Endocrinology* **80**, 99.

Malaisse, W. J., Malaisse-Lagae, F., Wright, P. H., and Ashmore, J. (1967c). *Endocrinology* **80**, 975.

Malaisse, W. J., Malaisse-Lagae, F., Mayhew, D. A., and Wright, P. H. (1967d). *In* "Tolbutamide—After Ten Years" (W. J. H. Butterfield and W. Van Westering, eds.), Int. Congr. Ser. No. 149, p. 49. Excerpta Med. Found., Amsterdam.

Malaisse, W. J., Malaisse-Lagae, F., and Wright, P. H. (1967e). *Amer. J. Physiol.* **213**, 843.

Malaisse, W. J., Malaisse-Lagae, F., and McCraw, E. F. (1967f). *Diabetes* **16**, 643.

Malaisse, W. J., Malaisse-Lagae, F., and Wright, P. H. (1967g). *Proc. Soc. Exp. Biol. Med.* **126**, 474.

Malaisse, W. J., Malaisse-Lagae, F., Lacy, P. E., and Wright, P. H. (1967h). *Proc. Soc. Exp. Biol. Med.* **124**, 497.

Malaisse, W. J., Malaisse-Lagae, F., and Coleman, D. L. (1968a). *Metab., Clin. Exp.* **17**, 802.

Malaisse, W. J., Like, A. A., Malaisse-Lagae, F., Gleason, R. E., and Soeldner, J. S. (1968b). *Diabetes* **17**, 752.

Malaisse, W. J., Malaisse-Lagae, F., and King, S. (1968c). *Diabetologia* **4**, 370.

Malaisse, W. J., Malaisse-Lagae, F., King, S., and Wright P. H. (1968d). *Amer. J. Physiol.* **215**, 423.

Malaisse, W. J., Lemonnier, D., Malaisse-Lagae, F., and Mandelbaum, I. M. (1969). *Horm. Metab. Res.* **1**, 9.

Manns, J. G., and Boda, J. M. (1967). *Amer. J. Physiol.* **212**, 747.

Manns, J. G., Boda, J. M., and Willes, R. F. (1967). *Amer. J. Physiol.* **212**, 756.

Marcker, K. (1960a). *Acta Chem. Scand.* **14**, 194.

Marcker, K. (1960b). *Acta Chem. Scand.* **14**, 2071.

Marglin, A., and Cushman, S. W. (1967). *Biochem. Biophys. Res. Commun.* **29**, 710.

Mariani, M. M. (1969). *Acta Diabetol. Latina* **6**, Suppl. 1, 256.

Markus, G. (1964). *J. Biol. Chem.* **239**, 4163.

Martin, J. M., and Bamber, G. (1964). *Fed. Proc., Fed. Amer. Soc. Exp. Biol.* **23**, 409.

Martin, J. M., Akerblom, H. K., and Garay, G. (1968). *Diabetes* **17**, 661.

Maske, H. (1957). *Diabetes* **6**, 355.

Matschinsky, F. M. (1970). Personal communication.

Matschinsky, F. M., and Ellerman, J. E. (1968). *J. Biol. Chem.* **243**, 2730.

Matschinsky, F. M., Rutherford, C. R., and Ellerman, J. E. (1968). *Biochem. Biophys. Res. Commun.* **33**, 855.

Mayhew, D. A., Goldberg, A. M., and Wright, P. H. (1968). *Diabetes* **17**, 308.

Mayhew, D. A., Wright, P. H., and Ashmore, J. (1969). *Pharmacol. Rev.* **21**, 183.

Mebane, D., and Madison, L. L. (1962). *J. Clin. Invest.* **41**, 1383.

Meek, J. C., Doffing, K. M., and Bolinger, R. E. (1968). *Diabetes* **17**, 61.

Mehnert, H., Schäfer, G., Kaliampetsos, G., Stuhlfauth, K., and Engelhardt, W. (1962). *Klin. Wochenschr.* **40**, 1146.

Meienhofer, J., Schnabel, E., Bremer, H., Brenkhoff, O., Zabel, R., Sroka, W., Klostermeyer, H., Brandenburg, D., Okuda, T., and Zahn, H. (1963). *Z. Naturforsch.* **18b**, 1120.

Miller, G. L., and Anderson, K. J. I. (1942). *J. Biol. Chem.* **144**, 465.

Milner, R. D. G. (1969a). *Lancet* **1**, 1075.

Milner, R. D. G. (1969b). *Biochim. Biophys. Acta* **192**, 154.

Milner, R. D. G., and Hales, C. N. (1967). *Diabetologia* **3**, 47.

Milner, R. D. G., and Hales, C. N. (1968). *Biochim. Biophys. Acta* **150**, 165.

Milner, R. D. G., and Hales, C. N. (1970). *In* "The Structure and Metabolism of the Pancreatic Islets" (S. Falkmer, B. Hellman, and I. B. Täljedal, eds.), p. 489. Pergamon Press, Oxford.

Mintz, D. H., Finster, J., and Strept, M. (1967). *J. Clin. Endocrinol. Metab.* **27**, 671.

Mintz, D. H., Finster, J. L., Taylor, A. L., and Fefer, A. (1968). *Amer. J. Med.* **45**, 187.

Mintz, D. H., Chez, R. A., and Horger, E. O. (1969). *J. Clin. Invest.* **48**, 176.

Mirsky, I. A., and Kawamura, K. (1966). *Endocrinology* **78**, 1115.

Mirsky, I. A., Jinks, R., and Perisutti, G. (1964). *Amer. J. Physiol.* **206**, 133.

Moloney, P. J., Aprile, M. A., and Wilson, S. (1964). *J. New Drugs* **4**, 258.

Mommaerts, W. F. H. M., and Neurath, H. (1950). *J. Biol. Chem.* **185**, 909.

Mondon, C. E., Burton, S. D., Grodsky, G. M., and Ishida, T. (1968). *Amer. J. Physiol.* **215**, 779.

Montague, W., and Taylor, K. W. (1968a). *Biochem. J.* **109**, 333.

Montague, W., and Taylor, K. W. (1968b). *Nature (London)* **217**, 853.

Montague, W., and Taylor, K. W. (1969). *Biochem. J.* **115**, 257.

Moody, A. J., Markussen, J., Sundby, F., Streenstrup, C., and Schaich-Fries, A. (1970). *In* "The Structure and Metabolism of the Pancreatic Islets" (S. Falkmer, B. Hellman, and I. B. Täljedal, eds.), p. 469. Pergamon Press, Oxford.

Morgan, C. R., Carpenter, A. M., and Lazarow, A. (1965). *Anat. Rec.* **153**, 49.

Narahara, N. T. (1968). Quoted in Rubenstein and Steiner (1970a).

Nicol, D. S. H. W. (1959). *Biochim. Biophys. Acta* **34**, 257.

Nicol, D. S. H. W. (1961). *Biochem. J.* **75**, 395.

Nicol, D. S. H. W., and Smith, L. F. (1960). *Nature (London)* **187**, 483.

Ogilvie, R. F. (1937). *Quart, J. Med.* **6**, 287.

Ogilvie, R. F. (1944). *J. Pathol. Bacteriol.* **56**, 225.

Ogilvie, R. F. (1964). *Ciba Found. Colloq. Endocrinol.* **15**, 49.

Ohneda, A., Parada, E., Eisentraut, A. M., and Unger, R. H. (1968). *J. Clin. Invest.* **47**, 2305.

Ohneda, A., Aguilar-Parada, E., Eisentraut, A. M., and Unger, R. H. (1969). *Diabetes* **18**, 1.

Oleesky, S., Bailey, I., Samols, E., and Bilkus, D. (1962). *Lancet* **2**, 378.

Orci, L., Stauffacher, W., Beaven, D., Lambert, A. E., Renold, A. E., and Rouillier, C. (1969). *Acta Diabetol. Latina* **6**, Suppl. 1, 271.

Parry, D. G., and Taylor, K. W. (1966). *Biochem. J.* **100**, 2C–4C.

Pavlatos, F. C., Karam, J. H., Grodsky, G. M., and Forsham, P. H. (1964). *Clin. Res.* **12**, 93.

Peake, G. T., McKeel, D. W., Mariz, I. K., Jarrett, L., and Daughaday, W. H. (1969). *Diabetes* **18**, 619.

Penhos, J. C., Wu, C. H., Basabe, J. C., Lopez, N., and Wolff, F. W. (1969). *Diabetes* **18**, 733.

Penttilä, I. M. (1966). *Ann. Med. Exp. Biol. Fenn.* **44**, Suppl. II.

Perkoff, G. T., and Simons, E. L. (1963). *Arch. Intern. Med.* **112**, 589.

Peters, B. H., and Samaan, N. H. (1969). *N. Engl. J. Med.* **281**, 91.

Petkov, P. E. (1966). *Ann. Histochim.* **11**, 79.

Petkov, P. E., Galabova, R. R., and Gospodinov, B. (1968). *Histochemie* **15**, 318.

Pfeiffer, E. F. (1969). *Acta Diabetol. Latina* **6**, Suppl. 1, 477.

Pfeiffer, E. F., Steigerwald, H., Sandritter, W., Bänder, A., Mager, A., Becker, U., and Retiene, K. (1957). *Deut. Med. Wochenschr.* **82**, 1568.

Pfeiffer, E. F., Pfeiffer, M., Ditschuneit, H., and Ahn, C. S. (1959). *Ann. N. Y. Acad. Sci.* **82**, 479.

Pfeiffer, E. F., Telib, M., Ammon, J., Melani, F., and Ditschuneit, H. (1965). *Deut. Med. Wochenschr.* **90**, 1663.

Pihl, E. (1968). *Diabetologia* **4**, 246.

Pollen, R. H., Grodsky, G. M., and Di Raimondo, V. C. (1961). *43rd Meet. Amer. Endocrine Soc.*

Porte, D., Jr. (1967). *Diabetes* **16**, 150.

Porte, D., Jr., and Pupo, A. A. (1969). *J. Clin. Invest.* **48**, 2309.

Porte, D., Jr., Graber, A. L., Kuzuya, T., and Williams. R. H. (1966). *J. Clin. Invest.* **45**, 228.

Rabinowitz, D., and Merimee, T. J. (1968). *In* "Human Growth" (D. B. Cheek, ed.), p. 207. Lea & Febiger, Philadelphia, Pennsylvania.

Rabinowitz. D., and Zierler, K. L. (1962). *J. Clin. Invest.* **41**, 2173.

Rabinowitz, D., Merimee, T. J., Maffezzoli, R., and Burgess, J. A. (1966). *Lancet* **2**, 454.

Randle, P. J., and Ashcroft, S. J. H. (1969). *Biochem. J.* **112**, 1P.

Raptis, S., Schröeder, K. E., Faulhaber, J. D., and Pfeiffer, E. F. (1968). *Deut. Med. Wochenschr.* **93**, 2420.

Raptis, S., Rau, R. M., Schröeder, K. E., Hartmann, W., and Pfeiffer, E. F. (1970). *Excerpta Med. Found.* No. 209, p. 13.

Rasmussen, H., and Tenenhouse, A. (1968). *Proc. Nat. Acad. Sci. U. S.* [N.S.] **59**, 1364.

R-Candela, J. L. (1964). *In* "The Structure and Metabolism of the Pancreatic Islets" (S. E. Brolin, B. Hellman, H. Knutson, eds.), p. 349. Macmillan, New York.

R-Candela, J. L., and Salinas, M. (1970). *In* "The Structure and Metabolism of the Pancreatic Islets" (S. Falkmer, B. Hellman, and I. B. Täljedal, eds.), p. 485. Pergamon Press, Oxford.

R-Candela, J. L., R-Candela, R., Martin-Hernandez, D., and Cortazar, T. C. (1962). *Nature (London)* **195**, 711.

R-Candela, J. L., Martin-Hernandez, D., and Castilla-Cortazar, J. (1963). *Nature (London)* **197**, 1304.

R-Candela, J. L., Castrillon, A. M., Martin-Hernandez, D., and Castilla-Cortazar, T. (1964). *Med. Exp.* **11**, 47.

R-Candela, J. L., R-Candela, R., Martin-Hernandez, D., Castilla-Cortazar, T. (1965). *In* "Perspectives in Biology" (C. F. Cori *et al.*, eds.). Elsevier, Amsterdam.

Reaven, G., and Dray, J. (1967). *Diabetes* **16**, 487.

Recant, L., and Fischer, G. L. (1957). *Ann. N. Y. Acad. Sci.* **71**, 62.

Reid, K. B. M., Grant, P. T., and Youngson, A. (1968). *Biochem. J.* **110**, 289.

Reitz, H. C., Ferrol, R. E., Fraenkel-Conrat, H., and Olcott, H. S. (1946). *J. Amer. Chem. Soc.* **68**, 1024.

Renold, A. E. (1970). *N. Engl. J. Med.* **282**, 173.

Rojas, J., Meneses, P., and R-Candela, J. L. (1964). *Nature (London)* **203**, 758.

Rommel, K., Melani, F., Burkhardt, H., and Grimmel, K. (1969). *Diabetologia* **5**, 309.

Rong-qing, J., Yu-cang, D., and Chen-lu, T. (1963). *Sci. Sinica* **12**, 452.

Rosa, U., Massaglia, A., Pennisi, F., Cozzani, I., and Rossi, C. A. (1967). *Biochem. J.* **103**, 407.

Roth, J., Gorden, P., and Pastan, I. (1968). *Proc. Nat. Acad. Sci. U. S.* **61**, 138.

Rubenstein, A. H., and Steiner, D. F. (1970a). *Med. Clin. N. Amer.* **54**, 191.

Rubenstein, A. H., and Steiner, D. F. (1970b). *In* "Early Diabetes" (R. A. Camerini-Davalos and H. S. Cole, eds.), Suppl. 1, p. 159. Academic Press, New York.

Rubenstein, A. H., Cho, S., and Steiner, D. F. (1968a). *Lancet* **1**, 1353.

Rubenstein, A. H., Cho, S., and Steiner, D. F. (1968b). *J. Lab. Clin. Med.* **72**, 1010.

Rubenstein, A. H., Steiner, D. F., Cho, S., Lawrence, A. M., and Kirsteins, L. (1969). *Diabetes* **18**, 598.

Ryan, W. G., and Robbins, P. (1969). *Clin. Res.* **17**, 394.

Sachs, H., and Haller, E. W. (1968). *Endocrinology* **83**, 251.

Samaan, N., Yen, S. C. C., Gonzalez, D., and Pearson, O. H. (1968). *J. Clin. Endocrinol. Metab.* **28**, 485.

Samols, E., Marri, G., and Marks, V. (1965). *Lancet* **2**, 415.

Samols, E., Tyler, J. M., and Mialhe, P. (1969). *Lancet* **1**, 174.

Sanbar, S. S., and Martin, J. M. (1967). *Metab., Clin. Exp.* **16**, 482.

Sandritter, W., Federlin, K., and Pfeiffer, E. F. (1964). *In* "The Structure and Metabolism of the Pancreatic Islets" (S. E. Brolin, B. Hellman, and H. Knutson, eds.), p. 67. Macmillan, New York.

Sanger, F. (1956). *Ciba Found. Colloq. Endocrinol.* **9**, 110.

Sanger, F. (1960). *Brit. Med. Bull.* **16**, 183.

Sanger, F., and Thompson, E. O. P. (1953). *Biochem. J.* **53**, 353.

Schätzle, W. (1958). *Acta Histochem.* **6**, 93.

Schlichtkrull, J. (1970). Excerpta Med. Found. No. 209, p. 3.

Schmidt, V. D. D., and Arens, A. (1968). *Hoppe-Seyler's Z. Physiol. Chem.* **349**, 1157.

Seidler, E., Rückert, A., Schöne, J., and Ditscherlein, G. (1964). *Klin. Wochenschr.* **42**, 406.

Seltzer, H. S. (1962). *J. Clin. Invest.* **41**, 289.

Semeijns de Vries van Doesburgh, J. T., and Havinga, E. (1964). *Biochim. Biophys. Acta* **82**, 96.

Shaw, W. N., and Chance, R. E. (1968a). *Diabetes* **17**, 737.

Shaw, W. N., and Chance, R. E. (1968b). *Diabetes* **17**, 310.

Sheldon, J., Taylor, K. W., and Anderson, J. (1966). *Metab., Clin. Exp.* **15**, 874.

Simpson, R. G., Benedetti, A., Grodsky, G. M., Karam, J. H., and Forsham, P. H. (1966). *Metab., Clin. Exp.* **15**, 1046.

Sluyterman, L. A. Æ. (1955). *Biochim. Biophys. Acta* **17**, 169.

Smith, C. H., and Lacy, P. E. (1962). *Lab. Invest.* **11**, 159.

Smith, E. L., Hill, R. L., and Borman, A. (1958). *Biochim. Biophys. Acta* **29**, 207.

Smith, L. F. (1964a). *Biochim. Biophys. Acta* **82**, 231.

Smith, L. F. (1964b). *Lilly Insulin Symp., 1964.*

Smith, L. F. (1966). *Amer. J. Med.* **40**, 662.

Sodoyez, J. C., Sodoyez-Goffaux, F., and Foà, P. P. (1969a). *Proc. Soc. Exp. Biol. Med.* **130**, 568.

Sodoyez, J. C., Sodoyez-Goffaux, F., Rossen, R. M., and Foà, P. P. (1969b). *Metab., Clin. Exp.* **18**, 433.

Sorenson, R. L., Lindall, A. W., and Lazarow, A. (1969). *Diabetes* **18**, 129.

Spellacy, W. N., Carlson, K. L., and Birk, S. A. (1967). *Diabetes* **16**, 590.

Spergel, G., Bleicher, S. J., Goldberg, M., Adesman, J., and Goldner, M. G. (1967). *Metab., Clin. Exp.* **16**, 581.

Springell, P. H. (1962). *Biochim. Biophys. Acta* **63**, 136.

Steiner, D. F. (1970). *In* "The Structure and Metabolism of the Pancreatic Islets" (S. Falkmer, B. Hellman, and I. B. Täljedal, eds.), p. 197. Pergamon Press, Oxford.

Steiner, D. F., and Clark, J. L. (1968). *Proc. Nat. Acad. Sci. U. S.* [N.S.] **60**, 622.

Steiner, D. F., and Oyer, P. E. (1967). *Proc. Nat. Acad. Sci. U. S.* **57**, 473.

Steiner, D. F., Cunningham, D., Spigelman, L., and Aten, B. (1967). *Science* **157**, 697.

Steiner, D. F., Hallund, O., Rubenstein, A. H., Cho, S., and Bayliss, C. (1968). *Diabetes* **17**, 725.

Steinke, J., Camerini, R., Marble, A., and Renold, A. E. (1961). *Metab., Clin. Exp.* **10**, 707.

Stork, H., Schmidt, F. H., Westman, S., and Hellerström, C. (1969). *Diabetologia* **5**, 279.

Stork, H., Schmidt, F. H., Hellerström, C., and Westman, S. (1970). *In* "The Structure and Metabolism of the Pancreatic Islets" (S. Falkmer, B. Hellman, and I. B. Täljedal, eds.), p. 331. Pergamon Press, Oxford.

Summerell, J. M., Osmand, A., and Smith, G. H. (1965). *Biochem. J.* **95**, 31.

Surmaczynska, B., and Metz, R. (1969). *Endocrinology* **85**, 368.

Sussman, K. E., and Vaughan, G. D. (1967). *Diabetes* **16**, 449.

Sussman, K. E., Vaughan, G. D., and Timmer, R. F. (1966). *Diabetes* **15**, 521.

Sussman, K. E., Stjernholm, M., and Vaughan, G. D. (1967). "Tolbutamide—After Ten Years" (W. J. H. Butterfield and W. Van Westering, eds.), Int. Congr. Ser. No. 149, pp. 22–33. Excerpta Med. Found., Amsterdam.

Sussman, K. E., Vaughan, G. D., and Stjernholm, M. R. (1969). *In* "Diabetes" (J. Östman and R. D. G. Milner, eds.), pp. 123–137. Excerpta Med. Found., Amsterdam.

Symposium (various authors). (1969). *Horm. Metab. Res.* Suppl. 1.

Tagg, J., Yasuda, D. M., Tanabe, M., and Mitoma, C. (1967). *Biochem. Pharmacol.* **16**, 143.

Täljedal, I. B. (1967). *Biochim. Biophys. Acta* **146**, 292.

Täljedal, I. B. (1969). *Biochem. J.* **114**, 387.

Tangford, C., and Epstein, J. (1954). *J. Amer. Chem. Soc.* **76**, 2163.

Tashima, L., and Cahill, G. F., Jr. (1968). *Gen. Comp. Endocrinol.* **11**, 262.

Taylor, K. W. (1968a). *Excerpta Med.* **184**, 220.

Taylor, K. W. (1968b). *Diabetologia* **4**, 179.

Taylor, K. W., and Parry, D. G. (1967). *J. Endocrinol.* **39**, 457.

Taylor, K. W., and Sheldon, J. (1964). *J. Endocrinol.* **29**, 99.

Taylor, K. W., Jones, V. E., and Gardner, G. (1962). *Nature (London)* **195**, 602.

Telfer, N. (1966). *Metab., Clin. Exp.* **15**, 502.

Théret, C., and Tamboise, E. (1963). *Ann. Endocrinol.* **24/2**, 169.

Tietze, F., and Neurath, H. (1952). *J. Biol. Chem.* **184**, 1.

Tietze, F., Mortimore, G. E., and Lomax, N. R. (1962). *Biochim. Biophys. Acta* **59**, 336.

Toreson, W. E. (1951). *Amer. J. Pathol.* **27**, 327.

Tung, A. K., and Yip, C. C. (1968). *Diabetologia* **4**, 68.

Tung, A. K., and Yip, C. C. (1969). *Proc. Nat. Acad. Sci. U. S.* [N.S.] **63**, 442.

Turner, D. S. (1968). *Diabetologia* **4**, 177.

Turner, D. S., and McIntyre, N. (1966). *Lancet* **1**, 351.

Turtle, J. R., and Kipnis, D. M. (1967). *Biochem. Biophys. Res. Commun.* **28**, 797.

Unger, R. H., and Eisentraut, A. M. (1969). *Arch. Intern. Med.* **123**, 261.

Unger, R. H., Lochner, J. de V., and Eisentraut, A. M. (1964). *J. Clin. Endocrinol. Metab.* **24**, 823.

Vance, J. E., Buchanan, K. D., Challoner, D. R., and Williams, R. H. (1968). *Diabetes* **17**, 187.

Varandani, P. T. (1968). *Diabetes* **17**, 547.

Vaughan, M., and Anfinsen, C. B. (1954). *J. Biol. Chem.* **211**, 367.

Vecchio, D., Luyckx, A., and Renold, A. E. (1967). *Helv. Physiol. Pharmacol. Acta* **25**, 134.

Virupaksha, T. K., and Tarver, H. (1964). *Biochemistry* **3**, 1507.

Volk, B. W., and Lazarus, S. S. (1963). *Diabetes* **12**, 162.

Volk, B. W., and Lazarus, S. S. (1964). *In* "The Structure and the Metabolism of the Pancreatic Islets" (S. E. Brolin, B. Hellman, and H. Knutson, eds.), p. 143. Macmillan, New York.

Waddell, R. W., Beck, J. C., and Dupré, J. (1969). *Diabetes* **18**, Suppl. 1, 375.

Wagle, S. R. (1965). *Biochim. Biophys. Acta* **107**, 524.

Walsh, D. A., Perkins, J. P., and Krebs, E. G. (1968). *J. Biol. Chem.* **243**, 3763.

Watkins, D., Cooperstein, S. J., Dixit, P. K., and Lazarow, A. (1968). *Science* **162**, 283.

Webb, J. L. (1966). "Enzyme and Metabolic Inhibitors," Vol. 3, p. 1. Academic Press, New York.

Wegman, R., and Petkov, P. (1965). *Ann. Histochim.* **10**, 93.

Weiniges, K. F., Wünsch, E., Biro, G., Kettl, H., and Mitzuno, M. (1969). *Diabetologia* **5**, 97.

Weitzel, G., Strätling, W. H., Hahn, J., and Martini, O. (1967). *Hoppe-Seyler's Z. Physiol. Chem.* **348**, 525.

Wellmann, K. F., Volk, B. W., Lazarus, S. S., and Brancato, P. (1969). *Diabetes* **18**, 138.

Wettermark, G., Tegnér, L., Brolin, S. E., and Borglund, E. (1970). *In* "The Structure and Metabolism of the Pancreatic Islets" (S. Falkmer, B. Hellman, and I. B. Täljedal eds.), p. 275. Pergamon Press, Oxford.

Whitney, J. E., and Massey, C. G. (1961). *J. Clin. Endocrinol. Metab.* **21**, 541.

Whitney, J. E., Cutler, O. E., and Wright, F. E. (1963). *Metab., Clin. Exp.* **12**, 352.

Willes, R. F., and Boda, J. M. (1968). *Fed. Proc., Fed. Amer. Soc. Exp. Biol.* **27**, 496.

Willes, R. F., Boda, J. M., and Stokes, H. (1969). *Endocrinology* **84**, 671.

Williamson, J. R., Lacy, P. E., and Grisham, J. W. (1961). *Diabetes* **10**, 460.

Wilson, S., and Dixon, G. H. (1961). *Nature (London)* **191**, 876.

Wilson, S., Dixon, G. H., and Wardlaw, A. C. (1962). *Biochim. Biophys. Acta* **62**, 483.

Wright, P. H., and Malaisse, W. J. (1968). *Amer. J. Phys.* **214**, 1031.

Yalow, R. S., and Berson, S. A. (1960). *J. Clin. Invest.* **39**, 1157.

Yalow, R. S., and Berson, S. A. (1961). *Amer. J. Med.* **31**, 882.

Yalow, R. S., and Berson, S. A. (1966). *Trans. N. Y. Acad. Sci.* **28**, 1033.

Yalow, R. S., Black, H., Villazon, M., and Berson, S. A. (1960). *Diabetes* **9**, 356.

Yalow, R. S., Goldsmith, S. J., and Berson, S. A. (1969). *Diabetes* **18**, 402.

Yip, C. C., and Logothetopoulos, J. (1969). *Proc. Nat. Acad. Sci. U. S.* [N.S.] **62**, 415.

Yokoh, S., Aoji, O., Matsuno, Z., and Yoshida, H. (1969). *Diabetologia* **5**, 137.

Yoshinaga, T., and Yamamoto, Y. (1966). *Endokrinologie* **50**, 87.

Young, F. G. (1961). *Brit. Med. J.* **2**, 1449.

Young, J. D., and Jenkinson, I. S. (1968). *Aust. J. Exp. Biol. Med. Sci.* **46**, 707.

Yu-cang, D., Rong-qing, J., and Chen-lu, T. (1965). *Sci. Sinica* **14**, 229.

Regulation of Calcium Transport in Bone by Parathyroid Hormone

ROY V. TALMAGE,* CARY W. COOPER,† AND HAN Z. PARK†

*Division of Biology and Medicine, Atomic Energy Commission, Washington, D. C.;
Department of Pharmacology, School of Medicine, University of North Carolina,
Chapel Hill, North Carolina; Department of Anatomy, School of Medicine,
University of Utah, Salt Lake City, Utah*

* On leave from Rice University. Present address: Orthopaedic Research Laboratory, Department of Surgery, School of Medicine, University of North Carolina, Chapel Hill, North Carolina.

† During preparation of this manuscript, C. W. C. was supported in part by a grant from the National Institute of Arthritis and Metabolic Diseases (AM10558) and by a Faculty Development Award from The Merck Company Foundation; H. Z. P. was supported in part by The Atomic Energy Commission.

I. Introduction

The last decade has been marked by a continued, perhaps even re-surgent, interest in research concerning calcium homeostasis in general and parathyroid hormone in particular. The convening of no less than three international conferences largely concerned with these topics (Greep and Talmage, 1961; Gaillard et al., 1965; Talmage and Bélanger, 1968) along with periodic review articles (Munson et al., 1963; Aurbach and Potts, 1964; Arnaud et al., 1967; Potts and Deftos, 1969; Copp, 1969) provide sufficient attestation to this interest. Undoubtedly, the advent of the calcitonin concept (Copp et al., 1962) and the discovery of thyro-calcitonin (Hirsch et al., 1963), which necessitated a reexamination of the control of calcium and skeletal metabolism, prompted much additional interest. This, coupled with increasingly sophisticated and diverse re-search approaches, has enabled considerable progress in the field.

We do not intend to provide a full, comprehensive review of the vast literature concerning the physiology of parathyroid hormone, the control of its secretion, or its chemistry. Rather, we have brought together selected, published contributions concerning the mode of action of parathyroid hormone—especially its action on bone—with the hope that this will provide for the reader a firmer basis for understanding and evaluating the model we propose to account for the actions and effects of parathyroid hormone on bone. The recent contributions cited are those that we feel have made the greatest impact on efforts in this field; how-ever, we should emphasize that evaluation of the true significance of many of the studies must await further progress. The mere fact that we must propose a model to account for the mode of action of parathyroid hor-mone signals the reader that complete understanding of this subject is lacking.

II. Recent Studies on the Mode of Action of Parathyroid Hormone

A. General Effects of Parathyroid Hormone

It is generally accepted that the principal function of parathyroid hormone is to promote the maintenance of a normal blood calcium level to assure the availability of this ion at concentrations optimal for the many metabolic activities it influences, including efficient neuromuscular activity and skeletal remodeling. Two important independent actions of the hormone appear to provide the basis for this function: (1) the primary action of parathyroid hormone is on bone to transfer calcium to the extracellular fluid phase; (2) the secondary action is an effect on the kidney to restrict urinary calcium excretion and to promote urinary phosphate excretion. In the absence of these effects, blood calcium levels fall rapidly. That parathyroid hormone promotes intestinal absorption of calcium by a direct action must presently be considered probable but not proved. The once popular theory of Albright and Reifenstein (1948) that the effect of parathyroid hormone on bone was secondary to, in fact mediated by, its phosphaturic effect on the kidney must now be considered untenable. Many studies over the past two decades, especially those show- ing characteristic effects of the hormone in the absence of the kidney (Stewart and Bowen, 1951; Talmage et al., 1953; Grollman, 1954) and on isolated bone, grafted or in tissue culture (Barnicot, 1948; Gaillard, 1955, 1961; Raisz, 1963) have amply demonstrated direct effects on bone. That the actions of the hormone on both target tissues act in concert to promote maintenance of the proper blood calcium concentration is an attractive concept. The effect on kidney may be considered an action designed to facilitate calcium reabsorption and, by causing phosphaturia, to prevent the blood phosphate levels from rising to such an extent that precipitation of calcium phosphate salts will occur [a phenomenon observed in the absence of proper kidney function (Talmage et al., 1960)]. The various means by which parathyroid hormone is thought to accomplish these general effects on bone and kidney will be considered in the following discussion prior to presentation of the model advanced to account for the mechanism of action of the hormone on bone.

B. Specific Effects of Parathyroid Hormone on the Kidney

Parathyroid hormone exerts a direct effect on the kidney to help control ion transport and excretion. The hormone appears to act directly on the proximal convoluted tubule to depress tubular reabsorption of phosphate and promote phosphaturia (Pullman et al., 1960; Lavender et al., 1961; Bartter, 1961; Hirsch and Munson, 1964). A direct influence of parathyroid hormone on renal transport of calcium has now become generally accepted. Such an effect was reported by Talmage in 1956. Subsequent studies in other species, including man, have confirmed this finding (Widrow and Levinsky, 1962; Eisenberg, 1968). Efforts to reveal the mechanisms involved in the renal effects of the hormone have been notably less than those devoted to understanding the action on bone. Possibly, the recent implication of cyclic AMP in the renal effect of parathyroid hormone (Chase and Aurbach, 1967, 1968a) will lend impetus to research in this area.

It is apparent that there is renewed interest in the importance of the renal effects of parathyroid hormone. Rasmussen *et al.* (1967a) have reported that lowering of plasma calcium in rats by infusion of a chelating agent causes phosphaturia and concomitantly promotes bone resorption. Nordin and Peacock (1969) have postulated that in adult man the kidney may be more important than bone for maintenance of calcium homeostasis. Rasmussen *et al.* (1967a) propose that their results are best explained by presuming that bone resorption is heavily dependent on and regulated by the ionic environment of osteolytic cells and that hormones, including parathyroid hormone, may exert their effects by altering this environment. Supportive data have also been provided by Pechet *et al.* (1967) and Raisz and Niemann (1969). The most attractive portion of these recent suggestions is, we feel, that osteolytic or osteoclastic bone resorption may be modified by changes in the ionic environment of bone cells. In this context, it would be wrong to consider that the actions of parathyroid hormone on the kidney are unimportant, since they contribute to overall electrolyte balance. It would seem most logical to conclude that all known effects of the hormone, whether on bone, kidney, or gut, and whether direct or indirect, should be considered of potential great importance for the maintenance of calcium homeostasis.

C. Specific Effects of Parathyroid Hormone on Bone

A true appreciation for the mode of action of parathyroid hormone on bone depends on recognition of the valuable contributions provided by multidisciplinary approaches to the problem. Investigations at the morphological, physiological, and biochemical levels have all provided pieces of the incomplete picture. Physiological and, especially, biochemical studies have generated considerable enthusiasm in recent years for the view that such studies will ultimately clarify the basic mechanisms of hormone action. However, bone as a target organ for parathyroid hormone, is a prime example of a complex target tissue. The diverse cellular topography and composition of bone exemplify the complex and often opposing forces (e.g., formation and resorption) at play in a given area of a given bone especially during growth and remodeling. While new and exciting findings emerge continually from increasingly sophisticated biochemical studies on extracts, homogenates, and slices of bone, such findings take on added dimensions only when the effects observed can be associated with specific areas and cell populations in the target tissue.

Attempts to classify particular studies according to discipline (e.g., histological, biochemical) are difficult at best and often arbitrary. However, we have, for purposes of organization, attempted such broad classification of the recent studies on bone.

1. *Histological and Cytological Studies*

In accordance with classical histological studies, the responsibilities for specific functions in the active bone processes of "formation" and "resorption" were assigned to the osteoblast and osteoclast, respectively. Except for its contribution to the sparse cellularity of bone, little concerning a possible functional role for the osteocyte could be deduced by usual histological methods. In the early 1950's, studies of the response of bone to parathyroid extract by Heller *et al.* (1950) and Heller-Steinberg (1951) suggested possible interconversion among the different cell populations, emphasized the apparent importance of osteoclasts for bone resorption, and promoted general interest in the origin of the osteoclasts found in large numbers following increased parathyroid activity. Subsequent elegant studies of bone in tissue culture clearly demonstrated the ability of the osteoclast to resorb bone. Gaillard (1961, 1965), using numerous histological criteria, was able to define the response of cultured bone to parathyroid hormone. Cinematographic techniques applied to living bone in tissue culture further indicated increased osteoclastic activity of bone under similar conditions (Goldhaber, 1965; Goldhaber *et al.*, 1968). During this same general period of time, numerous *in vivo* studies in the rat (Toft and Talmage, 1960; Talmage *et al.*, 1965a) unequivocally demonstrated a direct correlation between osteoclast numbers in bone and endogenous parathyroid activity. Indeed, by quantifying numbers of osteoclasts in metaphyseal regions of long bones, the parathyroid status of animals could be assessed (Talmage and Toft, 1961). Biochemical, histochemical, and electron microscopic studies have all indicated that osteoclasts possess the cellular enzymes and organization requisite for bone resorption (Doty *et al.*, 1968).

Although osteoclasts, under the influence of parathyroid stimulation, respond by increasing their numbers and activity, their possible physiological role in the return of calcium from bone salt to blood has recently been questioned. In studies over the past decade (Talmage *et al.*, 1965a; Talmage, 1967), considerable evidence has been amassed which suggests that rapid mobilization of calcium from bone is neither dependent on nor necessarily associated with increased osteoclastic activity. A recent review (Talmage, 1967) emphasizes three lines of evidence which support this conclusion: (1) experimental conditions have been found where numbers of osteoclasts cannot be associated with the level of parathyroid activity; (2) while the calcium-mobilizing response of bone to parathyroid stimulation is rapid, 6–8 hours of stimulation of the parathyroid glands are required before significant increases in numbers of osteoclasts can be demonstrated; (3) compact or "mature" diaphyseal bone appears most susceptible to parathyroid influence, while osteoclasts are most prevalent in trabecular or "newly formed" metaphyseal bone.

A possible, important role for the osteocyte in parathyroid-mediated bone resorption has recently emerged from the results of numerous histological and histochemical studies by Bélanger (1965) and supportive electron microscopic studies by Baud (1968). This cell type had long been considered of little importance in the response of bone to hormonal influence, and osteocytes were regarded simply as osteoblasts transformed in structure following entrapment in bone by the products of their own secretion. However, Bélanger has demonstrated rapid and dramatic changes in these cells associated with increased parathyroid activity. Characteristic alterations include evidence for increased production of lysosomal enzymes and noticeable enlargement of perilacunar borders (Bélanger and Migicovsky, 1963; Bélanger et al., 1963; Baud, 1968). These changes have led Bélanger (1965) to postulate the concept of "osteocytic osteolysis" and to theorize that this response represents the physiological resorptive response of bone to parathyroid hormone. Unquestionably the concept of osteocytic osteolysis has infused new enthusiasm into the studies concerned with delineation of bone cellular activities; however, it is important to point out that wide acceptance of this role for the osteocyte must await further evidence. Our own ideas concerning the role of the osteocyte in parathyroid-mediated bone resorption will be discussed in detail in Section IV.

Demonstrable changes in all bone cell types can be found following increased parathyroid activity. However, whether a given change results from a direct effect of the hormone or is secondary to changes in ionic environment or altered precursor cell activity remains to be determined. Nichols and associates (Flanagan and Nichols, 1964a; Vaes and Nichols, 1962), Johnston et al. (1962), Young (1963), and Cooper and Talmage (1965) all have demonstrated suppression of osteoblastic bone collagen synthesis following administration of large doses of parathyroid extract. A similar effect on bone in tissue culture was noted by Gaillard (1961, 1965). The possibility that this pharmacological effect would be insignificant at normal concentrations of circulating parathyroid hormone and does not represent exaggeration of a physiological action has been suggested (Cooper and Talmage, 1965).

The development and refinement of autoradiographic techniques useful at the cellular level and application of these techniques to the study of bone have allowed detailed investigation of the origins and activities of bone cells. Microautoradiographic studies by Young (1962a,b, 1963) using thymidine-^{3}H in "pulse-chase" type experiments suggested that the specialized bone cells arise by modulation from a common mesenchymal "progenitor" cell population in bone which renews itself by mitosis. Talmage *et al.* (1965a), in similar studies, suggested that the increased numbers of osteoclasts formed during parathyroid stimulation arise from the progenitor population, not by coalescence of osteoblasts as suggested earlier by Heller *et al.* (1950). Additional evidence for a parathyroid hormone effect on the endochondral mesenchyme cells of rat long bones was provided by a study showing increased incorporation of cytidine-^{3}H into the RNA of mesenchyme cells after parathyroid stimulation (Talmage *et al.*, 1965a). From similar studies on the compact bone of rabbits, Owen and Bingham (1968) have described an increase in RNA synthesis in osteoclasts and a decrease in RNA synthesis in osteoblasts following *in vivo* administration of parathyroid hormone. The results of these investigations, along with those showing effects of actinomycin D on the response of bone to parathyroid hormone (cited below), stimulated subsequent biochemical studies on RNA and DNA synthesis following increased parathyroid activity.

It is clear from numerous histological studies that the action of parathyroid hormone to promote bone resorption involves complex responses even at the cellular level. Future elucidation of the mechanism of action of parathyroid hormone on bone at the biochemical level will require correlation of observations with the cell type(s) involved before complete understanding is achieved.

2. *Physiological and Biochemical Studies*

Parathyroid hormone, whether acting on intestine, bone, or kidney, primarily promotes translocations of ionic calcium and inorganic phosphate resulting in the elevation of the blood calcium concentration. If the surface of bone is indeed covered by cell membranes (Neuman, 1969), then the effects of parathyroid hormone must involve intracellular as well as intercellular movement of calcium. Considerable study at the biochemical and physiological levels has explored the means by which parathyroid hormone acts. Numerous effects of parathyroid hormone on DNA and RNA synthesis, on membrane components of the cell, and on enzyme systems have recently been reported. It is difficult to estimate which, if any, of these numerous effects represents the primary mechanism of action of parathyroid hormone. If one effect is primary, is it primary for all target cells and tissues? Often it is assumed that perception of the most rapidly evoked response leads one closer to the primary action of a hormone. However, the experimental conditions employed and the sensitivity of analytical methods used both determine, to a large extent, the rapidity with which an effect appears to occur.

Although the action of parathyroid hormone on bone was long considered to be slower than its action on the kidney, it has become increasingly apparent that, under proper experimental conditions, administration or withdrawal of parathyroid hormone produces effects on bone rapidly. Talmage *et al.* (1965a) originally emphasized the rapidity with which a fall in extracellular calcium concentration occurs in rats after removal of autotransplanted parathyroid glands. Perfusion of parathyroid hormone through the isolated tibiae of cats or dogs (Parsons and Robinson, 1968), and injection or infusion of parathyroid hormone into thyrocalcitonin-deficient rats (Anast *et al.*, 1967; Cooper *et al.*, 1970) have provided more recent evidence for a rapid, direct action of the hormone on bone.

Even prior to a true appreciation of the rapid effect of parathyroid hormone on bone, there has been considerable interest in explaining, in biochemical terms, how parathyroid hormone mobilizes bone salt. The proposal of numerous theories to this effect over the past 15 years attests both to this interest and to the incompleteness of our understanding of how the hormone exerts its primary action. One of the more popular ideas, advanced by Neuman and associates (Neuman *et al.*, 1956; Firschein *et al.*, 1958) more than 10 years ago, proposed that cellular production and secretion of organic acids near the bone crystal surfaces might be instrumental in the calcium-mobilizing action of parathyroid hormone. Numerous subsequent studies in several laboratories demonstrated that increasing amounts of H^+, especially as citric and lactic acid, were indeed produced by bone cells under the influence of parathyroid hormone. While the popularity of this proposed mode of action has noticeably waned, the effects have been repeatedly and easily demonstrated. Recent studies of bone in tissue culture by Vaes (1968a) still suggest that sufficient acid may be produced under conditions of parathyroid stimulation to account for the amount of ^{45}Ca mobilized from prelabeled bone. However, Vaes (1968a) concluded that destruction of bone matrix, which he feels then allows solubilization of the mineral components, is of greater importance. Indeed, his exhaustive survey of the numerous hydrolytic enzymes present in bone cells prompted him to suggest that formation and release of these enzymes from cell lysosomes, are instrumental in parathyroid-mediated bone resorption. The studies of Bélanger (1965) also favor this idea of matrix solubilization preceding mineral dissolution, but concrete evidence concerning the order of these events is lacking. While both processes (matrix and mineral solubilization) are promoted by parathyroid hormone, they have appeared equally rapid in the hands of most investigators, and further studies will be required to clarify this issue.

At the time of the Second International Parathyroid Symposium in late 1964 (Gaillard *et al.*, 1965), considerable interest was still evident in studies on the effects of the hormone on organic acid production and on possible key enzymes and coenzymes in intermediary metabolism, particularly with regard to possible actions on nicotinamide nucleotides. Studies by Van Reen (1965), Hekkelman (1965a), and De Voogd van der Straaten (1965) left little doubt that such effects of parathyroid hormone could be demonstrated. However, enthusiasm for these studies was largely supplanted by that for another reported effect of parathyroid hormone.

Beginning in the early 1960's, DeLuca, Rasmussen, and associates, in a series of investigations (Sallis *et al.*, 1963; Rasmussen *et al.*, 1964a; Sallis and DeLuca, 1964), provided evidence that parathyroid hormone affected the movement of ions across the membranes of isolated mitochondria. They demonstrated that parathyroid hormone promoted the release of calcium and the uptake of phosphate and other ions by mitochondria. Additional effects on mitochondrial respiration and succinate oxidation were also demonstrated. What gradually evolved from these studies was the proposal that these effects reflected a primary effect of parathyroid hormone on membranes—perhaps on subcellular as well as cell membranes (DeLuca and Sallis, 1965; Aurbach *et al.*, 1965a; Rasmussen *et al.*, 1968a). Widespread enthusiasm for the concept can perhaps best be attributed to the idea that such a basic membrane effect could conveniently explain the myriad expressions of parathyroid hormone action, i.e., calcium, phosphate, and other ion movements as well as multiple secondary effects on intermediary metabolism. Many workers, including us, were hesitant to embrace this concept, particularly in view of the large amounts of hormone used to demonstrate these *in vitro* effects (Sallis *et al.*, 1965). Subsequently, further doubt concerning the physiological relevance of the results was raised when Aurbach *et al.* (1965b) demonstrated that several nonhormonal proteins mimicked the action of parathyroid hormone on mitochondria *in vitro*. Furthermore, Cohn *et al.* (1966) were unable to demonstrate metabolic alterations in mitochondria isolated from animals injected with parathyroid hormone. More recently Rasmussen *et al.* (1967b, 1968a), by employing intricate experimental conditions, have described results with isolated mitochondria which appear to be obtained only with parathyroid hormone. However, the significance of these findings and their relevance to *in vivo* action of the hormone remains obscure. Potts and Deftos (1969) have made three major criticisms of the mitochondrial studies: (1) much of the work has been performed using liver mitochondria, and liver is not known to be a target tissue for the hormone; (2) there is no assurance that the hormone *in vivo* ever penetrates the cell interior to contact the mitochondrial membrane; (3) whether the complex conditions used to demonstrate specific *in vitro* effects represent, or even approximate, those existing *in vivo* is uncertain. Despite many questions raised concerning this possible mode of action of parathyroid hormone, a most attractive portion of the concept remains the basic assumption that the hormone affects membranes.

Many recent studies indeed suggest that the primary effect of parathyroid hormone is somehow involved with an action on the cell membrane. Presumably the hormone, in order to exert its effects on bone and kidney, must initially make contact with membranes which comprise the exterior surface of the target cells. A possible mode of action of parathyroid hormone on the cell membrane was proposed by Borle (1968a,b; Borle and Herold, 1970). In a series of careful studies he examined the kinetics of calcium movement into and out of cultured HeLa and kidney cells; these cells appeared to allow entry of calcium by passive diffusion but rapidly extruded the ion by an active process ("active pump") apparently accounting for the extremely low intracellular calcium concentration found normally in most cells. According to his studies, parathyroid hormone, added *in vitro*, enhanced passive diffusion of calcium into the cell, and presumably secondarily caused more vigorous efflux out of the cell. More recently, Borle (1969) has proposed the existence of a calcium-carrier complex, sensitive to parathyroid hormone, to account for metabolically dependent calcium fluxes observed *in vitro*. These studies also point to an action of parathyroid hormone on cell membranes.

Among the most exciting recent studies on the possible mode of action of parathyroid hormone have been those suggesting that cyclic adenosine 3′,5′-monophosphate (cyclic AMP) somehow mediates the effects of the hormone. Since the initial implication of this nucleotide in the action of epinephrine on liver glycogenolysis, considerable evidence has accumulated pointing to a role for cyclic AMP in the mechanism of action and stimulation of secretion of a variety of hormones. From such studies, Sutherland and associates (Robison *et al.*, 1968) have postulated the concept of cyclic AMP as a "second messenger" which, by acting on intracellular target sites (enzymes?), evokes the physiological response of the particular hormone. Initial hormone action is thought to involve stimulation of membrane-bound adenyl cyclase which, in turn, catalyzes the formation of cyclic AMP from ATP. Various means of experimentally elevating intracellular cyclic AMP concentrations have been employed. Most pertinent in this regard have been studies showing that administration of cyclic AMP or its dibutyryl derivative, as well as administration of compounds inhibiting degradation of endogenous cyclic AMP (e.g., theophylline), may produce responses characteristically elicited by a particular hormone. Specificity of the physiological response is considered to reside with the individuality of the target cells for a given hormone. The studies of Chase and Aurbach have most directly demonstrated that the action of parathyroid hormone may be mediated through an action on cyclic AMP. In 1967 these authors reported that *in vivo* administration of parathyroid hormone to rats caused an impressive and rapid rise in the urinary excretion of cyclic AMP. Even more significant was their observation that the peak of excretion of cyclic AMP preceded that of the rapid phosphaturic effect of parathyroid hormone. Furthermore, suppression of endogenous parathyroid hormone secretion caused a fall in cyclic AMP excretion with a simultaneous decrease in phosphate excretion (Chase and Aurbach, 1967). Extension of these studies showed stimulation by parathyroid hormone of adenyl cyclase in renal cortex and led Chase and Aurbach to postulate that the mechanism of action of parathyroid hormone on the kidney is mediated by activation of the enzyme adenyl cyclase (Chase and Aurbach, 1968a,b). Additional subsequent studies by Chase *et al.* (1969), using bone, showed that hormonal activation of skeletal adenyl cyclase could also be demonstrated. Specificity of the effects of the hormone on the two well-recognized target tissues, bone and kidney, provided an attractive demonstration of a possible common, specific action of the hormone.

At approximately the same time, Wells and Lloyd (1967, 1968a,b) reported that *in vivo* administration of agents known to promote elevation of endogenous levels of cyclic AMP could imitate effects of administered parathyroid hormone. More specifically, these authors demonstrated that administration of theophylline, isoproterenol, or dibutyryl cyclic AMP to parathyroidectomized rats could cause elevation of the blood calcium concentration. Conversely, the hypercalcemic activity of these drugs, or of administered parathyroid hormone, could be decreased by imidazole (presumably because imidazole stimulates phosphodiesterase, thus favoring decreased levels of cyclic AMP). On the basis of such studies, these authors proposed that the mode of action of parathyroid hormone-mediated bone resorption involved an increase in the concentration of cyclic AMP in bone cells and that the level of cyclic AMP within bone cells in some manner directly determined the rate of bone resorption. Additional *in vivo* studies by Rasmussen *et al.* (1968a,b) showed that infusion of dibutyryl cyclic AMP into thyroparathyroidectomized rats appeared to duplicate many of the effects produced on bone and kidney by infusion of parathyroid hormone, including hypercalcemia, hypophosphatemia, and hyperphosphaturia. Further supportive evidence for *in vitro* effects of cyclic AMP which resemble those of parathyroid hormone have been reported by Raisz and co-workers (Raisz *et al.*, 1969; Raisz and Klein, 1969) and by Vaes (1968b). Both groups have independently reported stimulation of bone resorption in tissue culture by dibutyryl cyclic AMP; Vaes has further shown that this resorption is accompanied by release of lysosomal enzymes which, as previously mentioned, he feels are instrumental in causing the matrix dissolution required to permit resorption of bone mineral.

While a precise role for cyclic AMP in the mechanism of hormone action remains to be elucidated, the evidence for involvement of this nucleotide in parathyroid hormone action appears substantial. The available data are certainly compatible with a mediatory role for cyclic AMP, but such a role still remains to be conclusively demonstrated. It is important to note that this postulated mode of action of parathyroid hormone and the several others discussed above are not necessarily mutually exclusive, i.e., this new concept also implies that a primary action of the hormone involves an initial reaction with the cell membrane.

Numerous recent studies have indicated that the action of parathyroid hormone on bone is somehow related to RNA and protein synthesis. Early evidence for this was provided by Gaillard (1965), who showed that actinomycin D added *in vitro* could restrict the effects of parathyroid hormone on bone in tissue culture. Rasmussen *et al.* (1964b) reported that this antibiotic, known to inhibit DNA-directed RNA synthesis, could block the *in vivo* hypercalcemic action of parathyroid hormone in the parathyroidectomized rat. Subsequent studies from numerous laboratories (Eisenstein and Passavoy, 1964; Tashjian *et al.*, 1964; Raisz, 1965; Khoo and Kowalewski, 1965; Talmage *et al.*, 1965b), indeed suggested that parathyroid hormone was less effective in its actions on bone after prior administration of actinomycin D. However, from studies showing incomplete effectiveness of large doses of actinomycin D in blocking endogenous parathyroid hormone effects on bone and kidney, we concluded that inhibition by actinomycin D was somewhat nonspecific and merely indicated that normal RNA and protein synthesis were required for full expression of normal parathyroid activity (Talmage *et al.*, 1965b). These studies, along with those showing increased incorporation of cytidine-^{3}H into mesenchymal nuclei during parathyroid stimulation (Talmage *et al.*, 1965a), prompted more extensive investigations into possible effects of the hormone on DNA and RNA synthesis in bone.

Park and Talmage (1967, 1968) showed that following increased endogenous parathyroid activity, specific activities of both RNA and DNA, which had been extracted from rat bone incubated with labeled precursors of these nucleic acids, were elevated. Examination of both metaphyseal and diaphyseal areas of long bone revealed differences in the time course and magnitude of the responses in these areas which the authors suggested were illustrative of the complexity of bone as a tissue. Studies by Steinberg and Nichols (1968) also indicated that injection of parathyroid extract promoted DNA-directed RNA synthesis in bone cells. Park and Talmage (1968) extended their studies concerning the effect of endogenous parathyroid hormone on RNA synthesis in bone. They were able to demonstrate that aspects of the ability of parathyroid hormone to promote bone RNA synthesis could be simulated by experimental elevation of the circulating ionic calcium concentration. These results, along with the numerous other studies indicating effects of parathyroid hormone on the cell membrane, prompted them to propose that their observed hormonal effects on RNA synthesis, as well as many other metabolic expressions of increased parathyroid activity, might in fact be caused by an increased intracellular concentration of calcium. This implied that a primary action of parathyroid hormone is to permit a rise in intracellular calcium concentration. This concept will be discussed in detail along with a more critical examination of the effect promoted by both elevated calcium levels and increased parathyroid activity.

III. Comparison of Metabolic Effects Produced by Increased Calcium Ion Concentrations to Those Produced by Parathyroid Hormone

The purpose of this section is to compare effects of parathyroid hormone on a variety of biochemical parameters to those produced by *in vivo* administration of calcium or by its addition to incubation media. These comparisons are not always clear-cut due to difficulties arising from the different experimental procedures used by investigators who have administered parathyroid hormone to animals. The following observations illustrate some of the problems involved both in interpreting reports and in comparing effects of parathyroid hormone to those of calcium:

1. The parathyroid hormone preparations used in the studies, both early and recent, were often impure, containing nonspecific (nonhormonal) peptides (Potts *et al.*, 1965, 1966).

2. An effect observed with a large dose of hormone may not necessarily reflect an exaggerated physiological action of the hormone. Also, different doses of the hormone may produce qualitatively different responses, such as reported by Nagatsu and Hara (1966) for parathyroid hormone effects on leucine aminopeptidase activity and on aminopeptidase A.

3. The long duration of treatment with parathyroid hormone used by many investigators before studying biochemical responses suggests that many reported effects may have resulted from more than a simple, direct response to the hormone. While parathyroid hormone has been shown to produce changes in serum calcium and urine phosphate within minutes

after administration (Lavender *et al.*, 1961; Parsons and Robinson, 1968), many biochemical studies have been conducted following treatment periods with parathyroid hormone ranging from 20 minutes to several days. Biphasic responses to *in vivo* administration of parathyroid hormone have been shown for effects on RNA synthesis (Park and Talmage, 1967), on succinic dehydrogenase activity (Mills and Bavetta, 1965), and on collagen synthesis (Nichols *et al.*, 1965).

4. Many investigators attribute reported effects to only one cell type in bone, and others ignore the fact that this tissue consists of a heterogeneous mixture of cell types with different, and sometimes opposite, physiological activities. This problem has been emphasized by Park and Talmage (1968) and by Owen and Bingham (1968).

5. In a number of biochemical studies, effects of parathyroid hormone were demonstrated using tissues not known to be affected by the hormone under physiological conditions. For example, some investigators have studied liver, a tissue that is not known to be directly involved with control of calcium homeostasis.

6. There are the usual difficulties inherent in attempting to correlate *in vivo* and *in vitro* studies.

7. Because of the large amount of calcified intercellular material in bone, *in vitro* studies of cellular responses to parathyroid hormone are complicated by the problem of preparing adequate extracts or homogenates. Solubilization of calcified matrix in such homogenates may release sufficient mineral to cause either inhibition or activation of enzyme systems, thereby not accurately reflecting the *in vivo* situation. The work by Krane *et al.* (1961) on aconitase activity illustrates this problem.

Despite the many problems just outlined, there exists a marked similarity between the effects of parathyroid hormone administration on intact cells and the effects of increased calcium ion concentration on a variety of biochemical processes. Some of the more important similarities reported in the literature are summarized below.

A. Formation of Cyclic Adenosine 3′,5′-Monophosphate (Cyclic AMP)

The suggestion that parathyroid hormone acts through cyclic AMP has received considerable attention (Wells and Lloyd, 1967, 1968b; Chase and Aurbach, 1968a). Chase and Aurbach have demonstrated that parathyroid hormone produces a rapid and marked rise in urinary cyclic AMP and increased adenyl cyclase activity in membrane fractions of renal cortex. Recently, Chase and Aurbach (1968b) also reported an increased adenyl cyclase activity in homogenates of calvaria following parathyroid hormone treatment.

Epinephrine, which induces stimulation of liver adenyl cyclase, has also been reported to increase intracellular calcium concentrations (Ozawa, 1967). Ozawa suggested that the two simultaneous effects produced favorable conditions for stimulation by cyclic AMP of phosphorylase kinase B. It is possible that parathyroid hormone may function in a way similar to epinephrine, i.e., by increasing intracellular concentrations of cyclic AMP via changes in calcium ion concentrations. Bär and Hechter (1969) suggested that the calcium ion may play a general regulatory role in determining the rate of adrenal cyclic AMP formation in both the presence and absence of ACTH.

B. Influences on Glycolysis

Fairly extensive studies of the influence of parathyroid hormone on various stages of glycolysis have been reported. These range from early work showing decreased plasma glucose levels following administration of parathyroid extract (Seeling, 1931; Rappaport, 1938) to more recent studies reporting increased glucose utilization by calvaria in tissue culture (G. R. Martin et al., 1965). Effects of parathyroid hormone on steps in the glycolytic pathway have also been demonstrated. Borle et al. (1960a) reported that, under aerobic conditions, parathyroid hormone increased glucose utilization and lactic acid production. Dowse et al. (1963) described the reversal of the Pasteur effect by parathyroid hormone and also demonstrated increased lactate production. Schartum and Nichols (1961) noted that iodoacetate, which blocks the triosephosphate dehydrogenase reaction, also inhibited parathyroid hormone-like actions on bone. Stimulation by parathyroid hormone of lactic acid production was reported by Borle et al. (1960b), by Yates and Talmage (1965), and by Hekkelman and Herrmann-Erlee (1968). Nagata and Rasmussen (1968) reported that the activity of pyruvic kinase was inhibited by parathyroid hormone.

The effects of calcium ion on these biochemical processes has not necessarily been studied concurrently with parathyroid hormone or even in the same tissue. However, there appears to be a certain similarity in effects. For example: Calcium ion stimulates anaerobic glycolysis and the production of lactic acid (Adams and Quastel, 1956) while inhibiting aerobic glycolysis (Takagaki, 1968). Takagaki also reported that calcium inhibited the activities of such enzymes as hexokinase, phosphoglucoisomerase, phosphofructokinase, glyceraldehyde-3-phosphate dehydrogenase, enolase, and pyruvic kinase. Involvement of the calcium ion in feedback inhibition of glycolysis has been described by Bygrave (1966). He stressed the role of calcium ion in the glycolytic activity of Ehrlich ascites tumor cells showing that it inhibited pyruvic kinase activity in the supernatant and homogenates of these cells.

At least two groups have attempted to correlate parathyroid hormone actions on glycolysis with calcium entry into appropriate cells. Terepka *et al.* (1960), in a report proposing a unified concept for parathyroid hormone action, suggested that transfer of calcium ion, as well as inorganic phosphate, is stimulated by parathyroid hormone, thereby inducing changes in a variety of metabolic activities including glycolysis. Nagata and Rasmussen (1968) have also attempted to correlate the effect of calcium ion and the action of parathyroid hormone on glycolytic intermediates and enzymes in renal cells. Of particular interest was their observation that both parathyroid hormone and calcium ion inhibited the activity of pyruvic kinase.

C. Lipid Metabolism

Little work has been published relating parathyroid hormone activity to changes in lipid metabolism. However, Notario and Larriza (1956) reported that following parathyroid hormone treatment, both total lipid content and cholesterol content of plasma were elevated. It is possible to relate these changes to increased intracellular citrate production, which has been shown to stimulate malonyl-CoA and lipid formation (Matsuhashi *et al.*, 1962). Both parathyroid hormone and calcium ion have been reported to increase citrate production (see Section III, G, 6).

D. Collagen Biosynthesis

An observation that has been made repeatedly is that parathyroid hormone suppresses collagen synthesis in bone as judged by incorporation of radioactive proline or glycine. Supportive data have been reported by Gaillard (1961), De Voogd van der Straaten (1962), Vaes and Nichols (1962), Flanagan and Nichols (1964b), and Johnston *et al.* (1962). Nichols *et al.* (1965) suggested that the site of action of parathyroid hormone was related to the assembly of collagen molecules on the ribosomes.

Cooper and Talmage (1965), on the other hand, studying proline-^{3}H incorporation into bone collagen *in vitro*, noted an inverse relationship between the amount of proline incorporated and the calcium level of the incubation medium. Earlier, Everett and Holly (1961) had reported a general inhibition of amino acid incorporation into protein in the presence of excess calcium.

E. RNA Synthesis

Recent study has definitely demonstrated that parathyroid hormone influences RNA synthesis in bone cells. However, the effect observed depends upon the specific cell type. Increased hormone levels stimulate synthesis in mesenchyme cells and osteoclasts, but inhibit synthesis in osteoblasts and osteocytes (Park and Talmage, 1967; Owen and Bingham,

1968). In addition, Park and Talmage reported a biphasic response to parathyroid hormone in the diaphysis of the femur of rats; an immediate suppression of RNA synthesis was followed 4 hours later by stimulation of synthesis. Parathyroidectomy alone produced a minor increase. This biphasic response has been confirmed by Raisz and Niemann (1967).

Park and Talmage (1968) deliberately compared the effects of parathyroid hormone and calcium on RNA synthesis in bone cells. Under their experimental conditions, the two agents produced similar results, i.e., increased calcium concentrations mimicked the stimulation and inhibition pattern produced by parathyroid hormone on RNA synthesis in rat bone. In other tissues, Schwartz et al. (1966) reported that calcium ion stimulated RNA synthesis in mitochondria. Mallevais et al. (1966) reported that increased calcium ion concentration markedly inhibited the incorporation of ^{32}P into RNA of isolated hepatocytes.

F. Mitotic Rate and DNA Synthesis

The ability of parathyroid hormone or calcium to increase DNA synthesis and mitotic rates appears to depend upon the cell type in question and the experimental conditions employed. In recent studies, an increase in mitotic rate in HeLa cell cultures 24 hours after addition of parathyroid hormone was reported (Borle and Neuman, 1965), and an increase in DNA synthesis in bone in tissue culture was noted (G. R. Martin et al., 1965). Also, Rohr (1964) observed increased DNA synthesis in rat bone following parathyroid hormone administration. Park and Talmage (1967) reported that stimulation of endogenous parathyroid hormone secretion in the rat was followed 5 hours later by increased DNA synthesis in bone.

In marked contrast to the results of their studies on RNA synthesis, Park and Talmage (1968) did not observe increased DNA synthesis in rat bone after administration of calcium. However, an increase in mitotic rate of bone marrow cells was noted after raising plasma calcium concentrations by either administration of calcium or with injections of parathyroid hormone (Perris et al., 1967; Rixon, 1968; Whitfield et al., 1969). DNA synthesis in mammary epithelial cells did not respond to elevated ionic calcium (Turkington, 1968).

A possible explanation for some of the apparent discrepancies described above may be the resistance of different cell populations to the entry of Ca^{2+} into the cell. In some cells, such as bone marrow cells, the rate of entry of calcium may be proportional to the extracellular calcium concentration; other cells, such as the bone mesenchyme population, may require parathyroid hormone to facilitate increased intracellular calcium. Cells such as mammary epithelium could be both resistant to calcium entry (even in the presence of high extracellular calcium levels) and unresponsive to parathyroid hormone.

G. Influences on Enzyme Activities

Both parathyroid hormone and calcium ion have been implicated in the control of many enzymatic activities; in some cases effects appear stimulatory while, in others, inhibitory. Some of these are described briefly in the following reviews of published reports.

1. Transaminases and Proteolytic Enzymes

The following effects of parathyroid extract on proteolytic activity in bone cells have been reported: Bélanger and Migicovsky (1963) reported a stimulatory effect in osteocytes; Nagatsu and Hara (1966) noted that parathyroid hormone increased the activity of leucine aminopeptidase; Vaes (1968a) found an increase in the protease activity; and Striganova (1949) found enhancement of general proteolytic activity.

Buttara and Rattini (1950) reported a decreased total amino acid level in serum after parathyroid hormone administration. More recently, Tessari (1959, 1960) demonstrated increased activity of glutamic-oxaloacetic transaminase in metaphyseal bone and glutamic-pyruvic transaminase in secondary spongiosa following parathyroid hormone administration. Tessari suggested that parathyroid hormone stimulated protein catabolic processes. Finally, Rasmussen and DeLuca (1963) reported parathyroid hormone stimulation of glutamate oxidation in mitochondria while Herrmann-Erlee (1962) observed a relative increase in glutamic dehydrogenase activity.

On the other hand, calcium ion is known to activate proteolytic enzymes, such as trypsin (Sipos and Merkel, 1968). It is also known to stimulate production of glucose from amino acid sources (Rutman et al., 1965; Krebs and Bennett, 1963) and to activate transglutaminase (Folk et al., 1967). Calcium ion is considered both to activate breakdown of glutamic acid and to inhibit its formation (LeJohn, 1968).

2. Lysosomal Enzymes

In a series of papers, Vaes has suggested that activation and release of latent lysosomal enzymes in bone are influenced by parathyroid hormone (Vaes, 1965, 1968c). Increased acid phosphatase activity following parathyroid hormone treatment was also noted by Vaes (1968c) and described by Doty et al. (1968) in chemical and histochemical studies. Release of deoxyribonuclease (DNase) has been reported to be stimulated by parathyroid extract (Vaes, 1968c).

Calcium has also been reported to activate DNase (Miyasi and Greenstein, 1951), and Dabich and Neuhaus (1966) studied the activation of acid phosphatase by calcium ions. Finally, a study of the ability of calcium to release membrane-bound hydrolytic enzymes was reported by Verity *et al.* (1968). Acid phosphohydrolase and N-acetylglucosaminidase were released in parallel, and β-glucosaminidase was not affected.

3. *Collagenase*

There has been an intensive search recently for collagenase in bone. Walker *et al.* (1964) reported a collagenolytic factor in rat bone which was stimulated by parathyroid hormone administration. A similar type of collagenolytic activity was found in human, goat, and rat bone by Fullman and Lazarus (1967). A different, active collagenase responding to parathyroid hormone has been reported by Nichols and his colleagues (Woods and Nichols, 1963; Nichols *et al.*, 1965).

The interrelationship between calcium ion and bone collagenase was pointed out by Fullman and Lazarus (1967), who noted that the enzyme had an absolute requirement for calcium and was inactivated by EDTA.

4. *Pyrophosphatase*

Fleisch and his associates have not only related parathyroid hormone to pyrophosphatase activity but have also postulated that the primary action of the hormone is mediated through this enzyme (Fleisch and Neuman, 1961; Fleisch *et al.*, 1965; Fleisch, 1964). Their thesis is that changes in parathyroid hormone activity are reflected by parallel changes in the end product of the enzyme activity, inorganic pyrophosphatase. Others have presented evidence to suggest that parathyroid hormone inhibits the action of pyrophosphatase (Rasmussen and Tenenhouse, 1967; Avioli *et al.*, 1966).

Inhibition of pyrophosphatase activity by calcium has been demonstrated by Kunitz and Robbins (1961), by Soodsma and Nordlie (1966), and by Rasmussen and Tenenhouse (1967). From their study of pyrophosphatase in soft tissue, Nordlie *et al.* (1968) have suggested a feedback control of the enzyme activity by calcium ion. They postulated that a buildup of intracellular calcium ion would suppress hydrolysis of pyrophosphate by the enzyme which, in turn, would favor a decreased intracellular concentration of phosphate. Such a feedback mechanism would permit time for the removal of calcium before it could be precipitated by phosphate in the tissue.

5. CO_2 *Formation from Pyruvate*

A short report by DeLong and L'Heureux (1968) reported that parathyroid extract stimulated evolution of $^{14}CO_2$ from pyruvate-2-^{14}C in incubated bone tissue. A similar increase could be demonstrated by raising the calcium concentration of the medium to 14 mg/100 ml.

6. Citric Acid Utilization and Metabolism

Since Dickens (1941) first reported a high content of citric acid in bone, the relationship between the level of this organic acid and parathyroid hormone function has been emphasized (G. Martin et al., 1958; Talmage et al., 1965a).

The ability of calcium ion to inhibit citric acid oxidation in slices and homogenates of bone was reported by Krane et al. (1961). DeLuca et al. (1957) had previously demonstrated that the rate of oxidation of citrate by isolated mitochondria could be depressed by raising the calcium ion concentration of the incubation medium. A similar reduction in oxidation of citric acid by calcium was reported by Simpson (1967).

7. Aconitase

Hekkelman (1965b) suggested a possible role for aconitase-citrate-calcium interaction in the demineralization of bone by parathyroid hormone. Calcium ion inhibited the aconitase activity in extracts of bone. According to his postulate, the inhibition was caused by the formation of a calcium–citrate complex, thereby diminishing the substrate available to the enzyme.

8. Isocitric Dehydrogenase

Isocitric dehydrogenase has been reported to be inhibited by parathyroid hormone. However, De Voogd van der Straaten (1965) and Costello and Darago (1964) both suggested that this was due to a depletion of NADP as required cofactor rather than a specific inhibitory effect on the enzyme. On the other hand, Nagata and Rasmussen (1968) have reported that this enzyme is inhibited both by parathyroid hormone and by calcium.

9. Succinic Dehydrogenase

Mills and Bavetta (1965) attempted to explain earlier discrepancies in reports of the effect of parathyroid hormone on succinic dehydrogenase. They reported that following hormone treatment there was an early stimulation of enzyme activity but that this returned to normal within 24 hours. Stimulation of the activity of this enzyme by calcium has also been reported by Minato et al. (1966).

H. Summary: Explanation of Effects of Parathyroid Hormone on Enzyme Systems

Although we have not reviewed all enzyme systems affected by either calcium or parathyroid hormone, the discussion illustrates many similarities in the actions of these two agents (summarized diagrammatically in

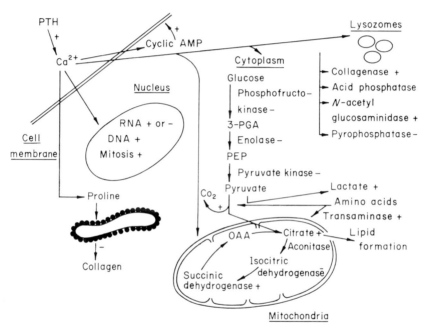

FIG. 1. Diagrammatic presentation of the influences of parathyroid hormone (PTH) and calcium on metabolic processes.

Fig. 1). The following general thesis is proposed to explain the stepwise action of parathyroid hormone on enzyme systems:

1. The primary effect of the hormone is on cellular and/or subcellular membranes to permit the entry of calcium into the cell and its subcellular compartments, resulting in a change in titer of calcium ions in these compartments.

2. Changes in intracellular calcium concentrations can lead to modifications of specific, calcium-sensitive enzymes and change patterns of intermediary metabolism which may eventually lead to functional and morphological changes in target cells.

3. Artificial changes in calcium concentrations of local milieu can

mimic some of the effects of parathyroid hormone even in tissues not normally influenced by the hormone.

IV. Calcium Homeostasis and Its Control by Parathyroid Hormone—A Model

In Sections II and III of this paper, we have reviewed many of the reported biochemical effects of parathyroid hormone. We feel that these effects can be largely explained by assuming a primary action of parathyroid hormone on the cell membrane which, in turn, allows an increased transport of calcium into the cell and its subcellular compartments.

This section will be concerned with a consideration of calcium transport into and out of bone. A model will be discussed that encompasses (1) the

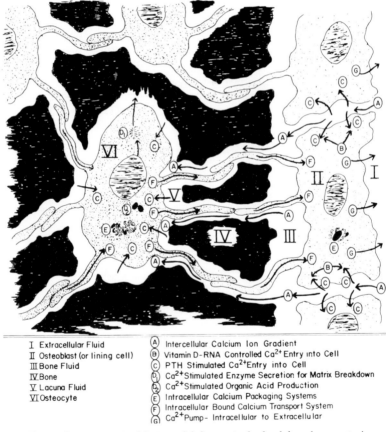

I   Extracellular Fluid
II Osteoblast (or lining cell)
III Bone Fluid
IV Bone
V   Lacuna Fluid
VI Osteocyte

(A) Intercellular Calcium Ion Gradient
(B) Vitamin D-RNA Controlled Ca^{2+} Entry into Cell
(C) PTH Stimulated Ca^{2+} Entry into Cell
(D) Ca^{2+} Stimulated Enzyme Secretion for Matrix Breakdown
(D₂) Ca^{2+} Stimulated Organic Acid Production
(E) Intracellular Calcium Packaging Systems
(F) Intracellular Bound Calcium Transport System
(G) Ca^{2+} Pump- Intracellular to Extracellular

Fig. 2. Osteocyte-osteoblast model for control of calcium homeostasis.

ability of parathyroid hormone to transfer calcium into bone cells, (2) the observed stimulation or suppression of numerous biochemical processes by both parathyroid hormone and calcium, and (3) the unique morphological structure of bone, which allows a relatively insoluble endoskeleton to exist within an organism which maintains a circulating ionic calcium level optimal for many complex physiological functions. The model itself is a revised version of that recently proposed (Talmage, 1969) and is shown in Fig. 2.

Before describing the model, we will briefly review several published reports which have provided scientific support for the concepts involved. However, our interpretation of the results of others is not meant to imply that they either agree or disagree with our concept of calcium homeostasis.

A. The Dual Role of Parathyroid Hormone in Bone Metabolism

It has been proposed that parathyroid hormone plays two rather different roles in bone metabolism (Talmage, 1966, 1967). One is to control calcium homeostasis, and the other is to influence rates of bone remodeling. We feel that both of these functions arise from the same basic action of the hormone, the transfer of calcium into the cell. Here, however, the similarity ends. The remodeling function evolves from stimulation of the internal machinery of the "progenitor" or mesenchyme cell by increased calcium. This increase in calcium, in turn, causes stimulation of RNA synthesis in mesenchyme cells and an increase in mitotic divisions in these cells, permitting an increase in numbers and activity of osteoclasts. It also produces a decrease in the collagen synthetic activity of osteoblasts (however, an increase in the numbers of active osteoblasts may also occur). These changes represent parathyroid stimulation of bone resorption in its classic sense, namely, the formation and stimulation of populations of osteoclasts which destroy bone and permit remodeling. The responses require changes in RNA synthesis, are relatively slow in onset, and are extremely important in the overall picture of bone metabolism.

The second function, that of control of calcium homeostasis, is that which is described by the proposed model. It involves the rapid, minute-by-minute control of plasma calcium levels and is regulated by the "osteocyte-osteoblast family" complex. This function will be considered in detail shortly.

B. Action of Parathyroid Hormone on Calcium Transport into Cells

We support the idea that parathyroid hormone stimulates movement of calcium into the cell and that this effect represents the primary or basic action of the hormone. This concept has been discussed repeatedly in this report. It is mentioned again here only to ensure that proper credit is given to Borle for his work in this area. While associated with Neuman at Rochester, he initiated his studies on calcium fluxes in HeLa cells (Borle and Neuman, 1965; Borle, 1968a,b). Here, too, we would like to emphasize the many important contributions, both intellectual and experimental, of Neuman and associates, which have promoted our understanding of bone physiology and biochemistry.

C. THE REDISCOVERY OF THE OSTEOCYTE

For many years the osteocyte was considered a dormant cell, imprisoned by its own metabolic activities, unimportant for calcium homeostasis and skeletal metabolism. Primary credit for rediscovery of the importance of this cell should go to Bélanger and co-workers (1963) and Baud (1962). Bélanger has formulated the theory of osteolysis and suggested that the primary action of parathyroid hormone is to stimulate secretion of hydrolytic enzymes by this cell. Upon release into the lacunae these enzymes solubilize the organic matrix and mobilize calcium for the extracellular fluid.

While we feel that Bélanger's observations outline secondary rather than primary effects of parathyroid hormone, it is obvious that the osteocyte must be considered an important contributor to the physiology of bone. As described by F. Wasserman and Yeager (1965), considered by Kashiwa (1968), and further illustrated by the electron microscopic studies of Doty (Doty and Robinson, 1970), this cell possesses many protoplasmic projections which radiate in all directions through canaliculi contacting both osteoblasts (or "lining cells") and other osteocytes. Doty (1970) has recently demonstrated that even a reasonably large protein molecule, horseradish peroxidase (presumably not present naturally in mammals) can penetrate to the lacunae of osteocytes within minutes after intravenous injection in rats and dogs. Only osteocytes not in contact with a functional blood supply were excluded.

D. THE "DIFFUSE FRACTION" IN BONE

Early autoradiographic studies of undecalcified bone unfortunately indicated only relative concentrations of the isotopes used, not the dynamics of their distribution. In a series of papers Marshall and Rowland studied the movement of ^{45}Ca into bone and pointed out (1) the rapidity of movement of the nuclide throughout compact bone, and (2) that approximately 60% of the nuclide in bone was in what they termed a "diffuse fraction" because it was not sharply defined in autoradiographs (Marshall *et al.*, 1959; Rowland, 1960, 1966; Marshall, 1969). It seems apparent, as they pointed out, that these findings could be attributed to an active and rapid movement of calcium throughout the canaliculi and lacunae of osteocytes.

E. Fluid Compartmentalization in Bone

The idea that bone extracellular fluid is somehow compartmentalized and, therefore, separated from the "primary" extracellular fluid compartment of the body was first reported by Howard (1959). This concept was reviewed recently by Baud (1968) and Vitalli (1968). Baud, from his electron microscopic studies of bone, emphasized the importance of the osteocyte for such a role. He concluded, however, that compartmentalization was essentially accomplished by a layer of cells, including osteoblasts, which lined the surface of bone. Vitalli based his conclusions on evidence derived from a mathematical model.

Most convincing data were presented in a series of papers by Neuman and his colleagues. They reported studies of the unique ionic composition of bone, especially concentrations of potassium. These investigators did not, however, concern themselves with the composition or nature of the "membrane" responsible for compartmentalization (Terepka et al., 1968; Canas et al., 1969; Geisler and Neuman, 1969; Neuman and Mulryan, 1969; Triffitt et al., 1968).

The model we are proposing is based on the thesis that an active cellular layer covers the surface of bone, enabling metabolic control of ion concentrations of the inner fluid space apposed to bone. This layer of cells, for want of a better name, has been called the "family of osteoblasts" (Talmage, 1969) because all of these bone cells are thought to be derived from a common progenitor cell and many, if not all, pass through a stage in which the cell actively synthesizes collagen. The properties and importance of this layer of cells is discussed later.

F. Transcellular Transport of Calcium

It is well recognized that there are cell layers across which calcium is rapidly transported. The mucosal layer lining the intestinal tract and that comprising metanephric tubules of the kidney are obvious, well-documented examples. In both of these tissues the barrier is a single layer of cells, and each cell is joined to adjacent cells by "tight junctions," anatomical structures which prevent intercellular transport. Muscle cells also exemplify cells which transport calcium rapidly. This is especially true for certain smooth muscle cells which require entry of calcium in order to contract and expulsion of calcium for relaxation.

Although calcium levels have been studied in only a limited number of cell types, it is generally accepted that the intracellular ionic calcium concentration is of the order of 10^{-7} M, as reported for the resting striated muscle cell (Ebashi and Endo, 1968). This assumption appears reasonable because many enzyme reactions are extremely sensitive to higher calcium ion concentrations (see Section III). The extracellular calcium level is of the order of 10^{-3} M; that in the milieu of the gut or in the kidney tubule is variable but probably rarely falls to the intracellular concentration.

This is important, for it means that for net movement of calcium across a cell layer, the first gradient is "downhill" into the cell, the second gradient is "uphill" out of the cell on the other side. It is assumed, therefore, that some sort of "pump" mechanism, possibly similar to the sodium pump, exists in every cell in the body as a means for maintaining the needed low ionic intracellular concentration. In a polarized situation such as in the gut or kidney, the "pump" mechanism must be limited primarily to one side of the cell.

On the other hand, cell membranes are relatively impervious to divalent cations, and calcium appears to accumulate in these membranes. Therefore, some metabolic effort must be required to actually move calcium into the interior of the cell. The possible role of vitamin D in this effect has been described in detail by DeLuca and his associates (1968, 1970; D. L. Martin and DeLuca, 1970) and by R. H. Wasserman (1968; R. H. Wasserman and Taylor, 1969). DeLuca feels that the action of the vitamin is a necessary prerequisite for the action of parathyroid hormone, which according to Borle (1968a), also promotes entry of calcium into the cell.

Once calcium enters the cell, the mechanism by which it is transported across the cell is unknown. However, it must exist intracellularly in some reactive state, if not as an ion, since it can affect enzyme processes.

G. The Intracellular Packaging and Transport of Calcium

Besides a rapid "pump" proposed for removal of calcium from the cell, mechanisms have been postulated for binding or packaging intracellular calcium ions to prevent increases in intracellular ionic concentrations. One suggested means is mitochondrial accumulation of calcium, a phenomenon demonstrated to occur in many cell types (J. H. Martin and Matthews, 1969). A second may involve ribosomes as suggested by Matthews (Matthews and Martin, 1970). The temporary storage of calcium in mitochondria has been particularly well demonstrated by Matthews at the electron microscopic level in gut mucosa, immediately after administration of vitamin D to vitamin D-deficient animals (Sampson et al., 1970). This ability of cells to render intracellular calcium unreactive can be considered a "defense mechanism."

Perhaps by a modification of such a defense mechanism, bone cells, particularly osteoblasts and osteocytes, and chondrocytes have the ability to "package" calcium internally, probably along with phosphate and an organic component. Following the early observations of Hancox and Boothroyd (1965), Matthews and his colleagues have postulated such an internal packaging system, and have suggested that transport of such a package to sites in a preformed collagen matrix may be the basis for both crystal nucleation in bone formation and calcification of cartilage (Matthews *et al.*, 1968). Nichols *et al.* (1969) have also reported that osteocytes package large amounts of calcium for transport out of bone.

H. The Unique Structure of the Cell Layer Lining Bone

Both Baud (1968) and Talmage (1969) have proposed that the cell layer separating the bone fluid compartment (adjacent to bone) from the extracellular fluid compartment is a single layer of cells made up of cells of the "family of osteoblasts" (see Fig. 2). Talmage suggested that this layer, like the mucosal layer of the gut or the epithelial lining of kidney tubules, "pumps" calcium toward the extracellular fluid compartment. However, Talmage (1969) pointed out that this layer of bone cells differed from the gut and kidney barriers by having open "channels" between the cells. That relatively large molecules can move down these channels in bone has been demonstrated by Doty, using horseradish peroxidase, a protein not known to cross cell membranes (Doty, 1970). Such a finding supports the concept of intercellular spaces between adjacent cells which permit movement of fluid and ions.

I. An Osteocyte-Osteoblast Model Explaining Control of Calcium Homeostasis

The proposed model is diagrammatically illustrated in Fig. 2. The following hypothesis is proposed: The bone fluid compartment consists of lacunar fluid, fluid surrounding cellular protoplasmic extensions in canaliculi, and spaces between the osteoblast layer and calcified matrix. This fluid is hypertonic compared to extracellular fluid, primarily because of its high potassium content. The calcium concentration in this fluid is, however, about one-third of that in extracellular fluid and is determined by its physical-chemical relationship with the bone salts. This provides a gradient of calcium movement toward bone through the "channels" separating the cells comprising the layer.

Parathyroid hormone works at two sites. The first is on the osteoblast layer allowing transfer of calcium into the cells through the membranes forming the walls of the "channels" and through the portion of the cell membrane adjacent to bone. This acquired calcium is rapidly "pumped" back out through the membrane bordering the extracellular fluid. Much of the calcium, therefore, is "short-circuited" by these cells in that it is returned to the extracellular fluid without actually entering into the bone fluid compartment. However, some calcium passes intercellularly to be transported through the lacunar system (Fig. 2, A). Without parathyroid hormone intercellular calcium movement toward bone would predominate until the two fluid compartments approach equilibrium with respect to calcium ion concentrations (e.g., in the parathyroidectomized state).

Even with parathyroid hormone, movement of calcium through the channels allows continuous loss of calcium to bone, and the second locus of action of parathyroid hormone must be brought into play. In contrast to the osteoblast, the osteocyte does not have a "polarized pump," and parathyroid hormone permits calcium to enter the interior of this cell from all directions. This calcium is "packaged" intracellularly both for protection of the cell and for subsequent transport. The package is transported intracellularly via the long protoplasmic extensions which contact similar extensions of the osteoblast cell layer. Reaching the osteoblast layer, the package can be disseminated for subsequent release to the extracellular fluid. If the action of parathyroid hormone is sufficiently intense, the rate of entry of calcium into the osteocyte exceeds the rate of packaging. In this condition the intracellular concentration of ionic or "reactive" calcium rises and stimulates metabolic processes which promote release of enzymes and organic acids into the lacunar space; these can solubilize calcified matrix thereby releasing additional calcium.

Since the osteoblast layer is functionally "polarized" for transfer of calcium ions to the extracellular fluid, an osteoblastic internal packaging system must also be proposed to account for the actions of osteoblasts engaged in forming new bone. Such packaged calcium could then be transported in the opposite direction, namely toward bone for nucleation of the collagen matrix (J. H. Martin and Matthews, 1969).

The proposed system is unique in that during periods of high extracellular concentrations of calcium, when parathyroid hormone secretion is suppressed, calcium passes primarily intercellularly toward bone and is rapidly spread throughout the "diffuse fraction" described by Rowland (1966). Conversely, when extracellular calcium concentrations are low and parathyroid hormone secretion is stimulated, transcellular transport of calcium into and then out of the osteoblast toward extracellular fluid is increased. At the same time, the hormone increases the entry of calcium into osteocytes for intracellular packaging and transport to the osteoblast as a further source of calcium for the extracellular fluid. By this system essentially the entire bone can act as a reservoir for deposition of excess calcium or a source for needed calcium. During periods of relative calcium balance, there would be little net transfer of calcium between the two fluid compartments; however, rapid ion exchange could still occur.

J. The Influence of Adrenal Hormones on Parathyroid Function

Talmage *et al.* (1970) and Talmage and Kennedy (1970) have recently published two papers demonstrating differences in parathyroid activity in adrenalectomized rats compared to cortisol-treated animals. In these reports, they emphasized that the ability of these rats to maintain normal plasma calcium levels was not affected either by adrenalectomy or by cortisol administration. However, the rates of removal from bone of radiocalcium, administered 2 weeks previously, were increased in the adrenalectomized rat and decreased in the cortisol-treated rat. The authors suggested that adrenal cortical hormone influenced the rate of intracellular transport of "packaged" calcium, presumably decreasing the rate of dissociation of the calcium complex and ultimate release of calcium into extracellular fluid, but had little effect on the recirculation of calcium in the osteoblast layer.

These results are cited here because they appear to support the idea of two separate processes, stimulated by parathyroid hormone, which effect movement of calcium into extracellular fluid. The two are normally "in balance," but if one process is affected, the other may undergo a compensatory change in an attempt to maintain the extracellular calcium concentration.

K. Calcium Transport in the Osteoclast

The osteoclast is also able to extrude calcium actively via a "pump." The cell membrane appears readily permeable to calcium; however, the cell also possesses the ability to rapidly secrete enzymes for dissolution of bone matrix. When an osteoclast approaches the bone surface, entry of calcium into the cell increases and stimulates enzymatic activity. The calcium released from bone by osteoclastic activity is not sufficient to influence calcium homeostasis significantly under normal conditions. However, since the numbers of these cells increase markedly with prolonged parathyroid stimulation, they may, in pathological situations, cause hypercalcemia since they are not under rapid feedback control by the hormone.

L. Unresolved Questions Concerning the Proposed Model

Unfortunately, a clear explanation for how thyrocalcitonin might act in this model system is not readily apparent. Talmage (1969) has postulated that this hormone may enhance phosphate transport through the osteoblast layer of cells toward bone fluid, and it thereby tends to suppress the transport of calcium toward extracellular fluid.

Many of the other problems attributable to this model for control of calcium homeostasis have been considered previously (Talmage, 1969). Only two observations will be made here. The first is that this model does not attempt to explain the biochemical mechanism for calcium entry into the cell or that required to pump it out of the cell. Also, it does not explain the assumed mediatory role of cyclic AMP, which may or may not be directly concerned with intracellular entry of this ion.

A second major unexplained problem is how intracellular packaged calcium might be transferred from osteocyte to osteoblast. Protoplasmic extensions of both cells appear to meet in the canaliculi, and electron micrographs have demonstrated protoplasmic extensions of these cells close together within a canaliculus. No obvious anatomical adaptations were evident at the ends of these extensions which might suggest a mechanism for transfer of packages sufficiently large to appear electron dense. However, until the tedious work is done of completely tracing, at the electron microscope level, a single canaliculus from osteocyte to osteoblast, one cannot exclude the possibility of protoplasmic continuity between the two cells—i.e., a syncytium.

V. General Summary

In this report we have attempted (1) to review current concepts concerning the mode of action of parathyroid hormone, (2) to point out apparent similarities between *in vivo* effects of this hormone on a variety of metabolic functions and those produced by elevated circulating calcium concentrations, and finally (3) to present a model to account for parathyroid control of calcium fluxes in bone. It is obvious that the proposals presented rest largely on our assumption that most, if not all, of the metabolic activities attributable to parathyroid hormone can be traced to the ability of the hormone to facilitate the movement of calcium across cell membranes into intracellular compartments.

We propose that, by enhancing entry of calcium into the interior of the cell, parathyroid hormone produces two divergent effects on the overall metabolism and physiology of bone and other target tissues:

1. By allowing increased intracellular ionic calcium levels, the hormone increases the amount of calcium transported across specific layers of target cells. This net movement of calcium is unidirectional or "polarized" and occurs against a concentration gradient via a "pump" mechanism. This effect of the hormone can be termed *stimulation of transcellular movement of calcium*.

2. If the intracellular concentration of ionic calcium is appreciably increased, many enzymatically controlled processes within the cell may in turn be affected. This secondary function of parathyroid hormone can

be termed *stimulation of calcium-influenced metabolic activities* and may occur in any cell which responds to the hormone by allowing increased entry of calcium.

The first postulated effect is important for target tissues in which a layer of cells functions as a "membrane" or barrier separating two fluid compartments differing in ionic composition. In all target tissues, the hormone appears to promote movement of calcium toward the primary extracellular fluid compartment of the body. In the gut, parathyroid hormone may abet the action of vitamin D in facilitating calcium transport from the lumen to extracellular fluid. In the kidney tubule it also enhances calcium transport from the lumen toward extracellular fluid while simultaneously restricting transport of phosphate in this direction. In bone also, parathyroid hormone increases the transport of calcium from the "bone fluid" compartment toward the extracellular fluid compartment. A similar effect of the hormone on calcium transport in other tissues may exist, e.g., in placenta and mammary gland; however, these possible sites of action have received inadequate attention at the present time.

The second proposed general effect of parathyroid hormone, its influence on intracellular metabolism, has been demonstrated only in bone tissue. A parathyroid hormone-induced increase in intracellular calcium concentration leads, not only to changes in biochemical processes, but also to the eventual morphological and cytological alterations observed in bone after intense or prolonged hormone treatment. These induced changes include: an increase in mitotic activity, changes in RNA synthesis, suppression of collagen synthesis, increased organic acid production, and stimulation of lysosomal enzyme activities. These are changes that mediate and reflect the influence of parathyroid hormone on bone remodeling and are primarily responsible for the classically described effects of the hormone on bone formation and resorption.

Previously, as well as in this report, we have emphasized the existence of two, separate primary effects of parathyroid hormone on bone which assist bone remodeling and concurrently permit continuous control of calcium homeostasis. The hormonal control of calcium homeostasis is exerted primarily by stimulation of transcellular transport of calcium. However, it also involves calcium-induced changes in cellular activity which may help liberate additional needed calcium from bone (e.g., osteolysis). Bone remodeling appears to result primarily from the ability of calcium to allow increased numbers and activity of the cells involved (e.g., osteoclasts).

Finally, we would like to suggest that in the normal individual these two hormonally influenced activities are in balance, allowing a normal rate of bone resorption to exist while simultaneously controlling plasma calcium levels. It is possible that many bone diseases of diverse etiologies may involve an imbalance between these activities.

VI. Conclusion

While numerous model theories have been proposed in the past to account for certain specific actions of parathyroid hormone on bone, we feel the virtue of the one presented here is that it attempts to account for a majority of the reported hormonal effects on bone. Rather than incorporating only our own observations, we have drawn on the diverse reports of many workers in the field and have attempted to comprise a comprehensive view of the mode of action of parathyroid hormone. We are well aware of the imperfections inherent in this proposed model. Many of the component concepts presented appear to have substantial basis in fact, while others are less well supported and, therefore, are subject to considerable uncertainty. Nevertheless, the ideas discussed provide a framework for future evaluation of studies on parathyroid hormone and skeletal metabolism.

We are also aware of the fact that knowledgeable colleagues in the field will disagree, wholly or in part, with the theories advanced here. This we welcome. Indeed, the three authors of this report are not in complete agreement on all of the basic concepts as they have been interpreted and discussed.

REFERENCES

Adams, D. H., and Quastel, J. H. (1956). *Proc. Roy. Soc.* **B145**, 472.

Albright, F., and Reifenstein, E. C., Jr. (1948). "The Parathyroid Glands and Metabolic Bone Disease." Williams & Wilkins, Baltimore, Maryland.

Anast, C., Arnaud, C. D., Rasmussen, H., and Tenenhouse, A. (1967). *J. Clin. Invest.* **46**, 57.

Arnaud, C. D., Jr., Tenenhouse, A. M., and Rasmussen, H. (1967). *Annu. Rev. Physiol.* **29**, 349.

Aurbach, G. D., and Potts, J. T., Jr. (1964). *Advan. Metab. Disord.* **1**, 46.

Aurbach, G. D., Houston, B. A., and Potts, J. T., Jr. (1965a). *In* "The Parathyroid Glands" (P. J. Gaillard, R. V. Talmage, and A. M. Budy, eds.), p. 197. Univ. of Chicago Press, Chicago, Illinois.

Aurbach, G. D., Houston, B. A., and Potts, J. T., Jr. (1965b). *Biochem. Biophys. Res. Commun.* **20**, 592.

Avioli, L. V., McDonald, J. E., Henneman, P. H., and Lee, S. W. (1966). *J. Clin. Invest.* **45**, 1093.

Bär, H., and Hechter, O. (1969). *Biochem. Biophys. Res. Commun.* **35**, 681.

Barnicot, N. A. (1948). *J. Anat.* **82**, 233.

Bartter, F. C. (1961). *In* "The Parathyroids" (R. O. Greep and R. V. Talmage, eds.), p. 388. Thomas, Springfield, Illinois.

Baud, C. A. (1962). *Acta Anat.* **51**, 209.

Baud, C. A. (1968). *Clin. Orthop.* **56**, 227.

Bélanger, L. F. (1965). In "The Parathyroid Glands" (P. J. Gaillard, R. V. Talmage, and A. M. Budy, eds.), p. 137. Univ. of Chicago Press, Chicago, Illinois.

Bélanger, L. F., and Migicovsky, B. B. (1963). J. Histochem. Cytochem. 11, 734.

Bélanger, L. F., Robichon, J., Migicovsky, B. B., Copp, D. H., and Vincent, J. (1963). In "Mechanisms of Hard Tissue Destruction," Publ. No. 75, p. 531. Am. Assoc. Advance. Sci., Washington, D. C.

Borle, A. B. (1968a). In "Parathyroid Hormone and Thyrocalcitonin (Calcitonin)" (R. V. Talmage and L. F. Bélanger, eds.), p. 258. Excerpta Med. Found., Amsterdam.

Borle, A. B. (1968b). J. Cell Biol. 36, 567.

Borle, A. B. (1969). Abstr. 51st Meet. Endocrine Soc. p. 104 (abstr.).

Borle, A. B., and Herold, E. (1970). J. Gen. Physiol. 55, 163.

Borle, A. B., and Neuman, W. F. (1965). J. Cell. Biol. 24, 316.

Borle, A. B., Nichols, N., and Nichols, G., Jr. (1960a). J. Biol. Chem. 235, 1206.

Borle, A. B., Nichols, N., and Nichols, G., Jr. (1960b). J. Biol. Chem. 235, 1211.

Buttara, C. A., and Rattini, E. (1950). Arch. Studio Fisiopatol. Clin. Ricamb. 14, 105.

Bygrave, F. L. (1966). Biochem. J. 101, 480.

Canas, F., Terepka, A. R., and Neuman, W. F. (1969). Amer. J. Physiol. 217, 117.

Chase, L. R., and Aurbach, G. D. (1967). Proc. Nat. Acad. Sci. U. S. 58, 518.

Chase, L. R., and Aurbach, G. D. (1968a). Science 159, 545.

Chase, L. R., and Aurbach, G. D. (1968b). In "Parathyroid Hormone and Thyrocalcitonin (Calcitonin)" (R. V. Talmage and L. F. Bélanger, eds.), p. 247. Excerpta Med. Found., Amsterdam.

Chase, L. R., Fedak, S. A., and Aurbach, G. D. (1969). Endocrinology 84, 761.

Cohn, D. V., Levy, R., and Eller, G. (1966). Endocrinology 79, 1001.

Cooper, C. W., and Talmage, R. V. (1965). Gen. Comp. Endocrinol. 5, 534.

Cooper, C. W., Hirsch, P. F., and Munson, P. L. (1970). Endocrinology 86, 406.

Copp, D. H. (1969). Annu. Rev. Pharmacol. 9, 327.

Copp, D. H., Cameron, E. C., Cheney, B. A., Davidson, A. G. F., and Henze, K. G. (1962). Endocrinology 70, 638.

Costello, L. C., and Darago, L. L. (1964). Arch. Biochem. Biophys. 108, 574.

Dabich, D., and Neuhaus, P. W. (1966). J. Biol. Chem. 241, 415.

DeLong, A. F., and L'Heureux, M. V. (1968). Fed. Proc., Fed. Amer. Soc. Exp. Biol. 27, 690.

DeLuca, H. F. (1969). In "Calcitonin" (S. Taylor and G. Foster, eds.), p. 205. Springer-Verlag, New York.

DeLuca, H. F., and Sallis, J. D. (1965). In "The Parathyroid Glands" (P. J. Gaillard, R. V. Talmage, and A. M. Budy, eds.), p. 181. Univ. of Chicago Press, Chicago, Illinois.

DeLuca, H. F., Gran, F. C., Steenbock, H., and Reiser, S. (1957). J. Biol. Chem. 228, 469.

DeLuca, H. F., Morii, H., and Melancon, M. J., Jr. (1968). In "Parathyroid Hormone and Thyrocalcitonin (Calcitonin)" (R. V. Talmage and L. F. Bélanger, eds.), p. 448. Excerpta Med. Found., Amsterdam.

De Voogd van der Straaten, W. A. (1962). Gen. Comp. Endocrinol. 2, 620.

De Voogd van der Straaten, W. A. (1965). In "The Parathyroid Glands" (P. J. Gaillard, R. V. Talmage, and A. M. Budy, eds.), p. 273. Univ. of Chicago Press, Chicago, Illinois.

Dickens, F. (1941). Biochem. J. 35, 1011.

Doty, S. B. (1970). Personal communication.

Doty, S. B., and Robinson, R. A. (1970). *In* "Biological Mineralization" (I. Zipkin, ed.). Wiley, New York (in press).

Doty, S. B., Schofield, B. H., and Robinson, R. A. (1968). *In* "Parathyroid Hormone and Thyrocalcitonin (Calcitonin)" (R. V. Talmage and L. F. Bélanger, eds.), p. 169. Excerpta Med. Found., Amsterdam.

Dowse, C. M., Neuman, M. W., Lane, K., and Neuman, W. F. (1963). *In* "Mechanisms of Hard Tissue Destruction," Publ. No. 75, p. 589. Am. Assoc. Advance. Sci., Washington, D. C.

Ebashi, S., and Endo, M. (1968). *Progr. Biophys. Mol. Biol.* **18**, 123.

Eisenberg, E. (1968). *In* "Parathyroid Hormone and Thyrocalcitonin (Calcitonin)" (R. V. Talmage and L. F. Bélanger, eds.), p. 465. Excerpta Med. Found., Amsterdam.

Eisenstein, R., and Passavoy, M. (1964). *Proc. Soc. Exp. Biol. Med.* **117**, 77.

Everett, G. A., and Holly, R. W. (1961). *Biochim. Biophys. Acta* **46**, 390.

Firschein, H., Martin, G., Mulryan, B. J., Strates, B., and Neuman, W. F. (1958). *J. Amer. Chem. Soc.* **80**, 1619.

Flanagan, B., and Nichols, G., Jr. (1964a). *Endocrinology* **74**, 180.

Flanagan, B., and Nichols, G., Jr. (1964b). *J. Biol. Chem.* **239**, 1261.

Fleisch, H. (1964). *Clin. Orthop.* **32**, 170.

Fleisch, H., and Neuman, W. F. (1961). *Amer. J. Physiol.* **200**, 1296.

Fleisch, H., Schibler, D., Maerki, J., and Frossars, I. (1965). *Nature (London)* **207**, 1300.

Folk, J. E., Malooly, J. P., and Cole, P. W. (1967). *J. Biol. Chem.* **242**, 1838.

Fullman, H. M., and Lazarus, G. (1967). *Isr. J. Med.* **3**, 759.

Gaillard, P. J. (1955). *Exp. Cell Res.* Suppl. 3, 154.

Gaillard, P. J. (1961). *In* "The Parathyroids" (R. O. Greep and R. V. Talmage, eds.), p. 20. Thomas, Springfield, Illinois.

Gaillard, P. J. (1965). *In* "The Parathyroid Glands" (P. J. Gaillard, R. V. Talmage, and A. M. Budy, eds.), p. 145. Univ. of Chicago Press, Chicago, Illinois.

Gaillard, P. J., Talmage, R. V., and Budy, A. M., eds. (1965). "The Parathyroid Glands." Univ. of Chicago Press, Chicago, Illinois.

Geisler, J. Z., and Neuman, W. F. (1969). *Proc. Soc. Exp. Biol. Med.* **130**, 608.

Goldhaber, P. (1965). *In* "The Parathyroid Glands" (P. J. Gaillard, R. V. Talmage, and A. M. Budy, eds.), p. 153. Univ. of Chicago Press, Chicago, Illinois.

Goldhaber, P., Stern, B. D., Glimcher, M. J., and Chao, J. (1968). *In* "Parathyroid Hormone and Thyrocalcitonin (Calcitonin)" (R. V. Talmage and L. F. Bélanger, eds.), p. 182. Excerpta Med. Found., Amsterdam.

Greep, R. O., and Talmage, R. V., eds. (1961). "The Parathyroids." Thomas, Springfield, Illinois.

Grollman, A. (1954). *Endocrinology* **55**, 166.

Hancox, N. M., and Boothroyd, B. (1955). *Clin. Orthop.* **40**, 153.

Hekkelman, J. (1965a). *In* "The Parathyroid Glands" (P. J. Gaillard, R. V. Talmage, and A. M. Budy, eds.), p. 221. Univ. of Chicago Press, Chicago, Illinois.

Hekkelman, J. (1965b). *Proc. St. Andrew Scat.* p. 356.

Hekkelman, J. W., and Herrmann-Erlee, M. P. M. (1968). *In* "Parathyroid Hormone and Thyrocalcitonin (Calcitonin)" (R. V. Talmage and L. F. Bélanger, eds.), p. 273. Excerpta Med. Found., Amsterdam.

Heller, M., McLean, F. C., and Bloom, W. (1950). *Amer. J. Anat.* **87**, 315.

Heller-Steinberg, M. (1951). *Amer. J. Anat.* **89**, 347.

Herrmann-Erlee, M. P. M. (1962). *Proc., Kon. Ned. Akad. Wetensch., Ser. C* **65**, 22.

Hirsch, P. F., and Munson, P. L. (1964). *Naunyn-Schmiedebergs Arch Exp. Pathol. Pharmakol.* **248**, 319.

Hirsch, P. F., Gauthier, G. F., and Munson, P. L. (1963). *Endocrinology* **73**, 244.

Howard, J. E. (1959). *Bone Struct. Metab., Ciba Found. Symp.* p. 207.

Johnston, C. C., Jr., Diess, W. P., Jr., and Miner, E. B. (1962). *J. Biol. Chem.* **237**, 3560.

Kashiwa, H. K. (1968). *Anat. Rec.* **162**, 177.

Khoo, E. C., and Kowalewski, K. (1965). *Proc. Soc. Exp. Biol. Med.* **119**, 946.

Krane, S. M., Shine, K. I., and Pyle, M. B. (1961). *In* "The Parathyroids" (R. O. Greep and R. V. Talmage, eds.), p. 298. Thomas, Springfield, Illinois.

Krebs, H. A., and Bennett, D. A. H. (1963). *Biochem. J.* **86**, 22.

Kunitz, M., and Robbins, P. W. (1961). *In* "The Enzymes" (P. D. Boyer, H. Lardy, and K. Myrbäck, eds.), Vol. 5, p. 169. Academic Press, New York.

Lavender, A. R., Pullman, T. N., Rasmussen, H., and Aho, I. (1961). *In* "The Parathyroids" (R. O. Greep and R. V. Talmage, eds.), p. 406. Thomas, Springfield, Illinois.

LeJohn, H. B. (1968). *J. Biol. Chem.* **243**, 5126.

Mallevais, J. P., Segard, E., and Mowtreuil, J. (1966). *C. R. Acad. Sci., Ser. D* **262**, 1892.

Marshall, J. H. (1969). *In* "Mineral Metabolism" (C. L. Comar and F. Bronner, eds.), Vol. 3, p. 1. Academic Press, New York.

Marshall, J. H., Rowland, R. E., and Jowsey, J. (1959). *Radiat. Res.* **10**, 258.

Martin, D. L., and DeLuca, H. F. (1970). *Biochim. Biophys. Acta* (in press).

Martin, G., Firschein, H., Mulryan, B. J., and Neuman, W. F. (1958). *J. Amer. Chem. Soc.* **80**, 6201.

Martin, G. R., Mecca, C. E., Schiffman, E., and Goldhaber, P. (1965). *In* "The Parathyroid Glands" (P. J. Gaillard, R. V. Talmage, and A. M. Budy, eds.), p. 261. Univ. of Chicago Press, Chicago, Illinois.

Martin, J. H., and Matthews, J. L. (1969). *Calcif. Tissue Res.* **3**, 184.

Martin, J. H., and Matthews, J. L. (1970). *Clin. Orthop.* **68**, 273.

Matsuhashi, M., Matsuhashi, S., Numa, S., and Lynen, F. (1962). *Fed. Proc., Fed. Amer. Soc. Exp. Biol.* **21**, 288.

Matthews, J. L., Martin, J. H., Lynn, J. A., and Collins, E. J. (1968). *Calcif. Tissue Res.* **1**, 330.

Mills, B. G., and Bavetta, L. A. (1965). *Proc. Soc. Exp. Biol. Med.* **118**, 273.

Minato, A., Ogisu, T., and Hoshiro, H. (1966). *Yakugaku Zasshi* **86**, 726.

Miyasi, T., and Greenstein, J. P. (1951). *Arch. Biochem. Biophys.* **32**, 414.

Munson, P. L., Hirsch, P. F., and Tashjian, A. H., Jr. (1963). *Annu. Rev. Physiol.* **25**, 325.

Nagata, N., and Rasmussen, H. (1968). *Biochemistry* **7**, 3728.

Nagatsu, I., and Hara, J. (1966). *Endocrinol. Jap.* **13**, 216.

Neuman, W. F. (1969). *Fed. Proc., Fed. Amer. Soc. Exp. Biol.* **28**, 1846.

Neuman, W. F., and Dowse, C. M. (1961). *In* "The Parathyroids" (R. O. Greep and R. V. Talmage, eds.), p. 310. Thomas, Springfield, Illinois.

Neuman, W. F., and Mulryan, B. J. (1969). *Calcif. Tissue Res.* **3**, 261.

Neuman, W. F., Firschein, H., Chen, P. S., Jr., Mulryan, B. J., and Di Stefano, V. (1956). *J. Amer. Chem. Soc.* **78**, 3863.

Nichols, G., Jr., Flanagan, B., and Woods, J. F. (1965). *In* "The Parathyroid Glands"

138   ROY V. TALMAGE, CARY W. COOPER, AND HAN Z. PARK

(P. J. Gaillard, R. V. Talmage, and A. M. Budy, eds.), p. 243. Univ. of Chicago Press, Chicago, Illinois.

Nichols, G., Jr., Flanagan, B., and van der Sluys Veer, J. (1969). *Arch. Intern. Med.* **124**, 530.

Nordin, B. E. C., and Peacock, M. (1969). *Lancet* **ii**, 1280.

Nordlie, R. C., Wright, S., Boyum, G. P., and Rohs, J. L. (1968). *Proc. Soc. Exp. Biol. Med.* **128**, 1039.

Notario, A., and Larriza, L. (1956). *Arch. Sci. Med.* **101**, 484.

Owen, M., and Bingham, P. J. (1968). *In* "Parathyroid Hormone and Thyrocalcitonin (Calcitonin)" (R. V. Talmage and L. F. Bélanger, eds.), p. 216. Excerpta Med. Found., Amsterdam.

Ozawa, T. (1967). *J. Biochem. (Tokyo)* **62**, 285.

Park, H. Z., and Talmage, R. V. (1967). *Endocrinology* **80**, 552.

Park, H. Z., and Talmage, R. V. (1968). *In* "Parathyroid Hormone and Thyrocalcitonin (Calcitonin)" (R. V. Talmage and L. F. Bélanger, eds.), p. 203. Excerpta Med. Found., Amsterdam.

Parsons, J. A., and Robinson, C. J. (1968). *In* "Parathyroid Hormone and Thyrocalcitonin (Calcitonin)" (R. V. Talmage and L. F. Bélanger, eds.), p. 329. Excerpta Med. Found., Amsterdam.

Pechet, M. M., Bobadilla, E., Carrol, E. L., and Hesse, R. H. (1967). *Amer. J. Med.* **43**, 696.

Perris, A. D., Whitfield, J. F., and Rixon, R. H. (1967). *Radiat. Res.* **32**, 550.

Potts, J. T., Jr., and Deftos, L. J. (1969). *In* "Duncan's Diseases of Metabolism" (P. K. Bondy, ed.), 6th ed., p. 904. Saunders, Philadelphia, Pennsylvania.

Potts, J. T., Jr., Sherwood, L. M., and Sandoval, A. (1965). *Proc. Nat. Acad. Sci. U. S.* **54**, 1743.

Potts, J. T., Jr., Aurbach, G. D., and Sherwood, L. M. (1966). *Recent Progr. Horm. Res.* **22**, 101.

Pullman, T. N., Lavender, A. R., Aho, I., and Rasmussen, H. (1960). *Endocrinology* **67**, 570.

Raisz, L. G. (1963). *Nature (London)* **197**, 1015.

Raisz, L. G. (1965). *Proc. Soc. Exp. Biol. Med.* **119**, 614.

Raisz, L. G., and Klein, D. C. (1969). *Fed. Proc., Fed. Amer. Soc. Exp. Biol.* **28**, 320 (abstr.).

Raisz, L. G., and Niemann, I. (1967). *Nature (London)* **214**, 486.

Raisz, L. G., and Niemann, I. (1969). *Endocrinology* **85**, 446.

Raisz, L. G., Brand, J. S., Klein, D. C., and Au, W. Y. W. (1969). *Proc. 3rd Int. Congr. Endocrinol., 1968* p. 696.

Rappaport, A. Y. (1938). *Prog. Endocrinol. (USSR)* **3**, 3.

Rasmussen, H., and DeLuca, H. F. (1963). *Ergeb. Physiol., Biol. Chem. Exp. Pharmakol.* **53**, 108.

Rasmussen, H., and Tenenhouse, A. (1967). *Amer. J. Med.* **43**, 711.

Rasmussen, H., Sallis, J., Fang, M., DeLuca, H., and Young, R. (1964a). *Endocrinology* **74**, 388.

Rasmussen, H., Arnaud, C., and Hawker, C. (1964b). *Science* **144**, 1019.

Rasmussen, H., Anast, C., and Arnaud, C. (1967a). *J. Clin. Invest.* **46**, 746.

Rasmussen, H., Shirasu, H., Ogata, E., and Hawker, C. (1967b). *J. Biol. Chem.* **242**, 4669.

Rasmussen, H., Nagata, N., Feinblatt, J., and Fast, D. (1968a). *In* "Parathyroid

Hormone and Thyrocalcitonin (Calcitonin)" (R. V. Talmage and L. F. Bélanger, eds.), p. 299. Excerpta Med. Found., Amsterdam.

Rasmussen, H., Pechet, M., and Fast, C. (1968b). *J. Clin. Invest.* **47**, 1843.

Rixon, R. H. (1968). *Car. Mod. Biol.* **2**, 68.

Robison, G. A., Butcher, R. W., and Sutherland, E. W. (1968). *Annu. Rev. Biochem.* **37**, 149.

Rohr, H. (1964). *Klin. Wochenschr.* **42**, 1209.

Rowland, R. E. (1960). *Clin. Orthop.* **17**, 146.

Rowland, R. E. (1966). *Clin. Orthop.* **49**, 233.

Rutman, J. Z., Meltzer, L. E., Kitchell, J. R., Rutman, R. J., and George, P. (1965). *Amer. J. Physiol.* **208**, 841.

Sallis, J. D., and DeLuca, H. F. (1964). *J. Biol. Chem.* **239**, 4303.

Sallis, J. D., DeLuca, H. F., and Rasmussen, H. (1963). *J. Biol. Chem.* **238**, 4098.

Sallis, J. D., DeLuca, H. F., and Martin, D. L. (1965). *J. Biol. Chem.* **240**, 2229.

Sampson, H. W., Matthews, J. L., Martin, J. H., and Kunin, A. S. (1970). *Calcif. Tissue Res.* (in press).

Schartum, S., and Nichols, G., Jr. (1961). *J. Clin. Invest.* **40**, 2083.

Schwartz, A., Johnson, C. L., and Safer, B. (1966). *Life Sci.* **5**, 243.

Seeling, S. (1931). *Z. Ges. Exp. Med.* **78**, 796.

Simpson, D. P. (1967). *Biochem. Med.* **1**, 168.

Sipos, T., and Merkel, J. R. (1968). *Biochem. Biophys. Res. Commun.* **31**, 522.

Soodsma, J. F., and Nordlie, R. C. (1966). *Biochim. Biophys. Acta* **122**, 510.

Steinberg, J., and Nichols, G., Jr. (1968). *In* "Parathyroid Hormone and Thyrocalcitonin (Calcitonin)" (R. V. Talmage and L. F. Bélanger, eds.), p. 226. Excerpta Med. Found., Amsterdam.

Stewart, G. S., and Bowen, H. F. (1951). *Endocrinology* **48**, 568.

Striganova, A. R. (1949). *Arkh. Patol.* **11**, 50.

Takagaki, G. (1968). *J. Neurochem.* **15**, 903.

Talmage, R. V. (1956). *Ann. N. Y. Acad. Sci.* **64**, 326.

Talmage, R. V. (1966). *In* "Abridged Proceedings of the Fourth European Symposium on Calcified Tissues," p. 99. Excerpta Med. Found., Amsterdam.

Talmage, R. V. (1967). *Clin. Orthop.* **54**, 163.

Talmage, R. V. (1969). *Clin. Orthop.* **67**, 210.

Talmage, R. V., and Bélanger, L. F., eds. (1968). "Parathyroid Hormone and Thyrocalcitonin (Calcitonin)." Excerpta Med. Found., Amsterdam.

Talmage, R. V., and Kennedy, J. W., III. (1970). *Endocrinology* **86**, 1075.

Talmage, R. V., and Toft, R. J. (1961). *In* "The Parathyroids" (R. O. Greep and R. V. Talmage, eds.), p. 224. Thomas, Springfield, Illinois.

Talmage, R. V., Kraintz, F. W., Frost, R. C., and Kraintz, L. (1953). *Endocrinology* **52**, 318.

Talmage, R. V., Toft, R. J., and Davis, R. (1960). *Tex. Rep. Biol. Med.* **18**, 298.

Talmage, R. V., Doty, S. B., Cooper, C. W., Yates, C., and Neuenschwander, J. (1965a). *In* "The Parathyroid Glands" (P. J. Gaillard, R. V. Talmage, and A. M. Budy, eds.), p. 107. Univ. of Chicago Press, Chicago, Illinois.

Talmage, R. V., Cooper, C. W., and Neuenschwander, J. (1965b). *Gen. Comp. Endocrinol.* **5**, 475.

Talmage, R. V., Park, H. Z., and Jee, W. (1970). *Endocrinology* **86**, 1080.

Tashjian, A. H., Jr., Ontjes, D. A., and Goodfriend, T. L. (1964). *Biochem. Biophys. Res. Commun.* **16**, 209.

Terepka, A. R., Dowse, C. M., and Neuman, W. F. (1960). *A.E.C. Rep. U. R.* **577**.

Terepka, A. R., Canas, F., Triffitt, J. D., and Neuman, W. F. (1968). *Calcif. Tissue Res.* **2**, 262.

Tessari, L. (1959). *Nature (London)* **84**, 904.

Tessari, L. (1960). *Endocrinology* **66**, 892.

Toft, R. J., and Talmage, R. V. (1960). *Proc. Soc. Exp. Biol. Med.* **103**, 611.

Triffitt, J. D., Terepka, A. R., and Neuman, W. F. (1968). *Calcif. Tissue Res.* **2**, 165.

Turkington, R. W. (1968). *Experientia* **24**, 226.

Vaes, G. (1965). *Biochem. J.* **97**, 393.

Vaes, G. (1968a). *In* "Parathyroid Hormone and Thyrocalcitonin (Calcitonin)" (R. V. Talmage and L. F. Bélanger, eds.), p. 318. Excerpta Med. Found., Amsterdam.

Vaes, G. (1968b). *Nature (London)* **219**, 939.

Vaes, G. (1968c). *Exp. Cell Res.* **39**, 470.

Vaes, G. M., and Nichols, G., Jr. (1962). *Endocrinology* **70**, 546.

Van Reen, R. (1965). *In* "The Parathyroid Glands" (P. J. Gaillard, R. V. Talmage, and A. M. Budy, eds.), p. 211. Univ. of Chicago Press, Chicago, Illinois.

Verity, M. A., Caper, R., and Brown, W. J. (1968). *Biochem. J.* **109**, 149.

Vitalli, P. H. (1968). *Clin. Orthop.* **56**, 213.

Walker, D. G., Lapier, C. M., and Gross, J. (1964). *Biochem. Biophys. Res. Commun.* **15**, 397.

Wasserman, F., and Yaeger, J. A. (1965). *Z. Zellforsch. Mikrosk. Anat.* **67**, 636.

Wasserman, R. H. (1968). *Calcif. Tissue Res.* **2**, 301.

Wasserman, R. H., and Taylor, A. N. (1969). *In* "Mineral Metabolism" (C. L. Comar and F. Bronner, eds.), Vol. 3, p. 322. Academic Press, New York.

Wells, H., and Lloyd, W. (1967). *Endocrinology* **81**, 139.

Wells, H., and Lloyd, W. (1968a). *Endocrinology* **82**, 468.

Wells, H., and Lloyd, W. (1968b). *In* "Parathyroid Hormone and Thyrocalcitonin (Calcitonin)" (R. V. Talmage and L. F. Bélanger, eds.), p. 332. Excerpta Med. Found., Amsterdam.

Whitfield, J. F., Perris, A. D., and Youdale, T. (1969). *J. Cell. Physiol.* **73**, 203.

Widrow, S. H., and Levinsky, N. C. (1962). *J. Clin. Invest.* **41**, 251.

Woods, J. F., and Nichols, G., Jr. (1963). *Science* **142**, 386.

Yates, C. W., and Talmage, R. V. (1965). *Proc. Soc. Exp. Biol. Med.* **119**, 88.

Young, R. W. (1962a). *Exp. Cell Res.* **26**, 562.

Young, R. W. (1962b). *J. Cell Biol.* **14**, 357.

Young, R. W. (1963). *In* "Mechanisms of Hard Tissue Destruction," Publ. No. 75. p. 471. Am. Assoc. Advance. Sci., Washington, D. C.

International Symposium on the Structures and Functions of Vitamin-Dependent Enzymes in Honor of Professor Hugo Theorell

A collection of invited papers presented at Lausanne-Ouchy, Switzerland on July 16, 17, and 18, 1970. This symposium was held in honor of Professor Hugo Theorell, and was supported by a grant from F. Hoffmann-La Roche Company.

First Session (E. C. Slater, Chairman)

Second Session (H. Aebi, Chairman)

Third Session (Esmond E. Snell, Chairman)

141

Fourth Session (Osamu Hayaishi, Chairman)

Introductory Remarks

ROBERT S. HARRIS

Massachusetts Institute of Technology, Cambridge, Massachusetts

It is a privilege and an honor for me to open this the Sixth Roche Symposium.*

On alternate years beginning in 1960, the Editors of *Vitamins and Hormones* have collaborated with a series of *ad hoc* committees in planning, producing, and publishing symposia that are critical evaluations of current knowledge concerning individual vitamins, vitamins in relation to anemias and to enzymes. The present symposium is concerned with enzymes that contain vitamins.

We take this occasion to thank F. Hoffmann-Le Roche and Co., Basel, Switzerland and Hoffmann-La Roche Co., Nutley, New Jersey for generously underwriting the costs of these symposia and contributing to the costs of publication of the proceedings in *Vitamins and Hormones.*

In the past, each symposium has been dedicated to a scientist who played a major role in the discovery of a selected vitamin and the elucidation of its metabolic functions. The honored scientist has been able to attend each symposium, to participate in the proceedings, and to recall the events that surrounded his discovery. At this symposium we meet to honor Professor Axel Hugo Theodor Theorell.

Dr. Theorell was born on July 6, 1903 in Linköping, Sweden. He is a son of Armida Bill and of Thure Theorell, who served as surgeon-major to the First Life Grenadiers, and practiced medicine in Linköping.

He attended a State Secondary School in Linköping for nine years and passed his student exam there on May 21, 1921. He received the Bachelor of Medicine degree in 1924 after three years at the Karolinska Institute, then studied bacteriology during three months at the Pasteur Institute in Paris under Professor Calmette. In 1930 he presented a thesis on the lipids of plasma and was awarded the M.D. degree.

Dr. Theorell served on the staff of the Medico-Chemical Institution

---

* The five previous symposia were: Vitamins A and Carotene, in honor of Professor Paul Karrer and published in Volume 18; Vitamins E, in honor of Professor Herbert E. Evans and published in Volume 20; Vitamin B₆, in honor of Professor Paul György and published in Volume 22; Vitamins K and Related Quinones, in honor of Professor Henrik Dam and published in Volume 24; and Vitamin-Related Anemias, in honor of Professor William B. Castle and published in Volume 26 of *Vitamins and Hormones.*

between 1924–28. During 1928–29, while temporary Associate Professor, he worked under Professor Einar Hammarsten on the influence of lipids on the sedimentation of blood corpuscles. During 1931–32 he was an associate of Professor Svedberg at Uppsala University, where he used the ultracentrifuge in determining the molecular weight of myoglobin. An appointment as Associate Professor in Medical and Physiological Chemistry at Uppsala University in 1932 enabled him to continue his research on myoglobin.

Between 1933 and 1935 he held a Rockefeller Fellowship that enabled him to work in Otto Warburg's laboratory at Berlin-Dahlem. While with Professor Warburg he developed an interest in oxidation enzymes, a subject which absorbed his attention during the next 35 years. It was while at Berlin-Dahlem that he identified for the first time "the yellow ferment," an oxidizing enzyme, and succeeded in splitting it reversibly into a coenzyme fraction (flavin mononucleotide) and a colorless fraction (protein). This was the first demonstration of the reversible separation of an enzyme into its prosthetic group (coenzyme) and a pure protein component (apoenzyme). It was his good fortune that the material he had isolated was essentially 95% carbohydrate and 5% riboflavin, and thus could readily be fractionated by electrophoresis.

Dr. Theorell returned to the Karolinska Institute in 1935. In 1937 he was appointed Head of the newly established Biochemical Department of the Nobel Medical Institute, which was located within the Karolinska Institute for ten years before moving into its own building in 1947.

During the past 35 years Dr. Theorell and his collaborators have conducted significant research on various oxidation enzymes, and have made important contributions to the knowledge of catalases, cytochrome c, flavoproteins, peroxidases, "pyridine" proteins, and especially alcohol dehydrogenases.

Dr. Theorell was awarded the Nobel Prize for Physiology and Medicine in 1955. He is a member of learned societies in Sweden, Norway, Denmark, Finland, Belgium, France, Italy, Poland, and India. He served as Chairman of the Swedish Medical Society during 1940–46, as member of the Swedish Society for Medical Research during 1942–50, also as a member of the State Research Council for the Natural Sciences during 1950–54, and as a member of the State Medical Research Council since 1958. He also served as Chairman of the Association of Swedish Chemists from 1947–49, as Chief Editor of the journal *Nordisk Medicin*, as Chairman of the Swedish National Committee for Biochemistry, and as Chairman of the Board of the Wenner-Gren Society and of the Wenner-Gren Center Foundation. He is currently President of the International Union of Biochemists.

Professor Theorell has been awarded honorary doctoral degrees by the Universities of Paris, Pennsylvania, Louvain, Brussels, and Rio de Janeiro, is a Foreign Member of the Royal Society of London and a Foreign Member of the National Academy of Sciences of the United States of America.

He married Elin Margit Elizabeth Alenius in 1931. They had one daughter, Eva Kristine, who died in 1935; and three sons: Klas Thure Gabriel (1935), Henning Hugo (1939), and Per Gunnar Töres (1942). Theo and Margit have remained deeply devoted to one another during years marked by great tragedy and great success.

Music has been a dominant interest throughout Professor Theorell's life. While he was a boy he traveled the 200 kilometers from Linköping to Stockholm each week to study under one of the best violin teachers in Sweden at that time. His interest in music was stimulated by his mother who joined him in presenting many concerts in the environs of Stockholm. It is likely also that his interest in music was further encouraged by a rather severe poliomyelitis paralysis that struck him when he was eight years old, for this crippling disease forced him to change from physical to artistic activities.

At the time of his matriculation he intended to become a professional musician. However, when several of his friends started to study medicine and when he noted that the medical university fee was only 50 öre (now approximately 10 cents), he suddenly decided on a medical career. While this decision was a great loss for music, it was an equally great gain for science.

During his student years he was a fanatic quartet player. It was natural, therefore, that he should select his wife from among those who shared his love for music. His wife is a professional harpsichord player who has taught at the Royal Academy of Music for many years.

Today Dr. Theorell is judged to be a fine violinist. He has played most of the first violin scores of the classical string quartet repertoire. His deep interest in providing fine music for others is evident from the fact that for many years he has been chairman of the Stockholm Academic Orchestra and the Stockholm Concert Association.

Dr. Theorell is well-endowed with a zest for living. Reports indicate that he is an intrepid boatman who seeks to fill his sails with a lusty wind until the sail-yards tremble. Many times he has been swept into the cold waters of the Stockholm archipelago as he struggled to learn the way of his vessel as it plowed through snarling seas. The many moods of the Baltic, the meeting of sky with earth, the aloneness of the expansive waters, the cadence of the heaving sea, and the quiet of the sun-sparkling calm are all music to his soul.

Professor Axel Hugo Theodor Theorell, scientist, musician, sailor, horticulturist, gastronomist, scholar, and friend, we your colleagues and friends salute you for your achievements and for what you are. We wish Margit and you many years of joyful health and satisfying achievement.

Tribute to Professor Theorell

E. C. SLATER

Professor Theorell,

It is a privilege and an honor to address you this evening on behalf of your fellow biochemists, particularly those interested in biological oxidations. Biological oxidoreductions—responsible as they are for the processes whereby the animal obtains energy from the food he eats and part of the air he breathes, and whereby the plant utilizes the energy of the sun to make food out of another part of the air and water—have long engaged the attention of great figures in biochemistry. Certainly one of the greatest, maybe the greatest of them all, Otto Warburg, was your teacher in Berlin-Dahlem more than 35 years ago.

You joined Warburg at a time when one of the glorious episodes in the history of the study of intracellular respiration—the discovery of the role of the hemoprotein electron carriers (the cytochromes)—was closing. The brilliant studies of Warburg on the photochemical absorption spectrum of the CO-compound of Atmungsferment, and the no less brilliant spectroscopic observations of Keilin on the cytochromes, had established the essential features of the oxygen end of the respiratory chain as we know it today. You arrived at Warburg's laboratory at the beginning of the period in which the second great series of discoveries were made. These discoveries form the basis of this symposium, the role of the nicotinamide- and flavin-containing nucleotides. Indeed, it was you who succeeded in crystallizing the old yellow enzyme, splitting it into its protein and nonprotein parts, and recombining them, and showing that the nonprotein prosthetic group is the phosphate ester of the vitamin riboflavin.

These findings, made during a short period in Berlin, were of tremendous importance. In the first place, the stoichiometry of the recombination—1 molecule of protein to 1 molecule of FMN—settled the long argument as to whether enzymes are protein or impurities adsorbed to protein. Secondly, FMN was the first example of a vitamin phosphoric ester being involved in an enzyme-catalyzed reaction. It was soon to be followed by the nicotinamide nucleotides, thiamine pyrophosphate, somewhat later by pyridoxal phosphate, and later still by coenzyme A. And of course the "old yellow enzyme," now called NADPH dehydrogenase, was only the first example of a whole class of oxidizing enzymes, the flavoproteins.

Since your return to Stockholm in 1935 there has been a continuous flow of papers of very high standard from the famous laboratory that you have led since 1936—the biochemical department of the Nobel Medical Institute. Although trained originally in medicine, your work is characterized by its rigorous chemical approach. Like all chemists, you like to work with purified, preferably crystalline, materials and to study a well-defined chemical reaction. You would not, I think, be happy to work with mitochondria or even submitochondrial particles that some of us are stuck with, by the very nature of the problem that we are investigating.

Your work falls naturally into three chapters—hemoproteins, flavoproteins, and alcohol dehydrogenase.

You had already crystallized and measured the molecular weight of myoglobin in Svedberg's laboratory in Uppsala before you joined Warburg, and after your return to Stockholm you extended your interest in hemoproteins to catalase, peroxidase, and cytochrome c. I know you best for your work on cytochrome c. You were the first to purify it thoroughly, removing a persistent impurity present in Keilin's preparation and your earlier preparations by electrophoresis, a procedure that you had used earlier and with great success in purifying the old yellow enzyme. You took grams of this purified preparation—unheard of in those days—to Linus Pauling's laboratory in California where you made one of the first detailed physical chemical examinations of an enzyme, published in a classical series of papers in the *Journal of the American Chemical Society*. You once told me an anecdote about this visit:

When you were entering America you had to declare several grams of cytochrome c with Customs. The difficulty was to classify it; for purified enzymes were something quite rare in those days. The Customs official patiently listened to a detailed description of how you made it—from so many hundred kilograms of heart tissue. The official entered it as *meat extract*.

Because of the deep color of hemoproteins, spectrophotometry is an obvious method of studying them, and you exploited this technique to the full in your work. But a unique feature of hemoproteins is that they contain iron. You and your student Anders Ehrenberg were the first to introduce magnetic methods into enzymology.

You were also the first to use fluorimetry in enzymology. You utilized the quenching of the fluorescence of FMN that occurs when it binds to the apoenzyme to study the binding of the prosthetic group.

But to return to cytochrome c: By studying the core left after pepsin digestion, you were able to determine the chemical structure of the protein in the region of the prosthetic group except for the methionine. Cytochrome c is a unique hemoprotein in that it is bound to the protein not only by coordinate bonds to the iron atoms, but by C—S covalent bonds between the vinyl side-chains and 2 cysteine molecules separated by two amino acids.

More recently, you have concentrated on alcohol dehydrogenase, an enzyme that is distinguished by heading the list drawn up by the Enzyme Nomenclature Commission of the International Union of Biochemistry and having as number EC 1.1.1.1. It also has a most interesting role in human affairs. In yeast it is the terminal catalyst in the series of reactions leading to the production of ethanol, the chemical that itself is so effective in catalyzing human interactions on an occasion like this. In liver its function is to get rid of the ethanol before its stimulating effect is replaced by a deadening effect. Finally, it is used by the police to determine whether we have consumed it more rapidly than our liver enzyme can cope with. *You* have used it as a model enzyme for studying the interactions between an enzyme and its two substrates, in this case ethanol (or acetaldehyde) and NAD^+ (or NADH). Here again you have used both spectrophotometric and fluorimetric methods, and Britton Chance introduced you to rapid-flow procedures. More recently, you have chosen alcohol dehydrogenase for a complete structural elucidation, which you promise to reveal at the International Congress of Biochemistry.

Naturally, what I have said about your work is not new to you, at least I hope that it is not, because that would mean that I have made a mistake. Perhaps you find it interesting, however, to hear what someone in the field, a good deal younger than yourself, considers to be the highlights of your work. Though some of the much younger ones here may perhaps be less familiar with some aspects of your work, they all know you as one of the great figures in biochemistry. As Otto Warburg's most distinguished student, you have carried on in his tradition, as well as in that of your great Swedish predecessors in physical chemistry and physical biochemistry—Berzelius, Svedberg, and Tiselius.

You and I have met far too seldom. Perhaps the old Warburg–Keilin controversy has something to do with this. But we have good friends in common—I am thinking particularly of Britton Chance—and so I know you well, from second hand. I have always greatly admired your achievements in biochemistry, and recently I have had reason to admire the way you are putting your warm personality and quiet humor to the cause of international cooperation in biochemistry as President of the International Union of Biochemistry.

After 34 years as head of the Department of Biochemistry of the Nobel

Medical Institute, you will soon retire. But a scientist is luckier than a banker, a doctor, a lawyer, or a dentist. He never really stops working, and retirement often means only a release from irksome administrative duties. Keilin worked in the laboratory for 12 years after his official retirement. I am sure that we shall hear from Hugo Theorell, both as biochemist and as President of the International Union of Biochemistry, long after his official retirement.

Dr. Harris has told us about your musical accomplishment. This surprised nobody. Anybody who has heard Hugo Theorell lecture knows that he is musical—because he sings rather than talks. But this is not the reason that you are a member of the Swedish Royal Academy of Music. You are a first-class violinist.

Professor Theorell, we wish you and Mrs. Theorell above all health during many active and happy years. Let us hear from you often as biochemist. May the time that you will win by being freed from administrative duties give you more opportunity to do also the other things you love, such as playing the violin. Let us hear this, too.

Historical Survey and Introductory Remarks

HUGO THEORELL

Medicinska Nobelinstitutet, Stockholm, Sweden

First, I would like to express my heartfelt and deep gratitude for the great honor you have bestowed upon me by inviting me to this symposium on a subject that has been my main interest for nearly 40 years. When in 1930 I defended my doctoral thesis in medicine at the Caroline Institute, it was still a matter of dispute whether the enzymes were proteins or comprised some other, still unknown, group. True enough, J. B. Sumner had crystallized urease from jack beans (1926) and had found the crystals to be of protein nature; but many, perhaps most, other biochemists had doubts about the enzymatic activity emanating from the colorless protein itself. The activity could have come from some minor impurity.

Even after Northrop's preparation (1930) of "a crystalline protein from a commercial pepsin preparation which appeared to be the enzyme pepsin" (quoted from Northrop's Nobel Lecture in 1946) the same objections were raised: How could enzymes be simply proteins produced in considerable quantities, when Willstätter had purified active peroxidase until the solutions gave *negative* analytical tests for proteins, carbohydrates, and iron? We found 15 years later in Stockholm that Willstätter's peroxidase actually contains all three of them.

Otto Warburg around 1925 had shown by his determinations of the photochemical activation spectrum of carbon monoxide-poisoned respiratory ferment that this was a hematin compound with an extra absorption band at 280 nm, indicating the functional participation of protein, but this was not regarded as definite proof that all enzymes are proteins or protein compounds. However, definite evidence was given in Warburg's institute in connection with his discovery of the "old yellow enzyme" in brewer's yeast. There is not time to go into details of the history of how the yellow dye was found by different groups of research workers in various biological materials (milk, egg white, yeast, and others), identified with vitamin B_2, and its constitution cleared up in the laboratories of Warburg, Karrer, and Kuhn. It is now called riboflavin.

The "old yellow enzyme" was prepared by Warburg and Christian from brewer's yeast and reported in 1933 to consist mainly of polysaccharides and some proteins. The yellow color was attached to some high molecular carrier and exerted a catalytic oxidoreduction function, being reduced to

151

the leuco form by a coenzyme–enzyme system from red blood cells and re-oxidized by oxygen. When I joined Warburg in the fall of 1933, I had had some previous experience in Sweden with electrophoresis methods, and I had some apparatus built in Dahlem—a smaller, analytical apparatus and a large preparative one. The chemical nature of the coenzyme from red blood cells was still unknown. I undertook to determine its electrophoretic mobility at different pH values by following the migration of the activity. The results proved it to be a phosphoric acid ester. We now call it "TPN," triphosphopyridine nucleotide. Warburg and Christian crystallized the active part as picrolonate in December, 1933. Because Warburg suspected that von Euler and Myrbäck were on the same track with their cozymase from yeast, he did not like my idea of going home to Stockholm for Christmas. He finally agreed, but advised me, "I am going to kill you if you mention the word 'picrolonic acid' in Stockholm." Warburg very soon had data on molecular weight, melting point, and elementary composition, but the structure remained difficult to determine because of the small amounts of material available. However, Warburg's friend, Professor Walter Schoeller, found the formula of nicotinic acid amide in a textbook; it had been synthesized some 50 years earlier, long before it was recognized as the antipellagra vitamin. How TPN interacts with enzymes remained unknown for some time.

Let us turn back to the "old yellow enzyme." In order to purify it, I submitted it to electrophoresis in a two-compartment apparatus, at a pH where the enzyme migrated cathodically into the next compartment, whereas neutral and acid polysaccharides remained in the anodic one. After repeated fractional precipitations with ammonium sulfate, we obtained a strongly yellow preparation that was nearly homogeneous in electrophoresis and showed signs of crystallizing. May I remind you that it took us 20 more years before we had really well-shaped crystals of practically 100% purity. The yellow color could be separated from the high molecular fraction after dialysis at slightly acid reaction and was found to be a colorless protein. The enzyme activity disappeared when the parts separated, but returned when they were recombined at neutral reaction. The yellow dye could not be riboflavin, which was much less active in restoring the activity than the natural dye, even though the absorption bands and fluorescence were identical. But there was one difference: the natural dye migrated as an acid in electrophoresis, whereas riboflavin was neutral. Could the "active group" of the old yellow enzyme be a phosphoric acid ester of riboflavin? I had no fresh material for an analysis except an old, heavily infected small quantity of solution that certainly no longer contained flavin—but I knew how much there had been. Yet, it could still be used for an elementary analysis of phosphorus.

I calculated how much there should be, assuming one P per mole of flavin. The result was 14 μg. I endured nervous hours until the result came from the analytical laboratory: 14 μg. There are golden moments in a scientist's life—but they are few.

The fact that enzymatic activity could be restored in a protein by the addition of *stoichiometric* quantities of a low molecular compound proved beyond doubt that at least this enzyme is a protein. We now know that this holds true for all other enzymes as well.

It was particularly interesting to notice that riboflavin, like nicotinic acid amide, is also a vitamin necessary for normal growth, and that both are functioning as "active groups" in enzymes. A great number of "pyridine" and flavin enzymes have since then been described. As a general, rule, pyridine enzymes take up hydrogen from substrates, and transfer the hydrogen to flavin enzymes. These often react with ferric hemin in cytochrome.

Very soon further members of the enzyme-cooperating vitamins group were found. Vitamin B_1 (the classical anti-beriberi factor) had been purified to some extent by Jansen and Donath in 1926, nearly purified by Windaus in 1931, and definitely characterized by crystallization, structure analysis, and synthesis in 1936 by R. R. Williams and Cline. In the following year Lohmann and Schuster proved that vitamin B_1 (or thiamine) in the form of pyrophosphate ester cooperates as active group, "cocarboxylase," with enzymes—for example, α-keto acid decarboxylases, α-keto oxidases, transketolases, and phosphoketolases.

Vitamin B_6 (pyridoxine) was purified, and its structure was established simultaneously in 1938 by five groups of research workers.

There are many enzymes that require pyridoxine, often as pyridoxal- or pyridoxamine phosphate, as coenzyme, as shown by the work, above all, of Braunstein in Soviet Russia and E. E. Snell in the United States. These enzymes are concerned with transaminations and oxidative decarboxylations.

Pantothenic acid was discovered and isolated as early as 1933 by R. J. Williams as a growth factor for yeast present in liver extracts. Most of the pantothenic acid in both animal tissues and microorganisms is built into a bigger molecule, coenzyme A, but it also occurs in other forms. Coenzyme A was discovered by Fritz Lipmann (1947). Snell demonstrated (1950) that its functional group is 2-mercaptoethylamine, which Feodor Lynen found in 1951 to form high energy thioesters with carboxylic acids; for example, acetic acid. The synthesis of fatty acids proceeds by the aid of fatty acid synthetases and acetyl coenzymes, adding the 2-carbon fragments stepwise to one another.

Other examples of vitamin compounds that function as prosthetic groups in enzymes: *Biotin* serves as a carrier of CO_2 in carboxylation reactions; in the holoenzymes the carboxyl group of biotin is bound by an amide link to ε-aminolysine in the protein. *Lipoic acid* is a coenzyme in reactions which generate or transfer acyl groups. *Folic acid* functions in transformylations, transmethylation, and transhydroxymethylation. *Cobalamin* (vitamin B_{12}), the most complicated of all vitamins, performs with its enzyme a most peculiar reaction, the rearrangement of methylmalonyl-CoA to its isomer succinyl-CoA. In addition, as we all remember, B_{12} is the specific cure of pernicious anemia.

It is obvious from this sketchy review that the old vitamin nomenclature —A, the vitamin against night blindness and xerophthalmia, fat soluble; B, against beriberi, water soluble; C, against scurvy, water soluble; and D, antirachitic, fat soluble—has proved itself unexpectedly realistic. A, C, and D are chemically remarkably homogeneous, in contrast to B, which contains a vast variety of chemical compounds that have one feature in common: they are all built into coenzymes that cooperate with enzymes in metabolic reactions. The A vitamins and the carotenes, like the B vitamins, cooperate with proteins, "opsins" in the retina, but are not completely analogous with the B vitamins.

The light-sensitive visual purple, rhodopsin, in the retina is a protein (opsin) conjugated with a carotenoid. Illumination converts it to a mixture of "retinene 1" and opsin. Retinene 1 is an aldehyde that can be reduced back to vitamin A_1 by an NADH-dependent dehydrogenase similar to liver alcohol dehydrogenase. Therefore, the vitamin A may be said to function as a substrate of a vitamin-B-dependent enzyme.

In summary, I think it is true to say that the topic of this symposium, "vitamin-dependent enzymes" could just as well have been called "vitamin B-dependent enzymes." If we now turn the question the other way around, asking: Are all the active groups in enzymes compounds of B vitamins?—the answer is, of course, "no."

Many reactions, for example hydrolytic ones, can be performed by pure proteins; others may require metal atoms in addition.

Among the hemoproteins we find a great variety of very important enzymes. What is the reason for porphyrins and hemins not being vitamins? I suppose the explanation is that hemin has not only catalytic functions that require only small quantities, which can comfortably be provided with the food, but also the transport function for oxygen in the hemoglobin, which requires larger quantities. I suppose some blood-sucking parasites may be dependent on an intake of heme; in this case it would be a B vitamin for them.

Let me take another example to illustrate how difficult it is to define a B vitamin as an essential nutrition factor used as building stone in the active group of an enzyme. In cytochrome *c* the electron transporting iron atom is attached by hexagonal bonds to the four pyrrole nitrogens of porphyrin, and by bond 5 to a histidine residue (No. 18) and bond 6 to a methionine residue (No. 80). This arrangement has been maintained throughout evolution from unicellular organisms to man, and it is therefore obviously indispensable for cytochrome c activity. In man methionine is an essential nutrition factor, histidine is not; in rat histidine is also essential. According to this, methionine should be regarded as a B vitamin for both man and rat, and histidine as a vitamin for rats but not for man.

Let us agree that it would be difficult to maintain the old terminology in such cases. It is, however, astonishing to remember that the old primitive alphabetic classification of vitamins B as the water-soluble ones has led to such a remarkable uniformity that all the classical B vitamins serve as active groups in coenzyme–enzyme systems, whereas this is not the case with vitamins A, C, or D.

Structure and Catalytic Role of the Functional Groups of Aspartate Aminotransferase

PAOLO FASELLA* AND CARLO TURANO†

Institute of Biochemistry, University of Parma, and Institute of Biological Chemistry, University of Perugia, and Center of Molecular Biology, C.N.R., Rome, Italy

I. INTRODUCTION

Aspartate aminotransferase (EC 2.6.1.1., L-aspartate:2-oxoglutarate aminotransferase; AAT) is a particularly interesting enzyme since its catalytic activity is duplicated, though with a much smaller efficiency, by its coenzyme moiety, even in the absence of the specific apoprotein (Snell, 1963). Available evidence (Jenkins and Sizer, 1957; Lis et al., 1960; Banks et al., 1963; Hammes and Fasella, 1962; Braunstein, 1964; Guirard and Snell, 1964) indicates that both the enzymatic and the model system operate according to the general mechanism proposed independently by Braunstein and by Snell for reactions involving pyridoxal phosphate (PLP). According to this hypothesis, transamination proceeds as shown in Fig. 1.

Extensive kinetic studies on the enzyme (Turano et al., 1960; Velick and Vavra, 1962; Hammes and Fasella, 1962; Banks et al., 1963; Henson and Cleland, 1964; Jenkins and D'Ari, 1966a; Fasella and Hammes, 1967) and on model systems (Snell, 1963; Jencks and Cordes, 1963; Bruice and Topping, 1963; Martell, 1963) indicate that, even though the general pattern is the same, the reaction rates are at least 10^6 times greater in the enzymatic than in the model system. Moreover, the enzy-

* Present address: Instituto di Biochimica, Università di Parma, Borgo Carissimi 10, Parma, Italy.
† Present address: Instituto di Chimica Biologica, Università, Perugia.

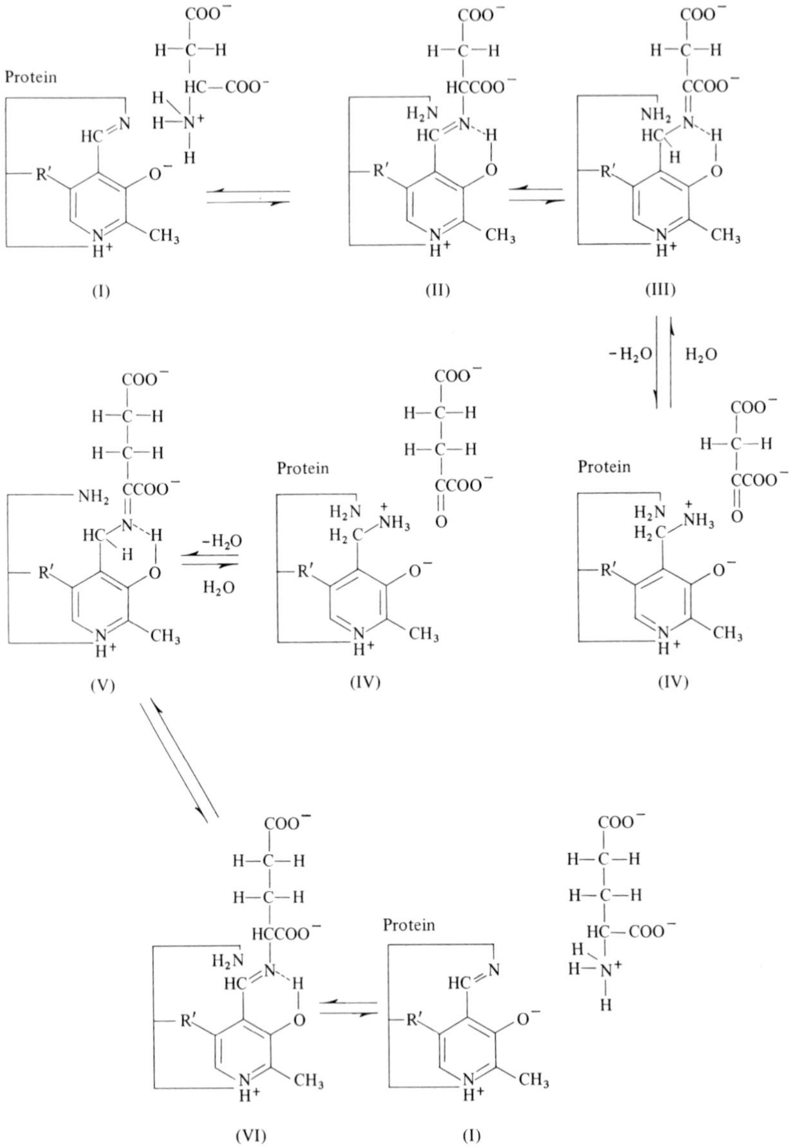

Fig. 1. Enzymic transamination. I = aldimine form of the free enzyme; II = aldimine complex between the enzyme and the four carbon substrate; III = ketimine complex between the enzyme and the four carbon substrate; IV = aminic form of the free enzyme; V = ketimine complex between the enzyme and the five carbon substrate; VI = aldimine complex between enzyme and the five carbon substrate.

matic reaction seems to proceed through a greater number of discrete steps (Fasella and Hammes, 1967; Jenkins and Taylor, 1965; Braunstein, 1970). Finally, the enzyme displays a marked substrate specificity, which is lacking in the model system (Novogrodsky and Meister, 1964; Jenkins and Sizer, 1959; Lis et al., 1960).

Evidently, it is the protein moiety that is responsible for both the specificity and the extreme efficiency of the holoenzyme.

In the present paper we shall first examine the mode of binding of the coenzyme to the apoprotein and discuss how binding may affect the functional properties of the coenzyme. We shall then deal with the reaction between the holoenzyme and the substrates and with the transformations undergone by the enzyme–substrate complex. For each step we shall consider the functional groups of the protein and of the coenzyme involved, the static and dynamic aspects of their disposition in space, and their role in catalysis.

It will not be possible to offer a complete survey of the evergrowing literature on AAT; however, the authors feel that this limitation is not serious in consideration of the many recent reviews of the field (Guirard and Snell, 1964; Ivanov and Karpeisky, 1969; Braunstein, 1970; Fasella, 1968).

Essentially all the material presented in this paper refers to the cytoplasmic isozyme of AAT from pig heart.

II. The Assembly of the Holoenzyme

A. The Binding of the Coenzyme to the Protein

The active site in AAT is formed by the union of the protein moiety and the coenzyme; the nature of the functional groups of each of these components, which participate in the assembling of the active site, is examined below.

As suggested by Koshland's induced-fit theory (1958) and as confirmed by extensive experimental evidence, enzymatic active sites assume their functioning conformations only when the substrates are bound to the enzyme; it is important to point out, therefore, that in this section we shall refer only to those functional groups responsible for the formation of the AAT-holoenzyme. In Section III we discuss the formation of the active site proper, formed by the interaction of holoenzyme and substrate.

The specific binding of the coenzyme to the apo-AAT confers on the coenzyme some characteristic chemical and physicochemical properties: typical UV and visible absorption spectra, a low quantum yield of fluorescence, optical rotatory activity, unusual pK's and a particular chemical reactivity; most of these properties have been exploited for the study of the active site structure; other information has been derived from the use of coenzyme analogs and from studying the effects of chemical modifications of the protein. However, the picture of the active site is still far from complete, and probably will be offered in all its details only by future X-ray diffraction analysis.

1. Coenzyme Groups Involved in the Binding

It has been known for several years (Meister et al., 1954) that both pyridoxal 5'-phosphate (PLP) and pyridoxamine 5'-phosphate (PMP) can act as coenzyme for AAT; these two forms of the coenzyme are interconverted during the normal catalytic process (Jenkins and Sizer, 1957; Lis et al., 1960). PLP and PMP differ uniquely for the substituent in position 4 on the pyridine ring, which is an aldehyde group for PLP and an aminomethyl group for PMP. This chemical difference is reflected, as will be discussed later, in the equilibrium constants for binding to the apoenzyme; however, both forms of the holoenzyme can be isolated, and neither of them can be appreciably resolved by acetone precipitation, dialysis, or gel filtration at pH values around neutrality (Lis et al., 1960; Jenkins and D'Ari, 1966a); this shows that the common part of the molecule of PLP and PMP is the one most important for binding to the apoprotein.

Actually, there is not a single functional group of the coenzyme that is solely responsible for the attachment of the coenzyme to the protein; binding results from a multiplicity of interactions, which jointly give origin to the active site, provided with full catalytic efficiency. As shown by the use of coenzyme analogs, the modification or the abolition of some of the coenzymatic functional groups does not always preclude binding to the apoenzyme; however, in many cases the resulting complex has a very low catalytic efficiency (Wada and Snell, 1962; Hullar, 1969; Furbish et al., 1969; Braunstein, 1970). In this connection, it is interesting that in at least one case an analog of PLP (2-nor-PLP) forms a holoenzyme that is appreciably more active than the natural one (Mühlradt et al., 1967; Braunstein, 1970).

The role of the phosphate group in the binding has long been recognized (Snell, 1958) not only for AAT, but for many other B6-dependent enzymes as well. Usually, the nonphosphorylated coenzyme derivatives are not bound by the apoenzymes, or are bound with a significantly decreased affinity (Snell, 1958). More recently it has been shown (Wada and Snell, 1962) that AAT binds the nonphosphorylated forms of the coenzymes, since a relatively slow transamination occurs between pyridoxal (PL) and an amino acid substrate, or between pyridoxamine (PM) and a keto acid substrate in the presence of apo-AAT. The energetic contribution of the phosphate group to the binding is difficult to calculate, because PL and PM have rather high dissociation constants, whereas PLP and PMP have such low ones that their binding seems practically irreversible, at least at moderate ionic strength and at pH around neutrality. The contribution of the phosphate group to the standard free energy of binding ($\Delta F°$), in the usual temperature range, has been estimated to be at least -4–5 kcal/mole (Braunstein, 1964; Snell and Ayling, 1968). According to gel filtration experiments (Turano et al., 1969), the dissociation constant for PL is higher than $2 \times 10^{-4} M$ at pH 8.4 in 0.04 M triethanolamine-HCl buffer, while under the same conditions the K_{diss} for PLP is probably less than 10^{-10} to $10^{-11} M$. It is therefore reasonable to assume that, under the above conditions, the lower limit of the energetic contribution of the phosphate group to the binding can be considered to be around -8 kcal/mole, even taking into account the fact that PL exists in solution partially as a poorly binding hemiacetal. A more accurate calculation of this value could be obtained in an enzyme, tyrosine aminotransferase (TAT) from rat liver, which is particularly suitable to this type of study because its coenzyme binding constants fall in a range amenable to accurate measurement. With this enzyme the contribution of phosphate to the $\Delta F°$ of binding, at 37°, is -6–7 kcal/mole (Turano et al., 1970a; Borri-Voltattorni and Turano, 1970).

The existence of a phosphate binding site in AAT (and in TAT) is confirmed by the fact that the inorganic phosphate competitively inhibits the recombination of the coenzyme with the apoprotein, apparently by combining at the active site (Banks et al., 1963; Hayashi et al., 1967); the $\Delta F°$ at 37° for the formation of the phosphate-apo TAT complex is -3.4 kcal/mole (Borri-Voltattorni and Turano, 1970).

Electrostatic effects are probably important in phosphate binding (Braunstein, 1964; Guirard and Snell, 1964). However, the formation of a covalent bond is not excluded, as will be discussed later.

The properties have been examined of a number of PLP derivatives having a modified side chain in position 5, e.g., phosphonic acid analogs, 5'-carboxymethyl-5-deoxypyridoxal, methylphosphonic acid of PLP, 5'-methyl-PLP (Bocharov et al., 1968; Hullar, 1969; Furbish et al., 1969).

All these compounds bind, but the resulting holoenzymes are inactive or much less active than the natural enzyme.

The importance of the aldehydic group of PLP for the binding to the apoenzyme is now well established, not only for AAT, but also for all the PLP enzymes that have been studied so far. The spectrum of enzyme-bound PLP, typical of a Schiff base of PLP, led Jenkins and Sizer (1957) to postulate the existence of an aldimine bond between the coenzyme and a group on the protein. This finding has been confirmed, and the nature of this bond has been proved by the identification of ϵ-N-pyridoxyllysine among the products of the complete acid hydrolysis of the enzyme that had been reduced with sodium borohydride (Fischer and Krebs, 1959). A partial enzymatic hydrolysis of the reduced enzyme has allowed the isolation of a pyridoxyl peptide, the sequence of which has been studied (Hughes et al., 1962; Polyanovsky and Keil, 1963; Morino and Watanabe, 1969).

An attempt to evaluate the energetic contribution of the aldimine bond to the binding can be made by comparing the relative affinities of PLP and PMP for the apoenzyme; this approach, however, is based on the nondemonstrated assumption that the aminomethyl side chain in position 4 of PMP does not contribute to binding.

Wada and Snell (1962) and Scardi et al. (1963) have shown that the resolution of the PMP-holoenzyme is achieved much more easily than that of the PLP-holoenzyme, as expected on the basis of the above considerations.

Also, it has been shown (Turano et al., 1964) that in modified preparations of AAT (i.e., with SH groups blocked), which have undergone a conformational change (Polyanovsky and Torchinsky, 1963), PMP dissociates from the holoenzyme at concentrations of about $1 \times 10^{-5} M$ or less, while under the same conditions PLP remains bound: this shows that the two coenzymes have a marked difference in affinity for the apoprotein.

An evaluation of the contribution of the aldimine bond to the ΔF° for coenzyme binding to the TAT apoenzyme can be made by comparing the affinity constants for PLP with those for PMP and for pyridoxine 5'-phosphate.* This value is of the order of about -2–3 kcal/mole at $37°$. Pyridoxine 5'-phosphate binds slightly better than PMP, possibly because in the latter case some electrostatic repulsion occurs between the positively charged amino groups of PMP and of the lysyl residue at the active site.

Various lines of evidence indicate that the coenzyme might bind to the protein also through the pyridine ring: (i) the coenzyme fluorescence is strongly quenched in the holoenzyme, suggesting an interaction between the protein and the chromophoric ring (Fasella et al., 1961); in this respect, it is important to note that the quantum yield of PM is lowered

---

* The true equilibrium binding constants of PLP and PMP to apoTAT have been calculated (Borri-Voltattorni and Turano, 1970) on the basis of the kinetic treatment proposed by Litwack and Cleland (1968). The equilibrium binding constant for pyridoxine 5'-phosphate has been calculated from competitive inhibition studies.

in a nonpolar solvent (Turano et al., 1970b). (ii) Wada and Snell (1962) have demonstrated that PM is capable of binding to the apoenzyme; (iii) finally, also pyridoxine has been shown to bind to the apoenzyme; a $\Delta F°$ at 37° for the formation of its complex with the apoenzyme of about —3 kcal/mole has been found (Turano et al., 1969).*

A desolvation of the aromatic ring, through the binding to a hydrophobic region of the protein, appears to be a logical explanation for this interaction, considering the positive $\Delta H°$ for the formation of the pyridoxine apoenzyme complex (4–5 kcal/mole) and the positive entropy change (20–30 e.u.) (Turano et al., 1969). A similar view has been expressed by Scardi and Marino (1968) in consideration of the strong affinity for apo-AAT displayed by other nonpolar compounds, i.e., estrogen derivatives. The possible existence of a hydrogen bond between the pyridine nitrogen and a group on the protein has been considered by Braunstein (1970) and is discussed later.

As far as the role of substituents on the pyridine ring is concerned, substituents in the 3 (phenolic OH) and the 2 (CH_3) positions do not seem to have a primary importance for binding: thus Furbish et al. (1969) have shown that O-methyl-PLP binds efficiently to the apoenzyme (although it gives origin to a scarcely active holoenzyme) while Mühlradt et al. (1967), Bocharov et al. (1968), and Ivanov and Karpeisky (1969) have demonstrated that coenzyme derivatives modified in position 2 bind very strongly to the apoenzyme forming active holoenzymes. Kinetic studies of the reaction between the apoenzyme and the coenzyme derivatives carrying aliphatic substituents of increasing length on carbon 2 are strongly suggestive of a hydrophobic interaction of these groups with the protein (Bocharov et al., 1968); however, also 2-nor-PLP, which lacks entirely a substituent in 2, binds very strongly to the apoenzyme (Mühlradt et al., 1967; Ivanov and Karpeisky, 1969).

2. Protein Groups Involved in the Binding

The first amino acid side chain to be identified with certainty as being present at the coenzyme binding site has been that of a lysine which, as mentioned in the previous section, forms a covalent bond with PLP, participating in the formation of a Schiff base. A chemical modification of the ε-amino group of this lysine (thereafter called the carbonyl-binding lysine) in the apoenzyme, which can be achieved by a mild treatment

---

* This has been calculated from the value of the equilibrium constant, determined as the competitive inhibition constant of pyridoxine relative to PM in the transamination reaction between PM and ketoglutarate catalyzed by the apoenzyme.

with acetic anhydride, not only leads to a complete inactivation of the enzyme, but prevents the formation of the PLP-apoenzyme complex (Torchinsky, 1963; Turano et al., 1967); since the aldimine bond, as mentioned before, is not essential for binding, this inhibition of recombination should be caused by steric reasons. In this connection, it is noteworthy that this critical ε-amino group, while very reactive in the apoenzyme, is partially masked toward many modifying reagents in the PMP form of the holoenzyme; e.g., it cannot be easily acetylated (Turano et al., 1967). It is conceivable that in the PMP enzyme the approach of the reagent to the lysyl amino group is sterically inhibited by the presence of the coenzyme.

The reduction of PLP-holoenzyme with borohydride, and the subsequent partial hydrolysis of the protein has allowed the study of the amino acid residues adjacent to the PLP-bound lysine. The studies of Hughes et al. (1962), Polyanovsky and Keil (1963), and Morino and Watanabe (1969) have revealed that a seryl residue and an asparaginyl residue are situated close to the lysine in the polypeptidic chain. Some uncertainty, however, remains about the exact sequence near the carbonyl binding lysine, which, according to Hughes et al. (1962), is

PLP
|
(Asp, Gly, Ala, Val, Ile, Lys, Lys) Gly-Ser-Asp-Phe

according to Polyanovsky and Keil (1963) is

PLP
|
Lys-Ser-Asn-Phe

and according to Morino and Watanabe (1969) is

PLP
|
Ser-Lys-Asn-Phe

The possible role of these amino acids in the constitution of active site is unknown; however, it is important to note that also in the mitochondrial isozyme of AAT an asparagine residue is contiguous to the PLP-binding lysyl residue (Morino and Watanabe, 1969).

Since different subforms of AAT have been separated (Martinez-Carrion et al., 1967a) it is known that the enzyme can exist also in an inactive form; this has the PLP bound in an abnormal way, which gives origin to an absorption band at 340 nm. Similar spectral and chemical characteristics are found in glycogen phosphorylase, for which the following mode of PLP binding has been postulated (Kent et al., 1958):

where X is a still unidentified nucleophilic group contributed by the protein.

A similar structure might be present in the inactive AAT fraction; also in this case, however, the identity of the hypothetical X group is unknown.

The resolution of the enzyme at high ionic strength and the findings that negatively charged side chains other than phosphate in position 5 of the coenzyme may contribute to the binding, suggest that electrostatic interactions between the coenzyme phosphate group and positively charged groups on the protein are important. A lysyl or an arginyl side chain should therefore be present at the active site, besides the previously mentioned carbonyl-binding lysyl residue. However, according to the latest results reported by Morino and Watanabe (1969), no positively charged residue is found adjacent to this lysine in terms of primary structure. The positively charged residues of the protein which presumably interact with the coenzyme phosphate group must therefore be brought into the active site by folding of the peptide chain.

Acetylation and dinitrophenylation experiments on AAT before and after removal of the coenzyme show that the only amino group that is unmasked upon resolution of the holoenzyme is the one that forms the Schiff base with PLP (Turano et al., 1967); this might indicate that, if an ionic bond is formed at the phosphate binding site, it should involve an arginine rather than a lysine residue of the protein.

The possible existence of a covalent ester bond between the phosphate and an amino acid side chain should also be considered, as first suggested by Vernon (1970). It is noteworthy that such an ester bond could co-exist with the electrostatic interactions mentioned above. In this connection it is interesting that when apo-AAT reacts with phosphopyridoxyl-glutamic acid, an analog of the coenzyme–substrate complex, the enzyme is irreversibly inhibited, one threonine residue on the protein becomes phosphorylated, and the bond between the phosphate group and pyridoxal glutamate is split (Khomutov et al., 1969). This finding is important because it shows that, at least under particular conditions, a phosphoric ester bond between the coenzyme and a protein residue at the active site can indeed be formed.

The positive standard enthalpy change for the binding of phosphate in TAT (Turano *et al.*, 1970a) is also consistent with an ester bond formation.

Besides the carbonyl-binding lysine residue and the threonine possibly interacting with the phosphate group, also a tyrosine residue appears to be involved in coenzyme binding. Chemical modifications which are known to affect the tyrosine side chains (iodination, acetylation with acetyl imidazole, nitration with tetranitromethane) completely inhibit the apoenzyme but have much less marked effects on the holoenzyme (Turano *et al.*, 1968a). The strongest evidence for the involvement of a tyrosine residue comes from the use of tetranitromethane, which, under particular conditions, modifies one tyrosine residue and one SH group of the apoenzyme; this modified apoenzyme is unable to bind PLP. Kinetic studies indicate that the latter effect is due to the modification of the tyrosine residue, since the inactivation of the apoenzyme parallels modification of the tyrosine group, while the —SH group loss occurs much faster (Turano *et al.*, 1968b, 1970c).

Further evidence for the presence of a tyrosine at the active site is provided by the finding that the attachment of PLP to the apoenzyme induces the appearance of a Cotton effect in the tyrosine absorption region, and that this Cotton effect is sensitive to changes in the functional state of AAT (Ivanov and Karpeisky, 1969). Moreover, nitration of a single tyrosine in the holoenzyme shifts the tyrosine Cotton effect to a longer wavelength, corresponding to the absorption band of nitrated tyrosine (Ivanov and Karpeisky, 1969). The nitration of a tyrosine in the holoenzyme is greatly accelerated in the presence of substrates (Christen and Riorden, 1969); under these conditions PLP is probably displaced from its original position; this could leave the tyrosine at the active site in an environment more favorable to chemical modification.

Finally, evidence for the presence of a tyrosine at the PLP-binding site comes from the use of a bifunctional reagent: in the apoenzyme, 1,5-difluoro-2,4-dinitrobenzene crosslinks the lysine amino group at the active site and the phenolic hydroxyl of a tyrosine (Turano *et al.*, 1968b).

According to Ivanov and Karpeisky (1969) and Braunstein (1970), the tyrosine at the active site is hydrogen bonded, through its phenolic OH, to the pyridine nitrogen of the coenzyme; an argument in favor of this view is the occurrence of a change in the previously mentioned tyrosine Cotton effect when PLP is replaced by its *N*-oxide derivative, which should be incapable of forming the postulated hydrogen bond (Ivanov and Karpeisky, 1969).

Chemical modification of one (or two) histidine residues inactivates the enzyme (Martinez-Carrion *et al.*, 1967b; Vorotniskaya *et al.*, 1968).

Evidence to be discussed later indicates that inactivation is due to an impairment of the transformation of the bound substrate and not to interference with coenzyme binding (Martinez-Carrion, 1969).

Blocking the sulfhydryl groups also inactivates AAT (Polyanovsky and Torchinsky, 1963; Turano et al., 1963); the inactivated enzyme is still capable of binding the coenzyme though much less tightly (Turano et al., 1964). This effect is probably connected with the conformational change induced by this treatment (Polyanosky and Torchinsky, 1963), rather than with a direct participation of the SH groups in the binding.

3. The Dynamics of Binding

The kinetics of the reaction between PLP and the apoenzyme are potentially very interesting but quite complicated.

Various factors contribute to this complexity, e.g., specific and nonspecific effects of the buffer ions (Banks et al., 1963), differences among the enzyme subforms (Martinez-Carrion et al., 1967a; Banks et al., 1968c), dependence upon enzyme concentration (Banks et al., 1968b), and the multiplicity of steps through which the reaction takes place (Churchirch, and Farrelly, 1968; Severin and Dixon, 1968; Arrio-Dupont, 1969). In general, available evidence indicates that the rates for the reaction between apo and coenzyme are much lower than those for the binding and transformation of the substrates.

B. STRUCTURAL AND FUNCTIONAL PROPERTIES OF THE BOUND COENZYME

It is evident from the preceding discussion that the picture of the coenzyme-apoenzyme interaction in AAT is still incomplete; some definite conclusions, however, can be drawn. The specific binding of the coenzymes to the protein takes place through multiple interactions, which cooperate to give a highly stable holoenzyme. The phosphate group has clearly an important role in binding, possibly through electrostatic interaction with a protein positive charge and/or through an ester bond with a protein hydroxyl. The pyridine ring probably fits in a hydrophobic pocket of the protein, and may form a hydrogen bond with a tyrosine side chain, the presence of which at the active site is indicated by a large number of experimental observations. Finally, the aldehydic group of one form of the coenzyme, PLP, is bound covalently, through an aldimine bond, to an amino group of a lysine side chain.

A tentative evaluation of the energetic contribution of these different interactions is summarized in Table I.

It is important to stress the approximate nature of the data reported in Table I, not only because most of them are derived from the study of another transaminase (TAT), but also because the $\Delta F°$ for the binding

TABLE I

STANDARD FREE ENERGY CHANGE FOR THE FORMATION OF THE COENZYME-
APOENZYME COMPLEX; CONTRIBUTION OF THE DIFFERENT
COENZYME FUNCTIONAL GROUPS

Group	$-\Delta F°$ (kcal/mole) at 37°C
Phosphate	7–8
Pyridine ring	2–3
Aldehydic group	2–3
PLP	11–14
PMP	9–11

of a single functional group is strongly dependent on the rest of the molecule of which it is a part.

However, the data listed in Table I give an idea of the relative importance of the different functional groups.

It has been noticed that many coenzyme analogs, capable of binding to the apoprotein, give origin to holoenzymes with poor or no catalytic activity (see Section III). This lack of activity is, in some cases, an obvious consequence of the absence of a group directly involved in catalysis (e.g., pyridoxine 5′-phosphate lacks the aldehydic function in position 4). With other analogs, the scarce activity of the resulting holoenzyme has suggested the possibility that coenzyme groups previously thought not to be important in catalysis, e.g., the phosphate group, could, to some extent, be involved in the transformation of the substrate (Furbish et al., 1969). In interpreting these results the possibility should also be considered that the inactivity of the holoenzyme obtained with a coenzyme analog may be due to geometrical factors such as an unfavorable relative orientation of the coenzyme and protein functional groups; even small structural changes in the coenzyme could impair its proper fitting to the protein. In this connection, some experimental evidence suggests that a conformational change of AAT upon coenzyme binding does indeed take place. Optical rotatory dispersion (Fasella and Hammes, 1965), hydrogen-deuterium exchange (Abaturov et al., 1968) and the postulated "two step" nature of the PLP binding reaction (Banks et al., 1963; Churchich and Farrelly, 1968), all seem to indicate the occurrence of a conformational change; similarly, in the case of TAT, the very large increase in standard entropy upon coenzyme binding (more than 70 e.u.) is rather difficult to explain without assuming a structural modification of the protein (Borri-Voltattorni and Turano, 1970).

The specific interactions taking place at the active center of AAT between the protein and the coenzyme provide the latter with some properties which are not found in the free coenzyme, and which undoubtedly contribute to the remarkable catalytic activity of the enzyme. The possible functional advantage of having the 4' carbon of the co-enzyme bound as a Schiff base to the protein is illustrated by Jencks' studies with model systems, showing that a Schiff base is more reactive than a carbonyl toward amino groups (Jencks and Cordes, 1963). The coenzyme-protein Schiff base has peculiar characteristics which make it in many respects different from the Schiff bases of model systems. The position of the absorption maxima [362 nm for the nonprotonated form, and 430 nm for the form with a protonated imino nitrogen hydrogen bonded to the phenolate group in the 3 position (Jenkins and Sizer, 1957; Martell, 1963)] is somewhat different from that of the corresponding model compounds, probably because of the particular environment provided by the protein or of a strain created by multiple binding. More-over, binding to the protein induces optical activity in the coenzyme ab-sorption bands (Torchinsky and Koreneva, 1963; Fasella and Hammes, 1965). Another pecularity is the exceptionally low pK of the imino nitrogen ($pK = 6.2$), which could be partly explained by a protonation of the ring nitrogen induced by the protein tyrosine residue at the active site (Braunstein, 1970); an additional factor could be the presence of a hypothetical positively charged group of the protein in the proximity of the phenolate in position 3 of the coenzyme (Braunstein, 1970). As will be discussed later, the lowering of the pK for the imino nitrogen may have important functional consequences.

In the holoenzyme, a steric strain might be exerted on the phosphate ester bond of the coenzyme, as suggested by Braunstein (1964) on the basis of the relatively easy splitting of this bond during the treatment of the enzyme with borohydride. Consistent with the hypothesis of a strained conformation of bound PLP are the slow, diphasic formation of the fully active PLP-holoenzyme described by Churchich and Farrelly (1968) and the finding that inorganic phosphate inhibits the reversible transamination between PL and amino acids catalyzed by cytoplasmic apo AAT (Wada and Snell, 1962). This strained conformation of the bound coenzyme could be relevant for catalysis, according to current ideas on the mech-anism of enzyme action (Jencks, 1966; Vallee and Williams, 1968). A conformational strain might also contribute to the movements or trans-locations that the coenzyme undergoes in the course of catalysis, accord-ing to the mechanism proposed by Ivanov and Karpeisky (1969).

III. The Interaction between the Holoenzyme and the Substrate

It is convenient to consider first the formation of the enzyme–substrate Schiff bases, compounds (II), (III), (V), and (VI) in Fig. 1, and then their interconversion. This distinction is, to some extent, arbitrary because in the enzyme system both the formation of the enzyme–substrate Schiff bases and their transformation are multistage processes and many of the enzyme functional groups are involved in both. However, a separate treatment helps in the recognition of the actual role of the various participating groups and in evaluating the importance of their spatial relationships.

A. FORMATION OF THE ENZYME–SUBSTRATE COMPLEXES

The formation of Schiff bases between the protein-bound coenzyme and the substrates, first postulated on theoretical grounds and by analogy with model reactions (Guirard and Snell, 1964; Braunstein, 1964) has been proved both by a study of the spectral properties of the enzyme-substrate complexes (Jenkins and Taylor, 1965; Jenkins and D'Ari, 1966a; Fasella and Hammes, 1967) and by the isolation of pyridoxyl-amino acid derivatives from the digests of enzyme preparations that had been treated with sodium borohydride when saturated with the substrates (Riva *et al.*, 1964; Malakhova and Torchinsky, 1965). According to Fig. 1, two cases should be considered, namely the formation of the aldimine complexes (II) and (VI) and that of the ketimine complexes (III) and (V). The former case has been studied in much greater detail, essentially because of the availability of suitable substrate analogs.

1. *Formation of the Enzyme–Substrate Aldimine Complexes*

This step has been studied by a variety of approaches: steady-state kinetics, study of the competitive inhibition by substrate analogs, spectral analyses of enzyme-substrate and enzyme–analog complexes at equilibrium and by fast reaction kinetics, specific chemical modifications of the coenzyme and protein molecule. The information relative to the substrate and enzyme groups involved in the reaction will be considered first. Successively, we shall deal with the dynamics of the process.

a. Substrate Groups Involved in Binding to the Active Site. The natural substrates for the aldimine enzyme are L-α-amino acids having a straight chain of 4 to 5 carbon atoms and a negatively charged group in the ω position. Studies with substrate analogs (for a review, see Fasella, 1968) indicate what all the characteristic groups of the substrates (i.e., the α-carboxylate, the α-amino, and the ω-carboxylate) contribute to the binding, though none of them is indispensable. Thus, for instance, hydroxylamine, cyanide, and thiosemicarbazide, which can be considered analogs of the substrate amino groups because of their capacity to react with the 4' carbon of the coenzyme, bind to the active site even though they do not possess the carboxylate groups (Sizer and Jenkins, 1963). Some amino acids, e.g., L-alanine (Jenkins, 1961a) and L-serine and L-methionine (Novogrodsky and Meister, 1964), which do not contain the ω-carboxyl-ate, do bind at the active site, forming a Schiff base with the coenzyme, even though their affinity constants are much lower than those for the real substrates.

That both carboxylate groups, however, contribute to binding is shown by the fact that dicarboxylic acids having a molecular geometry similar to that of the substrates act as powerful competitive inhibitors.

b. *Enzyme Groups Involved in Binding.* Although it is reasonable to suppose that each of the three substrate groups involved in binding inter-acts with a definite group on the enzyme molecule, only one of the bonds has been identified with precision, namely, the aldimine linkage between the substrate amino group and the coenzyme 4′ carbon. It is generally thought that the formation of the enzyme–substrate aldimine is facilitated by the fact that, in the holoenzyme, the 4′carbon is bound as a Schiff base to an amino group of the protein. However, Tate and Meister (1969) have recently shown that N-methylpyridoxal 5′-phosphate can bind to apo-L-aspartate-ω decarboxylase without forming this type of binding. The resulting holoenzyme is capable of catalyzing transamination slightly more efficiently than the natural aldiminic holoenzyme formed with PLP. The holoenzyme obtained with N-methylpyridoxal 5′-phosphate catalyzes also the decarboxylation of L-aspartate, but much less efficiently than the natural holoenzyme; moreover, the artificial enzyme catalyzes equally well the decarboxylation of the D and L stereoisomers of aspartate. This suggests that, at least in the case of L-aspartate-ω-decarboxylase, the formation of the coenzyme-protein Schiff base markedly contributes to specificity but is not an absolute requirement for catalytic activity. The evidence of the formation of the coenzyme-substrate aldimine bond has been discussed in a previous paragraph.

pH dependence studies show that carbonyl reagents (hydroxylamine, thiosemicarbazide, etc.) bind more strongly to the protein-bound co-enzyme when the latter is protonated (Jenkins and D'Ari, 1966b; Hammes and Fasella, 1963) ; conversely, the natural amino acid substrates and their analog α-methyl aspartate react preferentially with the non-protonated aldimine enzyme. The cause of this difference in the pH dependence of binding for the two classes of derivatives must probably be sought in the contribution to binding of the carboxylate groups of the dicarboxylic amino acid substrates and in the different pK's of the carbonyl reagents used. Some hypotheses have been made concerning the positively charged groups of the enzyme which are presumably interact-ing with the substrate carboxylates. Velick and Vavra (1962) have pro-posed that the ω-carboxylate of the substrate might form electrostatic interactions with the ring nitrogen of the coenzyme. Geometric reasons, however, make this seem unlikely, particularly for the 4-carbon substrates.

On the basis of studies with dicarboxylic acids analogs of the substrate, Jenkins and D'Ari (1966c) have suggested that one of the carboxylate groups of the substrate may bind to the protonated aldimine nitrogen, which corresponds to the ϵ-lysine amino group binding the pyridoxal phosphate. Fasella *et al.* (1966) have proposed that this electrostatic interaction with the substrate α-carboxylate might favor the transfer of a proton from the substrate amino group to the internal aldimine nitrogen. Ivanov and Karpeisky (1969) have postulated a similar but somewhat more complicated mechanism, which requires the existence of a positively charged protein residue in the proximity of the coenzyme–protein azomethinic nitrogen. This hypothetical positively charged group would be responsible for the unusually low pK of the azomethinic nitrogen in the holoenzyme ($pK = 6.2$ in the holoenzyme *vs.* $pK = 10$ in model Schiff bases between PLP and amino acids). The negatively charged carboxylate group of the substrate would bind to this positively charged group of the protein, and thus neutralize its effects on the pK of the neighboring coenzyme-protein azomethinic nitrogen. The latter would then acquire a proton assuming an electronic structure more suitable for a transaldimination reaction with the substrate amino group. This electrostatic interaction between the substrate carboxylate and the positively charged group on the enzyme would favor the transaldimination reaction also by another effect: the neutralization of the negative charge on the carboxylate group of the substrate should decrease the pK of the neighboring α-amino group, which, by losing a proton, would acquire a nonshared electron pair necessary for a nucleophilic attack on the coenzyme $4'$ carbon. This would lead to a situation which, according to Jencks and Cordes (1963), is the most suitable for transaldimination: i.e., a protonated azomethine and a nonprotonated amino group.

In support of this view is the finding that the binding of dicarboxylic acids to the holoenzyme does indeed raise the pK of the coenzyme–protein aldimine (Jenkins and Sizer, 1959; Velick and Vavra, 1962; Hammes and Fasella, 1963).

The amino group of a lysyl residue formerly thought to be adjacent to the pyridoxal binding lysine has often been considered as a possible site for binding one of the carboxylates of the substrate. However, as reported above, recent chemical analyses exclude the existence of this group (Morino and Watanabe, 1969).

In keeping with the interactions among the various substrate groups involved in binding, proposed by Fasella *et al.* (1966) and by Ivanov and Karpeisky (1969), is the fact that γ-aminobutyric acid, which differs from the real substrates only because it lacks the α-carboxylic group, is unable to react with the aldimine enzyme (Fasella, 1970).

A direct experimental approach to the problem of the interactions in the binding of the substrate carboxylate and amino groups has been attempted by Jenkins and D'Ari (1966b), who studied the binding of thiosemicarbazide (an analog of the substrate amino group) to the aldimine enzyme in the presence of a dicarboxylic acid (glutarate). It was found that, although thiosemicarbazone formation is favored when the enzyme is in the protonated form, the increase of pK for this protonation induced by the binding of glutarate does not increase the equilibrium constant for thiosemicarbazone formation. This would seem to indicate that the protonation of the coenzyme induced by the carboxylate moiety of the amino acid substrates does not necessarily favor the formation of the enzyme–substrate Schiff base. However, as pointed out by Jenkins and D'Ari (1966b), the possibility of steric hindrance between thiosemicarbazide and glutarate, as well as the difference in the pK of thiosemicarbazide and of the substrate amino group should be considered when interpreting these data.

A substrate analog which is very suitable to the study of the formation of the enzyme-substrate Schiff base is α-methyl aspartate, which closely reproduces the geometry and the chemistry of the substrate groups involved in the process. This compound reacts preferentially with the nonprotonated aldimine form of the enzyme, as the real substrates do (Torchinsky and Koreneva, 1963; Fasella et al., 1966), to form aldiminic enzyme–substrate complexes which, on the basis of their spectral properties, seem to be partially protonated. The finding that the ratio between the protonated and the nonprotonated forms of these complexes as judged by spectral properties is not appreciably affected by pH changes in the pH 6–9.5 region (Fasella et al., 1966; Hammes and Tancredi, 1967; Fonda and Johnson, 1970) suggests that the protonation occurs by internal proton transfer. On the whole the data obtained with α-methyl aspartate fit the scheme proposed by Ivanov and Karpeisky (1969) as well with the one proposed by Fasella et al. (1966).

An important aspect of the reaction between the negatively charged groups of the substrate and the positively charged groups of the protein has been raised by Jenkins and Tsai (1968), who pointed out that, in considering this interaction, one must take into account the negatively charged counterions from the medium which are replaced by the substrate carboxylate groups. Buffer ions behave as competitive inhibitors toward dicarboxylic substrates and analogs. A study of the pH dependence of this effect has shown that the binding of dicarboxylic compounds requires the displacement of two counterions at acidic pH and of only one counterion at alkaline pHs. Jenkins and D'Ari (1966c) concluded on the basis of these data that, as had been suggested by Mason (1959), dicarboxylic compounds bind to one positively charged group of the enzyme at high pHs and to two such groups at low pHs. This would account for the greater affinity of dicarboxylic acids for the enzyme at low pH.

The spectral changes observed when glutarate reacts with the aldimine enzyme at high pH would suggest that one of the carboxylate groups of the substrate binds first to the internal aldimine nitrogen, causing its protonation (formation of a transient intermediate absorbing at 430 nm); the second carboxylate of the substrate would then bind to a positively charged group on the protein, displacing a counterion; the first carboxylate group would then dissociate from the aldimine nitrogen, which thus would lose the proton, giving a glutarate–aldimine complex which absorbs at 360 nm. These observations suggest not only that enzyme substrate ligands are formed sequentially, but also that they need not be present simultaneously to account for the substrate specificity (Jenkins and D'Ari, 1966c).

The important effects that counterions from the medium may exert at the active site are also illustrated by the finding (Marino et al., 1966) that complete desalting of the aldimine enzyme lowers the pK of the bound coenzyme from 6.2 to less than 4.5.

In order to fit the results obtained by Marino et al. (1966) into the scheme of Ivanov and Karpeisky, it should be postulated that two protein positively charged groups are present in the neighborhood of the coenzyme dissociable group in question, i.e., of the azomethinic nitrogen of the coenzyme protein–Schiff base. One of the protein groups would normally bind very strongly a negative counterion from the medium and would exert an effect on the coenzyme dissociable group only in thoroughly desalted preparations, i.e., when the tightly bound counterion has been removed by thorough desalting (Marino et al., 1966). It is possible that this positively charged group of the protein is the one that interacts with the substrate ω-carboxylate. The other positively charged group of the protein would be the one which, according to Ivanov and Karpeisky, interacts with the α-carboxylate of the substrate and analogs. In the absence of the latter compounds, its positive charge would contribute to lowering the pK of the internal azomethine to 6.2. It is worth noting that, in order to exert this effect on the pK of the coenzyme, this positively charged group should not be normally neutralized by a counterion. A thorough discussion of the number and nature of the positively charged groups at the active site will be possible when more is known about the three-dimensional structure of the enzyme.

Some consideration should now be given to other enzyme groups involved in the formation of the enzyme-substrate complex.

According to the model proposed by Ivanov and Karpeisky (1969), the methyl group in the 2 position and the phosphate group in the 5' position of the coenzyme would exert an important role by providing the hinges around which the coenzyme ring would rotate during the transaldimination reaction. However, ω-methyl PLP and nor-PLP, which have an affinity for the apoenzyme as high as or higher than that of PLP, give origin to holoenzymes that approach or surpass the catalytic efficiency of the native enzyme (Snell and Ayling, 1968; Mühlradt et al., 1967; Braunstein, 1970). This indicates that the 2-methyl group of the coenzyme is not directly involved in the catalytic processes, although it may exert important conformational effects. It is possible, however, that the rotation of the plane of the coenzyme ring postulated by Ivanov and Karpeisky (1969) does occur even though the methyl group in the 2 position is not an indispensable hinge for it.

That the phosphate group in the 5' position is not essential for catalysis became evident when Wada and Snell (1962) showed that apo-AAT catalyzes the reversible transamination between nonphosphorylated PL and glutamate. The observed rates, however, were much lower than those for transamination between the aldimine enzyme and glutamate. It is therefore possible that the phosphate group, although not absolutely necessary for catalysis, may contribute to the reaction in a way other than by attaching the coenzyme to the protein.

Quite recently, a role of the coenzyme phosphate group in the formation of the enzyme–substrate aldimine complex has been proposed by Furbish et al. (1969). On the basis of a comparative study of the catalytic efficiency of holoenzymes obtained by coupling apotransaminase with several pyridoxal analogs having modified acidic substituents in the 5 position, these authors propose that the coenzyme phosphate group might be "more than a handle to bind the coenzyme to the protein" and that it might participate in the catalysis of the transaldimination reaction between the substrate and the aldimine enzyme by inducing modifications of the active site or, more directly, by promoting the transfer of a proton from the nitrogen of the substrate amino group to the nitrogen of the coenzyme–protein azomethine.

c. Geometric and Dynamic Aspects. The disposition in space of the three substrate groups and of the three protein groups involved in the formation of the enzyme–substrate aldimine should now be considered.

The geometry of the substrate binding groups on the enzyme surface is certainly important in establishing substrate specificity and may play a catalytic role by stabilizing a conformation of the bound substrate which is close to that of the transition state in the catalyzed reaction. In the case of the transaldimination reaction, in at least one of the steps, the transition state presumably approaches the conformation of a tetrahedral addition product of the substrate nitrogen to the 4' carbon of the coenzyme.

Direct knowledge on the three-dimensional structure of the protein at the active site is lacking; however, indirect information is offered by a study of the binding constants of substrate analogs provided with a rigid structure (Jenkins *et al.*, 1959; Khomutov *et al.*, 1967). Concerning the mutual orientation of the substrate carboxylate groups, the finding that fumarate does not bind to the enzyme, while maleate does, suggests that the substrate binds in the conformation having the carboxylic groups in proximity (Jenkins *et al.*, 1959). Khomutov's studies (Khomutov *et al.*, 1967) with cyclic analogs which reproduce the structure of the various rotamers of L-glutamate, support this view.

Linear chain dicarboxylic acids with 4–6 carbon atoms are capable of binding to the active site. A glance at the three-dimensional models of these molecules shows that the distance between the carboxylate groups is in succinate more than 1 Å longer, and in glutarate more than 2 Å longer than in maleate, if succinate and glutarate are in the extended conformation. Various hypotheses can be formulated to reconcile these geometric facts with the finding that all these molecules bind to the active site: (i) the long-chain dicarboxylic acids bind to the enzyme in a conformation which is not the extended one; (ii) the site for binding maleate and the 4-carbon substrates is at least partially different from the site which binds the 5- or 6-carbon substrates and analogs; the difference in the binding sites could involve only the protein group which interacts with the ω-carboxylate of the substrate, while the site interacting with the α-carboxylate could be common to all substrates: this type of difference between the sites for the 4- and 5-carbon atom substrates would not be detected by steady-state kinetic studies of the competition between substrates (Velick and Vavra, 1962); (iii) the enzyme undergoes a conformational change to adjust its geometry to that of the substrate; in this connection it might be significant that, while glutarate binds as well as maleate to the aldimine enzyme, the latter dicarboxylic acid binds much better than glutarate to the aminic enzyme (Banks *et al.*, 1963; Velick and Vavra, 1962; Jenkins, 1964; Michuda and Martinez-Carrion, 1970), the difference in conformational rigidity between the two analogs, however, could also come into play.

The strict specificity for L-amino acids suggests the existence of a fairly rigid geometric relations between the enzyme groups which bind the substrate carboxylate groups and the 4' carbon of the coenzyme, which reacts with the substrate amino group. The fact that D-aspartate and D-glutamate do not exert appreciable competitive inhibition, while the corresponding dicarboxylic acids lacking the α-amino group do, suggests that the space available for the substrate at the active site is limited and that steric hindrance prevents the α-amino acids of the D series from binding. Repulsive electrostatic effects may also play a part in the failure of D-amino acids to bind to the active site, since both the L- and D-isomers of malic acid, which are geometrically similar to L- and D-aspartate, seem to bind equally well to the active site (Evangelopoulos and Sizer, 1965).

When considering the various interactions between substrate and enzyme groups we have mentioned the possible occurrence of cooperative effects, such as the promotion of the binding of the substrate amino group to the 4' carbon of the coenzyme by electrostatic interactions between the substrate carboxylate and a positive group of the active site. Various studies have been made of the sequence of events which lead to the formation of the enzyme–substrate complex and these interactions between sites have been investigated by kinetic analyses. The reaction between the natural substrates and the enzyme at the high enzyme concentrations required for the detection of intermediates is too fast to be studied in detail by available methods: the apparent second-order rate constants for the formation of the enzyme-substrate aldimines is greater than 5×10^7 M^{-1} sec^{-1}. As previously mentioned, spectral measurements of the enzyme saturated by the substrates (Jenkins and D'Ari, 1966a; Jenkins and Taylor, 1965; Fasella and Hammes, 1967; Torchinsky et al., 1968) reveal the presence of absorption bands which have been attributed, respectively, to protonated and nonprotonated Schiff bases between the enzyme and the substrate. It is noteworthy that these spectral bands have little or no optical activity (Fasella and Hammes, 1965; Torchinsky et al., 1968) and therefore differ markedly in this respect from the absorption bands displayed at the same wavelengths by the aldiminic holoenzyme in the absence of substrates. This loss of the coenzyme optical activity upon reaction with the substrates has been taken as evidence for the occurrence of conformational changes at the active site (Fasella and Hammes, 1965) and has been related to the catalytic function (Ivanov and Karpeisky, 1969). The details of the mechanism proposed by the latter authors have been discussed in a recent review (Braunstein, 1970).

The multiplicity of the bands observed in spectral studies carried out at equilibrium suggests that various enzyme–substrate aldimine derivatives in rapid equilibrium with each other are formed. In order to study the sequence of the events leading to their formation, the kinetics of the reaction between the enzyme and various substrate analogs have also been studied. At neutral or slightly acidic pH values, the reaction between the enzyme and dicarboxylic acids is very fast and does not allow the detection of intermediates (Hammes and Fasella, 1963). At alkaline pH values, however, Jenkins and D'Ari (1966c) have observed a transient formation of a species absorbing at 430 nm when the aldimine enzyme is rapidly mixed with glutarate; these results have been discussed in a previous section.

Hammes and Haslam (1968) have shown that the reaction between the aldimine enzyme and α-methyl aspartate, which forms a Schiff base with the enzyme but cannot transaminate because of the methyl group attached to the α-carbon, involves at least three steps, some of which are related to conformational changes at the active site. According to these studies, each observed intermediate could exist as two rapidly equilibrating conformational species, possibly involving also intramolecular proton transfer, and having absorption maxima in the 360 nm and in the 430 nm region. These results are consistent with the previously discussed hypothesis on the role of the formation of protonated Schiff bases in the promotion of the transaldimination reaction (Fasella et al., 1966; Braunstein, 1970).

A kinetic study of the formation of the enzyme-substrate aldimine complexes has been possible with two other substrate analogs, namely erythro-β-hydroxyaspartate and threo-β-chloroglutamate. With the former analog, analyses carried out by the temperature jump and by the rapid-mixing technique have shown that at least three distinct intermediates, identified as aldimines on the basis of their spectral properties, are formed, probably in a sequential order (Hammes and Haslam, 1969). With threo-chloroglutamate, a study by the rapid-mixing technique (Antonini et al., 1970) has revealed the rapid formation of a single predominant enzyme–substrate complex, tentatively identified as a nonprotonated aldimine on the basis of its spectral properties.

The apparent second-order rate constant for the formation of complexes identified as aldimine between the enzyme and various substrates and analogs are the following: $10^7\ M^{-1}\ \text{sec}^{-1}$ for L-glutamate and L-aspartate (Fasella and Hammes, 1967); $3 \times 10^6\ M^{-1}\ \text{sec}^{-1}$ for β-hydroxy L-aspartate (Hammes and Haslam, 1969); $1.2 \times 10^4\ M^{-1}\ \text{sec}^{-1}$ for α-methyl L-aspartate (Hammes and Haslam, 1968); and $1.44 \times 10^{-3}\ M^{-1}\ \text{sec}^{-1}$ for threo-β-chloro-L-glutamate (Antonini et al., 1970).

When comparing these values it is important to remember that the evidence reported above indicates that, in many cases, various intermediates are involved in the formation of the enzyme substrate aldimine, so that the apparent second-order rate constants observed may actually be a combination of equilibrium and kinetic constants, relative to different steps in the process.

In conclusion, even though various reasonable hypotheses have been made concerning the possible sequence of events leading to the formation of enzyme–substrate complexes of aldiminic nature (Snell, 1963; Fasella et al., 1966; Jenkins and D'Ari, 1966c; Ivanov and Karpeisky, 1969; Braunstein, 1970), the evidence presently available conclusively proves only that the process of Schiff base formation on the enzyme involves many steps, but does not allow a detailed and comprehensive description of them all. From a general point of view, however, the very fact that enzymatic Schiff base formation is a multistage process is of some interest, since it seems to indicate that the enzyme achieves its extremely high catalytic efficiency [the rates are at least 10^6 times greater than in the corresponding model reactions (Banks et al., 1968a)] by breaking down the reaction into many steps, each of which has a very low activation energy.

2. Formation of the Enzyme–Substrate Ketimine Complex

Information relative to this process [i.e., formation of intermediates (III) and (V) in Fig. 1, starting from the aminic enzyme and a keto acid] is rather scanty. It is known, however, that with the real substrates, the second-order rate constants for the formation of the complex are quite large (greater than $10^7 \, M^{-1}sec^{-1}$). Specificity studies (Jenkins et al., 1959; Jenkins, 1961a; Velick and Vavra, 1962; Banks et al., 1963) show that dicarboxylic α-ketoacids bind to the aminic enzyme much more strongly than simple α-keto acids: this seems to suggest that both substrate carboxylates are involved in the binding. However, significant differences are found in the behavior of dicarboxylic acids toward the aminic and aldimine enzyme. Thus, for instance, oxaloacetate binds much more strongly than ketoglutarate to the aminic enzyme, but considerably less than ketoglutarate to the aldimine enzyme. Maleate and glutarate bind equally well to the aldimine enzyme (Jenkins et al., 1959), but maleate binds well also to the aminic enzyme (Velick and Vavra, 1962) whereas glutarate does not (Banks et al., 1963; Jenkins, 1964). These differences may reflect small changes in the geometry and charge distribution in the aminic enzyme respecting the aldimine enzyme. Studies of ketimine formation are scanty because of the difficulty of obtaining stable analogs of α-keto acids having suitable functional groups added to their molecule. However, Jenkins (1963) showed that β,β-difluoro-oxaloacetate reacts promptly with the aminic enzyme forming an intermediate absorbing in the 330 nm region, and identified tentatively as an enzyme–substrate ketimine.

Studies on the pH dependence of the formation of the ketimine enzyme–substrate complex would be very interesting, but have not been performed so far.

A stimulating hypothesis concerning the series of events leading to ketimine formation has been proposed by Braunstein (1970). According to this hypothesis the amino group of PMP is, in the aminic enzyme, in close proximity of two cationic groups at the active center, namely the ε-NH$_2$ of the lysine residue to which PLP was bound and the cationic group which, according to Ivanov and Karpeisky (1969), contributes to decreasing the pK of the internal aldimine. The pK of the PMP amino group is consequently decreased, the amino group remains nonionized and is therefore in the condition to perform a nucleophilic attack on the carbonyl of the keto acid substrates.

The previously mentioned work by Jenkins and D'Ari (1966c) on the role of the counterions from the buffer bears directly on the kinetics and thermodynamics of the dissociation of the product from the enzyme. According to Jenkins and Tsai (1968), under some conditions, the buffer counterions are necessary to allow the detachment of the keto acid product from the enzyme surface. When counterions from the medium are not available in sufficient concentration, the keto acid product can leave the aminic enzyme only if displaced by the keto acid substrate; e.g., in the transamination between aspartate and ketoglutarate, ketoglutarate would be necessary to remove from the enzyme the oxaloacetate produced during the first half of the reaction. This situation may mimic the kinetic behavior characteristic of mechanisms for two substrate reactions involving ternary complexes between the holoenzyme and both substrates.

B. THE INTERCONVERSION OF THE ENZYME–SUBSTRATE
   COMPLEXES

Chemical considerations and work with model systems suggest that in this step of the reaction the C—H bond in the α-position of the substrate is labilized; the bond electrons are attracted, through the conjugated bond system of the enzyme–substrate aldimine, by the positively charged ring nitrogen of the coenzyme: elimination of the α-proton results, leaving a quinoid intermediate (Metzler et al., 1954; Jenkins, 1964; Schirch and Slotter, 1966) [structure (VII), Fig. 2] with its mesomeric carbanionic form [structure (VIII), Fig. 2] (Perrault et al., 1961). This intermediate would then accept a proton on the 4′ carbon of the coenzyme to give the ketimine intermediate. According to Dunathan's hypothesis (1966), the labilization of the α-C—H bond by the above mechanism requires that the bond is oriented in a direction perpendicular to the plane of the double bonds conjugated to the coenzyme pyridine ring. This suitable conformation would be imposed by the geometry of the active site, which would thus be responsible not only for substrate specificity but also for the selection of the substrate bond to be labilized.

Evidence for the formation of carbanionic intermediates in the tautom-

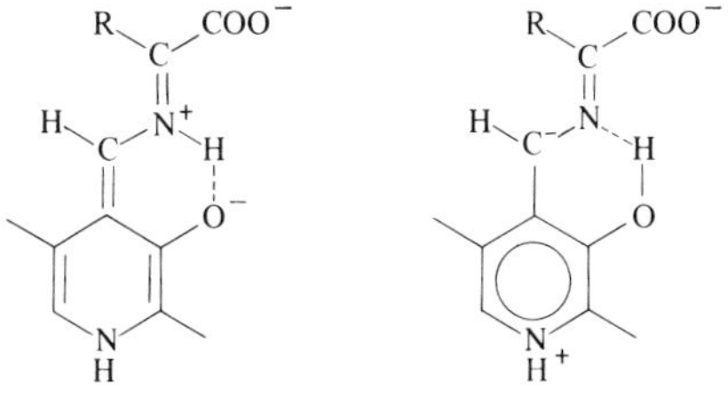

(VII)   (VIII)

FIG. 2. Mesomeric forms of the enzyme-substrate quinoid intermediate.

erization process in model systems has been obtained by Auld and Bruice (1967) and by Matsushima and Martell (1967). For what concerns the enzymatic system, Shlyapnikov and Karpeisky (1969) have suggested that the increased consumption of tetranitromethane by AAT in the presence of substrates can be taken as evidence for the formation of a carbanion intermediate during transamination. When interpreting these data, however, it is important to take into account the fact that, according to Christen and Riordan (1969), in the presence of substrates a tyrosine residue of the enzyme becomes exposed to nitration by tetranitromethane. Isolation of all the products of the reaction between the enzyme and tetranitromethane in the presence of substrates would be desirable.

The substrate, coenzyme, and protein groups which are thought to be involved in the catalysis of the tautomerization step will now be considered. This is, of course, a somewhat arbitrary analytical distinction, since catalysis is brought about by the concerted action of all groups involved. It may, however, be useful, just as the analytical study of the anatomy and physiology of muscles, bones, and joints is useful in understanding the performance of an athlete.

1. The Role of the Substrate Structure in the Tautomerization Step

In previous sections it has been shown how the geometry of the substrate groups interacting with the enzyme determines substrate and, to some extent, reaction specificity (Dunathan, 1966). It is worth noting that the selective orientation of the bond to be labilized at the active site not only confers reaction specificity, but also contributes to accelerating the reaction by selecting, among the possible rotamers around the nitrogen-carbon bond of the substrate, the one with a conformation that is the most similar to that of the transition state in the proton elimination reaction.

Studies with analogs show that the chemical structure of the amino acid substrate can greatly affect the events occurring at the active site after the formation of the enzyme–substrate aldimine complex. The aldimine complexes [(II) and (VI) in Fig. 1] formed by the natural substrates (L-aspartate and L-glutamate) are rapidly tautomerized to give the corresponding ketimine complexes [(III) and (V) in Fig. 1]. According to fast relaxation kinetics (Fasella and Hammes, 1967), the first-order rate constants for the slowest step in the transformation of bound substrates, a step which on the basis of spectral studies and chemical considerations is generally attributed to the tautomerization of the enzyme–substrate Schiff bases (Fasella and Hammes, 1967; Banks et al., 1968a), are, in the case of the 4-carbon substrates, 500 sec^{-1} for the aldimine to ketimine transformation and 1300 sec^{-1} for the reverse reaction; in the case of the 5-carbon substrates the figures are, respectively, 2900 and 1200 sec^{-1} (Fasella and Hammes, 1967). Comparable values have been obtained, by thorough steady-state kinetic studies that included the evaluation of the isotope effect of the replacement of the α-hydrogen by deuterium (Banks et al., 1968a). In absolute terms, the rates for the 5-carbon substrates are somewhat greater than those for the 4-carbon substrates; thus, the substrates which have a lower binding constant (glutamate and ketoglutarate) are those which are transformed more efficiently when bound. In Section III,A,1, when considering the geometry of the substrate binding groups, we pointed out that if the 4- and 5-carbon substrates bind by their carboxylate groups to the same protein groups which bind the carboxylates of the rigid maleate molecule, a greater conformational strain is imposed by binding on the 5-carbon than on the 4-carbon substrates. It is conceivable that this conformational strain is reflected both in the lower equilibrium binding constant and in the higher tautomerization rate constant observed with the 5-carbon substrates. The latter effect (increase of the tautomerization rate) would imply that the strained conformation would facilitate the release of the α-proton from the bound substrate, or the acceptance of a proton by the coenzyme 4' carbon in the quinoid intermediate.

It is also interesting that the rate constant for the aldimine to ketimine transformation is greater than the one for the reverse process in the case of the 5-carbon substrates, while the opposite is true for the 4-carbon substrates.

The introduction of a substituent in the β position of the substrate has marked effects on the transformation of the aldimine enzyme–substrate complex. *Threo-β*-hydroxyl-L-aspartate (Jenkins, 1961b) transaminates slowly (several orders of magnitude more so than the natural substrate L-aspartate). *Erythro-β*-hydroxy-L-aspartate transaminates more rapidly than the *threo* isomer (Jenkins, 1961b), the first-order rate constant for the slowest step being about 10 sec^{-1} (Hammes and Haslam, 1969). The reaction has been studied in detail both at equilibrium and kinetically (Jenkins, 1961b, 1964; Czerlinski and Malkewitz, 1964; Hammes and Haslam, 1969). Upon mixing *erythro-β*-hydroxy aspartate with the aldimine enzyme, a number of intermediates absorbing in the 360 nm and 430 nm regions (enzyme–substrate complexes of aldimine type) are rapidly formed and transformed into an intermediate having an absorption maximum in the 490 nm region. Chemical considerations (Metzler *et al.*, 1954; Jenkins, 1961b, 1964) and work with model systems (Schirch and Slotter, 1966) suggest that this compound has a quinoid character [structure (VII) of Fig. 2] and is formed by elimination of the proton from the substrate α-carbon. This compound would therefore be an intermediate in the tautomerization step. Spectral data (Jenkins and D'Ari, 1966a; Jenkins and Taylor, 1965; Fasella and Hammes, 1967) indicate that a compound absorbing at 490 nm is formed also during the transamination between the coenzyme and the natural substrates. However, when interpreting spectral data showing the appearance of small absorption bands in the 490 nm region upon addition of concentrated solutions of substrates or analogs, it is important to consider the possibility that contaminating traces of *erythro-β*-hydroxy aspartate present in the preparations used may be partly responsible. It is worth while remembering that the original discovery of the band at 490 nm was in part due to contaminating traces of *erythro-β*-hydroxy aspartate in a commercial glycine preparation (Jenkins, 1961b).

With the natural substrates the quinoid intermediate would rapidly be transformed into the ketimine intermediate, while in the case of β-hydroxy aspartate the presence of the hydroxyl group in the β position would hinder the protonation of the 4' coenzyme carbon of the quinoid intermediate and thus reduce the rate of tautomerization. Steric effects as well as charge distribution should be important in this phenomenon, considering that, as previously reported, the threo isomer of β-hydroxyaspartate transaminates even more slowly that the erythro isomer and does not form appreciable amounts of the quinoid intermediate (Jenkins, 1961b). In the case of the β-hydroxy derivatives of L-glutamate, the difference in behavior between the erythro and threo isomers is exactly the opposite (Fasella, 1968).

The introduction of a strongly electronegative group in the β position of the substrate substantially changes the course of events at the active site. *Threo-β*-chloroglutamate (Manning *et al.*, 1968) binds to the aldimine enzyme rapidly forming an enzyme–substrate Schiff base (Antonini *et al.*, 1970) and then undergoes a β elimination reaction:

chloride ions, ammonium ions, and ketoglutarate are the reaction products and the aldimine enzyme is regenerated at the end of each catalytic cycle. The first-order rate constant for the slowest step of this enzyme-catalyzed β elimination is about 100 times lower than that for the transamination of natural substrates.

When the substituent in the β position has leaving properties less pronounced than those of chlorine, as is the case of L-serine-O-sulfate, the Schiff base formed between the enzyme and the substrate undergoes two simultaneous, mutually competitive reactions: transamination to give aminic enzyme and β hydroxypyruvic-O-sulfate, and β elimination to give aldimine enzyme, pyruvate, sulfate, and ammonium ions (John and Fasella, 1969).

This multiplicity of reactions catalyzed by AAT can be explained by a common mechanism: specific binding of an L-amino acid with a negative charge at each end of the chain, formation of an enzyme substrate aldimine and labilization of the bond between the α carbon of the substrate and hydrogen to form a quinoid or anionic intermediate. Successive events depend upon the configuration and charge distribution in the substrate and can lead either to rapid transamination (as is the case with natural substrates), or to a fairly stable quinoid intermediate, which is slowly converted to the transamination products (as is the case with *erythro-β*-hydroxyaspartate and with *threo-β*-hydroxyglutamate) or to β elimination (as is the case with *threo-β*-chloroglutamate and with L-serine O-sulfate). It is noteworthy that, in the case of *threo-β*-chloroglutamate and of L-serine O-sulfate, no intermediates absorbing in the 490 nm region could be detected either as transients in rapid-mixing experiments or under steady-state conditions at high enzyme concentration and saturating substrate concentrations. This means that, if the species absorbing at 490 nm is indeed the postulated quinoid intermediate, an undetectable amount of it is formed with these substrates analogs, probably because its rate of decay by β elimination is fast relative to its formation by α proton elimination. Measurements of the rate of release of the α proton from the various substrates and analogs could help in defining the relationship between substrate structure and the relative speed of the various steps of the reaction. Preliminary studies (Kobayashi and Makino, 1969) indicate that such observation can suitably be carried out by nuclear magnetic resonance measurements.

2. The Role of the Coenzyme

An insight on this problem is provided by extensive studies carried out with coenzyme analogs. Various reviews of this subject are available (Snell, 1958; Snell and Ayling, 1968). The essential minimal requirements for the catalysis of transamination in model systems (Snell, 1963; Auld and Bruice, 1967) appear to be, besides the formyl group which forms the aldimine linkage with the substrate, an unsubstituted acidic hydroxyl group (phenolic or carboxylic), and an electron withdrawing group; all these functional groups should be in such a spatial relationship that in the Schiff base formed between the aldehyde and the amino acid a proton (or a metal ion) can form a 5- or 6-membered ring by chelation with the azomethine nitrogen and the acidic oxygen function, and the electrophilic group reduces the electron density about the formyl group, and hence about the α-carbon atom of the amino acid portion of the Schiff base. However, according to preliminary results by Maley and Bruice (quoted by Auld and Bruice, 1967) N-methylpyridine-4-aldehyde undergoes a transamination reaction with alanine in basic media. This shows that the 3-hydroxy group is not required for transamination if a positive charge can be maintained on the pyridine nitrogen at basic pH. That the functional requirements defined in the above paragraph hold not only for the model system but also for the enzyme is proved by the following findings. Pyridoxine phosphate and 4-deoxypridoxine phosphate, which lack the 4-formyl group, bind strongly to the protein but give inactive holoenzymes (Snell and Ayling, 1968); O-methyl PLP (Furbish et al., 1969) binds to the enzyme but gives a holoenzyme which has only 1% of the activity of the native enzyme, while N-methyl PLP (Furbish et al., 1969), which also binds to the protein, gives an inactive holoenzyme. PLP-N-oxide instead gives a fully active holoenzyme (Furbish et al., 1969; Ohishi et al., 1968; Braunstein, 1970).

3. The Protein Groups Involved in the Tautomerization Step

Information about this point comes essentially from a study of the effects of specific chemical modifications of the enzyme protein. We shall briefly review these studies and then discuss the active site as a whole, stressing the geometric and dynamic aspects of the catalytic process.

a. The —SH Group. Blocking of all the —SH groups present in the protein inactivates the enzyme (Polyanovsky and Torchinsky, 1963; Turano et al., 1963). At high enzyme concentration, it is possible to show that a modified enzyme with the SH groups blocked by N-ethylmaleimide or p-mercuribenzoate is still capable of catalyzing very effectively the transamination between the bound coenzyme and substrate, but, probably because of conformational changes (Torchinsky and Koreneva, 1963), has a greatly reduced affinity for the coenzyme (Turano et al., 1964). These data suggest that the —SH groups are not directly involved in catalysis, but may contribute to the stabilization of the conformation most suitable for coenzyme binding. Evidence suggesting the presence of an —SH group near the active site is provided by studies with a substrate analog (L-serine O-sulfate) which, when bound at the active site, can form a covalent bond with an enzyme group, tentatively identified as a cysteine residue (Fasella and John, 1969).

b. *The Carboxylate Groups.* Amidation of the available carboxylate groups (about 50% of the total) reduces considerably the specific activity of the holoenzyme; however, all-or-none tests show that each modified molecule is still capable of catalyzing transamination, though less efficiently than the native enzyme; this suggests that carboxylate groups are not directly involved in catalysis, but may contribute to stabilizing the proper conformation of the enzyme (Turano *et al.*, 1968c). The role of carboxylic groups in the maintenance of the quaternary structure is discussed in Section IV.

c. *The Amino Groups.* Extensive modification of the amino groups by acetylation (Turano *et al.*, 1962) or succinylation (Torchinsky and Koreneva, 1963; Braunstein *et al.*, 1965; Turano *et al.*, 1967) of the holoenzyme does not affect the activity, provided that care is taken to protect the —SH groups during the treatment. It is, in fact, possible to obtain a holoenzyme with more than 90% of its amino groups acetylated and a specific activity only 10% less than that of the native enzyme (Turano *et al.*, 1962).

These data make it seem unlikely that any of the protein amino groups available to acylating agents in the holoenzyme may constitute one or more of the positively charged groups involved in substrate binding or in substrate transformation. In the apoenzyme the ϵ-amino group of the lysine residue which in the aldimine enzyme is bound to the coenzyme 4' carbon, becomes exposed and very reactive toward amino group reagents: its blocking yields an apoenzyme which is unable to react with the coenzyme and to regenerate a holoenzyme (Turano *et al.*, 1967). It is not possible, therefore, to decide on the basis of these results whether this particular amino group is necessary only for binding the coenzyme or whether it also participates in the transformation of the bound substrate, as has often been suggested (Snell, 1963; Braunstein, 1970).

d. *The Histidine Groups.* Photooxidation in the presence of methylene blue or bengal rose (Martinez-Carrion *et al.*, 1967b; Vorotniskaya *et al.*, 1968) inactivates the enzyme; two histidine residues are destroyed at a rate identical to that of inactivation; all other photooxidizable groups are destroyed much more slowly. This suggests that one of the photooxidizable histidines is important for activity, or that, if both are important, the destruction of one histidine favors the destruction of the other. In fact, if both histidines were required for activity and if the photooxidation of one proceeded independently of that of the other, the rate of activity loss should be twice as high as the rate for histidine destruction. The finding that the destruction of one (or two) histidines causes the inactivation of the enzyme does not of course prove that a histidine is directly involved in the catalytic process.

The residue in question might in fact be distant from the active site, yet its destruction might affect the conformation of the enzyme. However, ultracentrifugation, optical rotatory dispersion, and microcomplement fixation experiments do not reveal major conformational changes in the photooxidized enzyme (Martinez-Carrion, 1969; Martinez-Carrion et al., 1970). On the other hand, circular dichroism shows that perturbation of the conformation near the active site may have occurred. By selective cross-linking experiments, Turano et al. (1966) have shown that in the apoenzyme at least one histidyl residue is positioned within a few angstroms from the ϵ-amino group which, in the holoenzyme, is bound to PLP. Apo-AAT, like holo-AAT, undergoes loss of activity and destruction of two histidine residues upon photooxidation (Martinez-Carrion et al., 1967b). The photooxidized apoenzyme is still capable of binding the coenzyme as the native apoenzyme does; moreover, the photooxidized holoenzyme is capable of reacting with amino acid substrates forming aldimine derivatives with them. The altered enzyme is unable, however, to form the quinoid type of intermediate absorbing at 490 nm with erythro-β-hydroxyaspartate, and incorporates tritium into the α-carbon of this amino acid at a reduced rate (Martinez-Carrion, 1969; Peterson and Martinez-Carrion, 1970; Martinez-Carrion et al., 1970). These results suggest that one of the photooxidizable histidines is involved in the catalysis of the elimination of the proton from the α-carbon of the bound substrate. In this connection it is interesting that the pH dependence for V_{max} (Velick and Vavra, 1962) is very similar to the pH dependence for photoinactivation (Martinez-Carrion et al., 1967b), which may suggest that the same histidine group is involved. This way of thinking is particularly attractive considering the extensive studies on model systems (Bruice and Benkovic, 1966; Auld and Bruice, 1967), showing that the rate-determining prototropic conversion of the aldimine into the ketimine intermediate can be catalyzed by imidazole. It must be remembered, however, that in model systems this tautomerization can be subject to general acid base catalysis and is in fact catalyzed by amino acids, water, formate, acetate, and phosphate (Auld and Bruice, 1967).

e. *The Tyrosine Groups.* The spectral and chemical evidence for the presence of a tyrosyl residue at the active site has been reviewed in a previous section. It has been suggested (Braunstein, 1970) that this tyrosyl residue may interact with the ring nitrogen of the coenzyme and thus facilitate the change of orientation of the coenzyme ring relative to the bound substrate as well as the movement of electrons from and to the substrate bond to be labilized. It is possible that a tyrosine at the active site may participate in catalysis also in other ways, e.g., by acid-base catalysis of one of the numerous steps of the reaction. In this connection, it is interesting that Christen and Riordan (1969) have observed that one tyrosyl residue of AAT becomes more readily attacked by tetranitromethane in the presence of substrates.

4. The Active Site as a Whole: Geometric and Dynamic Aspects

The evidence discussed above suggests that enzymatic transamination occurs through many steps, each of which is catalyzed by the concerted interaction of protein, coenzyme, and substrate groups. Since reaction schemes involving a various number of intermediates have already been proposed by various authors (Snell, 1963; Fasella et al., 1966; Ivanov and Karpeisky, 1969; Braunstein, 1970), it does not seem necessary to propose another one here. We wish, instead, to emphasize that, to be efficient, such a complicated system requires precise spatial relations among the groups involved. Some of these spatial relations can be inferred from available data and chemical considerations.

First of all, it is striking that several of the enzyme substrate interactions considered seem to promote catalysis by more than one mechanism. Thus, the previously discussed interaction between a positively charged group on the enzyme and the α-carboxylate group of the substrate may not only contribute to binding the substrate and to orienting it in the way most suitable for the interaction between the α-C—H bond electrons and the system of conjugated double bonds of the coenzyme, but, by neutralizing the negative charge of the α-carboxylate group, it may also facilitate the attack of a protein basic group of the substrate α-hydrogen (Auld and Bruice, 1967).

It has long been known that AAT is specific for L-amino acids; since transamination is reversible, this implies that the enzyme introduces the hydrogen into the α position of the substrate in a stereospecific way. Recently, Ayling et al. (1968) and Dunathan et al. (1968) have shown that stereospecificity occurs also in the enzyme-catalyzed introduction or removal of a proton at the 4' carbon of the bound coenzyme during the ketimine–aldimine tautomerization in pyridoxamine pyruvate transaminase and AAT. The stereospecificity of proton removal and introduction requires a precise geometry at the active site. A reasonable hypothesis is that proton removal and donation are catalyzed by suitably positioned basic and acidic groups. It is not possible yet to identify these groups with certainty. It is interesting, however, that Rose (1966), working with AAT, and Ayling et al. (1968), working with pyridoxamine pyruvate transaminase, found a small but significant direct transfer of deuterium from the substrate α-carbon atom to the methylene carbon of pyridoxamine phosphate. These results might suggest that a single enzyme group is involved in the tautomerization step, its function being that of transferring a proton from the substrate to the coenzyme carbon. The previously mentioned histidine residue related with activity could be a good candidate for the attribution of this important function. Another possible candidate is the amino group of the lysyl residue present at the active site.

Efficiency requires not only precise geometric relations, but also conformational changes to allow the geometry of the active site to be, at each step, optimal for catalysis. Evidence for the occurrence of conformational changes at the active site has been provided by the study of various physical and chemical properties of the enzyme in the presence of substrates or analogs (for reviews, see Fasella, 1968; Braunstein, 1970). Thus, for instance, the optical activity of the coenzyme absorption band is greatly reduced or abolished in some enzyme-substrate complexes such as the enzyme-substrate aldimines (Torchinsky *et al.*, 1968; Torchinsky and Koreneva, 1963; Fasella and Hammes, 1965) and inverted in others (e.g., in the quinoid intermediate formed by *erythro*-hydroxyaspartate) (Torchinsky and Koreneva, 1963).

These findings certainly prove that conformational changes do occur, but, unfortunately, they do not allow to describe these changes with precision.

A very suggestive and detailed description of the sequence of events that may occur at the active site during transamination has been presented by Ivanov and Karpeisky (1969). The dynamic model proposed by these authors is consistent with a large number of experimental findings and accounts for many of the structural and functional peculiarities of AAT. However, other models could also be proposed which fit the present knowledge.

IV. The Quaternary Structure of the Enzyme

Chemical and physicochemical evidence (for a review, see Fasella, 1968) indicates that cytoplasmic AAT is a dimer consisting of two identical subunits. Speculations could therefore be made on the possible interactions between the two active sites. However, all available data on the function of the enzyme can be interpreted assuming that each active site behaves independently of the other. Evidence for the dissociation of the native holoenzyme into subunits is controversial (Polyanovsky, 1968; Banks *et al.*, 1968b). It seems certain, however, that the monomer is capable of catalyzing transamination: modification of the net charge of the AAT protein either by succinylation of the amino groups (Braunstein *et al.*, 1965) or by amidation of the carboxylate groups with lysine methyl ester (Turano et al., 1970b) leads to the formation of monomeric forms of the modified enzyme which are active in all-or-none tests. The specific activity of this modified enzyme, however, is considerably less than that of the native enzyme. It is impossible to tell whether the decrease in specific activity is the result of monomerization in itself or of other chemical and conformational modifications induced by amidation.

Evidence has been obtained indicating that the apoenzyme may dissociate into subunits more readily than the holoenzyme (Banks et al., 1963), and that cooperation between the sites may occur in the recombination of the apoenzyme with PLP (Riva, 1965).

V. CONCLUSIONS

An impressive mass of information on the structure and function of AAT has been obtained in recent years. The general pattern of the chemical events occurring at the active site has been established; the reaction proceeds through a great number of discrete steps, each of which proceeds fast because it is catalyzed by a number of suitably disposed groups on the enzyme; conformational changes contribute to placing the various groups involved in the most appropriate position for the catalysis of each step. Many of the rate and equilibrium constants for the interconversion of the intermediates have been measured. However, some essential information is still lacking. In particular, not all the groups involved in catalysis have been identified and, most important, the three-dimensional structure of the active site is not known and can only be inferred from indirect evidence and clever thinking. What is probably most needed now is a knowledge of the three-dimensional structure of the enzyme and, possibly, of various enzyme substrate complexes. In this respect, AAT could offer great opportunities because, as we have seen, a series of substrate analogs are available, each of which forms predominantly a few of the intermediates of the overall process.

The formidable task of establishing the complete tridimensional structure of the enzyme seems justified considering that the data could lead to a good knowledge of an enzyme typical of a whole class (PLP dependent enzymes), which has been carefully characterized from the functional standpoint and which efficiently catalyzes a reaction quite different from the hydrolytic processes that are the object of the catalytic action of most of the enzymes thoroughly known today.

REFERENCES

Abaturov, L. V., Polyanovsky, O. L., Torchinsky, Yu. M., and Varshavsky, Ya. M. (1968). In "Pyridoxal Catalysis, Enzymes and Model Systems" (E. E. Snell et al., eds.), p. 171. Wiley (Interscience), New York.

Antonini, E., Brunori, M., Fasella, P., Khomutov, R., Manning, J. M., and Severin, E. S. (1970). *Biochemistry* **9**, 1211.

Arrio-Dupont, M. (1969). *Biochem. Biophys. Res. Commun.* **36**, 306.

Auld, D. S., and Bruice, T. C. (1967). *J. Amer. Chem. Soc.* **89**, 2098.

Ayling, J. E., Dunathan, H. C., and Snell, E. E. (1968). *Biochemistry* **7**, 4537.

Banks, B. E. C., Lawrence, A. J., Vernon, C. A., and Wootton, J. F. (1963). *In* "Chemical and Biological Aspects of Pyridoxal Catalysis" (E. E. Snell *et al.*, eds.), p. 197. Pergamon Press, Oxford.

Banks, B. E. C., Bell, M. P., Lawrence, A. J., and Vernon, C. A. (1968a). *In* "Pyridoxal Catalysis, Enzymes and Model Systems" (E. E. Snell *et al.*, eds.), p. 191. Wiley (Interscience), New York.

Banks, B. E. C., Doonan, S., Lawrence, A. J., and Vernon, C. A. (1968b). *Eur. J. Biochem.* **5**, 528.

Banks, B. E. C., Doonan, S., Gauldie, J., Lawrence, A. J., and Vernon, C. A. (1968c). *Eur. J.. Biochem.* **6**, 507.

Bocharov, A. L., Ivanov, V. I., Karpeisky, M. Ya., Mamaeva, O. K., and Florentiev, V. L. (1968). *Biochem. Biophys. Res. Commun.* **30**, 459.

Borri-Voltattorni, C., and Turano, C. (1970). Unpublished observations.

Braunstein, A. E. (1964). *Vitam. Horm. (New York)* **22**, 451.

Braunstein, A. E. (1970). *FEBS Symp.* **18**, 101.

Braunstein, A. E., Torchinsky, J. M., Malakhova, E. A., and Simcina, M. I. (1965). *Ukr. Biokhim. Zh.* **5**, 671.

Bruice, T. C., and Benkovic, S. J. (1966). "Bioorganic Mechanisms," Vol. II, Chapter 8. Benjamin, New York.

Bruice, T. C., and Topping, R. M. (1963). *J. Amer. Chem. Soc.* **85**, 1493.

Christen, P. L., and Riordan, J. E. (1969). *Fed. Proc., Fed. Amer. Soc. Exp. Biol.* **28**, 601.

Churchich, J. E., and Farrelly, J. G. (1968). *Biochem. Biophys. Res. Commun.* **31**, 316.

Czerlinski, G., and Malkewitz, J. (1964). *Biochemistry* **4**, 1127.

Dunathan, H. C. (1966). *Proc. Nat. Acad. Sci. U.S.* **55**, 712.

Dunathan, H. C., Davis, L., Kury, P. G., and Kaplan, M. (1968). *Biochemistry* **7**, 4532.

Evangelopoulos, A. E., and Sizer, I. W. (1965). *Chem. Chronika* **30**, 65.

Fasella, P. (1968). *In* "Pyridoxal Catalysis, Enzymes and Model Systems" (E. E. Snell *et al.*, eds.), p. 1. Wiley (Interscience), New York.

Fasella, P. (1970). Unpublished data.

Fasella, P., and Hammes, G. G. (1965). *Biochemistry* **4**, 801.

Fasella, P., and Hammes, G. G. (1967). *Biochemistry* **6**, 1798.

Fasella, P., and John, R. (1969). *Proc. 4th Int. Congr. Pharmacol. 1969*, p. 37.

Fasella, P., Turano, C., Giartosio, A., and Hammady, I. (1961). *Giorn. Biochim.* **10**, 175.

Fasella, P., Giartosio, A., and Hammes, G. G. (1966). *Biochemistry* **5**, 197.

Fischer, E. H., and Krebs, E. G. (1959). *Abstr. 136th Meet. Amer. Chem. Soc.* p. 24C.

Fonda, M., and Johnson, R. J. (1970). *J. Biol. Chem.* **245**, 2709.

Furbish, F. S., Fonda, M. L., and Metzler, D. E. (1969). *Biochemistry* **8**, 5169.

Guirard, B. M., and Snell, E. E. (1964). *Comp. Biochem.* **15**, 138.

Hammes, G. G., and Fasella, P. (1962). *J. Amer. Chem. Soc.* **84**, 4644.

Hammes, G. G., and Fasella, P. (1963). *J. Amer. Chem. Soc.* **85**, 3929.

Hammes, G. G., and Haslam, J. L. (1968). *Biochemistry* **7**, 1519.

Hammes, G. G., and Haslam, J. L. (1969). *Biochemistry* **8**, 1591.
Hammes, G. G., and Tancredi, J. (1967). *Biochim. Biophys. Acta* **146**, 312.
Hayashi, S., Granner, D. K., and Tomkins, G. M. (1967). *J. Biol. Chem.* **242**, 3998.
Henson, C. P., and Cleland, W. W. (1964). *Biochemistry* **3**, 338.
Hughes, R. C., Jenkins, W. T., and Fischer, E. H. (1962). *Proc. Nat. Acad. Sci. U.S.* **48**, 1615.
Hullar, T L. (1969). *J. Med. Chem.* **12**, 58.
Ivanov, V. I., and Karpeisky, M. Ya. (1969). *Advan. Enzymol.* **32**, 21.
Jencks, W. P. (1966). *In* "Current Aspects of Biochemical Energetics" (N. O. Kaplan and E. Kennedy, eds.), p. 273. Academic Press, New York.
Jencks, W. P., and Cordes, E. (1963). *In* "Chemical and Biological Aspects of Pyridoxal Catalysis" (E. E. Snell *et al.*, eds.), p. 57. Pergamon Press, Oxford.
Jenkins, W. T. (1961a). *J. Biol. Chem.* **236**, 474.
Jenkins, W. T. (1961b). *J. Biol. Chem.* **236**, 1121.
Jenkins, W. T. (1963). *In* "Chemical and Biological Aspects of Pyridoxal Catalysis" (E. E. Snell *et al.*, eds.), p. 139. Pergamon Press, Oxford.
Jenkins, W. T. (1964). *J. Biol. Chem.* **239**, 1742.
Jenkins, W. T., and D'Ari, L. (1966a). *J. Biol. Chem.* **241**, 2845.
Jenkins, W. T., and D'Ari, L. (1966b). *Biochemistry* **5**, 2900.
Jenkins, W. T., and D'Ari, L. (1966c). *J. Biol. Chem.* **241**, 5667.
Jenkins, W. T., and Sizer, I. W. (1957). *J. Amer. Chem. Soc.* **79**, 2655.
Jenkins, W. T., and Sizer, I. W. (1959). *J. Biol. Chem.* **234**, 1179.
Jenkins, W. T., and Taylor, R. T. (1965). *J. Biol. Chem.* **240**, 2907.
Jenkins, W. T., and Tsai, H. (1968). *In* "Symposium on Pyridoxal Enzymes" (K. Yamada *et al.*, eds.), p. 15. Maruzen Co., Ltd., Tokyo.
Jenkins, W. T., Yphantis, D. A., and Sizer, I. W. (1959). *J. Biol. Chem.* **234**, 51.
John, R. A., and Fasella, P. (1969). *Biochemistry* **8**, 4477.
Kent, A. B., Krebs, E. G., and Fischer, E. H. (1958). *J. Biol. Chem.* **232**, 549.
Khomutov, R. M., Kovaleva, G. K., Severin, E. S., and Vdovina, L. V. (1967). *Biokhimiya* **32**, 900.
Khomutov, R. M., Severin, E. S., Khurs, E. N., and Gulyaev, N. N. (1969). *Biochim. Biophys. Acta* **171**, 201.
Kobayashi, Y., and Makino, K. (1969). *Biochim. Biophys. Acta* **191**, 738.
Koshland, D. E., Jr. (1958). *Proc. Nat. Acad. Sci. U.S.* **44**, 98.
Lis, H., Fasella, P., Turano, C., and Vecchini, P. (1960). *Biochim. Biophys. Acta* **45**, 529.
Litwack, G., and Cleland, W. W. (1968). *Biochemistry* **7**, 2072.
Malakhova, E. A., and Torchinsky, Yu. M. (1965). *Dokl. Akad. Nauk SSSR* **161**, 1224.
Manning, J. M., Khomutov, R. M., and Fasella, P. (1968). *Eur. J. Biochem.* **5**, 199.
Marino, G., Greco, A. M., Scardi, V., and Zito, R. (1966). *Biochem. J.* **99**, 589.
Martell, A. E. (1963). *In* "Chemical and Biological Aspects of Pyridoxal Catalysis" (E. E. Snell *et al.*, eds.), p. 13. Pergamon Press, Oxford.
Martinez-Carrion, M. (1969). *FEBS Symp.* **18**, 35.
Martinez-Carrion, M., Turano, C., Chiancone, E., Bossa, F., Giartosio, A., Riva, F., and Fasella, P. (1967a). *J. Biol. Chem.* **242**, 2397.
Martinez-Carrion, M., Turano, C., Riva, F., and Fasella, P. (1967b). *J. Biol. Chem.* **242**, 1426.
Martinez-Carrion, M., Kuczenski, R., Tiemeier, D. C., and Peterson, D. L. (1970). *J. Biol. Chem.* **245**, 799.

Mason, M. (1959). *J. Biol. Chem.* **234**, 2770.

Matsushima, Y., and Martell, A. E. (1967). *J. Amer. Chem. Soc.* **89**, 1331.

Meister, A., Sober, A. H., and Peterson, E. A. (1954). *J. Biol. Chem.* **206**, 89.

Metzler, D., Ikawa, M., and Snell, E. E. (1954). *J. Amer. Chem. Soc.* **76**, 648.

Michuda, C. M., and Martinez-Carrion, M. (1970). *J. Biol. Chem.* **245**, 262.

Morino, Y., and Watanabe, T. (1969). *Biochemistry* **8**, 3412.

Mühlradt, P. F., Morino, Y., and Snell, E. E. (1967). *J. Med. Chem.* **10**, 341.

Novogrodsky, A., and Meister, A. (1964). *Biochim. Biophys. Acta* **81**, 605.

Ohishi, N., Nakai, Y., Shimizu, S., and Fukui, S. (1968). *In* "Symposium on Pyridoxal Enzymes" (K. Yamada *et al.*, eds.), p. 43. Maruzen Co., Ltd., Tokyo.

Perrault, A. M., Pullman, B., and Valdemoro, C. (1961). *Biochim. Biophys. Acta* **46**, 555.

Peterson, D. L., and Martinez-Carrion, M. (1970). *J. Biol. Chem.* **245**, 806.

Polyanovsky, O. L. (1968). *In* "Pyridoxal Catalysis, Enzymes and Model Systems" (E. E. Snell *et al.*, eds.), p. 155. Wiley (Interscience), New York.

Polyanovsky, O. L., and Keil, B. A. (1963). *Biokhimiya* **28**, 372.

Polyanovsky, O. L., and Torchinsky, Yu. M. (1963) *In* "Chemical and Biological Aspects of Pyridoxal Catalysis" (E. E. Snell *et al.*, eds.), p. 157. Pergamon Press, Oxford.

Riva, F. (1965). *8th Giorn. Biochim. Latine* Extract XIII.

Riva, F., Vecchini, P., Turano, C., and Fasella, P. (1964). *Proc. 6th Int. Congr. Biochem., 1964* Abstr., Sect. IV, pp. 140 and 329.

Rose, I. A. (1966). *Annu. Rev. Biochem.* **35**, 23.

Scardi, V., and Marino, G. (1968). *Corsi Semin. Chim.* **8**, 295.

Scardi, V., Scotto, P., Iaccarino, M., and Scarano, E. (1963). *Biochem. J.* **88**, 172.

Schirch, L., and Slotter, R. A. (1966). *Biochemistry* **5**, 3175.

Severin, E. S., and Dixon, H. B. F. (1968). *Biochem. J.* **110**, 19P.

Shlyapnikov, S. V., and Karpeisky, M. Ya. (1969). *Eur. J. Biochem.* **11**, 424.

Sizer, I. W., and Jenkins, W. T. (1963). *In* "Chemical and Biological Aspects of Pyridoxal Catalysis" (E. E. Snell *et al.*, eds.), p. 123. Pergamon Press, Oxford.

Snell, E. E. (1958). *Vitam. Horm. (New York)* **16**, 77.

Snell, E. E. (1963). *In* "Chemical and Biological Aspects of Pyridoxal Catalysis" (E. E. Snell *et al.*, eds.), p. 1. Pergamon Press, Oxford.

Snell, E. E., and Ayling, J. E. (1968). *In* "Symposium on Pyridoxal Enzymes" (K. Yamada *et al.*, eds.), p. 5. Maruzen Co., Ltd., Tokyo.

Tate, S. S., and Meister, A. (1969). *Biochemistry* **8**, 1056.

Torchinsky, Yu. M. (1963). *Biokhimiya* **28**, 731.

Torchinsky, Yu. M., and Koreneva, L. G. (1963). *Biokhimiya* **28**, 1087.

Torchinsky, Yu. M., Malakhova, E. A., Livanova, N. B., and Pikhelgas, V. Ya. (1968). *In* "Pyridoxal Catalysis: Enzymes and Model Systems" (E. E. Snell *et al.*, eds.), p. 269. Wiley (Interscience), New York.

Turano, C., Fasella, P., Giartosio, A., and Vecchini, P. (1960). *Boll. Soc. Ital. Biol. Sper.* **36**, 1968.

Turano, C., Giartosio, A., and Vecchini, P. (1962). *Arch. Biochem. Biophys.* **99**, 191.

Turano, C., Giartosio, A., Riva, F., and Vecchini, P. (1963). *In* "Chemical and Biological Aspects of Pyridoxal Catalysis" (E. E. Snell *et al.*, eds.), p. 149. Pergamon Press, Oxford.

Turano, C., Giartosio, A., and Fasella, P. (1964). *Arch. Biochem. Biophys.* **104**, 524.

Turano, C., Giartosio, A., Riva, F., Baroncelli, V., and Bossa, F. (1966). *Arch. Biochem. Biophys.* **117**, 678.

194 PAOLO FASELLA AND CARLO TURANO

Turano, C., Giartosio, A., Riva, F., and Baroncelli, V. (1967). *Biochem. J.* **104**, 970.
Turano, C., Giartosio, A., Riva, F., Bossa, F., and Baroncelli, V. (1968a). *In* "Pyridoxal Catalysis, Enzymes and Model Systems" (E. E. Snell *et al.*, eds.), p. 143. Wiley (Interscience), New York.
Turano, C., Giartosio, A., Riva, F., Barra, D., and Bossa, F. (1968b). *In* "Symposium on Pyridoxal Enzymes" (K. Yamada *et al.*, eds.), p. 27. Maruzen Co., Ltd., Tokyo.
Turano, C., Bossa, F., Barra, D., and Vecchini, P. (1968c). *Abstr. 5th Meet. Fed. Eur. Biochem. Soc. 1968* p. 225.
Turano, C., Giartosio, A., and Orlacchio, A. (1969). Unpublished observations.
Turano, C., Borri-Voltattorni, C., Orlacchio, A., and Bossa, F. (1970a). *FEBS Symp.* **18**, 123.
Turano, C., Giartosio, A., and Bossa, F. (1970b). Unpublished observations.
Turano, C., Ferraro, A., Giartosio, A., Barra, D., and Bossa, F. (1970c). Unpublished observations.
Vallee, B. L., and Williams, R. J. P. (1968). *Proc. Nat. Acad. Sci. U.S.* **59**, 498.
Velick, S. F., and Vavra, J. (1962). *In* "The Enzymes" (P. D. Boyer, H. Lardy, and K. Myrbäck, eds.), 2nd rev. ed., Vol. 6, p. 219. Academic Press, New York.
Vernon, C. A. (1970). Personal communication.
Vorotnitskaya, N. E., Lutovinova, G. F., and Polyanovsky, O. L. (1968). *In* "Pyridoxal Catalysis, Enzymes and Model Systems" (E. E. Snell *et al.*, eds.), p. 131. Wiley (Interscience), New York.
Wada, H., and Snell, E. E. (1962). *J. Biol. Chem.* **237**, 127.

Isoenzymes of NAD and NADP Dependent Dehydrogenases

G. PFLEIDERER

Ruhr Universität Bochum, Bochum, Germany

I. INTRODUCTION

The first description of a real isoenzyme concerned a dehydrogenase. Pfleiderer and Jeckel (1957) isolated two forms of lactate dehydrogenase (LDH) having strong differences in the biochemical and physical properties. These were obtained in crystalline form from mammalian heart and mammalian skeletal muscle. At the same time Wieland and Pfleiderer (1957) demonstrated by electrophoresis the existence of five multiple forms of LDH in mammalian organ extracts. These multiple forms have a characteristic distribution pattern in a variety of tissues. Apella and Markert (1961) and Markert (1963) gave an explanation for these multiple forms based on the results of dissociation and artificial hybridization experiments. Both the heart (H) and skeletal muscle (M) monomers are able to form five tetrametric LDH components (Fig. 1).

Markert and Møller (1959) proposed the term isoenzyme for iso-meric forms of an enzyme which have identical function and exist in a single cell of one organism. Since the detection of LDH isoenzymes was first published, numerous papers have appeared which report the exist-

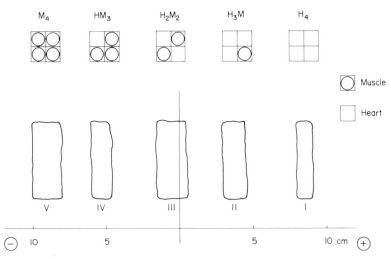

FIG. 1. Schematic configuration of the 5 multiple forms of LDH and the relationship to their electrophoretic mobility (on membrane foils, pH 8.6).

ence of multiple forms of enzymes occurring in the cells of microorganisms, plants, or animals. Before discussing further the structure and function of dehydrogenase isoenzymes, we must first consider the problem of artifacts and of genetic variations and microheterogeneity.

A. ARTIFACTS

Observations of the existence of multiple dehydrogenase forms—the first possible hint concerning isoenzymes—must be evaluated critically to eliminate the possibility of an artifact. Shaw and Koen (1965) used the term "nothing dehydrogenases." These are enzymes that catalyze the reduction of tetrazolium salts in the presence of NAD, but do not require the presence of substrate. Koen and Shaw (1964) presented evidence that several dehydrogenase activities are associated with the same protein zones in starch gel electrophoresis. Five components were identified and formed purple zones of formazan in exactly the same position as the LDH isoenzymes when glutamate, α-hydroxybutyrate, alanine, or α-glycerophosphate were used as substrates. The authors therefore postulated multiple dehydrogenase activities. Falkenberg *et al.* (1969) repeated this experiment. In a systematic investigation they demonstrated that there exists only one anionic migrating glutamate dehydrogenase component in human kidney, f.e. This result was also confirmed by ion exchange chromatography. The other formazane bands in gel electrophoresis mentioned above must originate from the five isoenzymes of LDH. Even after continuous washing before use, some gels contain water-

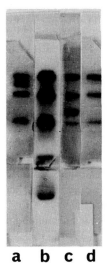

a b c d

Fig. 2. Electrophoresis of human kidney extract in 11.5% starch gel. Staining with tetrazolium salt was carried out (a) in presence of α-glycerophosphate, (b) in presence of lactate, (c) in presence of glutamate, (d) without substrate.

insoluble factors, which in the presence of sufficiently high LDH activity, form formazan bands in the absence of lactate. It appears impossible to exclude this effect (Fig. 2).

B. Genetic Variations and Microheterogeneity

It is now known that each polypeptide chain of an LDH subunit (heart = B, skeletal muscle = A) is controlled by a separate gene. Boyer *et al.* (1963) described a variant of the B subunit in red cell hemolysates from a Nigerian male. After starch gel electrophoresis, LDH I (B_4) was resolved into five enzymatically active components. LDH II, LDH III, and LDH IV were resolved into four, three, and two components, respectively. These findings can be explained by assuming that there is a mutant form of the normal B subunit. Since B and β can combine with A, the following isoenzyme combinations are possible and are found: B_4, $B_3\beta$, $B_2\beta_2$, $B\beta_3$, β_4, B_3A, $B_2\beta A$, $B\beta_2A$, β_3A, B_2A_2, $B\beta A_2$, β_2A_2, BA_3, βA_3 and A_4.

Numerous variants of genetically determined types of glucose-6-phosphate- and phosphogluconate-dehydrogenases are known (see Latner and Skillen, 1968). These multiple forms have very similar amino acid compositions, biochemical, and immunological properties (cf. liver alcohol-dehydrogenase). This phenomenon is not important for the present discussion because we cannot recognize any functional importance for the living cell. In many cases the genetic variants have not been confirmed as the cause of the existence of multiple enzyme forms which have the same kinetic and immunological properties. An example of this kind is provided by the detection of at least five glyceraldehyde-phosphate-dehydrogenase (GAPDH) forms distinguishable by electrophoresis (Krebs *et al.*, 1953). Kirschner and Voigt (1969) have found 13 or 14 components possessing GAPDH activity, after electrophoresis on 5% polyacrylamide gels of crude extracts from *Saccharomyces cerevisiae*. Each of the five major bands separates into 2 or 3 subbands. The authors excluded all artifacts caused by cell rupture, oxidation in the gel by ammonium persulfate, or differing contents of NAD. The crystalline enzyme consists of two GAPDH fractions that can be separated by ion exchange chromatography. The biochemical properties of the mixture and of the main pure component are identical.

The splitting of major bands into subbands by gel electrophoresis techniques is now quite well known. We isolated different dehydrogenases in crystalline form recently. In most cases conditions were found which promoted this splitting effect, even though the enzyme preparations were chromatographically uniform. The best resolving capacity has the method of electrofocusing. Another explanation often given as cause for existence of strong structural and catalytic similarity is a change in conformation.

C. Definition of Real Isoenzymes

In order to examine the structure and function of dehydrogenases or other isoenzymes, three conditions must be fulfilled as postulated previously (Pfleiderer, 1968):

1. Different biochemical and physical characteristics associated with the same qualitative substrate specificity and a similar molecular weight.

2. Different distribution patterns of an isoenzyme mixture in different functional organs or tissues. In the case of microorganisms, distinct distribution patterns appear under different metabolic conditions.

3. Different genetic control of the basic isoenzyme types, which, as we know in the case of LDH, can result in the occurrence of intermediate types by the process of hybridization.

With these conditions in mind, the discussion of the isoenzyme problem can be determined.

II. Structure of Dehydrogenase Isoenzymes

The most detailed research concerning the structure and function of dehydrogenase isoenzymes is that related to LDH. Knowledge about the other isoenzymes is limited. The only complete primary structure of a dehydrogenase published to date is that of glyceraldehyde-3-phosphate dehydrogenase (GAPDH). The excellent work of the Harris group (Davidson *et al.*, 1967; Harris and Perham, 1968) has elucidated the primary structure of the enzyme isolated from lobster and pig muscle. Unfortunately this enzyme possesses no isoenzymes. We are now awaiting the primary structure of the horse liver alcohol-dehydrogenase (E-E) and its isoenzyme (S-S) (Jörnvall, 1970). Study of the primary structure of pig heart and pig muscle LDH is in progress in our group, but is not completed (Mella, 1970). Dr. Rossmann and co-workers (Adams *et al.*, 1970) published a 2.8 Å electron density map of dogfish LDH M_4, and Bränden *et al.* (1970) have published a 5 Å electron density map of horse liver ADH.

A. Structure of LDH from Pig Heart and Pig Muscle

Wachsmuth *et al.* (1964) have isolated in a pure form LDH I, II, and III from human brain, LDH I and II from human kidney, LDH I and II from human heart, LDH V from human liver, LDH I from pig heart, and LDH V from pig skeletal muscle. These were isolated in order to test the nature of the high biochemical similarity between LDH components possessing identical electrophoretic mobilities even though isolated from different tissues of the same organism, as well as to test the strong differences in the properties of electrophoretically different components isolated from the same organ. Amino acid analyses have shown that the human LDH bands possessing the same electrophoretic mobilities have identical composition. Comparing human LDH I-V, an increase in content of arginine, glycine, tyrosine, and phenylalanine and a decrease in aspartic acid, glutamic acid, alanine, valine, and methionine were observed. Kaplan's group has prepared crystalline LDH from heart and skeletal muscle of different species and has analyzed the amino acid compositions (Pesce *et al.*, 1964). The authors also find more homology among H_4 or M_4 of different species than among H_4 and M_4 of one species.

Table I shows our recent amino acid analyses of pig heart and pig skeletal muscle LDH. Both enzymes have nearly identical amounts of lysine and of arginine. Tryptic digestion experiments revealed about 30 cleavages for both LDH-isoenzymes (H_4 and M_4). The fingerprint analysis of the two LDH-isoenzymes is significantly different, as Wieland *et al.* (1964) and Fondy *et al.* (1964, 1965) have already demonstrated. By separating the tryptic peptides of pig H_4 and pig M_4 it can be shown that only a small number of amino acid sequences are homologous (Mella, 1970).

The first homologies between heart and skeletal muscle LDH of a single species were discovered in essential cysteine peptides. Fondy *et al.* (1965) and our group (Holbrook *et al.*, 1966) have isolated a tryptic

Amino acid	Pig heart	Pig muscle
Carboxymethyl-cysteine	4	4
Aspartic acid	40	30
Threonine	18	13
Serine	26	20
Glutamic acid	38	30
Proline	12	12
Glycine	26	25
Alanine	19	19
Valine	36	29
Methionine	8	7
Isoleucine	24	26
Leucine	37	34
Tyrosine	8	7
Phenylalanine	5	7
Lysine	26	27
Histidine	8	13
Arginine	9	10

[a] Number of residues per subunit of MW 35,000.

cysteine peptide by applying different radioactive labels to one essential SH group. For both H_4 and M_4 this essential cysteine peptide has almost the same amino acid composition in different species. The exact sequence for pig heart, pig skeletal muscle, and chicken skeletal muscle according to Holbrook et al. (1967) and Mella et al. (1969) is: Val-Ile-Gly-Ser-Gly-Cys-Asn-Leu-Asp-Ser-Ala-Arg. Another homology exists in two additional arginine peptides with the sequence: Gln-Gln-Glu-Gly-Glx-Ser-Arg and Leu-Asn-Leu-Val-Gln-Arg (Pfleiderer and Mella, 1970). Further homologies in the structure of both pig LDH isoenzymes apparently exist in an essential histidine peptide containing 13 amino acid residues. This peptide was identified by Woenckhaus et al. (1969) after labeling with 3-(2-brom-1-[^{14}C]-acetyl)pyridine.

After blocking the ϵ amino groups by trifluoroacetylation, we found differences between the primary structure of pig H_4 and pig M_4. A fingerprint of the tryptic hydrolyzate of the trichloroacetic acid-soluble fraction showed that only three out of the ten possible heart muscle peptides contained C-terminal arginine. In contrast to the heart enzyme, we have found seven low molecular arginine peptides and free arginine in the fingerprint of pig muscle LDH. This means that almost all the arginine peptides are arranged in close proximity to each other in the sequence of muscle LDH. The fingerprint from chicken muscle LDH shows seven low molecular weight arginine peptides similar to those in the pig muscle enzyme. The last four amino acids in heart muscle LDH are Leu-Lys-Asp-Leu, and the carboxyl terminal peptide in muscle LDH has the sequence Glu-Leu-Gln-Phe (Mella *et al.*, 1969). Allison (1968) found a COOH-terminal of dogfish LDH, i.e., Phe, identical with the pig muscle terminal.

In summary, we find a homology in the essential parts of the primary structure of the two pig isoenzymes, but no identity exists in the remaining parts.

B. TERTIARY STRUCTURE

Many experiments carried out by our team have demonstrated that the differences in tertiary structure are least in the region of the active center of the two LDH isoenzymes. We suppose that there is a different conformation in the vicinity of the essential SH group, because this group reacts rapidly in pig heart LDH with various maleinimides and causes loss of enzyme activity. Under the same conditions, the pig muscle enzyme was not attacked (Holbrook *et al.*, 1966). The excellent work of Rossmann's group at Lafayette (Adams *et al.*, 1970) now give us exact data of the dogfish muscle peptide chain. It would be very interesting to examine the ternary and quaternary structure of the corresponding heart enzyme. Although the investigations are started, the production of large crystals of this isoenzyme for X-ray crystallography is very difficult (Rossmann, 1969).

C. IMMUNOLOGICAL INVESTIGATIONS

We also have information on differences in tertiary structure obtained by the immunotechnique. Nisselbaum and Bodansky (1959) examined the reactions of various rabbit LDH forms with a rooster antiserum to rabbit skeletal muscle LDH. Whereas the heart muscle enzyme was only slightly inhibited by the M_4 antibody, they observed a complete inhibition of the skeletal muscle and the liver enzyme.

In further experiments, the same authors (Nisselbaum and Bodansky, 1961) confirmed the nonidentity of the antibody to both isoenzymes. Many authors have been unable to detect any cross reaction when using rabbit antisera to M_4 or H_4 isoenzymes isolated from different species. Antibodies to beef M_4 LDH show a decreasing inhibitory effect on the five beef LDH components with $M_4 = 86\%$, M_3H 60%, M_2H_2 41%, M_1H_3 23%, and H_4 0% (Kaplan and White, 1963). On the other hand, Rajewsky *et al.* (1964) observed the cross reaction of anti-pig heart or anti-beef heart LDH with heart LDHs isolated from different, mam-

malian species. They used immunoelectrophoresis to reaffirm the immunological relation of the hybrid isoenzymes to both the nonhybrid isoenzymes. This experiment demonstrated again that skeletal muscle LDH
arising from different species are more closely related to each other than
are the heart and skeletal muscle enzymes from one single organism.
Furthermore, Rajewsky (1966) has been able to demonstrate an immunological relationship by using acetic anhydride-treated LDH for the im-
munization. Even the antibody against acetylated heart muscle LDH
yields a cross reaction with the appropriately treated enzyme of skeletal
muscle.

D. Molecular Weight

Many authors have examined the physicochemical characteristics of
LDH isoenzymes isolated from different species. All data indicate a
uniform molecular weight of approximately 140,000 (Pesce et al., 1964;
Jaenicke, 1970). Under conditions that favor dissociation, the molecular
weight of the subunits was found to be of the order of 35,000.

E. LDH-X from Testis and Sperm

In mature testis and sperm of many animals and of man, a new LDH
component has been detected by gel electrophoreses (Blanco and Zinkham, 1963; Goldbey, 1963). This component is in addition to the other
five. The new LDH isoenzyme (LDH-X or -C) is the most active form
of the enzyme in mature human and rat sperm (Zinkham et al., 1963).
It is found in the postpubertal testis, and is present in differentiating
spermatogonia and mature spermatozoa. LDH-X can be distinguished
from the other LDH forms by its different biochemical properties (Zinkham et al., 1963; Clausen and Øvlisen, 1965). In the middle piece fraction
of human sperm cells (the sediment obtained after centrifugation at $900g$
for 10 minutes in $0.25 M$ sucrose containing 1 mM EDTA), Clausen
found only LDH-X; this fraction also contains the mitochondrial
apparatus.

III. Function of the LDH Isoenzymes

A. Biochemical Properties

The metabolic role of both LDH isoenzymes is not yet completely
understood. In one of the first investigations of the biochemical properties
of heart and muscle LDH, we found a 2-fold higher turnover of the muscle
enzyme in the pyruvate hydrogenation reaction (Pfleiderer and Jeckel,
1957). Later Pesce et al. (1964) (see Table II) and Wachsmuth and
Pfleiderer (1963), published kinetic characteristics of pure H_4 and M_4
LDH isolated from different species. For LDH in chicken, beef, pig, and

TABLE II
KINETIC CHARACTERISTICS OF SOME CRYSTALLINE BEEF AND CHICKEN
LACTATE DEHYDROGENASES[a]

Characteristic	Beef H_4	Chicken H_4	Beef M_4	Chicken M_4
Optimal pyruvate concentration	$6 \times 10^{-4} M$	$4 \times 10^{-4} M$	$3 \times 10^{-3} M$	$3 \times 10^{-3} M$
K_m pyruvate[b]	$1.4 \times 10^{-4} M$	$8.9 \times 10^{-5} M$	$1 \times 10^{-3} M$	$3.2 \times 10^{-3} M$
Turnover number[c] with pyruvate at V_{max}	49,400	45,000	80,200	93,400
Optimal lactate concentration	$4 \times 10^{-2} M$	$3 \times 10^{-2} M$	$2 \times 10^{-1} M$	$2.5 \times 10^{-1} M$
K_m lactate[b]	$9 \times 10^{-3} M$	$7 \times 10^{-3} M$	$2.5 \times 10^{-2} M$	$4 \times 10^{-2} M$
NHXDH$_1$:NADH$_3$[d]	2.78	3.02	0.63	0.40
AcPyAD$_1$:TNAD$_1$[e]	0.17	0.26	1.0	4.3

[a] From Pesce et al. (1964).
[b] Determined by reciprocal plots.
[c] Represents moles of NADH oxidized per mole of enzyme per minute at 25°C at pH 7.5.
[d] Ratio of rates of reduced hypoxanthine analogue of NAD.
[e] Ratio of rates of acetylpyridine analogue of NAD:Thionicotinamide adenine dinucleotide.

human, the same 2-fold higher turnover number for the muscle enzyme is always found. Another physiologically interesting characteristic was published by Plagemann et al. (1960). At any given pH and temperature, the greater the electrophoretic mobility of an LDH isoenzyme the lower its K_m for pyruvate and the lower the concentration of pyruvate which inhibits the enzyme. Cahn et al. (1962) demonstrated that the heart muscle LDH was inhibited by much lower pyruvate concentrations than that from skeletal muscle. Wachsmuth and Pfleiderer (1963) confirmed the different inhibiting effect of increasing pyruvate or lactate concentrations toward the five multiple LDH forms. A further biochemical characteristic is the different capacity of heart and of muscle LDH to hydrogenate 2-oxobutyrate compared to pyruvate. The heart type enzyme shows the same activity with this homologous substrate or with pyruvate. In contrast, the skeletal muscle enzyme has less activity with the homologous substrate (Rosalki and Wilkinson, 1960; Wilkinson et al., 1961) (see Table III; decrease ratio oxobutyrate/pyruvate).

In the course of our study of the production of the five multiple LDH forms in human embryonal development, we have found that LDH V is more predominant in anaerobically metabolizing tissues (i.e., skeletal muscle epidermis), whereas LDH I is predominant in aerobically metabolizing tissues, (i.e., brain and heart) (Pfleiderer and Wachsmuth, 1961).

As shown in Table IV, the first group of organs consists of components

TABLE III

RATIOS OF THE ACTIVITIES OF HUMAN TISSUE LACTATE DEHYDROGENASE
ISOENZYMES WITH 3.3 mM 2-OXOBUTYRATE AND 0.7 M-PYRUVATE AT 25°[a]

Tissue	Isoenzyme				
	1	2	3	4	5
Heart	1.0[b]	1.0	0.67	0.29	—
Skeletal muscle	0.84	0.80	0.45	0.28	0.10
Liver	—	0.53	0.53	0.29	0.16

[a] Plummer et al. (1963).
[b] Values are expressed as ratio of activity with 2-oxobutyrate:activity with pyruvate.

with activity mainly associated with molecules that migrate most rapidly
to the anode during electrophoresis (I); in the second group the LDH
activity is mainly associated with the slowest moving components (V),
the activity in the third group is found mainly in the intermediate components (III).

It appears that in all organs the intermediate components predominate
at an earlier stage of fetal development. This observation can be explained by an equal production of H_4 and M_4 LDH in the cell, which
results in forming a maximal number of H_2M_2 hybrids. After the organ
or tissue starts to differentiate, the distribution pattern of the isoenzymes
changes to that found in the adult tissue caused by increase of H_4 or M_4
biosynthesis.

TABLE IV

DISTRIBUTION PATTERN OF LDH ISOENZYMES IN DIFFERENT HUMAN
ADULT TISSUES[a]

Tissue	I	II	III	IV	V
Group 1					
Heart	60	30	5	3	2
Kidney	28	34	21	11	6
Brain	28	32	19	16	5
Group 2					
Liver	0.2	0.8	1	4	94
Muscle	3	4	7.5	9.5	76
Epidermis	0	0	7	17	79
Group 3					
Esophagus	5	18	40	24	13
Uterus	8	24.5	39	24.7	7.7
Thyroid gland	12.5	29.6	30.8	20.3	6.6
Spleen	5	15	31	31	18
Lung	14	28	30	22	6

[a] Percent of total activity.

In the embryonic mouse (Markert and Ursprung, 1962), LDH IV and LDH V predominate. During development there is a gradual change to a pattern containing more anionic components. Numerous investigations in this field have shown that there are wide species variations in the developmental changes and, in addition, wide variations in the rate of development of different tissue patterns within a single species. The changes in the distribution pattern of LDH isoenzymes in embryonic and adult tissues can give important information about the metabolic regulation of isoenzyme biosynthesis. Further, it appears that substrate inhibition has less physiological importance than product inhibition. Stambaugh and Post (1966) demonstrated the great influence on pyruvate reduction effected by lactate. They found that (even in the resting state of an isolated cat muscle) a 21.9 mM concentration of lactate was sufficient to cause 55% product inhibition of pyruvate reduction by the LDH H$_4$ but only a 13% inhibition by the function LDH M$_4$.

The rate of synthesis of M$_4$ subunits appears to be specifically regulated by oxygen tension. Goodfriend et al. (1966) presented a detailed investigation of the control of LDH synthesis in tissue culture cells and chick embryos. In tissue cultured monkey heart cells the synthesis of M$_4$ was increased at very low oxygen tension (below 0.1 atm). This increase could be inhibited by adding actinomycin D or puromycin.

B. NATURAL SPECIFIC INHIBITORS

Another highly interesting form of regulation is typified by specific LDH inhibitors that occur in the human body. Schoenenberger and Wacker (1966) isolated two low molecular weight peptides from human urine and showed that they are present also in the liver, heart, skeletal muscle, and serum. Peptide No. I is a very potent inhibitor of LDH M$_4$, but has no effect on LDH H$_4$. Peptide No. II is effective only in inhibiting LDH H$_4$ and is inactive against LDH M$_4$. A concentration of $9 \times 10^{-9}\ M$ of Peptide I completely abolished the activity of LDH M$_4$. This inhibition is reversible by dilution.

C. CLINICAL ASPECTS

This is not the appropriate place to describe in detail the clinical aspects based on the results discussed above. Many successes have been obtained from studies of the appearance of tissue-specific distribution patterns of LDH isoenzymes in the sera of patients. In certain cases it is possible to explore the origin of a tissue disease. An important result is the discovery of a change of the distribution pattern of LDH forms in cancerous tissues. As we pointed out in preliminary experiments (Pfleiderer and Wachsmuth, 1961), it seems that malignant tumor cells contain mainly LDH III, LDH IV, and LDH V, irrespective of the tissue from which the tumor arises. Many authors have since made similar observations. In other cases (hepatoma) an increase of H_4 type LDH was detected. It is impossible for the author to select critically the different experiments done in this field. The purity and histological characterization of a cancerous tissue is of considerable importance. At present, the common idea exists that during cancerogenesis a dedifferentiation process occurs. During this process the distribution pattern of multiple LDH forms changes to a fetal-type pattern (Schapira et al., 1970). This effect is most likely explained as due to a shift to a more glycolytic metabolism.

IV. HORSE LIVER ALCOHOL-DEHYDROGENASE (LADH) ISOENZYMES

In recent years there has been increasing interest in the observation of multiple forms of liver ADH. At first Dalziel (1958) was able to separate the crystalline enzyme (Bonnichsen and Wassén, 1948) by free electrophoresis and chromatography into two distinct active fractions. More subfractions were demonstrated by the Swiss group (Papenberg et al., 1965) and by McKinley-McKee and Moss (1965). Papenberg et al. (1965) found that the two liver enzymes show marked differences in their catalytic properties. An improved chromatographic procedure now permits the separation of up to seven different fractions (see von Wartburg et al., 1970). By 1960, Ungar had observed the activity of commercial LADH on hydroxysteroid substrates. In systematic investigations Theorell et al. (1966) found more steroid-active fractions in the collected supernatants from many LADH crystallizations. In addition, an ADH (designated $LADH_s$) was crystallized that proved to be less active (2/3) on ethanol than ordinary LADH ($LADH_E$), but many times more active on steroids (S designates steroids, and E designates ethanol). Because of the dimeric structure, the most steroid-active enzymes is called S-S, the most ethanol-active is called E-E, and the hybrid is designated E-S. The additional components must be explained by the existence of gene variants in the E and S subunit genes. Inhibition experiments and estimation of the quotient of activity with acetaldehyde and 5β-androstan-17β-ol-3-one (5 dihydro-testosterone, DHT) show no significant differences between fractions I, IIa, b and c, but large differences between this group and components III, IV, and V (von Wartburg et al., 1970). After Theorell (1970), the relationship between different terminology starts from the cathode.

Stockholm	SS	SS'	SS"	ES	ES'	ES"	EE	EE'	EE"	—	—
Shrewsbury	—	—	—	1	2	2A	3	4	5	—	—
Bern	V	—	—	IV	—	—	III	IIc	IIb	IIa	I

The E-E enzyme is not active with DHT; the quotient of the velocity acetaldehyde/DHT is 50 for E-S and 2.3 for S-S.

Akesone and Lundquist (1970) have recently purified S-S (most basic). The amino acid composition of E-E, E-S, and S-S is very similar. Jörnwall (1969) has carefully studied the fingerprints of these three major components after carboxymethylation and tryptic digestion. A few differences between the digests were observed. Four peptides not detected in E-E were found in E-S. In each peptide only a single amino acid residue was substituted by another. He postulated a common genetic origin for the E and S chains, each of which have evolved into two different chains by a few mutations. The substitutions as numbered from the acetyl-N-terminal are the following:

No.	Theorell (1970) Position from N-terminal	E	S
1	17	Glu	Gln
2	92	Thr	Ile
3	99	Arg	Ser
4	108	Phe	Leu
5	362	Glu	Lys

The changes in substrate specificity can be explained by differences in the binding sites. Apparently the regions of mutation might be in close vicinity to the binding sites. Fluorometric titration experiments on E-E, E-S and S-S with NADH and kinetic investigations have demonstrated the difference between the isoenzymes and the hybrid. Enzyme S-S binds NADH more firmly than does E-E. The dissociation constant for the interaction of S-S with NADH is nearly independent of pH, whereas NADH affinity for E-E is diminished by a factor of 10 in going from pH 9.35 to 10.

We can expect that in the near future knowledge of the primary and the three dimensional structure of both isoenzymes E-E and S-S will develop. These results will give us very interesting information on the relationship between structure and function.

V. Cytoplasmic and Mitochondrial Malate Dehydrogenase (MDH)

Malate dehydrogenase (MDH) is distributed both in mitochondrial and cytoplasmic cell fractions. Wieland et al. (1959) have separated rat liver homogenate into mitochondrial and cytoplasmic fractions. From both fractions MDH was extracted. The MDH from the two fractions could be distinguished by their different electrophoretic mobilities and by their different sulfite inhibition ratios. The kinetic characteristics of the two isoenzymes were shown to be different by Delbrück et al. (1959a,b). Grimm and Doherty (1961) succeeded in separating two species of malate dehydrogenase from bovine heart and found immunological differences between them. On the other hand, Thorne *et al.* (1963) have demonstrated multiple forms of MDH in pig heart mitochondria. The latter were postulated to be conformational isomers of the same polypeptide chain in chicken heart (Kitto *et al.*, 1966). Mann and Vestling (1968) were successful in separating the major band of rat liver mitochondrial MDH by CM Sephadex chromatography. Three fractions were obtained which were partially overlapping, starting from the cathode, these are designated A, B, and C. Dissociation experiments with each component were carried out at pH 2 in 0.1 M mercaptoethanol, and renaturation was achieved by dilution with 0.5 M sodium citrate (pH 7). After this procedure there is no difference in the electrophoretic mobilities of A and C. Reversible dissociation of component B resulted in three components identical with A, B, and C. At least two isoenzymes may exist.

The most characteristic difference between mitochondrial and cytoplasmic MDH is the strong inhibiting effect of oxaloacetate on the mitochondrial enzyme at concentrations at which the cytoplasmic enzyme still shows maximal activity. Substrate inhibition by malate is more pronounced with the cytoplasmic enzyme. This observation would indicate that the mitochondrial enzyme is better employed for the oxidation of malate, while the cytoplasmic enzyme favors the reduction of oxaloacetate. Witt *et al.* (1966) also detected in *Saccharomyces cerevisiae* the existence of two forms of MDH distinguishable by different inhibition effects of oxaloacetate. One of these enzymes was only found in the mitochondria and was called A; the other one was observed in the extramitochondrial space and was called B. Only A could be detected in yeast grown on glucose, but after incubating cells on acetate as the only carbon source both isoenzymes were found. A repression of A synthesis is postulated as occurring in the glucose medium.

Murphy *et al.* (1967) have postulated an identical molecular weight for mitochondrial and cytoplasmic MDH isolated from higher animals (~70,000). Because of their different amino acid compositions (Kitto and Kaplan, 1966), the mitochondrial and cytoplasmic MDH isoenzymes yield a different tryptic fingerprint (Devenyi *et al.*, 1966).

VI. CONCLUDING REMARKS

In view of the initial critical remarks, further observations about the existence of other multiple dehydrogenase forms will not be discussed here. We do not have enough information concerning the isoenzymes of isocitrate dehydrogenase. As in the case of MDH, there appears to exist a mitochondrial and a cytoplasmic form distinguishable by immunotechniques (Lowenstein and Smith, 1962). Today we anxiously anticipate more information and understanding of the structure and the function of dehydrogenase isoenzymes. More detailed experiments with pure isoenzymes and further intensive genetic and metabolic investigations are necessary. In conclusion, we can state that the occurrence of true isoenzymes is an expression of a highly developed organism and represents a new regulatory mechanism for the complicated higher organisms.

REFERENCES

Adams, M. J., McPherson, A., Rossmann, M. G., Schevitz, R. W., Smiley, I. E., and Wonacott, A. J. (1970). In "Pyridine Nucleotide Dependent Dehydrogenases" (H. Sund, ed.), p. 157. Springer, Berlin.

Akeson, A., and Lundquist, I. (1970). In preparation.

Allison, W. S. (1968). Ann. N. Y. Acad. Sci. 151, 180.

Apella, E., and Markert, C. L. (1961). Biochem. Biophys. Res. Commun. 6, 171.

Blanco, A., and Zinkham, W. H. (1963). Science 139, 601.

Bonnichsen, R., and Wassén, A. (1948). Arch. Biochem. Biophys. 18, 361.

Boyer, S. H., Fainer, D. C., and Watson-Williams, E. J. (1963). Science 141, 142.

Brändén, C. I., Zeppezauer, E., Boiwe, T., Söderlund, G., Söderberg, B. O., and Nordström, B. (1970). In "Pyridine Nucleotide Dependent Dehydrogenases" (H. Sund, ed.), p. 129. Springer, Berlin.

Cahn, R. D., Kaplan, N. O., Levine, L., and Zwilling, E. (1962). Science 136, 962.

Clausen, J., and Øvlisen, B. (1965). Biochem. J. 97, 513.

Dalziel, K. (1958). Acta Chem. Scand. 12, 459.

Davidson, B. E., Sajgò, M., Noller, H. F., and Harris, J. I. (1967). Nature (London) 216, 1181.

Delbrück, A., Zebe, E., and Bücher, T. (1959a). Biochem. Z. 331, 27.

Delbrück, A., Schimassek, H., Bartsch, K., and Bücher, T. (1959b). Biochem. Z. 331, 297.

Devenyi, T., Rogers, S. J., and Wolfe, R. G. (1966). Nature (London) 210, 489.

Falkenberg, F., Lehmann, F. G., and Pfleiderer, G. (1969). Clin. Chim. Acta 23, 265.

Fondy, T. P., Pesce, A., Freedberg, I., Stolzenbach, F. E., and Kaplan, N. O. (1964). Biochem. Z. 3, 527.

Fondy, T. P., Everse, J., Priscoll, G. A., Castillo, F., Stolzenbach, F. E., and Kaplan, N. O. (1965). J. Biol. Chem. 240, 4219.

Goldbey, E. (1963). Science 139, 602.

Goodfriend, T. L., Sokol, D. M., and Kaplan, N. O. (1966). J. Mol. Biol. 15, 18.

Grimm, F. C., and Doherty, D. G. (1961). J. Biol. Chem. 236, 190.

Harris, J. I., and Perham, R. N. (1968). Nature (London) 219, 1025.

Holbrook, J. J., Pfleiderer, G., Schnetger, J., and Diemair, S. (1966). Biochem. Z. 344, 1.

Holbrook, J. J., Pfleiderer, G., Mella, K., Volz, M., Leskowac, W., and Jeckel, R. (1967). Eur. J. Biochem. 1, 476.

Jaenicke, R. (1970). In "Pyridine Nucleotide Dependent Dehydrogenases" (H. Sund, ed.), p. 71. Springer, Berlin.

Jörnvall, H. (1969). Biochem. Biophys. Res. Commun. 35, 542.

Jörnvall, H. (1970). Eur. J. Biochem. 16, 25 and 41.

Kaplan, N. O., and White, S. (1963). Ann. N. Y. Acad. Sci. 103, 835.

Kirschner, K., and Voigt, B. (1969). *Hoppe Seyler's Z. Physiol. Chem.* **349**, 632.

Kitto, G. B., and Kaplan, N. O. (1966). *Biochemistry* **5**, 3966.

Kitto, G. B., Wassermann, P. M., and Kaplan, N. O. (1966). *Proc. Nat. Acad. Sci. U. S.* **56**, 578.

Koen, A. L., and Shaw, C. R. (1964). *Biochem. Biophys. Res. Commun.* **15**, 92.

Krebs, E. G., Rafter, G. W., and Junge, J. M. (1953). *J. Biol. Chem.* **200**, 479.

Latner, A. L., and Skillen, A. W. (1968). "Isoenzymes in Biology and Medicine," pp. 92–118. Academic Press, New York.

Lowenstein, J. M., and Smith, S. R. (1962). *Biochim. Biophys. Acta* **56**, 385.

McKinley-McKee, J. S., and Moss, D. W. (1965). *Biochem. J.* **96**, 583.

Mann, K. G., and Vestling, C. S. (1968). *Biochim. Biophys. Acta* **159**, 567.

Markert, C. L. (1963). *Science* **140**, 1329.

Markert, C. L., and Møller, F. (1959). *Proc. Nat. Acad. Sci. U. S.* **45**, 753.

Markert, C. L., and Ursprung, H. (1962). *Develop. Biol.* **5**, 363.

Mella, K. (1970). Unpublished data.

Mella, K., Fölsche, E., Torff, H. J., and Pfleiderer, G. (1968). *Hoppe Seyler's Z. Physiol. Chem.* **349**, 891.

Mella, K., Torff, H. J., Fölsche, E., and Pfleiderer, G. (1969). *Hoppe Seyler's Z. Physiol. Chem.* **350**, 28.

Murphy, W. H., Kitto, G. B., and Kaplan, N. O. (1967). *Biochemistry* **6**, 603.

Nisselbaum, J. S., and Bodansky, O. (1959). *J. Biol. Chem.* **234**, 3276.

Nisselbaum, J. S., and Bodansky, O. (1961). *J. Biol. Chem.* **236**, 323.

Papenberg, J., von Wartburg, J. P., and Aebi, H. (1965). *Biochem. Z.* **342**, 65.

Pesce, A., McKay, R. H., Stolzenbach, F. E., Cahn, R. D., and Kaplan, N. O. (1964). *J. Biol. Chem.* **239**, 1753.

Pfleiderer, G. (1968). *6th Int. Congr. Clin. Chem., 1966* Vol. 2, pp. 10–20.

Pfleiderer, G., and Jeckel, D. (1957). *Biochem. Z.* **331**, 103.

Pfleiderer, G., and Mella, K. (1970). *FEBS Symp.* **18**, 151.

Pfleiderer, G., and Wachsmuth, E. D. (1961). *Biochem. Z.* **334**, 185.

Plagemann, P. G. W., Gregory, K. F., and Wroblewsky, F. (1960). *J. Biol. Chem.* **235**, 2288.

Plummer, D. T., Elliot, B. A., Cooke, K. B., and Wilkinson, J. H. (1963). *Biochem. J.* **87**, 416.

Rajewsky, K. (1966). *Biochim. Biophys. Acta* **121**, 51.

Rajewsky, K., Avrameas, S., Grabar, P., Pfleiderer, G., and Wachsmuth, E. D. (1964). *Biochim. Biophys. Acta* **92**, 248.

Rosalki, S. B., and Wilkinson, J. H. (1960). *Nature (London)* **188**, 1110.

Rossmann, M. G. (1969). Personal communication.

Schapira, F., Dreyfus, J. C., and Schapira, G. (1970). *FEBS Symp.* **18**, 305.

Schoenenberger, G. A., and Wacker, W. E. C. (1966). *Biochemistry* **5**, 1375.

Shaw, C. R., and Koen, A. L. (1965). *J. Histochem. Cytochem.* **13**, 431.

Stambaugh, R., and Post, D. (1966). *J. Biol. Chem.* **241**, 1462.

Theorell, H. (1970). In "Pyridine Nucleotide Dependent Dehydrogenases" (H. Sund, ed.), p. 121. Springer, Berlin.

Theorell, H., Tanaguchi, S., Akeson, A., and Shursky, L. (1966). *Biochem. Biophys. Res. Commun.* **24**, 603.

Thorne, C. J. R., Grossmann, L. I., and Kaplan, N. O. (1963). *Biochim. Biophys. Acta* **73**, 193.

Ungar. F. (1960). *Univ. Minn. Med. Bull.* **31**, 226.

von Wartburg, J. P., Kopp, P. M., and Lutstorf, V. M. (1970). *FEBS Symp.* **18**, 195.

Wachsmuth, E. D., and Pfleiderer, G. (1963). *Biochem. Z.* **336**, 545.

Wachsmuth, E. D., Pfleiderer, G., and Wieland, T. (1964). *Biochem. Z.* **340**, 80.

Wieland, T., and Pfleiderer, G. (1957). *Biochem. Z.* **329**, 112.

Wieland, T., Pfleiderer, G., Haupt, I., and Wörner, W. (1959). *Biochem. Z.* **332**, 1.

Wieland, T., Georgopulos, D., Kampe, H., and Wachsmuth, E. D. (1964). *Biochem. Z.* **340**, 483.

Wilkinson, J. H., Cooke, K. B., Elliot, B. A., and Plummer, D. T. (1961). *Biochem. J.* **80**, 29P.

Witt, J., Kronau, R., and Holzer, H. (1966). *Biochim. Biophys. Acta* **128**, 6.

Woenckhaus, C., Berghäuser, J., and Pfleiderer, G. (1969). *Hoppe Seyler's Z. Physiol. Chem.* **350**, 473.

Zinkham, W. H., Blanco, A., and Kupchyk, L. (1963). *Science* **142**, 1303.

Role of Acetyl Coenzyme A Carboxylase in the Control of Fatty Acid Synthesis

S. NUMA, S. NAKANISHI, T. HASHIMOTO, N. IRITANI, AND T. OKAZAKI

Department of Medical Chemistry, Kyoto University Faculty of Medicine, Kyoto, Japan

I. INTRODUCTION

The main route of *de novo* synthesis of long-chain fatty acids proceeds via malonyl-CoA as an intermediate (Wakil, 1958; Formica and Brady, 1959; Lynen, 1959, 1961; cf. reviews of Vagelos, 1964; Stumpf, 1969) as follows:

$$\text{Acetyl-CoA} + \text{HCO}_3^- + \text{ATP} \underset{}{\overset{\text{Mg}^{2+}}{\rightleftarrows}} \text{malonyl-CoA} + \text{ADP} + \text{P}_i \quad (1)$$

$$\text{Acetyl-CoA} + 7 \text{ malonyl-CoA} + 14 \text{ NADPH} \rightarrow$$
$$\text{palmitic acid} + 7 \text{ CO}_2 + 8 \text{ CoA} + 14 \text{ NADP} + 6 \text{ H}_2\text{O} \quad (2)$$

Malonyl-CoA is formed by carboxylation of acetyl-CoA catalyzed by acetyl-CoA carboxylase [acetyl-CoA:CO₂ ligase (ADP), EC 6.4.1.2] [Eq. (1)] and is converted to fatty acids through a series of reactions catalyzed by fatty acid synthetase [Eq. (2)].

Acetyl-CoA carboxylase contains biotin as prosthetic group (Wakil,

1958; Wakil *et al.*, 1958), and the carboxylation is achieved in two steps as follows:

$$\text{ATP} + \text{HCO}_3^- + \text{biotin enzyme} \overset{\text{Mg}^{2+}}{\rightleftharpoons} \text{carboxybiotin enzyme} + \text{ADP} + \text{P}_i \quad (3)$$

$$\text{Carboxybiotin enzyme} + \text{acetyl-CoA} \rightleftharpoons \text{biotin enzyme} + \text{malonyl-CoA} \quad (4)$$

This reaction sequence was demonstrated first by exchange experiments with labeled substrates (Lynen *et al.*, 1963; Matsuhashi *et al.*, 1964). The carboxybiotin enzyme intermediate was then isolated, and the active carboxyl was shown to be bound to the 1′-*N*-atom of biotin, which is amide-linked to the ε-amino group of a lysine residue in the enzyme protein (Fig. 1) (Numa *et al.*, 1964). The role of biotin-dependent carboxylations in biosynthetic reactions was reviewed thoroughly by Lynen (1967a).

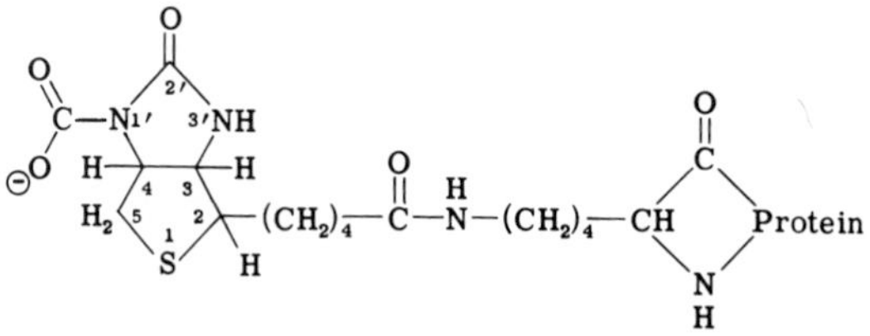

Fig. 1. Structure of the carboxylated active site of acetyl-CoA carboxylase. From Numa *et al.* (1964).

II. Acetyl-CoA Carboxylase as Key Enzyme for Fatty Acid Synthesis

In order to study the control mechanisms of a metabolic sequence consisting of several steps catalyzed by different enzymes, it is of importance to know which step is rate-limiting in the overall process. Shortly after the discovery of the fatty acid-synthesizing pathway via malonyl-CoA, evidence was presented which indicated that the carboxylation step is rate-limiting in overall synthesis from acetyl-CoA in tissue extracts (Ganguly, 1960; Numa *et al.*, 1961). Subsequent investigations revealed that carboxylase was not fully activated under the conditions employed in these experiments. It was shown, namely, that the activity of carboxylase is affected by a variety of substances and conditions as discussed in more detail in Section IV. Above all, carboxylase is activated markedly by tri- and dicarboxylic acids, especially by citrate (Matsuhashi *et al.*, 1962; Martin and Vagelos, 1962; Waite, 1962; Kallen and Lowenstein, 1962). In order to fully activate carboxylase from rat liver as well as from rat adipose tissue, it is required to preincubate enzyme with citrate, and the degree of activation varies largely with the conditions of the preincubation (Vagelos *et al.*, 1963; Numa and Ringelmann, 1965; Greenspan and Lowenstein, 1967, 1968). Furthermore, Swanson *et al.* (1968) showed that carboxylase in rat liver extract is activated following preincubation even without citrate. It was also found that the activity of carboxylase in liver extract, when fully activated, is as high as one-third to one-half that of synthetase (Chang *et al.*, 1967; Majerus *et al.*, 1968).

Our data pertinent to this are presented in Fig. 2 showing comparative effects of preincubation at 37°C on overall fatty acid synthesis from acetyl-CoA, acetyl-CoA carboxylase, and fatty acid synthetase in rat liver extract. It is evident that carboxylase was activated in parallel with overall fatty acid synthesis during preincubation with or without citrate (10 mM) and Mg^{2+} (10 mM), whereas synthetase activity was not increased but rather decreased by preincubation. Thus, stimulation of overall fatty acid synthesis in liver extract following preincubation is ascribed to activation of carboxylase. It is also seen from Fig. 2 that, although carboxylase activity, when assayed without preincubation, was far lower than synthetase activity, it attained a level comparable to that of synthetase following preincubation.

Table I shows the effects of addition of either purified carboxylase, purified synthetase, or both on overall fatty acid synthesis by preincubated or nonpreincubated rat liver extract. Addition of carboxylase to nonpreincubated extract increased fatty acid synthesis by an amount corresponding roughly to the amount of the enzyme added, whereas addition of purified synthetase exhibited no significant effect. In contrast to this, addition of either carboxylase or synthetase to preincubated extract hardly elevated fatty acid synthesis, as compared with the amounts of the enzymes added. Since addition of both carboxylase and synthetase resulted in a rise in fatty acid synthesis corresponding roughly to the amounts of the enzymes added, inhibition of added carboxylase or synthetase by some factors present in the extract was excluded. These results indicate that carboxylase is rate-limiting in overall fatty acid synthesis in nonpreincubated rat liver extract, whereas carboxylase and synthetase exhibit comparable activities in preincubated extract.

The mechanisms by which activation of carboxylase in crude rat liver extract occurs following preincubation with citrate are probably similar to those established for purified enzyme, i.e., citrate-induced aggregation of enzyme molecules as described in Section IV,A. It is possible, however, that the activation following preincubation without citrate may occur somewhat differently. This activation cannot be ascribed to endogenous citrate or other low-molecular components, since preincubation of gel-filtered liver extract likewise resulted in activation of carboxylase. In this

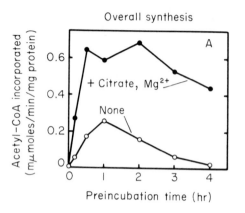

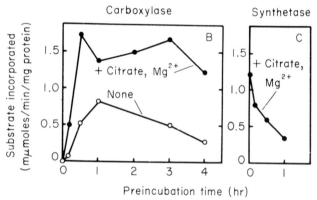

FIG. 2. Effect of preincubation on overall fatty acid synthesis from acetyl-CoA (A), acetyl-CoA carboxylase (B), and fatty acid synthetase (C) in rat liver extract. Carboxylase was assayed at 37°C by measuring incorporation of acetyl-CoA-^{14}C into fatty acids in the presence of excess synthetase, and synthetase by measuring incorporation of malonyl-CoA-2-^{14}C into fatty acids. Since different liver extracts were employed for the three types of assays, the values obtained cannot be compared with each other. In another experiment, in which the same extract was used for all the assays, the maximal values found for overall synthesis, carboxylase, and synthetase were 0.41, 0.56, and 1.21 mμmoles/min/mg protein, respectively. Under the experimental conditions employed, preincubation with 10 mM citrate alone activated carboxylase to the same extent as that with 10 mM citrate and 10 mM Mg^{2+}. The data were presented at a seminar. "Control of Fatty Acid Synthesis and Oxidation in Higher Animals," under the U. S.–Japan Cooperative Science Program, at Waltham, Massachusetts in October, 1968.

regard, it is of interest that carboxylase is activated by trypsin treatment (cf. Section IV,C).

The question, to what extent carboxylase is activated *in vivo*, is of great interest in relation to the physiological regulation of fatty acid

TABLE I

EFFECT OF ADDITION OF PURIFIED CARBOXYLASE OR PURIFIED SYNTHETASE
ON OVERALL FATTY ACID SYNTHESIS IN RAT LIVER EXTRACT

Assay conditions	Addition (mμmoles/min)	Acetate or acetyl-CoA incorporated (mμmoles/min)
Without preincubation[a] (liver extract protein, 2.0 mg)	None	0.16
	Carboxylase 0.46	0.49
	Carboxylase 0.91	0.86
	Synthetase 6.85	0.30
	Carboxylase 0.91 ⎱ Synthetase 6.85 ⎰	1.28
With preincubation[b] (liver extract protein, 1.0 mg)	None	0.37
	Carboxylase 0.88	0.40
	Carboxylase 4.80	0.88
	Synthetase 0.59	0.36
	Synthetase 3.04	0.69
	Carboxylase 4.80 ⎱ Synthetase 2.30 ⎰	2.49

[a] From Numa et al. (1961). Acetate-^{14}C incorporation was measured.

[b] Preincubated at 37°C for 30 minutes with 10 mM potassium citrate and 10 mM MgCl$_2$. Acetyl-CoA-^{14}C incorporation was measured. Data presented at a seminar, "Control of Fatty Acid Synthesis and Oxidation in Higher Animals," under the U.S.–Japan Cooperative Science Program, at Waltham, Massachusetts in October, 1968.

synthesis in cells. Indeed, it is not possible at present to answer this question, but some speculations can be made as follows: Carboxylase is activated by citrate and subjected to end-product inhibition by long-chain fatty acyl-CoA derivatives (Bortz and Lynen, 1963a; Numa et al., 1965a). The apparent Michaelis constant (K_m) for citrate and the apparent inhibition constant (K_i) for palmityl-CoA are 2–6 mM and 0.8–1.1 μM, respectively (Numa et al., 1965b). The contents of citrate (Lynen, 1967b; Start and Newsholme, 1968) and long-chain acyl-CoA derivatives (Bortz and Lynen, 1963b; Tubbs and Garland, 1963, 1964) in liver are about 0.3 and 0.015–0.05 μmole/gm wet weight, respectively. From comparison of the cellular concentrations of these effectors with the K_m and K_i values, it appears reasonable to assume that carboxylase is not fully activated in cells, although the circumstances in vivo are hard to assess on account of cellular compartmentation and of interactions with various proteins. These considerations suggest that acetyl-CoA carboxylase represents a key enzyme for cellular control of fatty acid synthesis. This would be of teleonomic significance, since the carboxylation reaction is the first step in the biosynthetic sequence leading specifically to fatty acids. In the following sections, control mechanisms of the amount as well as the activity of this regulatory enzyme will be discussed.

III. CONTROL MECHANISMS FOR THE AMOUNT OF ACETYL-CoA CARBOXYLASE

It is well known that the level of acetyl-CoA carboxylase activity in liver extract is lowered in fasted or alloxan-diabetic rats and elevated upon refeeding fasted animals a fat-free diet (Numa *et al.*, 1961; Wieland *et al.*, 1963; Allmann *et al.*, 1965). Previous studies on the regulation of the carboxylase were based exclusively on measurements of catalytic activity, which do not differentiate between changes in catalytic efficiency per enzyme molecule and changes in the number of enzyme molecules, i.e., enzyme quantity. Recently, an immunochemical approach has been undertaken independently by our group (Numa *et al.*, 1969; Nakanishi *et al.*, 1969; Nakanishi and Numa, 1970) and by Majerus and Kilburn (1969) to elucidate the mechanisms by which the level of acetyl-CoA carboxylase activity is changed following the dietary and hormonal variations. We developed a procedure to purify rat liver acetyl-CoA carboxylase to homogeneity and prepared antibody by injecting this enzyme to rabbits. By means of this antibody, the quantity of carboxylase protein was estimated in liver extracts from rats under the different dietary conditions and in diabetes. Furthermore, the rates of synthesis and degradation of this enzyme under these conditions were assessed by immunochemical techniques with the use of isotopic leucine in order to explore the mechanisms of variations in enzyme quantity. Majerus' group, employing antibody against homogeneous chicken liver enzyme, which cross-reacted with rat liver enzyme, made similar studies with rats under the different dietary conditions. The results obtained by both groups were in general agreement. Our results including those on diabetes will be presented below.

A. PURIFICATION OF RAT LIVER ACETYL-CoA CARBOXYLASE AND ITS IMMUNOLOGICAL CHARACTERIZATION

Table II summarizes the procedure of purification of rat liver acetyl-CoA carboxylase. The enzyme was purified 1,700-fold over crude liver extract, the yield being 17%. The specific activity of purified rat liver carboxylase (6.2–7.5 units/mg protein at 25°C) was comparable to that of pure chicken liver enzyme, i.e. 3–5 units/mg protein at 25°C (Numa *et al.*, 1966; Goto *et al.*, 1967; Numa, 1969) or 8–11 units/mg protein at 37°C (Gregolin *et al.*, 1966a, 1968a). Figure 3 shows that the rat liver enzyme preparation sedimented as a single, sharp, symmetrical boundary in the analytical ultracentrifuge with no evidence of impurity.

Figure 4A represents an Ouchterlony double diffusion pattern of anti-

TABLE II

PURIFICATION OF ACETYL-CoA CARBOXYLASE FROM RAT LIVER[a]

Fraction	Volume (ml)	Protein (mg)	Total activity[b] at 25°C (units)	Specific activity[b] at 25°C (units/mg)
Crude extract	2,440	105,000	465[c]	0.0044[c]
First (NH₄)₂SO₄	815	43,400	330[c]	0.0076[c]
Ca₃(PO₄)₂ gel + second (NH₄)₂SO₄	105	1,530	227	0.15
Dialysis at 24°C	112	1,120	364	0.32
DEAE-cellulose	104	134	225	1.68
Sepharose-2B	55	10.2	77	7.55

[a] From 1,660 gm of livers obtained from rats fasted for 48 hours and subsequently refed a fat-free diet for 48 hours. From Nakanishi and Numa (1970).

[b] Assayed at 25°C spectrophotometrically by coupling with the fatty acid synthetase reaction except for crude extract and first (NH₄)₂SO₄ fraction. One unit of enzyme is defined as that amount which catalyzes the carboxylation of 1 μmole of acetyl-CoA per minute.

[c] Assayed at 37°C by the ¹⁴CO₂-fixation method and corrected to the conditions for the spectrophotometric assay at 25°C by multiplying by a factor of 0.5.

body made against purified rat liver carboxylase in the center well and carboxylase preparations of widely differing specific activities. A single connecting band of precipitation was observed, indicating that the carboxylase preparation employed as antigen was homogeneous. Figures 4B, C, D, and E show Ouchterlony double diffusion analyses in the absence and the presence of citrate with the first ammonium sulfate fractions derived from livers of normal, fasted, refed, and diabetic rats. As discussed in more detail in Section IV,A, acetyl-CoA carboxylase is known to exist

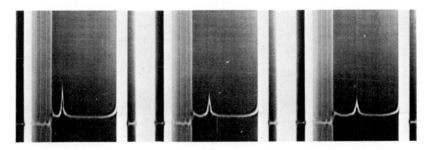

FIG. 3. Sedimentation pattern of rat liver acetyl-CoA carboxylase. Purified enzyme (specific activity, 7.5 units/mg protein at 25°C) dissolved in a phosphate medium containing citrate was centrifuged at 23.9°C in the Spinco Model E ultracentrifuge. Sedimentation is shown from left to right at 4-minute intervals, the first picture being taken 4 minutes after the full speed of 31,410 rpm was reached.

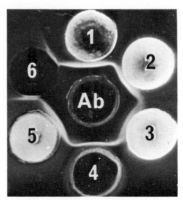

A. No citrate

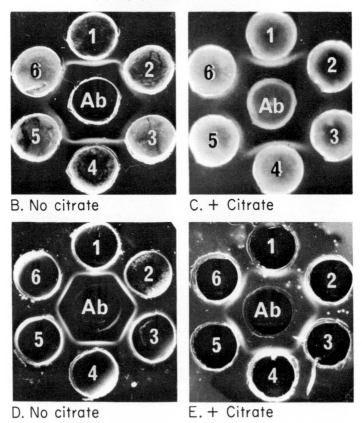

B. No citrate   C. + Citrate

D. No citrate   E. + Citrate

FIG. 4. Ouchterlony double diffusion patterns of rat liver acetyl-CoA carboxylase. The center wells contained antiacetyl-CoA carboxylase γ-globulin. (A) Well *1*, first $(NH_4)_2SO_4$ fraction from refed rats; well *2*, first $(NH_4)_2SO_4$ fraction from normal rats;

both as an inactive protomeric form and as an active polymeric form, the former being converted to the latter in the presence of citrate. The appearance of a single precipitin band in the presence and the absence of citrate indicates therefore that both forms of carboxylase can be precipitated by antibody. The band of precipitation under addition of citrate was located more closely to the antigen wells, corresponding to slower diffusion of aggregated carboxylase molecules in the presence of citrate. Furthermore, the completeness of connections of the precipitin bands shows that carboxylase molecules obtained from livers of fasted, refed, and diabetic rats are immunologically similar to those from normal animals.

B. LIVER ACETYL-CoA CARBOXYLASE CONTENT UNDER DIFFERENT DIETARY AND HORMONAL CONDITIONS

Figure 5 represents immunochemical titrations of liver extracts obtained from normal, fasted, refed, and diabetic rats. Despite the fact that

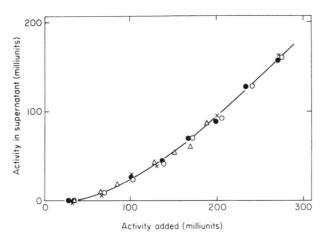

FIG. 5. Immunochemical analysis of levels of liver acetyl-CoA carboxylase activity of normal, fasted, refed, and diabetic rats. To 50 μg of antiacetyl-CoA carboxylase γ-globulin were added increasing amounts of liver extracts. Following completion of precipitation, the supernatant fluids were assayed for carboxylase activity at 37°C by the $^{14}CO_2$-fixation method. ○, normal rats; △, rats fasted for 48 hours; ×, rats fasted for 48 hours and subsequently refed a fat-free diet for 48 hours; ●, diabetic rats. From Nakanishi and Numa (1970).

well *3*, first (NH₄)₂SO₄ fraction from fasted rats; well *4*, carboxylase of the Sepharose-2B step from refed rats; well *5*, second (NH₄)₂SO₄ fraction from refed rats; well *6*, NaCl. (B and C) Wells *1* and *4*, refed; wells *2* and *5*, normal; wells *3* and *6*, fasted. (D and E) Wells *1*, *3*, and *5*, normal; wells *2*, *4*, and *6*, diabetic. From Nakanishi and Numa (1970).

the level of carboxylase activity derived from 1 gm of liver fell 4.5-fold and 2.7-fold in starvation and diabetes, respectively, and rose 2.0-fold following refeeding, the equivalence point, i.e., the point at which enzyme activity first appeared in the supernatant fluid, was the same for all four types of liver extracts when based on the amount of enzyme activity added. This finding showed that the changes in the level of carboxylase activity resulting from the dietary and hormonal variations are accompanied by proportionate changes in the quantity of immunochemically reactive protein.

In these studies, the amount of antibody was held constant. Another titration procedure, in which the amount of liver extract was kept constant, was carried out in an experiment represented in Fig. 6. The amount of antibody required to precipitate completely the carboxylase activity in a given amount of liver extract, as estimated by extrapolations of the linear portions of the titration curves to zero carboxylase activity, was decreased 2.2-fold by fasting and increased 2.7-fold by refeeding. Since the levels of carboxylase activity in normal, fasted, and refed rats were

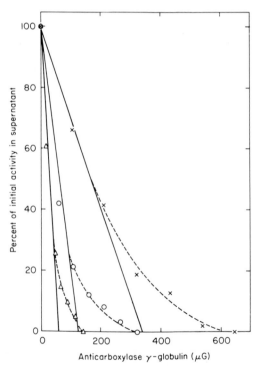

FIG. 6. Immunochemical titration of liver acetyl-CoA carboxylase from normal, fasted, and refed rats. The amount of liver extracts used was 1.0 ml. The symbols represent the same as in Fig. 5. From Nakanishi and Numa (1970).

95, 43, and 241 mU per milliliter of liver extract, respectively, the proportionality between catalytic activity and immunochemically estimated enzyme protein was confirmed. Thus, the catalytic efficiency per acetyl-CoA carboxylase molecule is not changed despite the 9-fold variations in the level of carboxylase activity derived from 1 gm of liver of rats under the different alimentary and hormonal conditions. The changes in the level of enzyme activity in liver extract are actually determined by changing quantities of enzyme protein.

C. Synthesis and Degradation of Liver Acetyl-CoA Carboxylase

In order to assess whether changes in the quantity of acetyl-CoA carboxylase following dietary manipulation or in diabetes are due to changes in the rate of enzyme synthesis or in that of enzyme degradation, studies on the incorporation of isotopic leucine into enzyme were undertaken. As a measure of the rate of enzyme synthesis, the extent of leucine-^{3}H incorporation into protein precipitated by antiacetyl-CoA carboxylase following pulse-labeling was determined. The results of such experiments with normal, fasted, refed, and diabetic rats are shown in Table III. The

TABLE III

Relative Rate of Liver Acetyl-CoA Carboxylase Synthesis in Normal, Refed, Fasted, and Diabetic Rats[a]

	Acetyl-CoA carboxylase in liver extract[c]			Leucine-^{3}H incorporation[d]		
				(a) Acetyl-CoA carboxylase total[e] (cpm)	(b) Total soluble protein (cpm/mg)	a/b
Treatment[b]	Mean weight (gm)	Specific activity (mU/mg)	Total activity[e] (units)			
None	180	8.58	8.36	38,013	9,253	4.1
Fasted for 48 hours and subsequently refed a fat-free diet for 72 hours	180	26.9	31.4	130,302	7,846	16.6
Fasted for 48 hours	180	3.16	2.32	29,110	13,454	2.2
Alloxan-diabetes	250	3.79	4.41	11,695	4,857	2.4

[a] From Nakanishi and Numa (1970).
[b] Two rats of each group were employed, except that three fasted rats were used.
[c] $^{14}CO_2$-fixation assay at 37°C.
[d] Incorporation in 3 hours after intraperitoneal injection of 0.9 mCi of L-leucine-4,5-^{3}H (57.6 Ci/mmole).
[e] Per two rats.

specific radioactivity of total soluble liver protein precipitated with tri-chloroacetic acid differed considerably in the four types of rats due prob-ably in part to different free amino acid pools present in the various ani-mals. Since the extent of labeling of total soluble protein is reflected in carboxylase labeling, the ratio of the radioactivity incorporated into enzyme to that incorporated into total soluble protein (a/b) was calcu-lated as a measure of the rate of enzyme synthesis. The data indicate that this relative rate of enzyme synthesis is decreased 1.9-fold and 1.7-fold by fasting and diabetes, respectively, and increased 4.0-fold by re-feeding.

As a measure of the rate of enzyme degradation, the rate of loss of radioactivity from prelabeled carboxylase was determined after injection of leucine-[3]H. Figure 7 represents the results of such experiments with normal, refed, and diabetic rats, which exhibited different steady state contents of carboxylase. The decay of specific radioactivity of carboxy-lase followed a first-order reaction. The rate of loss of isotope, expressed as half-life, was essentially the same under all three conditions, i.e., 59, 55, and 59 hours in normal, refed, and diabetic animals, respectively.

In Fig. 8 are shown the results of studies on enzyme degradation in fasted animals. In contrast to steady state conditions, the rate of degrada-tion of protein under conditions of changing contents is given by the change in total radioactivity in the protein, not by the change in specific

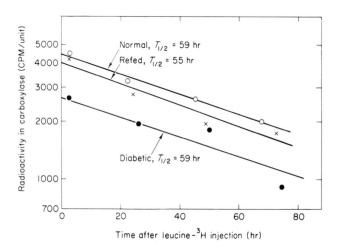

Fig. 7. Turnover of liver acetyl-CoA carboxylase in normal, refed, and diabetic rats. At zero time, 0.9 mCi of L-leucine-4,5-[3]H (57.6 Ci/mmole) was injected intra-peritoneally to rats treated as indicated in Table III. Two rats from each group were killed at the indicated times to measure the radioactivity incorporated into enzyme. O—O, normal; X—X, refed; ●—●, diabetic. From Nakanishi and Numa (1970).

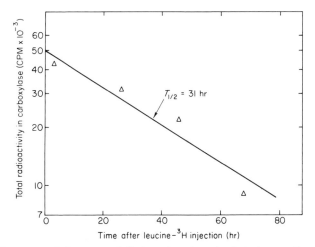

Fig. 8. Turnover of liver acetyl-CoA carboxylase in fasted rats. Experimental conditions were the same as in Fig. 7, except that three fasted rats were killed at the indicated times. From Nakanishi and Numa (1970).

radioactivity (Koch, 1962). The decay of total radioactivity precipitated by antiacetyl-CoA carboxylase followed a first-order reaction, the half-life being 31 hours.

In experiments like these, reutilization of leucine-^{3}H may lead to an overestimation of the half-life (Koch, 1962). However, this appears not to be of major significance in our experiments for the following reasons: The half-life for total soluble liver protein estimated simultaneously by means of this isotope was 3.8 days, 3.7 days, 3.4 days, and 2.9 days in normal, refed, diabetic, and fasted rats, respectively, whereas the half-life found by the use of guanido-labeled arginine, which is not reutilized, is 5.1 days in normal rats (Arias et al., 1969).

Under steady state conditions, the content of an enzyme is related to the rates of its synthesis and degradation as follows:

$$E = k_s/k_d \qquad (5)$$

where E is the content of enzyme per mass, k_s is a zero-order rate constant of synthesis per mass, and k_d is a first-order rate constant of degradation expressed as time^{-1} (cf. Arias et al., 1969). Normal rats maintained on a balanced diet, those refed a fat-free diet for more than 72 hours, and animals suffering from prolonged diabetes can be assumed to be in a steady state, and the level of liver acetyl-CoA carboxylase activity can be taken as the content of enzyme as concluded above. Since the rate constant of enzyme degradation is essentially the same in these three types of animals (Fig. 7), the 3.8-fold increase in enzyme content observed in refed rats and the 1.9-fold decrease in it seen in diabetic rats (Table III) should be reflected by changes in the rate constant of enzyme synthesis. In fact, the isotopic leucine incorporation studies shown in Table III indicate that the relative rate of enzyme synthesis (a/b) rises 4.0-fold in refed animals and falls 1.7-fold in diabetic animals. Thus, the changes in carboxylase content in refed and diabetic rats can be ascribed to changes in the rate of enzyme synthesis. Since the specific activity of homogeneous rat liver acetyl-CoA carboxylase is 15 units/mg protein at 37°C (Table II), the rate constant of enzyme synthesis can be calculated according to Eq. (5) to be 3.3 μg per hour per normal rat (mean body weight, 180 gm), 13.2 μg per hour per refed rat (180 gm), and 1.7 μg per hour per diabetic rat (250 gm).

Under the experimental conditions employed, fasted rats were not in a steady state, since both the weight of liver and the content of carboxylase per rat were diminished gradually during the experimental period. It is seen from Table III and Fig. 8 that the 3.6-fold decrease in enzyme content after 2 days' starvation is accompanied by a 1.9-fold rise in the rate of enzyme degradation and a 1.9-fold fall in the relative rate of enzyme synthesis. Although quantitative discussions according to Eq. (5) cannot be made in this instance, it is concluded that the decrease in enzyme content following fasting is due both to diminished enzyme synthesis and to accelerated enzyme degradation.

It is of interest to note that synthesis and degradation of liver acetyl-CoA carboxylase are controlled independently. In refed and diabetic rats, the rate of enzyme synthesis is increased or decreased, whereas the rate of enzyme degradation remains unchanged. On the other hand, in fasted rats not only the rate of enzyme synthesis is decreased, but also the rate of enzyme degradation is increased. Of particular interest is a comparison of the situations in diabetic and fasted animals. Although the enzyme content is diminished in both types of animals, an increased rate of enzyme degradation is encountered in fasted rats, but not in diabetic rats. Diabetic animals, like normal and refed animals, are presumably in a steady state, each type of animal exhibiting different steady state carboxylase contents, whereas fasted animals are not in a steady state. The above findings are consistent, therefore, with the assumption that control of enzyme content by changes in the rate of enzyme degradation may play an important role only when the animal deviates from a steady state for adjustment to a new environment. This view is supported also by the following findings of Schimke (1964) on liver arginase. Rats maintained on diets containing 8, 30, and 70% casein show different steady state arginase contents but essentially the same rates of arginase degradation. Upon changing rats from a diet containing 70% protein to one containing 8% protein, the rate of arginase degradation is increased during the first 3 days. However, it then gradually approaches the rate seen in the steady state, as the enzyme content attains a new steady state level lower than the initial one. When rats are fasted, the arginase degradation ceases, and the enzyme content rises concomitantly.

The factors responsible for independent controls of the synthesis and degradation of acetyl-CoA carboxylase are unknown. In this connection, Allmann et al. (1965) showed that addition of linoleate to fat-free diet tends to suppress the elevation of fatty acid synthesis seen when fat-free diet alone is fed. Moreover, the relative linoleate content was found to fall progressively during refeeding of fat-free diet coincidently with a rise in fatty acid synthesis. It remains to be elucidated, however, whether linoleate or a substance related to it acts as a corepressor for enzyme synthesis. The finding of the same group (Hicks et al., 1965) that actinomycin D or puromycin prevents the rise in the level of carboxylase activity upon refeeding is consistent with the present results indicating an increase in the rate of enzyme synthesis in refed rats.

One of the striking features of minimum deviation hepatomas is their loss of control of fatty acid synthesis following dietary alterations (Sabine et al., 1968; Elwood and Morris, 1968). Majerus et al. (1968) demonstrated that the acetyl-CoA carboxylase from hepatomas is essentially identical with that derived from liver. Preliminary results indicate that the level of enzyme activity in the tumors parallels the content of immunologically reactive protein and that no change in the rate of enzyme synthesis occurs in the tumors after fat-free feeding (Majerus and Kilburn, 1969). These results suggest that the defect of control of fatty acid synthesis is due to the failure of the tumors to change the amount of enzyme rather than to structural alteration of enzyme. It is of great interest to explore the mechanisms by which the control of the amount of enzyme is lost in hepatomas, since this defect may be related to the malignancy of the tumor cells.

IV. Control Mechanisms for the Activity of Acetyl-CoA Carboxylase

In Section III, it was concluded that the changes in the level of acetyl-CoA carboxylase activity in liver extract seen under the different dietary and hormonal conditions studied are determined by changing quantities of enzyme protein. However, this finding in vitro excludes by no means that control by changes in catalytic efficiency per enzyme molecule may be also involved in the regulation of the rate of acetyl-CoA carboxylation in vivo. In fact, the activity of liver acetyl-CoA carboxylase is affected by various metabolites. Tri- and dicarboxylic acids including citrate (cf. Section II) and long-chain acylcarnitine compounds (Fritz and Hsu, 1967; Greenspan and Lowenstein, 1968) activate carboxylase, whereas long-chain acyl-CoA derivatives (cf. Section II) and malonyl-CoA (Matsuhashi et al., 1964; Gregolin et al., 1966b) are inhibitors. The inhibition by long-chain acyl-CoA derivatives can be regarded as a negative feedback mechanism due to end-product inhibition. The effectors are more concentrated in liver cells than in their extract and may possibly be localized in certain cellular compartments. In addition, in such metabolic conditions associated with depressed fatty acid synthesis as fasting or diabetes, the citrate content of liver is lowered to about one half (Lynen, 1967b; Start and Newsholme, 1968), while the content of long-chain acyl-CoA derivatives is elevated 2- to 4-fold (Bortz and Lynen, 1963b; Tubbs and Garland, 1963, 1964). Moreover, Korchak and Masoro (1962) and Wieland and Eger-Neufeldt (1963) demonstrated that in an earlier stage of fasting, i.e., after 24 hours' fasting or in acute decompensated diabetes, the fatty acid-synthesizing capacity of liver slices is more depressed than can be accounted for by the level of acetyl-CoA carboxylase activity in liver extract. It is evident from the half-lives of carboxylase given in Section III,C that the enzyme content cannot fall very rapidly. Therefore, control mechanisms by inhibition or activation of enzyme activity may play an important role, when the rate of fatty acid synthesis must be adjusted promptly. On the other hand, control mechanisms by changes in enzyme quantity may contribute more to the long-term regulation of fatty acid synthesis.

Recently, two hypolipidemic agents, 2-methyl-2-[p-(1,2,3,4-tetrahydro-1-naphthyl)phenoxy]propionate and ethyl 2-(p-chlorophenyl)-2-methylpropionate, have been demonstrated to inhibit liver acetyl-CoA carboxylase (Maragoudakis, 1969). Kinetic analysis showed that both drugs act on a site different from the site of inhibition by palmityl-CoA. It is suggested that the effect of these compounds as lipid-lowering agents may be accounted for by inhibition of acetyl-CoA carboxylase in vivo.

A. MOLECULAR BASIS FOR CHANGES IN CATALYTIC ACTIVITY OF ACETYL-COA CARBOXYLASE

In order to understand the mechanisms by which the catalytic efficiency per acetyl-CoA carboxylase molecule is changed, detailed studies on the relationship between structure and activity of this carboxylase are required. The correlation found between catalytic activity and sedimentation coefficient of acetyl-CoA carboxylase suggested that activation and inhibition of the carboxylase is accompanied by association and dissociation of enzyme molecules, respectively (Vagelos et al., 1963; Numa et al., 1965b; Numa and Ringelmann, 1965). The subsequent isolation of homogeneous enzyme preparations from chicken liver permitted more definite characterization of the molecular properties of the enzyme (Gregolin et al., 1966a,b, 1968a,b; Numa et al., 1966, 1967; Ryder et al., 1967; Henniger, 1969). The protomeric ("small") form has a sedimentation coefficient ($s_{20,w}$) of 13–14 S and a molecular weight of 409,000 and represents the molecular unit containing 1 molecule of biotin. The polymeric ("large") form is composed of 10–20 protomers, exhibiting a sedimentation coefficient of 40–55 S and a molecular weight of 4–8 millions. A characteristic feature of the polymeric form is its filamentous structure revealed by electron microscopy (Gregolin et al., 1966a; Kleinschmidt et al., 1969). Work of our group, measuring light scattering at various angles, showed that the polymeric form assumes a rodlike shape also in its solution (Henniger, 1969). The protomeric and polymeric forms are in an association-dissociation equilibrium which is influenced not only by the allosteric effectors mentioned above but also by a variety of factors including carboxylation of enzyme to produce carboxybiotin enzyme, protein concentration, pH, ionic strength, and composition of medium. Extensive studies under various conditions demonstrated that there is always a correlation between catalytic activity and aggregational state of liver acetyl-CoA carboxylase; the "large" (40–55 S) and the "intermediary" (27–33 S) polymeric forms are catalytically active, whereas the protomeric form (13–14 S) is practically inactive. This is true even when sucrose density gradient centrifugation and activity measurements are carried out under conditions as comparable as possible, especially with regard to enzyme concentration; the aggregational state of the enzyme depends largely upon its concentration as mentioned above. The problem, whether alterations in catalytic activity are caused primarily by a subtle conformational change or related directly to the aggregational state, remains to be solved.

Knowledge of the subunit structure of acetyl-CoA carboxylase is of great importance to elucidate its allosteric characters. Gregolin et al. (1968b) found that further dissociation of the protomer of chicken liver enzyme with sodium dodecyl sulfate gives rise to subunits with a molecular weight of 114,000. The presence of nonidentical subunits is indicated by the fact that there is a single biotinyl prosthetic group and there are single binding sites for both citrate and acetyl-CoA on the protomer. An important advance in this regard is recent work on Escherichia coli acetyl-CoA carboxylase (Alberts and Vagelos, 1968; Alberts et al., 1969; Nervi and Alberts, 1970). This enzyme is composed of three functionally dissimilar proteins. One, designated on the basis of its catalytic activity as biotin carboxylase, catalyzes ATP-dependent carboxylation of biotin which is covalently bound to a low molecular weight protein, carboxyl carrier protein. The third protein catalyzes the transfer of the carboxyl

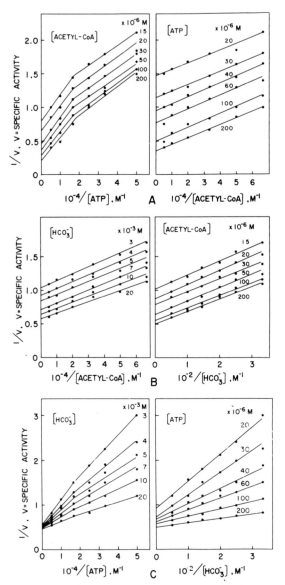

FIG. 9. Lineweaver-Burk plots of initial velocities of the forward reaction. (A) ATP and acetyl-CoA were varied at a fixed concentration of KHCO₃ (5 mM). (B) KHCO₃ and acetyl-CoA were varied at 0.05 mM ATP. (C) ATP and KHCO₃ were varied at 0.03 mM acetyl-CoA. Enzyme activity was assayed at 37°C spectrophotometrically by coupling with the pyruvate kinase and lactate dehydrogenase reactions; the citrate concentration was 10 mM. From Hashimoto et al. (1970).

group from the carboxyl carrier protein to acetyl-CoA, thus forming malonyl-CoA. The carboxyl carrier protein resembles acyl carrier protein in many respects. The *E. coli* system, which can be dissociated more readily than the animal enzyme, is not activated by citrate. Thus, the acetyl-CoA carboxylase from animal sources appears to be a complex of tightly bound subunits corresponding to the three proteins of the bacterial enzyme, therefore exhibiting allosteric properties.

B. Kinetic Analysis of Reaction Mechanism of and Citrate Action on Acetyl-CoA Carboxylase

As described in Section I, isotope exchange studies as well as the isolation of the carboxylated enzyme intermediate support the reaction mechanism of acetyl-CoA carboxylase involving two partial reactions as expressed by Eqs. (3) and (4); both these steps are activated by citrate (Matsuhashi *et al.*, 1964; Gregolin *et al.*, 1968a; Stoll *et al.*, 1968). However, a detailed study of reaction kinetics which might corroborate the two-step mechanism has been lacking. It is obviously important to analyze kinetically the reaction mechanism of acetyl-CoA carboxylase and the stimulatory effect of citrate, in order to understand the control mechanisms for the activity of this enzyme. We therefore have undertaken the following studies.

Figures 9 and 10 represent the results of initial velocity studies for the forward and reverse reactions of rat liver acetyl-CoA carboxylase. Reciprocal initial velocities are plotted against reciprocal concentrations of one of the three substrates at various fixed concentrations of a second substrate. In these experiments, the concentration of the third substrate was held at a constant value close to its Michaelis constant, not at a saturating level. When the concentrations of acetyl-CoA and either ATP or HCO_3^- were varied for the forward reaction, the plots gave families of parallel lines (Figs. 9A and 9B). On changing the concentrations of ATP and HCO_3^-, however, nonparallel lines were obtained (Fig. 9C), and the lines intersected to the left of the $1/v$ axis. In the reverse reaction, variations in the concentrations of malonyl-CoA and either ADP or P_i resulted in families of parallel lines (Figs. 10A and 10B). The lines obtained with ADP and P_i as varied substrates, however, intersected to the left of the vertical axis (Fig. 10C). These results indicate that the mechanism as expressed by Eqs. (3) and (4) represents the main pathway for the overall reaction. It is also indicated that the first partial reaction [Eq. (3)] proceeds either through the "ordered" mechanism or through the "rapid equilibrium random" mechanism as designated by Cleland (1963).

Table IV summarizes the results of product inhibition studies. Inhi-

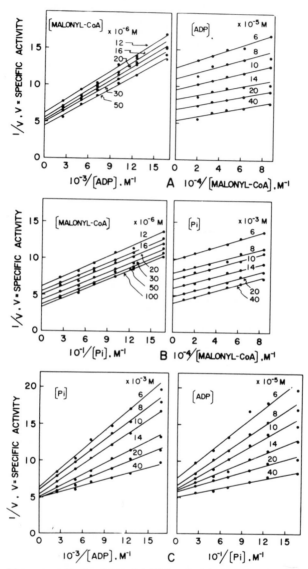

FIG. 10. Lineweaver-Burk plots of initial velocities of the reverse reaction. (A) Malonyl-CoA and P_i were varied at a fixed concentration of ADP (0.14 mM). (B) Malonyl-CoA and ADP were varied at 10 mM P_i. (C) P_i and ADP were varied at 0.02 mM malonyl-CoA. Enzyme activity was assayed at 37°C spectrophotometrically by coupling with the hexokinase and glucose-6-phosphate dehydrogenase reactions; the citrate concentration was 10 mM. From Hashimoto et al. (1970).

TABLE IV
PRODUCT INHIBITION PATTERNS FOR THE FORWARD REACTION[a]

Inhibitory product	Substrate varied		Inhibition
Malonyl-CoA	ATP	lower concentrations	Noncompetitive
		higher concentrations	Competitive
	HCO_3^-	lower ATP concentrations	Noncompetitive
		higher ATP concentrations	Noncompetitive
	Acetyl-CoA		Noncompetitive
ADP	ATP	lower concentrations	Noncompetitive
		higher concentrations	Competitive
	Acetyl-CoA		Uncompetitive

[a] From Hashimoto et al. (1970).

bition by malonyl-CoA of the forward reaction showed a noncompetitive pattern with HCO_3^- as varied substrate at both low and high concentrations of ATP, and likewise a noncompetitive pattern with acetyl-CoA as varied substrate. The inhibition by malonyl-CoA was indeed competitive with ATP as varied substrate at its higher concentrations, but noncompetitive at its lower concentrations. Inhibition by ADP of the forward reaction exhibited similar patterns with ATP as varied substrate, i.e., noncompetitive at lower concentrations of ATP but competitive at its higher concentrations. The inhibition by ADP was uncompetitive when the acetyl-CoA concentration was varied. These results are generally consistent with the "ordered" mechanism of the first partial reaction [Eq. (3)], ATP being the first substrate to add and P_i being the last product to be released (cf. Cleland, 1963). Gregolin et al. (1966b) reported that inhibition by malonyl-CoA of the forward reaction of chicken liver acetyl-CoA carboxylase was competitive with respect to acetyl-CoA. This apparent discrepancy from our results may be due to the high ATP concentration employed by these authors, since the inhibition pattern is likely to appear to be of competitive type in the presence of a large excess of ATP (cf. Cleland, 1963).

On the basis of the results of the initial velocity and product inhibition studies described above, the acetyl-CoA carboxylase reaction is most likely to proceed through the "bi bi uni uni ping pong" mechanism as outlined by the scheme below (cf. Cleland, 1963). The apparent Michaelis constants (K_m) as well as the apparent dissociation constants (K_i) for substrates at infinite concentrations of the other two cosubstrates were determined by replotting the data of the initial velocity and product inhibition studies (Cleland, 1963; Rudolph and Fromm, 1969; Dalziel, 1969). These values, together with the apparent dissociation constant for

TABLE V

APPARENT KINETIC CONSTANTS FOR ACETYL-CoA CARBOXYLASE

	K_m (M)	K_i (M)
ATP	1.5×10^{-5a}	8.0×10^{-4a}
HCO_3^-	2.5×10^{-3}	
Acetyl-CoA	2.5×10^{-5}	2.8×10^{-7}
Malonyl-CoA	1.6×10^{-5}	8.7×10^{-5}
P_i	7.0×10^{-3}	4.5×10^{-2}
ADP	1.0×10^{-5}	
Citrate		
Forward reaction	4.5×10^{-3}	
Reverse reaction	3.2×10^{-3}	

[a] Determined from the linear portion of the plots for lower ATP concentrations.

citrate (K_i (citrate)) determined from the data of Figs. 11 and 12, are listed in Table V.

As described in Section II, rat liver acetyl-CoA carboxylase requires preincubation with citrate for full activation, and the degree of activation depends on various factors including citrate concentration, temperature and time of preincubation, and enzyme concentration (Numa and Ringelmann, 1965). In order to minimize the complexities of the activation effect, enzyme preincubated with 10 mM citrate for sufficiently long periods of time was employed in all experiments, so that only the citrate effect during catalysis was analyzed. The initial velocities of the forward and reverse reactions were determined with changing concentrations of a substrate at various fixed concentrations of citrate. Plots of reciprocal initial velocities against reciprocal concentrations of either citrate or substrate are shown in Figs. 11 and 12. In the forward reaction, the plots for citrate and either ATP or HCO_3^- as varied substrate yielded families of parallel lines (Figs. 11A and 11B), whereas those for citrate and acetyl-CoA as varied substrate intersected on the $1/v$ axis (Fig. 11C). In the reverse reaction, families of parallel lines resulted from the plots for citrate and malonyl-CoA as varied substrate (Fig. 12A). On the other hand, the plots for citrate and P_i as varied substrate intersected on the $1/v$ axis (Fig. 12B), whereas those for citrate and ADP as varied substrate to the left of the vertical axis (Fig. 12C).

These data on the effect of citrate on the initial velocities of the forward and reverse reactions indicate that the site of citrate action during catalysis lies predominantly on the carboxylated enzyme (cf. Cleland, 1963). Previous results with the chicken liver carboxylase (Gregolin et al., 1966b, 1968b; Numa et al., 1967; Ohtsu et al., 1968) showed that

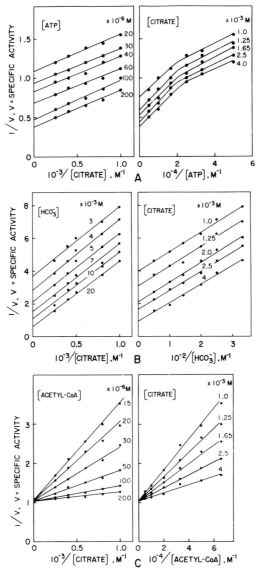

FIG. 11. Lineweaver-Burk plots of forward reaction velocity and citrate concentration as function of one of the three substrates. (A) Initial velocities were determined as functions of citrate and ATP at fixed concentrations of KHCO₃ (5 mM) and acetyl-CoA (0.05 mM). (B) Effects of citrate and KHCO₃ at 0.05 mM ATP and 0.03 mM acetyl-CoA. (C) Effects of citrate and acetyl-CoA at 0.05 mM ATP and 5 mM KHCO₃. For assay of enzyme activity, see Fig. 9. From Hashimoto et al. (1970).

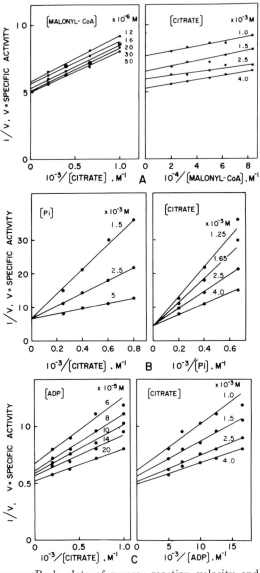

Fig. 12. Lineweaver-Burk plots of reverse reaction velocity and citrate concentration as function of one of the three substrates. (A) Initial velocities were determined as functions of citrate and malonyl-CoA at fixed concentrations of P_i (5 mM) and ADP (0.1 mM). (B) Effects of citrate and ADP at 0.02 mM malonyl-CoA and 5 mM P_i. (C) Effects of citrate and P_i at 0.02 mM malonyl-CoA and 0.14 mM ADP. For assay of enzyme activity, see Fig. 10. From Hashimoto et al. (1970).

the carboxylated enzyme form (E-biotin $\sim CO_2$) has a greater tendency to be dissociated than the uncarboxylated enzyme form (E-biotin) and that citrate prevents this dissociation or reassociates the dissociated protomers. At the same time, citrate increases the rate of decarboxylation of the carboxylated enzyme, enhancing the reactivity of the $1'$-N-carboxyl group of carboxybiotinyl enzyme (Ryder et al., 1967; Ohtsu et al., 1968). We propose therefore that there exists an equilibrium between active E-biotin $\sim CO_2$ and inactive E_0-biotin $\sim CO_2$ and that this equilibrium is shifted toward the active form by binding of citrate to the carboxylated enzyme. Thus, the reaction mechanism of citrate-dependent liver acetyl-CoA carboxylase may be outlined as follows:

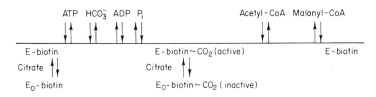

As described in Section IV,A, citrate acts also on the uncarboxylated enzyme to induce polymerization of protomeric carboxylase molecules. Binding experiments of Gregolin et al. (1968b) revealed that the chicken liver carboxylase (uncarboxylated form) has one tight binding site per protomer for citrate, the dissociation constant ($K_{i\ (citrate)}$) being 2–3 × $10^{-6}\ M$. This value is about 10^3 times lower than the $K_{i\ (citrate)}$ value found by our kinetic experiments, which indicate that citrate acts on the carboxylated enzyme as described above. The effect of citrate on the uncarboxylated enzyme would not manifest itself in the present studies, since the citrate concentrations used ranged from 1 to 5 mM.

Previous studies showed that the citrate activation of acetyl-CoA carboxylase was due to an elevation of the V_{max} values for substrates (Numa et al., 1965b; Gregolin et al., 1968a). The present results disagree in part with the previous ones. The main difference is that the present data give double reciprocal plots intersecting on the $1/v$ axis, when the concentration of acetyl-CoA was changed at various fixed concentrations of citrate, indicating an effect of citrate on the apparent K_m value for acetyl-CoA. This discrepancy may be ascribed to different experimental conditions employed in both studies. In the present investigation, enzyme was fully activated before use for assay of catalytic activity by preincubation with 10 mM citrate for more than 30 minutes, whereas in our previous experiments preincubation of enzyme was conducted for 10 minutes at various citrate concentrations corresponding to its final concentrations during catalysis. It was found that under these conditions of preincubation, enzyme was not fully activated. Moreover, in the present experiments, the citrate concentration was kept lower than 4–5 mM, whereas previously citrate concentrations up to 10 mM were used; higher citrate concentrations were found to result in excessive activation by changing the concentration of free Mg^{2+} (Hashimoto et al., 1970).

C. Modification of Acetyl-CoA Carboxylase by Trypsin

Another aspect of interest in relation to the allosteric nature of rat liver acetyl-CoA carboxylase is its modification by trypsin treatment. Trypsin-treated carboxylase exhibits altered sensitivities toward allosteric effectors, suggesting some modification of the citrate site or a site related closely to it. This phenomenon will be discussed below in some detail.

Using crude and partially purified rat liver enzyme preparations, Swanson et al. (1967) showed that the citrate-effect during preincubation is replaced by trypsin treatment of carboxylase. Subsequently, we demonstrated that homogeneous rat liver enzyme, when treated with trypsin, exhibits considerable activity even in the assay mixture without citrate (Iritani et al., 1969). In the experiment shown in Fig. 13, carboxylase was preincubated either with citrate, with trypsin, or with both, and the

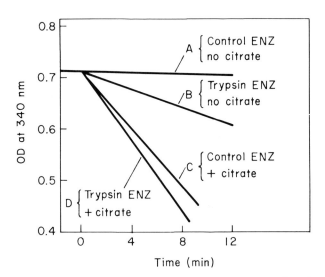

Fig. 13. Effects of trypsin and citrate on rat liver acetyl-CoA carboxylase. Enzyme was preincubated at 25°C for 10 minutes either with 4 µg/ml trypsin, with 10 mM citrate, or with both when indicated, and then assayed at 25°C spectrophotometrically by coupling with the pyruvate kinase and lactate dehydrogenase reactions. From Iritani et al. (1969).

reaction was initiated by adding the preincubated enzyme to the assay mixture. The extent of activation attained by trypsin treatment was 30–50% of that induced by citrate.

Table VI shows the inhibitory effects of varying concentrations of palmityl-CoA on trypsin-treated enzyme and control enzyme. Trypsin-treated enzyme was less sensitive toward inhibition by palmityl-CoA than control enzyme. Detailed kinetic studies on the reaction mechanism of the modified enzyme are in progress.

TABLE VI

EFFECT OF PALMITYL-CoA ON TRYPSIN-TREATED CARBOXYLASE[a]

| Palmityl-CoA (μM) | Relative activity[b] | |
	Trypsin-treated carboxylase (%)	Control carboxylase (%)
0	100	100
2	94	68
5	86	44
10	71	39
20	68	34

[a] From Iritani et al. (1969).
[b] Assay method as in Fig. 13.

In view of the close relationship between catalytic activity and aggregational state of liver acetyl-CoA carboxylase as described above, the sedimentation behavior of trypsin-treated carboxylase was studied under different conditions by means of sucrose density gradient centrifugation. Trypsin-treated enzyme sedimented as the "large" form even in the medium without citrate, whereas control enzyme sedimented as the "small" form in the absence of citrate and as the "large" form in its presence (Fig. 14A). In the presence of palmityl-CoA (Fig. 14B) or of ATP plus Mg^{2+} (Fig. 14C) which is known to inhibit carboxylase (Gregolin et al., 1966b; Greenspan and Lowenstein, 1967, 1968; Numa et al., 1967), trypsin-treated enzyme assumed the "large" form, whereas control enzyme assumed the "small" form. Thus, the catalytic activity is well correlated with the sedimentation coefficient in these instances, too. The trypsin treatment appears to result in conformational changes of enzyme protein similar to those induced by citrate and to lead to an aggregation of enzyme molecules. This finding, together with preliminary kinetic evidence (Hashimoto et al., 1970), suggests that the modification by trypsin of carboxylase might shift the equilibrium between E-biotin $\sim CO_2$ and E_0-biotin $\sim CO_2$ as well as that between E-biotin and E_0-

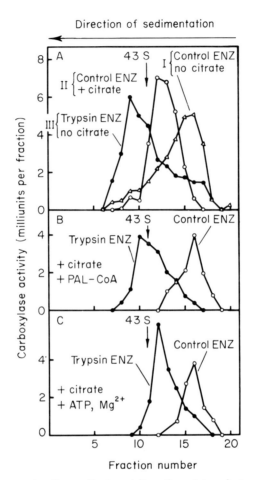

FIG. 14. Sucrose density gradient centrifugation of trypsin-treated rat liver acetyl-CoA carboxylase. Partially purified enzyme (second $(NH_4)_2SO_4$ fraction), with or without trypsin treatment, was centrifuged for 80 minutes at 38,000 rpm and 25°C in a gradient from 5 to 20% sucrose under the additions as indicated. From Iritani *et al.* (1969).

biotin toward the E-form (see the scheme in Section IV,B). Further studies are required to identify the molecular basis of this modification.

V. CONCLUSIONS

This paper concerns recent advances in studies on the regulatory mechanisms of a biotin enzyme, liver acetyl-CoA carboxylase, which plays a critical role in the control of fatty acid synthesis. Evidence is presented which indicates that the regulation of this carboxylation step *in vivo* is achieved both by changes in the amount of acetyl-CoA carboxylase, i.e., the number of enzyme molecules, and by changes in the activity of carboxylase, i.e., catalytic efficiency per enzyme molecule. The former mechanisms appear to be more responsible for the long-term control, while the latter for the short-term one. The question, how the action of hormones and the nervous system is exerted upon this enzymic control system, remains to be answered in the future.

REFERENCES

Alberts, A. W., and Vagelos, P. R. (1968). *Proc. Nat. Acad. Sci. U. S.* **59**, 561.

Alberts, A. W., Nervi, A. M., and Vagelos, P. R. (1969). *Proc. Nat. Acad. Sci. U. S.* **63**, 1319.

Allmann, D. W., Hubbard, D. D., and Gibson, D. M. (1965). *J. Lipid Res.* **6**, 63.

Arias, I. M., Doyle, D., and Schimke, R. T. (1969). *J. Biol. Chem.* **244**, 3303.

Bortz, W. M., and Lynen, F. (1963a). *Biochem. Z.* **337**, 505.

Bortz, W. M., and Lynen, F. (1963b). *Biochem. Z.* **339**, 77.

Chang, H. C., Seidman, I., Teebor, G., and Lane, M. D. (1967). *Biochem. Biophys. Res. Commun.* **28**, 682.

Cleland, W. W. (1963). *Biochim. Biophys. Acta* **67**, 104.

Dalziel, K. (1969). *Biochem. J.* **114**, 547.

Elwood, J. C., and Morris, H. P. (1968). *J. Lipid Res.* **9**, 337.

Formica, J. V., and Brady, R. O. (1959). *J. Amer. Chem. Soc.* **81**, 752.

Fritz, I. B., and Hsu, M. P. (1967). *J. Biol. Chem.* **242**, 865.

Ganguly, J. (1960). *Biochim. Biophys. Acta* **40**, 110.

Goto, T., Ringelmann, E., Riedel, B., and Numa, S. (1967). *Life Sci.* **6**, 785.

Greenspan, M. D., and Lowenstein, J. M. (1967). *Arch. Biochem. Biophys.* **118**, 260.

Greenspan, M. D., and Lowenstein, J. M. (1968). *J. Biol. Chem.* **243**, 6273.

Gregolin, C., Ryder, E.. Kleinschmidt, A. K., Warner, R. C., and Lane. M. D. (1966a). *Proc. Nat. Acad. Sci. U. S.* **56**, 148.

Gregolin, C., Ryder, E., Warner, R. C., Kleinschmidt, A. K., and Lane, M. D. (1966b). *Proc. Nat. Acad. Sci. U. S.* **56**, 1751.

Gregolin, C., Ryder, E., and Lane, M. D. (1968a). *J. Biol. Chem.* **243**, 4227.

Gregolin, C., Ryder, E., Warner, R. C., Kleinschmidt, A. K., Chang, H. C., and Lane, M. D. (1968b). *J. Biol. Chem.* **243**, 4236.

Hashimoto, T., Iritani, N., Nakanishi, S., and Numa, S. (1970). *Proc. Jap. Conf. Biochem. Lipids Meet.* **12**, 21.

Henniger, G. (1969). Ph.D. Thesis, University of Munich.

Hicks, S. E., Allmann, D. W., and Gibson, D. M. (1965). *Biochim. Biophys. Acta* **106**, 441.

Iritani, N., Nakanishi, S., and Numa, S. (1969). *Life Sci.* **8**, 1157.

Kallen, R. G., and Lowenstein, J. M. (1962). *Arch. Biochem. Biophys.* **96**, 188.

Kleinschmidt, A. K., Moss, J., and Lane, M. D. (1969). *Science* **166**, 1276.

Koch, B. L. (1962). *J. Theor. Biol.* **3**, 283.

Korchak, H. M., and Masoro, E. J. (1962). *Biochim. Biophys. Acta* **58**, 354.

Lynen, F. (1959). *J. Cell. Comp. Physiol.* **54**, Suppl. 1, 33.

Lynen, F. (1961). *Fed. Proc., Fed. Amer. Soc. Exp. Biol.* **20**, 941.
Lynen, F. (1967a). *Biochem. J.* **102**, 381.
Lynen, F. (1967b). *Progr. Biochem. Pharmacol.* **3**, 1.
Lynen, F., Matsuhashi, M., Numa, S., and Schweizer, E. (1963). *In* "The Control of Lipid Metabolism" (J. K. Grant, ed.), pp. 43–56. Academic Press, New York.
Majerus, P. W., and Kilburn, E. (1969). *J. Biol. Chem.* **244**, 6254.
Majerus, P. W., Jacobs, R., Smith, M. B., and Morris, H. P. (1968). *J. Biol. Chem.* **243**, 3588.
Maragoudakis, M. E. (1969). *J. Biol. Chem.* **244**, 5005.
Martin, D. B., and Vagelos, P. R. (1962). *Fed. Proc., Fed. Amer. Soc. Exp. Biol.* **21**, 289.
Matsuhashi, M., Matsuhashi, S., Numa, S., and Lynen, F. (1962). *Fed. Proc., Fed. Amer. Soc. Exp. Biol.* **21**, 288.
Matsuhashi, M., Matsuhashi, S., and Lynen, F. (1964). *Biochem. Z.* **340**, 263.
Nakanishi, S., and Numa, S. (1970). *Eur. J. Biochem.* **16**, 161.
Nakanishi, S., Ohtsu, E., and Numa, S. (1969). *Seikagaku* **41**, 492.
Nervi, A. M., and Alberts, A. W. (1970). *Fed. Proc., Fed. Amer. Soc. Exp. Biol.* **29**, 333 Abs.
Numa, S. (1969). *Methods Enzymol.* **14**, 9.
Numa, S., and Ringelmann, E. (1965). *Biochem. Z.* **343**, 258.
Numa, S., Matsuhashi, M., and Lynen, F. (1961). *Biochem. Z.* **334**, 203.
Numa, S., Ringelmann, E., and Lynen, F. (1964). *Biochem. Z.* **340**, 228.
Numa, S., Bortz, W. M., and Lynen, F. (1965a). *Advan. Enzyme Regul.* **3**, 407.
Numa, S., Ringelmann, E., and Lynen, F. (1965b). *Biochem. Z.* **343**, 243.
Numa, S., Ringelmann, E., and Riedel, B. (1966). *Biochem. Biophys. Res. Commun.* **24**, 750.
Numa, S., Goto, T., Ringelmann, E., and Riedel, B. (1967). *Eur. J. Biochem.* **3**, 124.
Numa, S., Nakanishi, S., and Iritani, N. (1969). *Proc. Jap. Conf. Biochem. Lipids Meet.* **11**, 235.
Ohtsu, E., Akagami, H., Okazaki, T., and Numa, S. (1968). *Seikagaku* **40**, 278.
Rudolph, F. B., and Fromm, H. J. (1969). *J. Biol. Chem.* **244**, 3832.
Ryder, E., Gregolin, C., Chang, H. C., and Lane, M. D. (1967). *Proc. Nat. Acad. Sci. U. S.* **57**, 1455.
Sabine, J. R., Abraham, S., and Morris, H. P. (1968). *Cancer Res.* **28**, 46.
Schimke, R. T. (1964). *J. Biol. Chem.* **239**, 3808.
Start, C., and Newsholme, E. A. (1968). *Biochem. J.* **107**, 411.
Stoll, E., Ryder, E., Edwards, J. B., and Lane, M. D. (1968). *Proc. Nat. Acad. Sci. U. S.* **60**, 986.
Stumpf, P. K. (1969). *Annu. Rev. Biochem.* **38**, 159.
Swanson, R. F., Curry, W. M., and Anker, H. S. (1967). *Proc. Nat. Acad. Sci. U. S.* **58**, 1243.
Swanson, R. F., Curry, W. M., and Anker, H. S. (1968). *Biochim. Biophys. Acta* **159**, 390.
Tubbs, P. K., and Garland, P. B. (1963). *Biochem. J.* **89**, 25P.
Tubbs, P. K., and Garland, P. B. (1964). *Biochem. J.* **93**, 550.
Vagelos, P. R. (1964). *Annu. Rev. Biochem.* **33**, 139.
Vagelos, P. R., Alberts, A. W., and Martin, D. B. (1963). *J. Biol. Chem.* **238**, 533.
Waite, M. (1962). *Fed. Proc., Fed. Amer. Soc. Exp. Biol.* **21**, 287.

Wakil, S. J. (1958). *J. Amer. Chem. Soc.* **80,** 6465.

Wakil, S. J., Titchener, E. B., and Gibson, D. M. (1958). *Biochim. Biophys. Acta* **29,** 225.

Wieland, O., and Eger-Neufeldt, I. (1963). *Biochem. Z.* **337,** 349.

Wieland, O., Eger-Neufeldt, I., Numa, S., and Lynen, F. (1963). *Biochem. Z.* **336,** 455.

Binding of Pyridoxal Phosphate to Apoenzymes as Studied by Optical Rotatory Dispersion and Circular Dichroism

OSAMU HAYAISHI AND YUTAKA SHIZUTA

Department of Medical Chemistry, Kyoto University Faculty of Medicine, Kyoto, Japan

I. Introduction

The enzyme-catalyzed reactions are, in general, stereospecific in contrast to the nonenzymatic reactions or reactions catalyzed by inorganic or simple organic catalysts, because the active centers of an enzyme are so organized as to bind and react with substrate in terms of stereochemical specificity. In order to understand the nature of the binding forces involved in the formation of the enzyme-substrate complex and also the nature of the specific loci responsible for the catalytic function, it is necessary to elucidate the mode of interaction between apoenzymes and coenzymes.

At present, X-ray crystallographic analysis appears to be the best method by which the three-dimensional structure of an enzyme can be determined in detail. But it is a laborious and time-consuming technique, and it can be used only with enzymes of relatively small molecular weights and those which can be prepared in large and homogeneous crystals. Since all the pyridoxal enzymes so far described in the literature have molecular weights of at least 38,000, none of these enzymes has been subjected to X-ray crystallographic analysis. Until this is accomplished, optical rotatory dispersion (ORD) and circular dichroism (CD) would be the most fruitful approach to the elucidation of three-dimensional mechanism of the enzyme catalysis involving pyridoxal phosphate (PLP).

In this paper we would like first briefly to review the principle of ORD and CD and then discuss some of our experimental results in regard to the binding of PLP and its analogs with bovine serum albumin (BSA) as a model system and also with biodegradative threonine deaminase. The remainder of this article briefly summarizes spectropolarimetric studies from several laboratories on other pyridoxal enzymes. For theoretical aspects of ORD and CD as well as their application and general use, the readers are referred to recent review articles and monographs (Djerassi, 1960; Urnes and Doty, 1961; Blout, 1964; Ulmer and Vallee, 1965; Beychok, 1966, 1968; Snatzke, 1967).

II. General Considerations

The optical rotatory power of an asymmetric molecule is best understood by considerations of the Cotton effect. If one considers that a beam of plane-polarized light is made up of two circularly polarized vibrations rotating in opposite directions with the same frequency and if the beam of light passes through a medium which has a different index of refraction for the left and right components, the left and right circular vibrations are transmitted with unequal velocities, and the plane of polarization is rotated (optical rotation). Since refractive indexes are expressed as functions of wavelength, the rotatory power varies with the wavelength of light, and this phenomenon is called rotatory dispersion (ORD).

When an optically active medium is traversed by a plane polarized light in the spectral range in which an optically active chromophore absorbs, not only does the plane of polarization rotate, but the resulting light is also elliptically polarized. In this case, a difference is observed between extinction coefficients for left and right circularly polarized light, i.e., there exists circular dichroism (CD), which is usually expressed as molar ellipticity. The combined phenomena for left and right circularly polarized light are known as the Cotton effect which is illustrated schematically in Fig. 1.

When a sample of enzyme protein is subjected to analysis by ORD and CD, the observed effect can be classified into intrinsic and extrinsic Cotton effects (Blout, 1964). The former is due to asymmetricity of the protein conformation. The latter, in contrast, is generated by an asymmetric chromophore on the protein or by a chromophoric molecule interacting with an asymmetric site of the protein. Alternatively, neither the chromophore nor the protein per se exhibits asymmetricity and yet they may be rendered asymmetric upon binding to each other through multiple ligand forces. In the case of chromophores with induced asymmetry, the dissymmetry factor g of Kuhn (1958) is considered to be a measure of the effect of the asymmetric environment. This factor g is equal to $\Delta\epsilon/\epsilon$, where $\Delta\epsilon$ is the difference in molar extinction coefficients between left- and right-handed circularly polarized light, and ϵ is the usual molar extinction

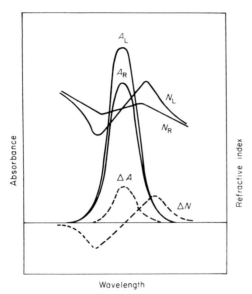

Wavelength

Fig. 1. Schematic illustration of the Cotton effect. A is the absorption coefficient, N the index of refraction, R the right and L the left circular component. $\Delta N = N_L - N_R$ is the optical activity (rotation) and $\Delta A = A_L - A_R$ is the ellipticity or circular dichroism (CD). The combined phenomena of unequal absorption (CD) and unequal velocity of transmission of the left and right circularly polarized light constitute the Cotton effect.

coefficient. If the observed CD (ΔA) and the observed absorbance (A) are measured with the same sample using equal path length, then $\Delta \epsilon / \epsilon$ is equal to $\Delta A / A$. Extrinsic Cotton effects thus present direct evidence for the asymmetry of an active site, affording a physical basis for the characteristic stereochemical specificity of enzymatic catalysis. In this paper we confine ourselves to the discussion of extrinsic Cotton effects, which provide valuable information as to the binding of PLP with the enzyme protein as well as the reaction mechanism of these enzymes.

III. Interaction between Bovine Serum Albumin and Pyridoxal Derivatives: A Model System

PLP itself is optically inactive, but recent reports from several laboratories indicated that PLP exhibits optical activity when it is bound to various apoenzymes. In order to elucidate the reason for this induced optical activity, we decided to study the mode of interaction between BSA and PLP and its analogs as a model system.

In 1962 Dempsey and Christensen reported that BSA forms three types of complexes with PLP. Two of these are characterized by relatively

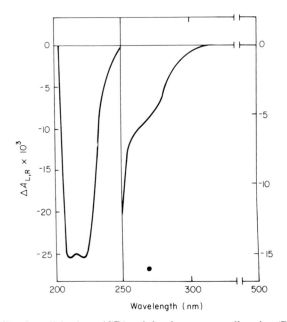

Fig. 2. Circular dichroism (CD) of bovine serum albumin (BSA). BSA was purchased from Sigma. CD measurements were performed at 24°C with a Jasco ORD/UV-5 recording spectropolarimeter with a CD attachment. The left-hand figure shows the CD of BSA plotted as ΔA in the wavelength region between 200 and 250 nm. In this case the protein was 0.22 mg/ml in 0.1 M potassium phosphate, pH 7.5, and a 2-mm silica cell was used. The right-hand figure is the CD of BSA in the wavelength region between 250 and 500 nm when the protein was 11 mg/ml in the same cell. The illustrated smooth curve was drawn from the experimental trace.

high affinity toward PLP, association constants being above 10^6 and about 10^5, respectively, and one of each site is present per molecule of BSA. The third type has relatively poor affinity for PLP, association constants being in the order of 10^3 to 10^4, and several sites are present in a molecule of the protein. The two more stable complexes seem to be rather specific for PLP and show principal absorbancy maxima at 332 nm (site I) and 415 nm (site II), respectively, at neutral pH. The third type (site III) binds not only PLP but also pyridoxal (PAL), and exhibits absorption maximum at 415 nm. All seem to be formed with ϵ-amino groups of lysine residues. The structure of the most stable complex (site I) remains undetermined, but it appears that PLP is bound to the protein as a substituted aldamine as in the case of muscle glycogen phosphorylase (see below), since this chromophore is not reduced by $NaBH_4$. On the other hand, those of other two types (site II and site III) seem to be hydrogen-bonded Schiff bases (aldimine linkages). More recently Johnson and Graves (1966) investigated CD and ORD of muscle glycogen phosphorylase and described in the same paper that the BSA-PLP complex which absorbs at 332 nm, exhibits a positive CD band but that which absorbs at 415 nm does not exhibit extrinsic Cotton effect.

In an attempt to investigate further the interaction between BSA and PLP, we have employed several analogs of PLP and determined induced optical activity under the conditions described by Dempsey and Christensen (1962). Since a better resolution of various optically active chromophores is obtained by CD, this technique is almost exclusively employed for the present investigation. As shown in Fig. 2, BSA did not exhibit any Cotton effect above 320 nm, but exhibited a negative CD band with a minimum at around 210–220 nm. This CD band is due to intrinsic Cotton effect as a result of ordered structure of the protein. When each one molecule of PLP was added to the site I and site II of BSA, new absorption bands appeared at around 330 nm and 410 nm with two distinct CD bands, indicating that the binding of PLP at both sites induced optical activity (Fig. 3). The appearance of a CD band

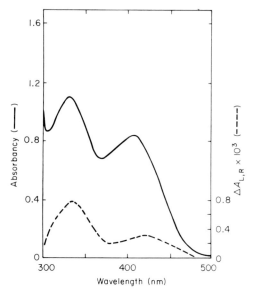

Fig. 3. Absorption spectrum and circular dichroism (CD) of BSA (0.167 mM) in the presence of 0.33 mM pyridoxal phosphate (PLP) and 0.1 M potassium phosphate, pH 7.5. The molecular weight of bovine serum albumin was taken to be 65,000. PLP was a product of Sigma. Absorption spectrum was determined at 24°C with a Cary model 14 spectrophotometer. CD was measured with the same instrument as in Fig. 2. Both measurements were performed in a 1-cm silica cuvette at about 15 hours after mixing.

near 410 nm, which has not been reported by previous investigators, is in good agreement with the finding that the PLP enzymes with absorption maxima at around 410 nm are optically active (Torchinsky and Koreneva, 1963; Fasella and Hammes, 1964; Breusov *et al.*, 1964; Huntley and Metzler, 1967; Nakazawa *et al.*, 1967; Bocharov *et al.*, 1968; Shizuta *et al.*, 1969).

In order to investigate the role of the formyl group of PLP, pyridoxamine phosphate or pyridoxine phosphate was added to a solution of albumin in a molar ratio of 2:1. Neither distinct absorption bands nor CD were observed in the entire visible range (Fig. 4). When the binding of pyridoxal phosphate was determined in the presence of an equimolar quantity of pyridoxamine phosphate or pyridoxine phosphate, no inhibition was observed. These results, taken together, indicate that neither pyridoxamine nor pyridoxine phosphate is bound to the serum albumin and that the 4-formyl group of PLP is essential for the binding with serum albumin and the appearance of CD bands.

We then studied the effect of the phosphate group of PLP on the optical activity by determining CD of a mixture of BSA and PAL. It can be seen from Fig. 5 that this complex exhibits an absorption maximum at

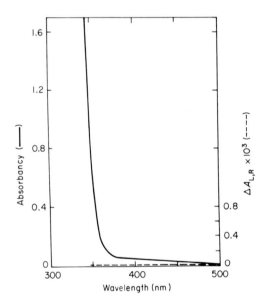

FIG. 4. Absorption spectrum and circular dichroism of bovine serum albumin (0.167 m*M*) in the presence of 0.33 m*M* pyridoxamine phosphate. Pyridoxamine phosphate was purchased from Nakarai Chemical Company (Kyoto). Other experimental conditions were the same as in Fig. 3.

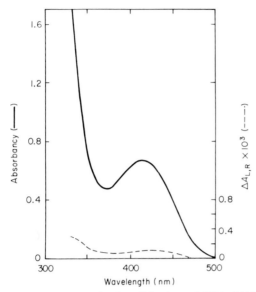

F<small>IG</small>. 5. Absorption spectrum and circular dichroism of BSA (0.167 mM) in the presence of 0.33 mM pyridoxal (PAL). PAL was purchased from Nakarai Chemical Company. Other experimental conditions were the same as in Fig. 3.

410 nm with a weak CD band in the same region. Furthermore, there exists a weak CD near 330 nm. These results were interpreted to mean that PAL is bound to both site I and II (or III) of BSA but the phosphate linkage contributes significantly to the appearance of extrinsic Cotton effect. When 3-methoxy analog of pyridoxal phosphate was used in the next experiment, neither distinct absorption bands nor CD were observed in the visible range (Fig. 6). Furthermore, this compound did not compete with the binding of PLP to BSA, as in the case of pyridoxamine phosphate or pyridoxine phosphate. Thus, these results suggest that the 3-hydroxyl group of PLP is essential both for the binding with BSA and the manifestation of CD bands.

In the next experiment PLP-N-oxide was mixed with BSA in order to elucidate the role of the heterocyclic nitrogen. Two absorption maxima were observed at 320 nm and 410 nm, and two CD bands also appeared in these regions indicating that this compound was bound to site I as well as site III (Fig. 7). It is interesting to note that the dissymmetry factor at site II is higher than that of the BSA-PLP complex shown in Fig. 3. On the other hand, the absorption at site I is considerably higher than that of the BSA-PLP complex and the dissymmetry factor appears to be lower than that of the BSA-PLP complex. These results suggest that the

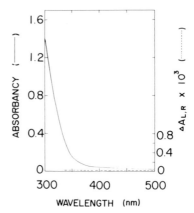

FIG. 6. Absorption spectrum and circular dichroism of bovine serum albumin (0.167 mM) in the presence of 0.33 mM 3-methoxy analog of PLP, which is a gift of Dr. Helmreich. Other experimental conditions were the same as in Fig. 8.

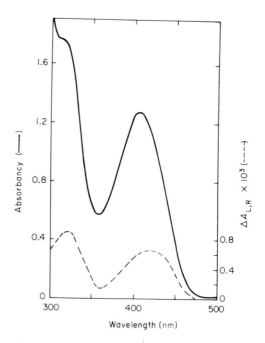

FIG. 7. Absorption spectrum and circular dichroism of bovine serum albumin (0.084 mM) in the presence of 0.167 mM pyridoxal phosphate (PLP) N-oxide. PLP-N-oxide was a gift from Dr. S. Fukui. Other experimental conditions were the same as in Fig. 3.

heterocyclic nitrogen of PLP plays a significant role in the asymmetricity of this coenzyme.

In order to study the effect of 2-methyl group of PLP, we then examined the absorption spectrum and CD of an ω-methyl PLP (3-hydroxy-5-(hydroxymethyl)-2-ethyl-isonicotinaldehyde 5-phosphate) and BSA complex. The profile of absorption spectrum as well as CD bands was essentially similar to that of the BSA-PLP complex (Fig. 8). In contrast, when ω-hydroxy PLP (3-hydroxy-5-(hydroxymethyl)-2-hydroxymethyl-isonicotinaldehyde 5-phosphate) was used, two absorption maxima were observed at 330 nm and 410 nm both having approximately the same extinction coefficients (Fig. 9). It should be noted that the dissymmetry factor at site II near 410 nm is considerably higher than that of the BSA-PLP complex. On the other hand, the dissymmetry factor at site I is about the same order of magnitude as that of the BSA-PLP complex. These results taken together indicate that the 2-methyl group does not significantly contribute to the asymmetricity of the binding at site I and that the substitution by hydroxymethyl group would increase the affinity of site II with the coenzyme analog.

The above results with BSA as a model system clearly demonstrate

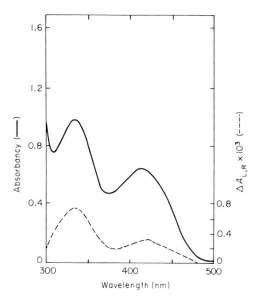

FIG. 8. Absorption spectrum and circular dichroism of bovine serum albumin (0.167 mM) in the presence of 0.33 mM ω-methyl pyridoxal phosphate (PLP). ω-Methyl PLP was a gift from Dr. E. E. Snell. Other experimental conditions were the same as in Fig. 4.

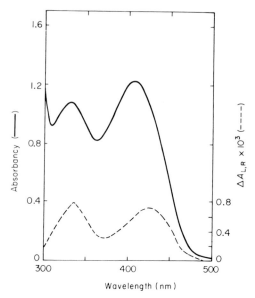

FIG. 9. Absorption spectrum and circular dichroism of bovine serum albumin (0.167 mM) in the presence of 0.33 mM ω-hydroxy pyridoxal phosphate (PLP). ω-Hydroxy PLP was a gift from Dr. S. Fukui. Other experimental conditions were the same as in Fig. 4.

that the formyl group, the phosphate group as well as the hydroxy group of PLP are essential for the binding and the manifestation of the extrinsic Cotton effect and, in addition, the heterocyclic nitrogen atom and the 2-methyl group play a significant role in the asymmetricity of the chromophore. In other words, the specific loci of the protein which bind PLP must be sterically organized in such a way that they interact closely with all the ligands of PLP.

IV. BIODEGRADATIVE THREONINE DEAMINASE

The L-threonine deaminases of microorganisms catalyze the deamination of L-threonine to form α-ketobutyrate and ammonia and have contributed a great deal to the understanding of the allosteric behavior of enzymes and metabolic regulation by feedback inhibition as well as activation. Our interest in this particular enzyme stems from the observation published at the Symposium on Pyridoxal Catalysis in Rome in 1962 that the ADP activation of the *Clostridium tetranomorphum* threonine deaminase resulted from an ADP-induced decrease in K_m for L-threonine of 3- to 7-fold (Hayaishi *et al.*, 1963). General properties and allosteric nature of various threonine deaminases have recently been reviewed in detail in an excellent review article by Wood (1969).

In this chapter, we would like to review some of our results with bio-degradative threonine deaminase of *E. coli*. This enzyme, which was originally described by Gale and Stephenson in 1938 to be activated by AMP, has recently been the subject of intensive investigation by Wood and his co-workers in the United States and in our laboratory in Kyoto. In contrast to the biosynthetic threonine deaminase which is pre-dominantly formed under aerobic conditions and in a glucose-rich medium (Umbarger and Brown, 1957), this enzyme is produced in large quantities when cells are grown anaerobically in a medium containing high amino acids and no glucose (Wood and Gunsalus, 1949). AMP causes a decrease in K_m for L-threonine of about 10-fold with the V_{max} value being increased almost 6-fold (Hirata *et al.*, 1965). On the other hand, L-isoleucine which is a potent inhibitor of the biosynthetic deaminase, does not influence the enzyme activity. Recently we were able to obtain this enzyme in a homogeneous crystalline form and investigated various properties in de-tail (Shizuta *et al.*, 1969), the results of which are summarized in Table I. It can be seen that AMP not only increases the affinity of substrate toward enzyme protein but also stabilizes the activity and accelerates the asso-ciation of protein subunits. The enzyme appears to be composed of four identical monomers each containing 1 mole of PLP and one AMP binding site.

The visible absorption spectrum of the native enzyme shows a single prominent peak at 415 nm, which is not altered by the presence of AMP (Fig. 10). The peak at 415 nm does not change in the pH range of 6.0 and 9.0. It seems that the binding of PLP to this enzyme is similar to that of site II in the case of the BSA-PLP complex, namely the hydrogen-bonded

TABLE I
Properties of Biodegradative Threonine Deaminase of *Escherichia coli*[a]

Property	+AMP	−AMP
Optimal pH	7.4–9.2	>9.0
Stability	Stable	Unstable
K_m for threonine	11 mM	91 mM
K_m for serine	5 mM	40 mM
K_a for AMP	0.07 mM	—
$s_{20,w}^{\circ}$	8.16 S	8.0 S
		4.4 S
$D_{20,w}^{\circ}$	5.20×10^{-7}	—
Molecular weight	147,000	147,000
		70,000
AMP	4	—
PLP	4	4

[a] Hirata *et al.* (1965) and Shizuta *et al.* (1969).

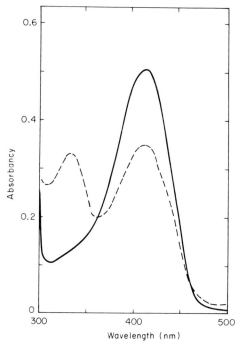

Fɪɢ. 10. Absorption spectra of native and spontaneously denatured threonine deaminase (2.86 mg per milliliter of protein in 50 mM potassium phosphate, pH 6.8,
containing 2 mM 2-mercaptoethanol). ——, Native; ‑ ‑ ‑ ‑ ‑, denatured. From Shizuta
et al. (1969).

Schiff base. When the enzyme is kept in the absence of AMP, the activity
is slowly lost with the concomitant disappearance of the peak at 415 nm
and the appearance of a new absorption band at 333 nm similar to the
site I of the BSA-PLP complex. Judging from the height of both peaks and
the remaining activity, it was concluded that the enzyme with the peak
at 333 nm was inactive and that with the peak at 415 nm was the active
form.

The CD curve of the native enzyme is shown in Fig. 11. A positive CD
band is observed at around 415 nm with the dissymmetry factor of 1.5 ×
10^{-3} (Nakazawa *et al.*, 1967; Shizuta *et al.*, 1969). This value is in the
same order of magnitude as those of other PLP enzymes having absorption maxima at 410 nm but is about four times as much as that of the
BSA-PLP complex. The result indicates that the binding of PLP to the
apothreonine deaminase is probably tighter than that of the BSA-PLP
complex and the chromophore is more strongly twisted by multiple attachment to the enzyme protein. When the enzyme is treated with NaBH$_4$,

NH$_2$OH, or urea, the CD band completely disappears indicating that the aldimine linkage and the conformational integrity of enzyme protein are essential for the optical activity.

In order to see whether the addition of substrate could cause any change in the extrinsic Cotton effect, L-threonine (50 mM) was added to a concentrated solution of enzyme. As can be seen from Fig. 12, the CD band disappeared almost instantaneously and then gradually reappeared in several minutes. After about 10 minutes, when the substrate was completely used up, the CD band went back to the original level. When D-threonine, a substrate analog and a competitive inhibitor, was added to the enzyme solution under the same conditions, CD at 415 nm decreased to the extent of about 40% and remained unchanged. L-Valine, which is neither a substrate nor a competitive inhibitor, did not cause any change in the CD band under these conditions.

The absorption in the visible region is also significantly altered by the addition of substrate. When L-threonine was added to the enzyme solution,

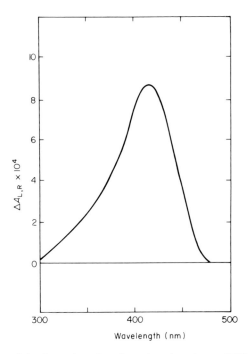

Fig. 11. Circular dichroism of native threonine deaminase (3.26 mg per milliliter of protein in 50 mM potassium phosphate, pH 6.8, containing 2 mM 2-mercaptoethanol and 10 mM AMP). The dissymmetry factor of the enzyme is 1.5×10^{-3} (Shizuta *et al.*, 1969).

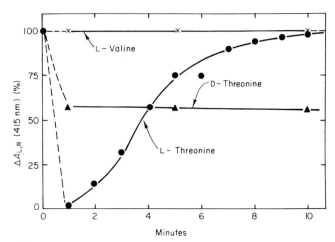

Fig. 12. Time course of circular dichroism (CD). The reaction mixture contained the enzyme (8.0 mg), 25 mM potassium phosphate, pH 7.4, 5 mM AMP, 5 mM 2-mercaptoethanol, and 50 mM each of amino acids in a total volume of 1.0 ml. CD is expressed as percentage of the original value. The details are described in the text (Nakazawa *et al.*, 1967).

the peak at 415 nm shifted to the longer wavelength, with the peak of difference spectra at 450 nm (Fig. 13). The time course of the appearance and disappearance of this peak at 450 nm is shown in Fig. 14. The peak at 450 nm appeared in less than a minute and thereafter it gradually disappeared as the reaction proceeded. On the other hand, the addition of D-threonine under these conditions caused a slight shift of the absorption band, but this change was again irreversible.

From the above experimental results, it is reasonable to postulate the following sequence of reactions as a plausible mechanism of threonine deaminase of *E. coli* (Fig. 15). Since the disappearance of CD could be observed with either L- or D-threonine, it seems reasonable to assume that this phenomenon is due to the binding of substrate or substrate analog to the formyl group of PLP by transaldimination (Hayaishi *et al.*, 1967). On the other hand, the appearance of a peak of difference spectrum at 450 nm did not take place in the presence of D-threonine and therefore seems to represent an intermediate of the reaction, for example, pyridoxyl aminocrotonate. Similar, if not exactly identical reaction mechanism, has now been proposed independently by Wood and his co-workers (Phillips and Wood, 1965; Rabinowitz *et al.*, 1969; Niederman *et al.*, 1969). In order to elucidate the reaction mechanism and in particular to find out the exact site of AMP activation, further studies are now in progress in our laboratory.

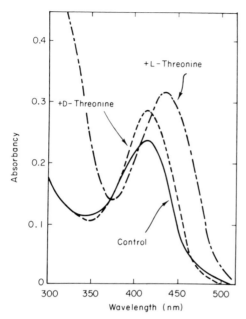

Fɪɢ. 13. Absorption spectra of threonine deaminase upon addition of ʟ- and ᴅ-threonine. Measurements were performed 1 minute after additions of ʟ-threonine at 10 mM and ᴅ-threonine at 20 mM. Protein concentration was 1.36 mg/ml. Other experimental conditions are as described for Fig. 9 (Tokushige *et al.*, 1968; Shizuta *et al.*, 1969).

V. OTHER PYRIDOXAL ENZYMES

All the PLP enzymes so far investigated exhibit optical activity in the region of absorption maxima in the visible spectral range.

Aspartate aminotransferase of swine heart muscle was the first PLP enzyme to be investigated by ORD and CD. Studies by Torchinsky and Koreneva (1963), Fasella and Hammes (1964), Breusov *et al.* (1964), and Bocharov *et al.* (1968) were recently reviewed in detail in an excellent review article by Ivanov and Karpeisky (1969). This enzyme exhibits extrinsic Cotton effect at 430 nm at pH 5.2, and at 360 nm at pH 8.1 and the dissymmetry factors were 2.8×10^{-3} and 1.9 to 2.8×10^{-3}, respectively (Breusov *et al.*, 1964; Bocharov *et al.*, 1968). These values are the highest among those of the PLP enzymes ever reported, indicating that the binding force of each ligand is stronger and the molecular dissymmetry is more extensive than the other cases of PLP enzymes. The pyridoxamine type enzyme also exhibits Cotton effect at 330 nm with a dissymmetry factor 1.4×10^{-3} (Breusov *et al.*, 1964).

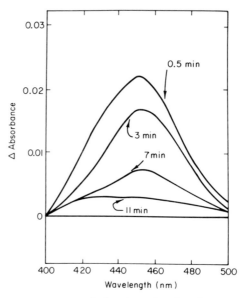

FIG. 14. Difference spectrum of the threonine deaminase reaction. The reaction mixture contained the enzyme (0.7 mg), 25 mM potassium phosphate, pH 7.4, 5 mM AMP, 5 mM 2-mercaptoethanol, and 50 mM of L-threonine in a total volume of 1.0 ml (Tokushige et al., 1968).

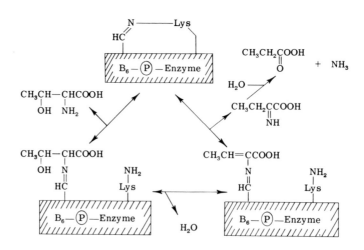

FIG. 15. A possible mechanism of threonine deaminase reaction (Hayaishi et al., 1967).

Studies on the optical activity of glutamate decarboxylase of *E. coli* were carried out independently by Sukhareva and Torchinsky (1966) and Huntley and Metzler (1967). This enzyme exhibits positive CD with maxima at 420 nm at pH 4.6 and 340 nm at pH 6.5, with dissymmetry factors of 0.89×10^{-3} and 0.09×10^{-3} (Huntley and Metzler, 1967). It appears that at pH 6.5 the apoenzyme is bound to PLP in a manner similar to the site I of the BSA-PLP complex but the dissymmetry factor is rather low and the mode of binding appears to be somewhat loose. This observation is consistent with the fact that the optimum pH of the reaction lies around pH 5.5 and the enzyme is essentially inactive around neutrality. In other words, the molecular strain of PLP makes it most reactive at acidic pH range.

ORD and CD of rabbit muscle phosphorylase was investigated by Torchinsky *et al.* (1965) and Johnson and Graves (1966). Native enzyme exhibits Cotton effect at 333 nm with a dissymmetry factor of 1.1×10^{-3}. When this enzyme was treated with acid (pH 2.0) or detergents, the absorption maximum shifted to 415 nm but the optical activity is no longer observed, indicating that the aldamine linkage in the native phosphorylase is converted to the aldimine linkage and other ligands are destroyed by these treatments (Johnson and Graves, 1966). It is interesting to note that the treatment of this enzyme with sodium borohydride did not alter the enzyme activity (Fischer *et al.*, 1958), but the magnitude of CD band decreased by about 40% by the reduction (Johnson and Graves, 1966).

Wilson and Meister (1966) investigated aspartate β-decarboxylase of *Alcaligenes faecalis* by ORD. This enzyme exhibits Cotton effect at

TABLE II

CIRCULAR DICHROISM MAXIMA AND DISSYMMETRY FACTORS OF
PROTEIN PYRIDOXAL PHOSPHATE COMPLEXES

Complex	λ_{max} (nm)	$\Delta\epsilon/\epsilon$	References
BSA-PLP	410–420	0.37×10^{-3}	This paper
	330	0.68×10^{-3}	
Threonine deaminase	415	1.5×10^{-3}	Shizuta *et al.* (1969)
			Nakazawa *et al.* (1967)
Aspartate β-decarboxylase	360	—	Wilson and Meister (1966)
Glutamate decarboxylase	420	0.89×10^{-3}	Huntley and Metzler (1967)
	340	0.09×10^{-3}	
Phosphorylase	415	0	Johnson and Graves (1966)
	333	1.1×10^{-3}	
Aspartate aminotransferase	420–450	2.8×10^{-3}	Bocharov *et al.* (1968)
	360	$1.9–2.8 \times 10^{-3}$	Breusov *et al.* (1964)
	330	1.4×10^{-3}	

around 360 nm but dissymmetry factor is not exactly known; the amplitude of the Cotton effect was reported to be in the order of 60–80% of
that of aspartate aminotransferase. Rotatory dispersion titration of the
apoenzyme with PLP indicates that about 15.5 moles of PLP are bound
to 800,000 g of enzyme, a value in close agreement with spectrophotometric, chemical, and microbiological experiments.

The position of CD bands and dissymmetry factors of these four PLP
enzymes together with threonine deaminase and the BSA-PLP complex
are summarized in Table II.

VI. SUMMING UP

In the past, the binding of PLP with various kinds of apoenzymes has
been investigated in detail mainly by spectrophotometric means. In addition to these results (Jenkins, 1961), the data obtained by CD and ORD
indicate that PLP enzymes may be classified into four types as shown
below.

(I)   Threonine deaminase type ----- (A)
(II) Aspartate β-decarboxylase type ----- (B)
(III) Glutamate decarboxylase or phosphorylase type ----- (A) $\rightleftarrows$ (C)
(IV) Aspartate aminotransferase type ----- (B) $\rightleftarrows$ (A)

Type I exhibits absorption maximum and Cotton effect at around 415
nm, which is independent of pH values (state A in Fig. 16). Threonine
deaminase is an example of type I. Type II exhibits absorption maximum
and Cotton effect at around 360 nm, which is also independent of pH
change (state B). Aspartate β-decarboxylase is an example of type II.
Type III exhibits absorption maxima and Cotton effects at 330 nm (state
C) and at 410 nm (state A) depending on the pH values. Phosphorylase
is active in the state of (C), whereas glutamate decarboxylase is active
in the state of (A). Type IV resembles a pH indicator and absorption
maxima as well as Cotton effects gradually change depending on pH
values. For example, aspartate aminotransferase is yellow (state A) at

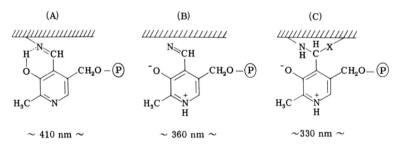

Fig. 16. Modes of binding of pyridoxal phosphate to apoenzymes.

acidic pH's but gradually fades to become colorless (state B) at alkaline pH values.

It may be concluded that in the binding of PLP to apoenzymes, the formyl group plays a major role, but the phosphate group, 2-methyl group, 3 hydroxyl groups, and the heterocyclic nitrogen atom also play significant roles in the binding as well as in the appearance of Cotton effect. Since PLP is an inherently symmetric chromophore but is asymmetrically perturbed by being connected with the active site of enzyme protein, CD and ORD would be a useful means of investigating not only the mode of binding, but also the three-dimensional mechanism of catalytic function as well. More quantitative analysis of the contribution of each ligand must await further studies.

ACKNOWLEDGMENTS

The authors are grateful to Dr. E. E. Snell for the sample of ω-methyl PLP, to Dr. Helmreich for the sample of 3-methoxy PLP, and to Dr. S. Fukui for the samples of PLP-N-oxide and ω-hydroxy PLP. We are indebted to Drs. M. Nozaki, H. Wada, Y. Morino, and M. Okamoto for critically reading the manuscript and valuable discussions. The original work in our laboratory was in part carried out in collaboration with Drs. M. Tokushige, A. Nakazawa, and M. Hirata and was supported by Public Health Service Research Grants No. CA-04222 from the National Cancer Institute and No. AM-10333 from the National Institute of Arthritis and Metabolic Diseases, and by grants from the Jane Coffin Childs Memorial Fund for Medical Research, the Squibb Institute for Medical Research, the Scientific Research Fund of the Ministry of Education of Japan, and the Toyo Rayon Science Foundation.

REFERENCES

Beychok, S. (1966). *Science* **154**, 1288.
Beychok, S. (1968). *Annu. Rev. Biochem.* **37**, 437.
Blout, E. R. (1964). *Biopolym. Symp.* **1**, 397.
Bocharov, A. L., Ivanov, V. I., Karpeisky, M. Ya., Mamaeva, O. K., and Florentiev, V. L. (1968). *Biochem. Biophys. Res. Commun.* **30**, 459.
Breusov, Yu. N., Ivanov, V. I., Karpeisky, M. Ya., and Morozov, Yu. V. (1964). *Biochim. Biophys. Acta* **92**, 388.
Dempsey, W. B., and Christensen, H. N. (1962). *J. Biol. Chem.* **237**, 1113.
Djerassi, C., ed. (1960). "Optical Rotatory Dispersion." McGraw-Hill, New York.
Fasella, P., and Hammes, G. G. (1964). *Biochemistry* **3**, 530.
Fischer, E. H., Kent, A. B., Snyder, E. R., and Krebs, E. G. (1958). *J. Amer. Chem. Soc.* **80**, 2906.
Gale, E. G., and Stephenson, M. (1938). *Biochem. J.* **32**, 392.
Hayaishi, O., Gefter, M., and Weissbach, H. (1963). *Proc. Symp. Chem. Biol. Aspects Pyridoxal Catal., 1962,* p. 467.
Hayaishi, O., Tokushige, M., Nakazawa, A., and Shizuta, Y. (1967). *Vitamins (Kyoto)* **36**, 473.
Hirata, M., Tokushige, M., Inagaki, A., and Hayaishi, O. (1965). *J. Biol. Chem.* **240**, 1711.

Huntley, T. E., and Metzler, D. E. (1967). *Biochem. Biophys. Res. Commun.* **26**, 109.
Ivanov, V. I., and Karpeisky, M. Ya. (1969). *Advan. Enzymol.* **32**, 21.
Jenkins, W. T. (1961). *Fed. Proc., Fed. Amer. Soc. Exp. Biol.* **20**, 978.
Johnson, G. F., and Graves, D. J. (1966). *Biochemistry* **5**, 2906.
Kuhn, W. (1958). *Annu. Rev. Phys. Chem.* **9**, 417.
Nakazawa, A., Tokushige, M., and Hayaishi, O. (1967). *Biochem. Biophys. Res. Commun.* **29**, 184.
Niederman, R. A., Rabinowitz, K. W., and Wood, W. A. (1969). *Biochem. Biophys. Res. Commun.* **36**, 951.
Phillips, A. T., and Wood, W. A. (1965). *J. Biol. Chem.* **240**, 4703.
Rabinowitz, K. W., and Piperno, J. R., and Niederman, R. A. (1969). *Fed. Proc., Fed. Amer. Soc. Exp. Biol.* **27**, 341.
Shizuta, Y., Nakazawa, A., Tokushige, M., and Hayaishi, O. (1969). *J. Biol. Chem.* **244**, 1883.
Snatzke, G., ed. (1967). "Optical Rotatory Dispersion and Circular Dichroism in Organic Chemistry." Heyden, London.
Sukhareva, B. S., and Torchinsky, Yu. M. (1966). *2nd Int. Union Biochem. Symp.* Abstr., p. 86.
Tokushige, M., Nakazawa, A., Shizuta, Y., Okada, Y., and Hayaishi, O. (1968). *In* "Symposium on Pyridoxal Enzymes" (N. Katsunuma and H. Wada, eds.), p. 105. Maruzen Co. Ltd., Tokyo.
Torchinsky, Yu. M., and Koreneva, L. G. (1963). *Biokhimiya* **28**, 1087.
Torchinsky, Yu. M., Livanova, N. B., and Pikhelgas, V. Ya. (1965). *Biochim. Biophys. Acta* **110**, 619.
Ulmer, D. D., and Vallee, B. L. (1965). *Advan. Enzymol.* **27**, 37.
Umbarger, H. E., and Brown, B. (1957). *J. Bacteriol.* **73**, 105.
Urnes, P., and Doty, P. (1961). *Advan. Protein Chem.* **16**, 401.
Wilson, E. M., and Meister, A. (1966). *Biochemistry* **5**, 1166.
Wood, W. A. (1969). *In* "Current Topics in Cellular Regulation" (B. L. Horecker and E. R. Stadtman, eds.), p. 161. Academic Press, New York.
Wood, W. A., and Gunsalus, I. C. (1949). *J. Biol. Chem.* **181**, 171.

Analogs of Pyridoxal or Pyridoxal Phosphate: Relation of Structure to Binding with Apoenzymes and to Catalytic Activity*

ESMOND E. SNELL

Department of Biochemistry, University of California, Berkeley, California

I. INTRODUCTION

Among the vitamins and coenzymes, pyridoxal (PL)† and pyridoxal 5'-phosphate (PLP) are almost unique in that they slowly catalyze in dilute aqueous solutions at ambient temperatures or above, and at physiological pH values many of the same reactions of amino acids for which PLP-enzymes are required *in vivo*. Model studies with pyridoxal analogs permitted delineation of the structural features required for catalysis of such nonenzymatic reactions; in the pyridine series these features are supplied by either 3-hydroxypyridine-2-aldehyde or 3-hydroxypyridine-4-aldehyde; i.e., substituents at the 2- and 5-positions of pyridoxal are not essential, whereas the formyl group at position 4, the phenolic group at position 3, and the heterocyclic nitrogen at position 1 are required (Snell, 1958). Schiff's base formation between these aldehydes and amino acids is greatly enhanced by the phenolic group (French *et al.*, 1965), and in the resulting complex, both the heterocyclic nitrogen atom and the azomethine nitrogen provide electrophilic groups so placed as to weaken each

---

* This article is based upon a lecture delivered in Lausanne, Switzerland, at the International Symposium on the Structures and Functions of Vitamin-Dependent Enzymes, July 16–18, 1970, and does not provide a complete review of the topics covered.

† Abbreviations used in the text and tables are to compounds having structures derived from pyridoxal 5'-phosphate (PLP) as indicated in the table on the following page. Unphosphorylated compounds are abbreviated in a corresponding fashion.

ABBREVIATIONS AND STRUCTURES OF PYRIDOXAL PHOSPHATE ANALOGS

Abbreviation	x	y	Abbreviation	x	y
2-NorPLP	2	H	PL-5'-sulfate	5	$CH_2OSO_3^-$
2'-MePLP	2	CH_2CH_3	5'-MePLP	5	$CHOPO_3^{2-}$
					$\quad\mid$
					CH_3
2'-PropylPLP	2	$CH_2(CH_2)_2CH_3$	5'-CM-5 deoxyPLP	5	$CH_2CH_2COO^-$
2',2'-diMePLP	2	$CH(CH_3)_2$			
2'-HydroxyPLP	2	CH_2OH	PL-5'-methylene phosphonate	5	$CH_2CH_2PO_3^{2-}$
					CH_3
					$\quad\mid$
2-Nor-6-MePLP	2, 6	H, CH_3	PL-5'-Mephosphonate	5	$CH_2OPO_2^-$
6-MePLP	6	CH_3			
					O
					$\parallel$
N-MePLP	1	CH_3	PL-5'-(β-cyanoethyl phosphate)	5	$CH_2OP{-}O^-$
					$\quad\mid$
					$CNCH_2CH_2O$
PNP	4	CH_2OH			
PMP	4	CH_2NH_2	5-DeoxyPL-5'-phosphonate	5	$CH_2PO_3^{2-}$
4-DeoxyPNP	4	CH_3			

Column headers for both halves: "Replace side chain at position x in PLP by y"

of the bonds about the α-carbon atom of the amino acid (as shown for the α-hydrogen by the transition I → II) and thus activate the amino acid for the variety of reactions catalyzed by pyridoxal. This is especially true when the structure is appropriately stabilized in a planar conformation by a catalytic metal ion (as in compound III), or, in PLP-enzymes, by the

(I)   (II)   (III)

enzyme itself. These concepts, derived largely from studies of non-enzymatic reactions of pyridoxal with amino acids, provided the basis for a general mechanism for participation of PLP in enzymatic reactions of amino acids (Braunstein and Shemyakin, 1953; Metzler *et al.*, 1954; Snell, 1958, 1963) which has been confirmed in general outline and further elaborated by detailed studies of many individual nonenzymatic and enzymatic reactions (for reviews, see Snell, 1958; Braunstein, 1960; Guirard and Snell, 1964; Ivanov and Karpeisky, 1969; Snell and DiMari, 1970).

One might assume that the same structural features that permit PL or PLP to catalyze a given model reaction would be prerequisite to catalysis of the corresponding enzymatic reaction, but that additional features, necessary for binding to the enzyme, might also be necessary. Although useful as a guiding principle, such an assumption ignores the major and largely unidentified contribution of the enzyme protein to catalysis. The recent demonstration that covalently bound pyruvate in a bacterial histidine decarboxylase provides a functional replacement for the PLP of other amino acid α-decarboxylases (Riley and Snell, 1968; Recsei and Snell, 1970) emphasizes the dangers in an overly rigid application of the principle. A closer definition of those structural features of PL and PLP that are necessary for catalysis, as opposed to binding, in enzymatic reactions would aid in understanding the mechanism of these reactions, and can be derived in part from a study of the activity of analogs of PL in various enzymatic reactions. This review will discuss briefly (1) the effect of structure on enzymatic transamination of unphosphorylated compounds related to PL and PM; (2) the effect of binding of PLP upon the conformation of PLP enzymes; and (3) the activity of analogs of PLP in duplicating the effects of this coenzyme on conformation and activity of several PLP enzymes.

II. Enzymatic Transamination of Free Pyridoxal and Its Analogs

A. Pyridoxamine-Pyruvate Transaminase

This inducible bacterial transaminase, which is readily available in crystalline form, catalyzes a reaction (Eq. 1)

$$\text{Pyridoxamine} + \text{pyruvate} \underset{r}{\overset{f}{\rightleftharpoons}} \text{pyridoxal} + \text{L-alanine} \tag{1}$$

analogous to those studied in model system (Wada and Snell, 1962a). The enzyme contains no PLP; a detailed study of its kinetics (Ayling and Snell, 1968a) showed that Eq. (1) proceeds by a mechanism that requires a compulsory sequence of addition of substrates to enzyme with formation of rate-determining ternary complexes, EXY, as indicated in Eq. (2), where E, PM, Pyr, PL, and Ala represent enzyme and the several substrates of Eq. (1), respectively.

$$E \xrightleftharpoons{\overset{\text{PM}}{}} E.PM \xrightleftharpoons{\overset{\text{Pyr}}{}} EXY \xrightleftharpoons{\overset{\text{Ala}}{}} E.PL \xrightleftharpoons{\overset{\text{PL}}{}} E \qquad (2)$$

$$\underbrace{\hspace{6cm}}_{A}$$

Segment A of Eq. (2) is precisely analogous to each of the two half-reactions catalyzed by PLP-dependent transaminases such as aspartate aminotransferase (E'), which are shown by segments

$$E'.PLP \xrightleftharpoons{\overset{\text{Glu}}{}} E'XY \xrightleftharpoons{\overset{\alpha\text{-KG}}{}} E'PMP \xrightleftharpoons{\overset{\text{OA}}{}} E'X'Y' \xrightleftharpoons{\overset{\text{Asp}}{}} E'.PLP \qquad (3)$$

$$\underbrace{\hspace{4cm}}_{C} \quad \underbrace{\hspace{3cm}}_{B}$$

B and C of Eq. (3) where Glu, α-KG, OA, and Asp represent glutamate α-ketoglutarate, oxalocetate, and aspartate, respectively. We assume on this basis that the interconversions within segments A, B, and C of Eqs. (2) and (3) occur by similar mechanisms. Since Eqs. (2) and (3) have similar overall rates, it immediately appears that the 5'-phosphate group of PLP is not a general requirement for enzymatic transamination, although as discussed later it plays a very important role in binding and positioning of PLP on PLP-dependent enzymes.

Determination of the specificity of PL and PM as substrates for pyridoxamine pyruvate transaminase yielded results shown in Fig. 1. Substituents at the 2 and 5 positions of PL are unnecessary for enzymatic transamination, as shown by the activity of 2-norpyridoxal, 2'-methyl-pyridoxal, and, most strikingly, 3-hydroxy-4-pyridine aldehyde, whereas a free phenolic group at position 3 is required. The formyl group at position 4 is also required, since it participates in the reaction, and since both PN and 4-deoxyPN are good inhibitors (Dempsey and Snell, 1963). In short, the minimum structural requirements for enzymatic and for non-enzymatic transamination within this series are identical. More detailed investigation (Table I) showed that any alteration in the structure of PL or PM reduced their affinities for the enzyme, as shown by values for K_{diss} (Table I), and usually increased the Michaelis constants for both these compounds and the cosubstrate. However, the maximum velocity of the forward (V_f) or reverse (V_r) reactions was remarkably

Structure	Name	Substituents			Active as substrate
		R	R'	R"	
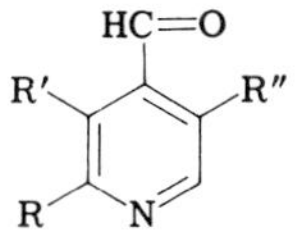 HC=O (structure I–IX)	(I) Pyridoxal	CH$_3$	OH	CH$_2$OH	Yes
	(II) ω-Methylpyridoxal	CH$_3$CH$_2$	OH	CH$_2$OH	Yes
	(III) Norpyridoxal	H	OH	CH$_2$OH	Yes
	(IV) 5-Deoxypyridoxal	CH$_3$	OH	CH$_3$	Yes
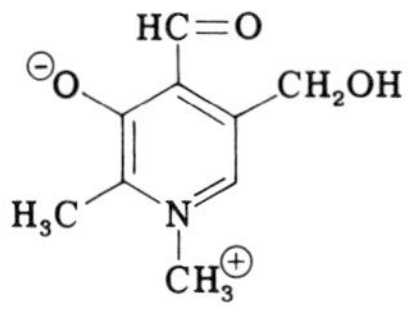	(V) 3-Hydroxy-4-pyridine aldehyde	H	OH	H	Yes
	(VI) Pyridoxal phosphate	CH$_3$	OH	CH$_2$OPO$_3^{2-}$	(Yes)
	(VII) 3-Deoxypyridoxal	CH$_3$	H	CH$_2$OH	No
	(VIII) Pyridine-4-aldehyde	H	H	H	No
	(IX) O-Methylpyridoxal	CH$_3$	OCH$_3$	CH$_2$OH	No
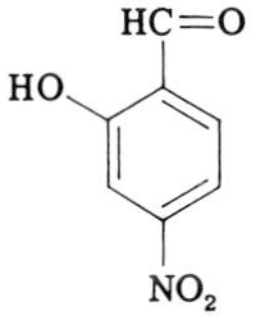 (X) structure	(X) N-Methylpyridoxal	(See column I)			No
(XI) structure	(XI) 4-Nitrosalicylaldehyde	(See column I)			No

Fig. 1. Structure of pyridoxal analogs and their activities as substrates of pyridoxamine pyruvate transaminase. Compounds (I)–(V) are excellent substrates, compound (VI) is a very poor substrate, and (VII)–(XI) are inactive as substrates. Reproduced from Ayling and Snell (1968b) with consent of the publisher.

high for all of these compounds when sufficiently high concentrations were tested.

Both N-MePL (Johnston et al., 1963) and 4-nitrosalicylaldehyde (Metzler et al., 1954) undergo nonenzymatic transamination, but are not substrates of pyridoxamine pyruvate transaminase (Fig. 1). Appropriate trials showed that they also were not inhibitors of the enzyme, i.e., their inactivity was a consequence of their inability to bind at the active site. 3-DeoxyPL, O-MePL, and pyridine 4-aldehyde also were neither substrates nor inhibitors. Apparently, therefore, both the 3-phenolic group and a free pyridine nitrogen are required for binding at the active site of this enzyme; indirect evidence indicated that the 3-phenolic group, like the heterocyclic N, may also participate in catalytic events within the enzyme substrate complex (Ayling and Snell, 1968b).

The most effective inhibitor of this enzyme so far found is N-pyridoxyl-alanine (IV), which combines the structural characteristics of its

TABLE I
KINETIC PARAMETERS FOR EQ. (1) CATALYZED BY
PYRIDOXAMINE PYRUVATE TRANSAMINASE[a]

Kinetic parameter, Eq. (1f)[b]	PM	2'-MePM	5-Deoxy-PM	2-NorPM	3-OH-4-CH$_2$NH$_2$-pyridine
K_{pm} (mM)	0.013	0.48	0.014	0.16	0.35
K_{pyr} (mM)	0.35	0.4	0.42	0.52	7.4
$K_{pm,pyr}$ (μM^2)	0.024	8.5	0.082	5.9	45.0
V_f (sec^{-1})	12.6	18.3	4.9	19.7	2.6
K_{diss} (mM)	0.07	21	0.20	12	6.0

Kinetic parameter, Eq. (1r)[b]	PL	2'-MePL	5-Deoxy-PL	2-NorPL	3-OH-4-CHO-pyridine
K_{pl} (mM)	0.012	1.3	0.009	0.59	0.89
K_{ala} (mM)	1.6	0.58	1.9	2.7	65.0
$K_{pl,ala}$ (μM^2)	0.032	4.3	0.036	5.9	390.0
V_r (sec^{-1})	10.5	5.95	7.95	10.0	24.0
K_{diss} (mM)	0.02	7.5	0.019	2.2	6.1
$K_{eq} = \dfrac{VP \cdot K_{PL,al}}{V_r \cdot K_{PM,pyr}}$	1.58	1.53	0.27	1.96	0.96

[a] From Ayling and Snell (1968b).

[b] These constants (e.g., K_{pm}, $K_{pm,pyr}$, etc.) refer to the values for the analog listed at the head of each column, not only for PM or PL. The subscripts f and r indicate, respectively, forward and reverse of Eq. (1) in text.

(IV)

pyridine substrates with those of its cosubstrates, alanine and pyruvate. Pyridoxylalanine is closely related to the intermediate Schiff bases involved in this transamination reaction; its K_I value (1.8×10^{-4} mM) is far lower than the K_M values for PL (0.015 mM), PM (0.031 mM), alanine (2.0 mM), or pyruvate (0.3 mM), and is also much lower than that for several related pyridoxylamino acids which do not include the 3-carbon skeleton of alanine (Dempsey and Snell, 1963).

B. Aspartate Aminotransferase (AAT)

Apo-AAT (extramitochondrial) but not the holoenzyme, was found by Wada and Snell (1962b) to catalyze transamination reactions with free PM or PL [Eqs. (4) and (5)] at a slow rate. The two

$$\text{Oxaloacetate} + \text{PM} \rightleftharpoons \text{PL} + \text{L-aspartate} \tag{4}$$

$$\text{L-Glutamate} + \text{PL} \rightleftharpoons \text{PM} + \alpha\text{-ketoglutarate} \tag{5}$$

reactions were completely inhibited by PLP, and since summation of Eqs. (4) and (5) represents the normal reaction catalyzed by the holo-enzyme [Eq. (3)], PL and PM were assumed to serve as poorly bound, and readily dissociable analogs of PLP and PMP which replaced these coenzymes inefficiently in catalyzing the overall reaction of Eq. (3), and were excluded from the active site by the firmly bound phosphorylated coenzymes. These results again demonstrate that the 5′-phosphate group is not required for enzymatic transamination. At the same time the relatively low rate of these apoenzyme-catalyzed reactions [Eqs. (4) and (5)] and the high K_M value for PM (2.4 mM) are in marked contrast to the relatively much higher rate of the overall reaction catalyzed by the holoenzyme [Eq. (3)], and the very low dissociation constant of the holoenzyme for PLP (<0.2 μM). These findings emphasize the overriding importance of the 5′-phosphate group in permitting interaction of co-enzyme and apoenzyme to occur in a way that permits its firm binding and produces a maximally effective juxtaposition of catalytic groups supplied by the coenzyme with those supplied by the enzyme protein.

III. Binding and Coenzymatic Activity of Analogs of Pyridoxal Phosphate

A. Nature and Effects of Coenzyme Binding

Binding of PLP to its conjugate apoenzymes is a complex process, which is not at present well understood. It involves multipoint attachment via the labile covalent azomethine linkage, ionic linkages via phosphate and probably via the phenolic oxygen and heterocyclic nitrogen, and perhaps hydrogen bonding and physical bonding through interaction of aromatic rings as well. These interactions vary somewhat from one PLP enzyme to another, as indicated by differences in their spectral (Table II) and fluorescent properties, in the ease of resolution of different holoen-

TABLE II

SOME COMPARATIVE PROPERTIES OF ENZYMES TESTED FOR ACTIVITY AGAINST ANALOGS OF PYRIDOXAL OR PYRIDOXAL PHOSPHATE[a]

Enzyme	Mol. wt. $\times 10^{-3}$	Subunits	Binding sites	λ_{max} (nm) of holoenzyme at pH 7.0[b]	Sequence of isolated pyridoxyl peptide
Arginine decarboxylase	820	10	10	420	—
Aspartate β-decarboxylase	600	12	12	358	—
Aspartate aminotransferase (soluble)	90	2	2	362, 420	Ser.Lys.Asn.Phe (Pxy on Lys)
Pyridoxamine-pyruvate aminotransferase	150	4	2	325, 415	Val.Thr.Gly.Pro.Asp.Lys.Cys.Leu (Pxy on Lys)
Phosphorylase a	370	4	4		Met.Lys.Phe.Met (Pxy on Lys)
Serine dehydratase	45	1	1	330, 410	—
Tryptophanase	220	4	4	337, 420	Ser.Ala.Lys.Lys.Asp.Ala.Met.Val.Pro.Met. (Pxy on Lys)

[a] For references to the original literature, see Snell and DiMari (1970).

[b] "Holoenzyme" refers to the PLP enzyme in all instances except pyridoxamine–pyruvate aminotransferase, which binds pyridoxal as substrate and contains no PLP.

zymes, in the extent of conformational change induced by the interaction, in the structure of isolated segments of the coenzyme binding sites (Table II), in the nature and extent of the optical activity induced in the coenzyme by binding (circular dichroism), and in the effectiveness of various PLP analogs as substitutes for the parent coenzymes. Almost all these property changes have been used to study binding of PLP or its analogs; unfortunately, in no case have several such criteria been applied systematically to several different enzymes. Some of the fragmentary studies that have appeared are discussed briefly in the following sections.

1. *Resolution of PLP-Enzymes*

Early studies (review, Snell, 1958) showed that binding of PLP by its conjugate apoenzymes occurred rather slowly; once bound, the coenzyme did not dissociate readily, even at high dilutions, and was not readily displaced by added coenzyme analogs, such as 4-deoxyPLP. Similarly, the conditions necessary for resolving different PLP-holoenzymes vary enormously. For example, alanine aminotransferase is resolved with great difficulty, losing its coenzyme (with substantial irreversible inactivation) only after treatment with p-chloromercuribenzoate (Matsuzawa and Segal, 1968). Aspartate aminotransferase, on the other hand, is readily resolved by ammonium sulfate precipitation from acidic media (Wada and Snell, 1962b). Phosphorylase b, which resisted early attempts at resolution, is rapidly resolved in the presence of cysteine and a "deforming buffer," imidazole-citrate (Shaltiel *et al.*, 1966); tryptophanase is readily resolved by crystallization from high concentrations of ammonium sulfate at pH 7.0 (Newton *et al.*, 1965), especially in the presence of cysteine or penicillamine (Morino and Snell, 1967a). Recent studies of D-serine dehydratase from *E. coli* show that the holoenzyme does in fact lose its coenzyme very slowly on incubation near its pH optimum at very high dilutions (20 nM); over 24 hours was required to achieve equilibrium and no observable losses occurred at these dilutions during time periods necessary for assay (Dowhan and Snell, 1970). The measured dissociation constant was 35 nM. Association of coenzyme with apoenzyme was also very slow, over 5 minutes being required for reconstitution of a maximally active holoenzyme when 35 nM enzyme was incubated with excess (1500 nM) PLP. The holoenzyme is resolved rapidly by dialysis against cysteine in the presence of imidazole-citrate buffer (Dowhan and Snell, 1970).

In each of these cases, it appears that rapid resolution is obtained only under conditions that distort the protein structure (e.g., changes in pH, crystallization, reaction with pCMB, presence of a deforming buffer) and in the presence of reagents (e.g., cysteine) that add to and weaken the azomethine link between PLP and protein. These observations, and the slow time course of reactivation of apoenzymes by added PLP, indicate that reaction between coenzyme and protein is a multistage process, involving one or more slow reactions such as a conformational change in the protein.

2. *PLP-Induced Conformational Changes in Protein Structure*

Rather extensive conformational changes accompany resolution of several PLP-enzymes. With tryptophanase, for example, substantial decreases occur in the sedimentation coefficient (cf. curves a and d Fig. 2) with corresponding increases in the reduced viscosity (from 3.80 to 5.55 ml/g) both without change in molecular weight (Morino and Snell, 1967a). These changes are reflected also in the dissociation behavior of this polymeric enzyme (Table II): no dissociation of the tetrameric holoenzyme ($s^{\circ}_{20,w} = 10.55$ S, curve a, Fig. 2) into dimers occurs even at low temperature and protein concentration, whereas the apoenzyme readily dissociates to the dimer ($s^{\circ}_{20,w} = 6.0$ S) under these conditions (curve f, Fig. 2). With aspartate β-decarboxylase, too, dissociation of the poly-subunit holoenzyme ($s_{20,w} = 19$ S) to a much smaller molecule ($s_{20,w} = 6$ S) occurs at room temperature upon resolution; reassociation occurs upon addition of pyridoxal-P or several of its analogs (Tate and Meister, 1968, 1969). Apophosphorylase b and a also represent associating-dissociating systems; in both cases aggregation to the monodisperse higher molecular weight form accompanies combination with PLP (Shaltiel *et al.*, 1969). With each of these enzymes, reactivation with PLP was accompanied by reaggregation; however, certain coenzyme analogs (e.g., pyridoxine-5'-P) produced reaggregation without reactivation, thus demonstrating that azomethine formation is not always prerequisite to the conformational effects.

In the single subunit enzyme, D-serine dehydratase (Table II), no effect of PLP on the hydrodynamic behavior of the enzyme was observed. However, whereas only a single —SH group is titrated by DTNB in the holoenzyme, three —SH groups (none of which are required individually for activity) titrate in the apoenzyme (Dowhan and Snell, 1970). The result, together with the greatly increased temperature stability of the holoenzyme, indicates that localized conformational changes induced by PLP occur in this and perhaps in most instances, even though the magnitude of the change, as reflected by hydrodynamic parameters, is small. Such changes would explain the almost general observation that PLP holoenzymes are more stable to heat and other denaturants than the corresponding apoenzymes (e.g., Morino and Snell, 1967a; Blethen *et al.*, 1968; Shaltiel *et al.*, 1969; Dowhan and Snell, 1970; Chatagner,

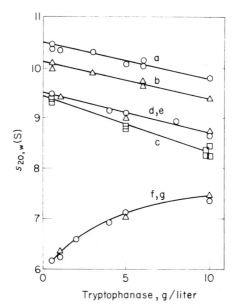

Fig. 2. Variation in sedimentation rate of apo- and holotryptophanase as a function of concentration, ionic environment, and temperature. All experiments were performed at pH 8.0 in buffer containing 0.02 M imidazole-HCl, 2 mM EDTA, and 5 mM β-mercaptoethanol, with the additions and temperature as follows. Curves: a, holoenzyme, 0.1 M KCl, 5° and 24°; b, holoenzyme, 0.1 M NaCl, 5° and 24°; c, holoenzyme and apoenzyme, 0.1 M imidazole-HCl 5° and 24°; d, (○), apoenzyme, 0.1 M KCl, 22°; e, (△), apoenzyme, 0.1 M NaCl, 24°; f and g, apoenzyme, 0.1 M KCl (○) or 0.1 M NaCl (△), 5°. Reproduced from Morino and Snell (1967a) with consent of the publisher.

1970), and also are in accord with the slow rate of resolution and reactivation discussed in the preceding section.

B. Effect of Structure on Activity of Pyridoxal
    Phosphate Analogs in Different Enzyme Systems

1. D-Serine Dehydratase

D-Serine dehydratase contains only one peptide chain, and therefore provides a system in which the activities of PLP analogs can be tested without complications arising from their separate effects on quaternary structure. Dowhan and Snell (1970) used kinetic methods under equilibrium conditions to obtain the true dissociation constants of both coenzymatically active analogs (Fig. 3) and inactive analogs which competed with PLP for binding (Fig. 4). All active and inhibitory analogs showed

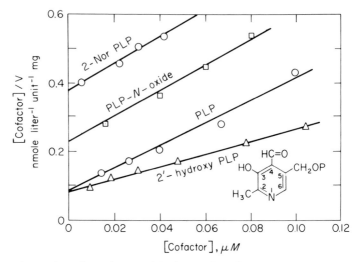

Fig. 3. Activation of D-serine apodehydratase by PLP and certain of its analogs. Each cofactor was incubated with apoenzyme (0.05–0.1 μg/ml) at pH 7.8 for 3 hours at 25° in the presence of dithiothreitol and acetylated serum albumin as stabilizing agents. The slope gives $1/V_{max}$ and the intercept on the ordinate is equal to K_p/V_{max}, where K_p is the dissociation constant for the added cofactor. Modified from Dowhan and Snell (1970) and reproduced with the permission of the *Journal of Biological Chemistry*.

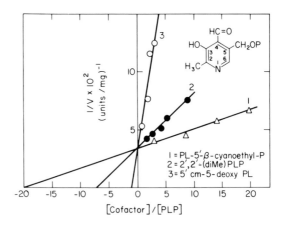

Fig. 4. Effect of inhibitory analogs on the activation of D-serine apodehydratase by PLP. Incubations were performed as in Fig. 3 in the presence of 0.42 μg of apoenzyme and 0.4 μM PLP. Modified from Dowhan and Snell (1970) and reproduced with permission of the publisher.

spectral shifts to longer wavelengths upon interaction with the apoenzyme (Table III) similar to those shown by PLP; quantitative study showed that the stoichiometry of binding was the same for PLP and 2'-propyl-PLP, two compounds with widely different affinities and activities.

The results (Table III) show clearly that the 2-methyl group and the unsubstituted 6-position of PLP are not essential for its activity; the former can be replaced by either H- (cf. 2-norPLP), CH_3CH_2- (2'-MePLP), or $HOCH_2$- (2'-hydroxyPLP) without inactivation—indeed, the latter compound combines with the enzyme as readily as PLP itself to yield an analog holoenzyme with a higher V_{max}. As the 2-substituent increases in size beyond an ethyl group (i.e., to 2'-propylPLP or 2'2'-diMePLP), ability of the analog to combine efficiently with the enzyme is retained, but all catalytic effectiveness is lost. This result probably indicates a sufficient displacement of the analog on the enzyme surface by the bulky side chain to either prevent formation of the enzyme-substrate complex or, more likely, to prevent the proper juxtaposition of catalytic groupings within that complex. It should be noted that no indication that a given complex is catalytically ineffective is provided by the spectral shifts. Insertion of a CH_3 group at position 6 decreases the affinity of the analog coenzyme for the apoenzyme but does not prevent formation of a catalytically effective complex. Although the bulkier 6-MePLP shows lower affinity for the apoenzyme than 2-nor-6-MePLP, the complex formed is a more efficient catalyst, as indicated by values of both K_m and V_{max}. These results suggest that the combining site for this portion of the coenzyme has limited spatial tolerances, and the presence of the 2-methyl group in PLP prevents displacement of the ring by the 6-methyl group toward a catalytically less productive position. Although modification of the 5'-position (cf. 5'-methylPLP) is possible without inactivation of the analog holoenzyme, no active analog in which the phosphate has been replaced by a monovalent anion has so far been found, although such compounds (e.g., 5'-CM-5-deoxyPL) bind very well. However if the 5'-oxygen is replaced by a —CH_2— group (cf. PL-5'-methylenephosphonate, which like PLP is a dibasic acid), a catalytically effective complex results. Apparently interaction of two appropriately placed anionic groups with protein is essential for orienting the coenzyme in a catalytically effective position; alternatively and less likely, one ionizable group of the dianion plays a catalytic role in the reaction.

Although at the concentrations tested neither 3-O-MePLP nor N-MePLP reactivated serine apodehydratase, they also did not inhibit its reactivation by PLP, and no spectral shift occurred upon their addition to apoenzyme solutions. As with pyridoxamine pyruvate aminotransferase, therefore, a free 3-phenolic group and probably an unsubstituted hetero-

TABLE III

INTERACTION OF PYRIDOXAL PHOSPHATE ANALOGS WITH D-SERINE APODEHYDRATASE AND APOTRYPTOPHANASE AS DETERMINED BY SPECTROPHOTOMETRIC AND ACTIVITY MEASUREMENTS

Analog	λ_{max} (nm)			D-Serine apodehydratase[a]			Apotryptophanase[b]		
	Alone	+ApoDH[a]	+ApoTPase[b]	$K_p{}^a$ (μM)	K_m (mM)	V_{max} (rel)	$K_{Co}{}^b$ (μM)	K_m (mM)	V_{max} (rel)
A. Active									
PLP	388	415	337, 420	0.035	0.37	1.00	0.71	0.27	1.00
2-NorPLP	382	410	330, 420	0.075	0.23	0.80	3.8	0.7	0.6
2'-MePLP	390	410	330, 420	0.11	0.40	0.25	11	0.2	0.04
2'-HOPLP	370	405		0.04	0.79	1.85	59	0.22	0.6
6-MePLP	370	415		13	0.32	0.20	7.7	0.57	0.2
2-Nor-6-MePLP	325	410		1.3	1.8	0.13	80	2.7	0.06
5'-MePLP	388	405		0.035	0.45	0.25	(not tested)		
PL-5'-methylene phosphonate	385	425		0.24	1.0	0.30	(not tested)		
B. Inhibitory									
2'-PropylPLP	390	420		9.1			20		
2',2'-DiMePLP	382	410		0.23			360		
PL-5'-Me phosphonate	390	420–440		7.2					
PL-5'-(β-cyanoethyl) phosphate	390	420–440		0.95					
5'-CM-5-deoxyPL	382	420		0.034					

[a] From Dowhan and Snell (1970). K_p designates dissociation constants for the PLP analogs determined under equilibrium conditions for PLP.

[b] Entries for PLP, 2-NorPLP, and 2'-MePLP are from Morino and Snell (1967b); other entries are unpublished data of Kagamiyama and Snell. In these cases K_{Co} represents the concentration of PLP analog necessary to obtain half maximum activity after an arbitrary period of incubation (30 minutes); or K_i values calculated under similar conditions in the presence of PLP; equilibrium conditions were not defined.

cyclic N are essential for efficient binding of the coenzyme. The role of the latter group is not entirely clear, however, since the N-oxide of PLP apparently reactivates the enzyme (Fig. 3). This compound, however, decomposes in part under the conditions of such assays and probably is not active per se.* 5-Deoxypyridoxal also is not bound by the enzyme, indicating the importance of an anionic grouping in the side chain for binding.

2. Tryptophanase

Results with this tetrameric enzyme (Table III) are very similar to those for the monomeric D-serine dehydratase with respect to classification of analogs into active and inactive categories. On closer comparison, however, it becomes apparent that structural variations affect the affinity of certain analogs for these two enzymes quite differently. A striking instance of such differences is provided by 2'-hydroxyPLP, which has nearly the same affinity as PLP for D-serine apodehydratase, but is very much less firmly bound by apotryptophanase, and once bound is a less effective coenzyme. Similar but less marked differences occur in other kinetic parameters of the two reactions. Such differences must reflect still unidentified differences in the coenzyme binding sites of various PLP-dependent enzymes, as concluded also from earlier studies (Snell, 1958; Morino and Snell, 1967b) and emphasized in an earlier part of this review.

3. Aspartate Aminotransferase (AAT)

Spectral shifts similar to those observed for D-serine apodehydratase and apotryptophanase (Table III) also occur on interaction of PLP analogs with apoAAT, as shown in Fig. 5A. As originally shown by Jenkins and Sizer (1959), holoAAT is a pH indicator; data of Fig. 5B show that the pK_a of the ionizing group (probably a hydrogen bond between the phenolic oxygen and the azomethine N) is substantially different in holoenzymes reconstituted with PLP (pK 6.3), 2-norPLP (pK 5.8), or 2'-MePLP (pK 6.5), all of which show substantial catalytic activity (Morino and Snell, 1967b). These observations have been confirmed and extended to additional 2-substituted analogs by Bocharov et al. (1968), who also showed that each of the active analogs upon binding to the apoenzyme produced circular dichroism at 365 nm (Table IV). With this enzyme, too, both the 2- and the 6-positions of PLP can be modified with only minor reductions in coenzymatic activity (Table IV); indeed, relatively high transaminase activity is retained even with 2'-propylPLP,

---

* Private communication from Professors E. Fischer and E. Helmreich.

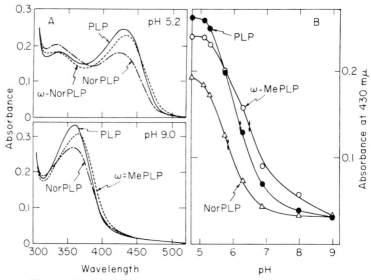

Fig. 5. pH-dependent variation of spectra of aspartate aminotransferase reconstituted with PLP, norPLP, or 2′-MePLP. The arrows (panel B) indicate the pK value for the spectral change. The apoenzyme preparation (22 mg) was incubated for 15 minutes at 25° with 0.4 µmole of the specified analog in 1 ml of 0.02 M potassium phosphate buffer, pH 7.0. One-tenth milliliter of this solution was then transferred to 0.9 ml of buffer solution of the desired pH: 0.1 M potassium acetate (pH 4.8–5.2) 0.1 M potassium phosphate (pH 5.8–8.0), or 0.1 M potassium carbonate (pH 9.0). From Morino and Snell (1967b); reproduced with the permission of the publishers.

which is an inhibitory analog for both D-serine dehydratase and tryptophanase (Table III). This wide latitude in spatial tolerance at the 2-position, together with the high catalytic activity of 2-norPLP, seems difficult to reconcile with the rather specific role postulated for the 2-methyl group (as one pivot of a stationary axis upon which the coenzyme rocks during transamination) by Ivanov and Karpeisky (1969). Unlike pyridoxamine-pyruvate aminotransferase and D-serine dehydratase, considered earlier, apoAAT also binds both N-MePLP and 3-O-MePLP, as shown both by ultraviolet and circular dichroic spectra (Furbish et al., 1969). Binding of N-MePLP occurred very slowly, however, and the adduct transaminated very slowly on addition of glutamate (Table V), so that catalytic activity for the overall transamination reaction was essentially zero. The catalytic activity reported for the AAT-O-MePLP complex (about 1% that of PLP-AAT, Table V) was low, but, if real, it would indicate that although the 3-phenolic group contributes to the high catalytic activity of the bound coenzyme, it is not essential for a de-

TABLE IV

SOME PROPERTIES OF ASPARTATE AMINOTRANSFERASES RECONSTITUTED WITH
VARIOUS 2-SUBSTITUTED ANALOGS OF PYRIDOXAL PHOSPHATE[a]

Property measured	Apoenzyme reconstituted with					
	PLP	2-NorPLP	2'-MePLP	2'-PropylPLP	6-MePLP	2-Nor-6-MePLP
λ_{max}, pH 5.2 (nm)	430	425	435	440	455	455
λ_{max}, pH 8.1 (nm)	360	360	365	370	370	370
pK_a	6.25	5.8	6.5	6.4	6.3	—
$\Delta D/D \times 10^4$ at 360 nm[b]	19	21	—	15	15	—
V_{max}, relative	1	1.2 (1.8)	(0.32)	0.5	0.56	0.47
K_m, α-ketoglutarate (mM)	0.1 (0.16)	0.24 (0.5)	(0.05)	0.08	0.14	—
K_m, L-aspartate (mM)	2.0 (3.0)	1.8 (5.0)	(0.5)	0.6	1.0	—
K_{co} (μM)[c]	(0.15)	(0.07)	(1.5)	—	—	—

[a] Values in parentheses are from Morino and Snell (1967b); all other values are from Bocharov et al. (1968).

[b] A measure of the magnitude of the induced optical activity at 360 nm.

[c] Concentration of analog required for half-maximum activity of the reconstituted enzyme under arbitrary nonequilibrium conditions.

TABLE V

TIMES FOR COMPLETION OF REACTION OF PYRIDOXAL PHOSPHATE (PLP) AND ANALOGS WITH APOTRANSAMINASE IN CUVETTE[a]

Compound	Binding to Apoenzyme pH 8.3	Reaction with Glutamate pH 8.3	Reaction with α-ketoglutarate, pH about 6.5	Activity (% of activity of native enzyme)
PLP	<2 min	<2 min	<2 min (pH 7.1)	100
5'-CM-5-DeoxyPL	<2% change after 2 min	<2 min except for slow loss of 420 nm band	Slow, faster at pH 8.3	<0.2
PL-5'-Mephosphonate	6–7% change after 2 min	80% complete in 2 min	*Very slow*	<0.2
PL-5'-(β-cyanoethyl)-P	>20 min	Slow	Slow except for a small portion reacting fast	Variable
PL-5'-phosphonate	<2 min	Slow, 430 nm intermediate	*Very slow*	<0.2
5'-MePLP	<2 min	<2 min	<2 min (pH 8.3)	3.0
N-MePLP	~10 min	Slow	Very slow	0
3-O-MePLP		5 min	5 min	1.0

[a] Reproduced (with slight modification in form) from Furbish *et al.* (1969) with permission of the authors. Abbreviations: 5'-CM-5-deoxy PL, β-(2-methyl-3-hydroxy-4-formyl-5-pyridyl)propionic acid; 5'-phosphono-5-deoxypyridoxal, α-(2-methyl-3-hydroxy-4-formyl-pyridyl-5)methylphosphonic acid.

creased rate of catalysis that is still very much higher than the non-enzymatic rate. α^5-PL-acetate binds to apoAAT effectively—as it does to serine apodehydratase and apotryptophanase (Table III)—but slowly, then undergoes a half reaction with glutamate to yield the corresponding amine, which is very poorly bound (Furbish et al., 1969). As a result it (and other PLP analogs with a monovalent cationic group in the 5'-position) is a very poor catalyst of the overall reaction. Furbish et al. (1969) point out that one of the two acid groups of the 5'-phosphate group of PLP can occupy a position that would permit it to act as a general acid-base catalyst in transamination. However, in view of the efficiency of catalysis of other transamination reactions in which a 5'-phosphate cannot be involved (see Section II,A and B) and other factors discussed previously, it seems unnecessary to invoke such a role for the phosphate group at this time.

4. *Arginine Decarboxylase*

Limited tests of various PLP analogs with this apoenzyme (Table VI) yield results in accord with those already discussed for tryptophanase and D-serine dehydratase: both the 2- and the 6-positions can be modified without loss in activity, although large variations (e.g., 2'-propylPLP) yield compounds which bind at the active site in a catalytically ineffective way, thus inhibiting reactivation with PLP. The high catalytic effectiveness of the 2-norPLP-enzyme relative to the PLP enzyme is notable. The tremendous increase in affinity ($>10,000$-fold) produced by presence of the 5'-phosphate group (cf. PLP vs PL or 5-deoxyPL), and its essential role in permitting formation of a catalytically active complex, are noteworthy.

5. *Aspartate β-Decarboxylase*

This polysubunit enzyme catalyzes both the decarboxylation of L-aspartate to L-alanine, and (at a rate $<0.1\%$ that of the decarboxylation reaction) a transamination reaction between L-aspartate and pyruvate. Binding of PLP to the 6 S apoenzyme causes association of subunits to yield 19 S holoenzyme (Tate and Meister, 1968, 1969). Structural variations in PLP affect these various activities differently (Table VI). All analogs that bind specifically (1 mole/50,000 g of enzyme) produce the conformational effect necessary for the 6 S to 19 S transformation, and these include several compounds that lack the 4-formyl group. The latter compounds, however, are devoid of catalytic activity for both decarboxylation and transamination. Both N-MePLP and O-MePLP bind and catalyze both decarboxylation and transamination reactions at rates 3 to 6% those of the PLP-catalyzed reactions. No spectral evidence

TABLE VI

INTERACTION OF PYRIDOXAL 5'-PHOSPHATE (PLP) ANALOGS WITH ARGININE APODECARBOXYLASE AND ASPARTATE APO-β-DECARBOXYLASE AS DETERMINED BY SPECTROPHOTOMETRIC AND ACTIVITY MEASUREMENTS

| Analog | λ_{max} (nm) | Aspartate β-decarboxylase[a] | | | V_{max} (relative)[d] for | | Arginine decarboxylase[b] | | |
		Moles bound/ 50,000 g of enzyme	Activity in 6S → 19S reaction	K_{Co}^{c} (μM)	Decarboxylation[d]	Transamination[d]	K_{Co}^{e} (μM)	K_m (mM)	V_{max} (relative)[f]
PLP	358	0.93	+	→0	1.0	1.0	0.027	0.95	1.0
2-NorPLP	358	0.94	+	→0	0.58	2.4	0.40	2.6	2.4
2'-MePLP	358	0.94	+	→0	0.11	1.5	0.14	2.1	0.36
6-MePLP							0.94	2.3	0.38
2'-PropylPLP	370	0.91	+	→0	0.05	0.76	0.54	(Inhibitor vs PLP)	0
3-O-MePLP	299	1.1	+	→0	0.05	0.03			
N-MePLP	398[g]	(1.0)[h]	+	3.3	0.06	0.03			
PMP	322	1.0	+	2.8	0[i]	—			
PNP	—	(1.0)[h]	+	0.7	0[i]	0[i]			
4-deoxyPNP	314[g]	0.93	+	→0	0	0			
PL			−				330	(Inhibitor vs PLP)	0

5-DeoxyPL	300 (Inhibitor vs PLP)		0
5'-CM-5-deoxyPL	>1000 (Inhibitor vs PLP)		0
PL-5'-sulfate	0	—	0	0

[a] From Tate and Meister (1969).

[b] From Blethen et al. (1968).

[c] →0 signifies "approaching zero," i.e., not measured because essentially complete binding occurred between stoichiometric amounts of enzyme subunit (mol. wt. 50,000) and coenzyme analog. Equilibrium conditions for association of apoenzyme and coenzyme have not, in general, been defined. It is not certain, therefore, that K_{Co} values listed represent true dissociation constants.

[d] Maximum velocity for the PLP enzyme was 122 units/mg for the decarboxylation reaction (micromoles of CO_2 formed per minute in the reaction: L-aspartate → L-alanine + CO_2). The transamination reaction catalyzed by this enzyme (L-aspartate + pyruvate ⇌ oxaloacetate + L-alanine) proceeds at less than 0.1% of this rate (V_{max} = 9.2 nmoles of oxaloacetate formed min⁻¹ mg⁻¹).

[e] Measured as amount of cofactor required for half-maximum velocity; because of slow reversibility K_{Co} is not a true dissociation constant.

[f] V_{max} for the PLP enzyme was 530 μmoles of CO_2 min⁻¹ mg⁻¹ in the reaction: L-arginine → agmatine + CO_2.

[g] These absorption maxima are unchanged upon binding to the enzyme.

[h] An assumed value: because of relatively loose binding, more than stoichiometric amounts of the analog coenzyme were required for reconstitution. In the case of PMP, actual binding was measured by use of the radioactive compound.

[i] Since these compounds bind at the active site and are coenzymatically inactive, they would inhibit recombination with PLP, presumably competitively, as is the case for arginine decarboxylase.

of azomethine formation between N-MePLP and apoenzyme was obtained; despite this fact, the complex is catalytically active. This finding indicates that intramolecular azomethine formation, which occurs in all PLP-enzymes thus far examined, may enhance their catalytic activity but is not essential for it (Tate and Meister, 1969). Several analogs (e.g., 2-norPLP, 6-MePLP) are relatively much more effective in promoting transamination than in promoting decarboxylation; converse variations in activity also occur (e.g., N-MePLP) but are less pronounced. Such relationships are not unexpected if, as appears likely, the transamination reaction catalyzed by this enzyme results only when the spatial relationships within the holoenzyme-substrate complex occasionally vary from those optimal for decarboxylation. In that event, a slightly altered position of the analog coenzyme within the complex could affect one of two alternative catalytic steps preferentially. In view of the wide latitude for the binding reaction, the complete inactivity of pyridoxal 5'-sulfate is surprising. This analog is also ineffective as a substitute for PLP in aspartate aminotransferase and tryptophanase as well as in phosphorylase, results which emphasize once more the unique effectiveness of the divalent phosphate (or phosphonate) ion in producing a catalytically effective coenzyme-apoenzyme complex.

6. *Phosphorylase*

PLP plays a unique role in phosphorylase, since no amino acid substrates of this enzyme are known (Hedrick and Fischer, 1965) and reduction with sodium borohydride does not inactivate the enzyme (Kent *et al.,* 1958). Just as in other PLP enzymes, however (see Section III,B,2), PLP induces profound conformational changes on combination with apophosphorylase *b* which are reflected by a change in quaternary structure [cf. the increase in sedimentation coefficient from about 6.7 to 8.3 S (Table VII)]. In an attempt to delineate the structural features of PLP necessary for its separate effects, Shaltiel *et al.* (1969) conducted a careful comparison of the effects of PLP analogs on both apophosphorylase *a* and *b*. Their results, some of which appear in Table VII, indicate that (a) positions 2, 3 and 6 of PLP are not essential for catalysis since 2-norPLP, 3-*O*-MePLP and 6-MePLP all reactivate both apoenzymes; (b) reactivation requires a divalent anion on the 5' side chain, since PL, PL-5'-sulfate, and 5'-CM-5-deoxyPL, although bound, are all inactive, whereas PL-5'-methylenephosphonate is active; (c) all the compounds tested that reactivate phosphorylase *b* also promote aggregation of the enzyme; however, several compounds (e.g., PL, 5'-CM-5-deoxyPL, PL-5'-sulfate) are bound and cause reaggregation without producing catalytic activity; (d) presence of an *N*-methyl group greatly reduces or eliminates binding; and

TABLE VII
EFFECT OF ANALOGS OF PYRIDOXAL PHOSPHATE ON CATALYTIC ACTIVITY
OF APOPHOSPHORYLASES a AND b^a

Analog	Reactivation (%)		Aggregation state of apophosphorylase b
	Apophosphorylase a	Apophosphorylase b	
None	0	0	6.7
PLP	50–60	95–100	8.3
2-NorPLP	42	65	8.3
2'-MePLP	0	0	—
3-O-MePLP	40	25	8.5
6-MePLP	4	8	—
N-MePLP	0	0	7.5
PL-5'-methylene phosphonate	~25[b]	~25[b]	8.2[b]
PL-5'-sulfate		0	8.2
5'-CM-5-deoxyPL		0	8.2
PNP	0	0	6.5
PMP	0	0	6.5
PL	0	0	8.2
3-Hydroxypyridine-4-aldehyde	0	0	8.4

[a] From Shaltiel et al. (1969). 2 mM analog (or 0.1 mM PLP) was tested in each case.
[b] From Fischer (1970).

(e) an aldehyde group at position 4 strongly promotes binding (as evidenced by both catalytic activity and reaggregation measurements) even though, once the coenzyme is bound, this group is not required for activity. The latter finding correlates with the observation that PLP binds only as its thiazolidine with L-cysteine (Hedrick et al., 1966). To the extent that this is also true of PLP analogs, binding of compounds lacking the aldehyde group would not be expected. PLP binds to apophosphorylase slowly, as it does to other PLP-dependent enzymes, and the rate of binding is slowed even further by certain structural modifications, e.g., in 3-O-MePLP (Fig. 6).

These results suffice to establish that PLP in phosphorylase, as in other PLP-enzymes, plays an important conformational or structural role, but do not establish whether it also plays an essential catalytic role. If it does play a catalytic role, then clearly the 2-methyl group, the 3-phenolic group, the 4-formyl group, the 5-phosphate ester oxygen and the 6-hydrogen atom are not essential participants, since each can be modified either before or after binding without inactivating the enzyme. The pK of the pyridine nitrogen of pyridoxal and its derivatives is greatly lowered by replacing the 3-phenolic group by the 3-O-methyl group (pK for PL ~ 8.6; for O-MePL ~ 4.8; Metzler and Snell, 1955); the fact that the pH

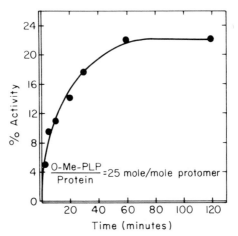

Fig. 6. Rate of reconstitution of apophosphorylase b with 3-O-MePLP. Solution contained apophosphorylase b $(1 \times 10^{-5}\,M)$, O-MePLP $(2.5 \times 10^{-4}\,M)$, 0.025 M sodium glycerophosphate, and 0.025 M β-mercaptoethanol (pH 7.0). Reactivation was allowed to proceed at 37°C for the period indicated. From Shaltiel et al. (1969); reproduced with the permission of authors and publishers.

optimum of phosphorylase does not change when 3-O-MePLP replaces PLP as coenzyme (Shaltiel et al., 1969) argues against the role for this nitrogen atom postulated by Bresler and Firsov (1968). If PLP plays a catalytical role, its ionizable phosphate group thus becomes the prime suspect as a participant in catalysis (cf. Kastenschmidt et al., 1968), since it is required for formation of a catalytically active enzyme, but not for aggregation (Table VII).

IV. General Comments and Conclusions

The results cited in this review confirm and extend the conclusions drawn from an earlier summation (Snell, 1958) of the effects of PLP analogs on catalytic activity of PLP-enzymes. It is now clear that catalytically productive binding of PLP and its analogs is a slow and poorly understood process, accompanied by conformational changes in the protein that produce in turn changes in the quaternary structure of polysubunit enzymes. Such conformational changes appear prerequisite for enzyme activity, but are not sufficient for it, since they frequently accompany binding of catalytically inactive analogs. These complexities complicate meaningful comparison of structural analogs, since structural changes affect not only the catalytic effectiveness of the bound analog, but also the binding capacity, the rate of binding, and the capacity to produce the essential conformational changes, and do so independently. Only occasionally have activity comparisons been made under equilibrium conditions of binding necessary for a proper comparison of affinities. Despite such deficiencies, it is clear that appropriate modifications in the 2- and 6-positions of PLP do not inactivate the coenzyme for any of the enzymes studied; the corresponding groups of PLP therefore play no catalytic role. Modification of these substituents does alter the affinity of the analog coenzymes for various apoenzymes, the affinity of the resulting analog holoenzymes for their substrates, and the maximal velocity of the reactions catalyzed, apparently as a result of deformations at the active site. These effects vary from enzyme to enzyme, thus indicating differences in their active sites; extensive modification renders such analogs catalytically inactive for some enzymes without preventing binding and without significantly modifying the spectral properties of the adducts. Such results indicate that very slight changes in the orientation of the coenzyme on the apoenzyme are sufficient to inactivate the complex as a catalyst.

Modification at the 1, 3, and 5 positions of PLP greatly reduces the affinity of such analogs for those enzymes with amino acid substrates, and greatly reduces the catalytic efficiency of those analog holoenzymes which are formed. The extent to which this reduction in catalytic efficiency reflects incorrect orientation of the coenzyme on the holoenzyme, as opposed to catalytic inefficiency of the modified coenzyme, is not generally known, and may vary from enzyme to enzyme. An intact 4-formyl group is essential for catalytic activity of all PLP enzymes with amino acid substrates, but is not essential for binding; in phosphorylase, this group is required for binding, but not for catalytic activity.

REFERENCES

Ayling, J. E., and Snell, E. E. (1968a). *Biochemistry* **7**, 1616.
Ayling, J. E., and Snell, E. E. (1968b). *Biochemistry* **7**, 1626.
Blethen, S. L., Boeker, E. A., and Snell, E. E. (1968). *J. Biol. Chem.* **243**, 1671.
Bocharov, A. L., Ivanov, V. I., Karpeisky, M. Ya., Mamaeva, O. K., and Florentiev, V. L. (1968). *Biochem. Biophys. Res. Commun.* **30**, 459.
Braunstein, A. E. (1960). *In* "The Enzymes" (P. D. Boyer, H. Lardy, and K. Myrbäck, eds.), 2nd ed., Vol. 2 pp. 113–184. Academic Press, New York.
Braunstein, A. E., and Shemyakin, M. M. (1953). *Biokhimiya* **18**, 393.
Bresler, S., and Firsov, L. (1968). *J. Mol. Biol.* **35**, 131.
Bresler, S., Firsov, L., and Glazunov, E. (1968). *In* "Pyridoxal Catalysis: Enzymes and Model Systems" (E. E. Snell *et al.*, eds.), I.U.B. Symp. Ser. No. 35, p. 581. Interscience Press, New York.
Chatagner, F. (1970). *Vitam. Horm. (New York)* **28**, 291.
Dempsey, W. B., and Snell, E. E. (1963). *Biochemistry* **2**, 1414.
Dowhan, W., Jr., and Snell, E. E. (1970). *J. Biol. Chem.* **245**, 4629.
Fischer, E. H. (1970). Private communication.
French, T. C., Auld, D. S., and Bruice, T. C. (1965). *Biochemistry* **4**, 77.
Furbish, F. S., Fonda, M. L., and Metzler, D. E. (1969). *Biochemistry* **8**, 5169.

Guirard, B. M., and Snell, E. E. (1964). In "Comprehensive Biochemistry" (M. Florkin and E. H. Stotz, eds.), Vol. 15, pp. 138–199. Elsevier, New York.

Hedrick, J. L., and Fischer, E. H. (1965). Biochemistry 4, 1337.

Hedrick, J. L., Shaltiel, S., and Fischer, E. H. (1966). Biochemistry 5, 2117.

Ivanov, V. I., and Karpeisky, M. Ya. (1969). Advan. Enzymol. 32, 21.

Jenkins, W. T., and Sizer, I. W. (1959). J. Biol. Chem. 234, 1179.

Johnston, C. C., Brooks, H. G., Albert, J. D., and Metzler, D. E. (1963). In "Chemical and Biological Aspects of Pyridoxal Catalysis" (E. E. Snell et al., eds.), I.U.B. Symp. Ser. No. 30. p. 69. Pergamon Press, Oxford.

Kastenschmidt, L. L., Kastenschmidt, J., and Helmreich, E. (1968). Biochemistry 7, 3590.

Kent, A. B., Krebs, E. G., and Fischer, E. H. (1958). J. Biol. Chem. 232, 549.

Matsuzawa, T., and Segal, H. L. (1968). J. Biol. Chem. 243, 5929.

Metzler, D. E., and Snell, E. E. (1955). J. Amer. Chem. Soc. 77, 2431.

Metzler, D. E., Ikawa, M., and Snell, E. E. (1954). J. Amer. Chem. Soc. 76, 648.

Morino, Y., and Snell, E. E. (1967a). J. Biol. Chem. 242, 5591.

Morino, Y., and Snell, E. E. (1967b). Proc. Nat. Acad. Sci. U.S. 57, 1692.

Newton, W. A., Morino, Y., and Snell, E. E. (1965). J. Biol. Chem. 240, 1211.

Recsei, P. A., and Snell, E. E. (1970). Biochemistry 9, 1492.

Riley, W. D., and Snell, E. E. (1968). Biochemistry 7, 3520.

Shaltiel, S., Hedrick, J. L., and Fischer, E. H. (1966). Biochemistry 5, 2108.

Shaltiel, S., Hedrick, J. L., Pocker, A., and Fischer, E. H., (1969). Biochemistry 8, 5189.

Snell, E. E. (1958). Vitam. Horm. (New York) 16, 77.

Snell, E. E. (1963). In "Chemical and Biological Aspects of Pyridoxal Catalysis" (E. E. Snell et al., eds.), I.U.B. Symp. Ser. No. 30, pp. 1–12. Pergamon Press, Oxford.

Snell, E. E., and DiMari, S. (1970). In "The Enzymes" (P. D. Boyer, ed.), 3rd ed.. Vol. 2, pp. 335–370. Academic Press, New York.

Tate, S. S., and Meister, A. (1968). Biochemistry 7, 3240.

Tate, S. S., and Meister, A. (1969). Biochemistry 8, 1056.

Wada, H., and Snell, E. E. (1962a). J. Biol. Chem. 237, 133.

Wada, H., and Snell, E. E. (1962b). J. Biol. Chem. 237, 127.

Influences of Pyridoxine Derivatives on the Biosynthesis and Stability of Pyridoxal Phosphate Enzymes

FERNANDE CHATAGNER

Laboratoire de Chimie Biologique, Faculté des Sciences, Paris, France

I. INTRODUCTION

The main purpose of the present article is to survey and to discuss the results so far obtained related to the involvement of pyridoxal phosphate and other pyridoxine derivatives on the biosynthesis and stability of pyridoxal phosphate-dependent enzymes. Many attempts have been made in recent years to explain the function of pyridoxal phosphate at the molecular level. The main questions to be resolved were the following:

Is pyridoxal phosphate necessary to the biosynthesis of the proteins for which it participates as coenzyme?

Is the stability of these proteins modified whether pyridoxal phosphate is or is not bound to them?

Is the coenzyme implicated in the structure of these proteins?

Various investigators have suggested possible roles for pyridoxal phosphate and pyridoxine derivatives in these areas. Some information was obtained on the one hand from the extensive studies of the change of level of enzymatic activities in response to pyridoxine deficiency, and on the other hand from the data dealing with the effect on enzyme activities of pyridoxine injection into animals. Likewise, there have been many reports on the protective effects of pyridoxal phosphate when added at several stages during purification of a number of pyridoxal phosphate-dependent enzymes. It was previously pointed out (Greengard, 1963, 1964; Williams, 1964; Wiss and Weber, 1964) that interrelations may exist between pyridoxine and apoenzymes. Moreover, the results of recent experiments concerned with the protective effect of pyridoxal phosphate and pyridoxine derivatives when added to purified enzymes in the presence of urea, of other denaturing agents, of proteolytic enzymes, as well as during inactivation by heat, have been consistent with the concept that pyridoxal phosphate affects the stability of these enzymes and is involved in the conformation and the structure of pyridoxal phosphate-dependent enzymes. The question of a regulation of the biosynthesis of apoenzymes by pyridoxal phosphate remains open since there is as yet no evidence of a *direct* relationship between coenzyme availability and the rate of biosynthesis of pyridoxal phosphate enzymes.

These results taken as a whole indicate some similarities and some remarkable differences, depending upon the specific enzyme being considered as well as upon the inducing or denaturing agent involved. This survey reveals that pyridoxal phosphate and pyridoxine derivatives have interesting properties that afford some insight into the still rudimentary knowledge of the mechanism involved in the physiological biosynthesis and degradation of enzymes (Arias *et al.*, 1969).

II. Effects of Pyridoxine Deficiency

In discussing this subject, one must keep in mind the interesting results obtained when the activities of crude pyridoxal phosphate enzymes are measured in the presence or the absence of pyridoxal phosphate added to the assay system, even when the enzymes were extracted from the tissues of animals fed on standard "nutritionally complete" diets (such as pellets), or from bacteria grown on complete media. Some enzymes seemed saturated with coenzyme and had the same activity whether the determinations were carried out in presence or the absence of pyridoxal phosphate, whereas the activities of other enzymes were stimulated by the addition of the coenzyme. This observation has led to concepts concerning (1) the "endogenous activity," in other words, the activity estimated in the absence of coenzyme; (2) the "coenzyme-stimulated activity" or total activity, which is the activity measured with excess of coenzyme and seems to reflect the apoenzyme level of the extract; (3) the "percentage of saturation" or

$$\frac{\text{endogenous activity}}{\text{coenzyme-stimulated activity}} \times 100$$

(4) the "percentage of stimulation by the coenzyme," or

$$\frac{\text{coenzyme-stimulated activity minus endogenous activity}}{\text{endogenous activity}} \times 100$$

It is important to recall that many pyridoxal phosphate enzymes are included in the second group. For example, tyrosine decarboxylase from *Streptococcus faecalis* (Gunsalus *et al.*, 1944), various transaminases from pig heart, liver, and kidney (Cammarata and Cohen, 1950), glutamic acid decarboxylase from rat brain (Roberts and Frankel, 1951), diaminopimelic acid decarboxylase from *Escherichia coli* (Dewey *et al.*, 1954).

Enzymes of the first group include cysteinesulfinic acid decarboxylase from either rat liver (Bergeret *et al.*, 1955) or rabbit liver (Bergeret *et al.*, 1956), also glutamic-oxaloacetic transaminase and glutamic-pyruvic transaminase from brain and liver (Rosen and Milholland, 1960).

Stimulation of various enzyme activities by pyridoxal phosphate has been observed *in vitro,* suggesting that a similar mechanism may be operative *in vivo* whenever the availability of pyridoxal phosphate is increased.

It is not appropriate to present here a systematic compilation of all the published data on the behavior of each specific pyridoxal phosphate enzyme in response to pyridoxine deficiency. Detailed information on this can be found elsewhere (Meister, 1965). Enzymatic studies carried out with preparations extracted from the tissues of animals that had been fed pyridoxine-depleted diets, as well as studies with bacteria grown on deficient culture media, have revealed differential effects rather than uniform decreases of pyridoxal phosphate enzymes during pyridoxine deprival. Some enzymes are altered at early stages of deficiency at a time when other enzymes are not impaired (Wiss and Weber, 1964). This survey will be limited to a consideration of relatively few selected and significant enzymes.

Pyridoxine deficiency in rats causes decreases in the endogenous value of a number of pyridoxal phosphate enzymes: tyrosine-α-ketoglutarate and tryptophan-α-ketoglutarate transaminases, phenylalanine-pyruvate and histidine-pyruvate transaminases from rat liver (Lin *et al.*, 1958), glutamic acid decarboxylase from brain (Bergeret *et al.*, 1955), and cystathionase from liver (Chatagner and Durieu-Trautmann, 1965). The activity of cysteinesulfinic acid decarboxylase in the liver decreased rapidly in response to pyridoxine deficiency and soon disappeared (Chatagner *et al.*, 1954; Hope, 1955), whereas the activity of glutamic-pyruvic transaminase from liver was not altered even after long periods of depletion (Rosen and Milholland, 1960). On the other hand, the addition of pyridoxal phosphate to the assay system restored more or less completely, depending upon the degree of deficiency, when compared to normal value, the coenzyme-stimulated activity of these enzymes.

Cysteinesulfinic acid decarboxylase from liver was an exception, however, since its activity was not restored.

Surprisingly, several investigators have observed rises in the concentrations of some apoenzymes in response to pyridoxine deficiency: diaminopimelic acid apocarboxylase and lysine apodecarboxylase from a mutant of *E. coli* (Denman *et al.*, 1955), glutamic-oxaloacetic apotransaminase and pyridoxamine-oxaloacetic apotransaminase from *E. coli* (Wada and Morino, 1964), and tyrosine-α-ketoglutarate apotransaminase from rat liver (Lin *et al.*, 1958).

Except for those enzymes whose endogenous activities are suppressed by pyridoxine deficiency, these results indicated that pyridoxine deprivation did not affect the biosynthesis of various apoenzymes.

It has been reported also that in pyridoxine-deficient rats the induction of tyrosine apotransaminase and tryptophan apotransaminase by hydrocortisone in the liver was not impaired (Lin *et al.*, 1958), that cortisone injections increased the endogenous level of tyrosine decarboxylase (Davis, 1963), and that the increase of apocystathionase in rat liver in response to thyroidectomy was not eliminated (Chatagner and Durieu-Trautmann, 1965). Thus, the data obtained to date are consistent with the suggestion (Schimke *et al.*, 1965) that substrates and cofactors stabilize the existing enzymes, while hormonal factors alter the rate of biosynthesis of the apoenzymes. The decreases in activity reflect an increased instability of these proteins due to a limited availability of the coenzyme. The adaptive increases of apoenzymes, when observed, in response to hormonal treatments suggest also that depletion of pyridoxal phosphate did not impair the mechanisms involved in biosynthesis of these proteins.

However, in attempting to construct a framework consistent with most available data, and on which most of the observations dealing with the effect of pyridoxine deficiency on the level of enzymes in animals could be fitted, it cannot be ignored that some of the biochemical symptoms of vitamin-B_6 deficiency might be mediated, at least in part, by alterations in hormonal factors in response to pyridoxine deficiency. Thus, it has been reported that in pyridoxine-deficient rats the metabolic effects of follicle-stimulating and interstitial cell-stimulating hormones were greatly reduced (Wooten *et al.*, 1958), that the pituitary metabolism and more especially the growth hormone activity in the pituitaries was markedly altered, and that an insufficiency of insulin activity was observed (Gershoff, 1968). A general review devoted to the interrelations between pyridoxine and hormones has already appeared (Hsu, 1963). Therefore, one must keep in mind the possibility that hormonal alterations might take a part in the effects of pyridoxine deficiency, and that the amount of protein present in the diets of the animals under examination must be considered since a high protein intake increases the needs in pyridoxine (Canham *et al.*, 1969). Finally, it was observed that substances such as cysteine and histidine (Heyl *et al.*, 1948; Buell and Hansen, 1960), and norepinephrine (Black and Axelrod, 1969) act as "trapping" agents of pyridoxal phosphate.

On the other hand, it should be noted that, in the experiments conducted until now, the activity of the tyrosine transaminase was measured on the supernatant obtained by ultracentrifugation of a liver homogenate. Recently it was shown (Fellman *et al.*, 1969) that both soluble and mitochondrial forms of tyrosine transaminase are to be found in rat liver.

III. EFFECTS OF INJECTION OF PYRIDOXINE

From the results observed in pyridoxine deficiency, the idea developed that increasing the level of pyridoxal phosphate in an organism changes the level of its pyridoxal phosphate enzymes. Two kinds of experimental data were obtained in this field, the first dealt with the increase of the percentage of saturation of apoenzymes relative to the cofactor, while the second was concerned with the levels of appropriate apoenzymes.

A. EFFECT ON THE PERCENTAGE OF SATURATION OF APOENZYMES

It has been reported that injection of large doses of pyridoxine into rats increased the percentage of saturation of glutamic acid decarboxylase in the brain (De Marco, 1957), of tyrosine transaminase (Greengard and Gordon, 1963) and of cystathionase (Durieu-Trautmann *et al.*, 1964) in the liver.

B. EFFECT ON THE LEVEL OF APOENZYMES

Greengard and Gordon (1963) have observed that the injection of very high doses of pyridoxine into rats induces a significant increase in the level of apotyrosine transaminase in the liver. This increase exceeds that of the pyridoxal phosphate level. This observation led to the assumption that the cofactor concentration within the cell may regulate the biosynthesis of appropriate apoenzymes. However, since the induction of apotyrosine transaminase was inhibited by actinomycin, it has been suggested that the effect of pyridoxine may be mediated through hormonal factors (Holten *et al.*, 1967). Corticoids and thyroid hormones were excluded as possible mediators since pyridoxine is effective in adrenalectomized rats (Greengard and Gordon, 1963) and in thyroidectomized rats (Chatagner *et al.*, 1968c). Since pyridoxine did not evoke an increase of the apotyrosine transaminase in the liver of the alloxan diabetic rat, it has been suggested that insulin may be a repressor of tyrosine transaminase (Chatagner *et al.*, 1968c). Recent findings (Levitan and Webb, 1969) support the hypothesis that tyrosine transaminase turnover is dependent on the continued synthesis of a degradative enzyme of short half-life. Tyrosine transaminase purified from a homogenate of rat liver has a molecular weight of 115,000, contains 4 moles of pyridoxal phosphate and also 1 mole of pyridoxal phosphate so tightly bound to the protein that it is not resolved by dialysis (Valeriotte *et al.*, 1969).

Since the injection of pyridoxine increased the level of serine dehydrase in rat liver, it was suggested that this increase reflects a stabilizing effect of pyridoxal phosphate on this enzyme (Khairallah and Pitot, 1968). On the other hand, the injection of pyridoxine did not raise the level of another enzyme, not saturated in coenzyme, the cystathionase of rat liver (Durieu-Trautmann *et al.*, 1964). In addition, the levels of two decarboxylases of rat liver, fully saturated with coenzyme [a nonspecific aromatic amino acid decarboxylase (Greengard, 1964) and cysteinesulfinic acid decarboxylase (Durieu-Trautmann *et al.*, 1964)] did not change as a result of pyridoxine treatment.

Thus, at the present time, the available data do not provide clear evidence that the biosynthesis of apoenzymes is directly regulated by the pyridoxal phosphate level in animals; the increased stability of apoenzymes *in vivo* when in presence of the coenzyme, is presumably responsible for most of the effects observed to date.

IV. Effects of Pyridoxal Phosphate and Other Pyridoxine Derivatives on the Stability of Purified Enzymes

A. Protective Effects against Denaturing Agents

A number of enzymes have been described, the stabilities of which are influenced by the coenzyme that participates in the reaction. In most instances, the hypothesis of increased stability of holoenzymes has been tested by comparison with apoenzymes. Purified preparations of apoenzymes were submitted to denaturing treatments, with or without prior addition of coenzyme and the residual activities of both samples were measured after suitable dilution. It was reported that biosynthetic threonine dehydrase from yeast was protected against inactivation by pyridoxal phosphate and pyridoxamine phosphate (Holzer *et al.*, 1963). The inactivation of aspartic β-decarboxylase which occurs when the enzyme is incubated with L-aspartate, was delayed by initial addition of α-keto-acids, and reversed by the addition of pyridoxal phosphate. Since the protective effect was also demonstrated by 4'-deoxypyridoxine 5'-phosphate, it was suggested that the coenzyme analog may bind some of the active sites of the enzyme that normally bind the coenzyme (Novogrodsky and Meister, 1964). The data so far obtained suggest that when the enzyme molecule is supplied with coenzyme and coenzyme analog it is more stable than the corresponding apoenzyme. Thus, the coenzyme contributes to the structural integrity of the enzyme and is also necessary for the binding with the substrate (Wilson-Miles *et al.*, 1968; Tate and Meister, 1969a,b). It was reported also that the concentration of dodecyl sulfate necessary for irreversible inactivation of tryptophanase was much higher when holoenzyme was treated in comparison with apoenzyme (Morino and Snell, 1967a,b).

Pyridoxamine pyruvate transaminase isolated from a soil organism (Ayling and Snell, 1968a,b) did not contain pyridoxal phosphate, but the substrates of this enzyme, pyridoxal and pyridoxamine, play the same role as has been ascribed to pyridoxal phosphate and pyridoxamine phosphate in the usual transaminases. This enzyme was partially protected against urea denaturation by excess pyridoxal, but not by excess pyridoxamine (Kolb *et al.*, 1968). These data may indicate that the enzyme–pyridoxal complex assumes a physical structure that is resistant to denaturation. Pyridoxal and pyridoxamine also protected the enzyme against inhibition by *p*-chloromercuribenzoate (Fujioka and Snell, 1965).

The inactivation of partially purified tyrosine transaminase extracted from rat liver (Litwack *et al.*, 1966) and of cystathionase and cysteine-sulfinic acid decarboxylase from the same source (Chatagner *et al.*, 1968a,b) by urea and guanidine hydrochloride was prevented or delayed by the simultaneous addition of pyridoxal phosphate prior to incubation of the systems. Similar results were obtained when tyrosine transaminase (Holten *et al.*, 1967) cystathionase and cysteinesulfinic acid decarboxylase (Chatagner *et al.*, 1968a,b) were inactivated by heat. Pyridoxamine phosphate afforded as complete protection to tyrosine transaminase as pyridoxal phosphate. Other derivatives such as pyridoxine, pyridoxal hydrochloride and pyridoxamine hydrochloride did not protect the three enzymes against urea inactivation. These observations are in agreement with a report (Churchich and Farrelly, 1969) that the phosphate group of pyridoxal phosphate is necessary for the binding of the coenzyme to the apoprotein of aspartate transaminase. In this connection, Furbish *et al.* (1969) has suggested that the phosphate group of pyridoxal phosphate has a greater function than simply as a "handle" for binding the coenzyme to the protein.

Pyridoxal phosphate has also been shown to protect tyrosine transaminase against inhibition by *p*-chloromercuribenzoate (Holten *et al.*, 1967). Since this enzyme was readily inhibited by substances reacting with protein-SH groups, this result suggests that some of the SH groups of the enzyme were protected by the coenzyme and that those not protected were not essential for enzymatic activity. Furthermore, the observation that the addition of pyridoxal phosphate to apoenzyme led to inaccessibility of mercurial reagents to some SH groups, was taken as indicating that the binding of the coenzyme afforded a significant conformational change of the protein. Other results by Chatagner *et al.* (1970) indicated that cystathionase was far more susceptible to degradation by proteolytic enzymes (trypsin, α-chymotrypsin, pronase) when in the form of apoenzyme than in the form of holoenzyme. This observation also supports the claim that the conformational properties of holoenzymes are very different than those of apoenzymes. On the other hand, partially purified cysteinesulfinic acid decarboxylase from rat liver, obtained as holoenzyme, was not protected against proteolysis by the addition of pyridoxal phosphate to the mixture prior to the proteolytic enzyme (Chatagner *et al.*, 1970), whereas this enzyme was protected by pyridoxal phosphate against heat inactivation and urea denaturation.

Glutamate decarboxylase from Lupin seeds was protected by pyridoxal phosphate against inactivation (Luque *et al.*, 1970).

These various data taken all together support the concept that the stability of the pyridoxal phosphate enzymes is deeply modified when either apoenzymes or holoenzymes are under examination, and that a looser structure is to be attributed to the apoenzymes.

B. Effects on the Conformation and Structure of Enzymes

All the enzymes examined until now are implicated in amino acid metabolism. The presence of pyridoxal phosphate in an enzyme involved in carbohydrate metabolism was first reported for rabbit muscle glycogen phosphorylase (Baranowski *et al.*, 1957; Cori and Illingworth, 1957; Kent *et al.*, 1958). Pyridoxal phosphate has been found in all the phosphorylases so far prepared (Fischer *et al.*, 1963; Sevilla and Fischer, 1969). Detailed reviews of the properties of muscle phosphorylases a and b have already appeared (Fischer *et al.*, 1963, 1968). The finding that reduction of the phosphorylase by sodium borohydride did not suppress its enzymatic activity indicates that pyridoxal phosphate is not involved in the catalysis, although removal of pyridoxal phosphate led to a total loss of enzymatic activity. In addition, it was observed that muscle phosphorylase was decreased in rats deficient in pyridoxine (Illingworth *et al.*, 1960; Eisenstein, 1962).

The evidence is clear that pyridoxal phosphate participates in controlling the structure of the molecule by maintaining the enzyme in the conformation required for enzymatic activity. Indeed, recent studies (Hedrick and Fischer, 1965; Hedrick *et al.*, 1966, 1969; Shaltiel *et al.*, 1966, 1969) have shown that in the native phosphorylase, the cofactor (pyridoxal phosphate) is "buried" into the protein molecule. Treatment of the enzyme with deforming agents promotes dissociation of the enzyme into monomers, and this process unmasks the cofactor; as a result the cofactor which is still bound to the protein, becomes "exposed" to some reagents of the surrounding medium. Thus, L-cysteine (but not D-cysteine) reacts with the cofactor to form a thiazolidine, thereby removing the cofactor from the protein. The complete removal of the cofactor is associated with some irreversible denaturation of the protein.

Morino and Snell (1967a,b) have reported that apotryptophanase from a mutant of *E. coli* is a tetramer having a molecular weight of 220,000. At low temperature, and when the concentration of protein is low, the tetramer is dissociated into dimers of 110,000. In the presence of $8\,M$ urea or sodium dodecyl sulfate, or $5\,M$ guanidium chloride, inactive monomers of 55,000 appeared. In addition, the holoenzyme that was formed by binding 4 moles of pyridoxal phosphate to the tetramer was not dissociated at low temperature. Thus, a pronounced conformational change accompanied the binding of pyridoxal phosphate, as evidenced by an increased sedimentation velocity and a decreased viscosity. These results strongly support the idea that the holoenzyme has a more compact form than the apotryptophanase.

Inactivation of pyridoxamine pyruvate transaminase by $8\,M$ urea accompanied the dissociation of the enzyme into subunits (Kolb *et al.*, 1968). The delay of this inactivation by pyridoxal indicates that the binding of pyridoxal to the protein led to a structure more resistant to denaturation.

Various vitamin B_6-5′-phosphate derivatives promoted the association of the 6 S apoenzyme of aspartate β-decarboxylase to a 19 S form of the enzyme (Tate and Meister, 1969a).

Biodegradative AMP-dependent threonine dehydrase from *E. coli* (Phillips *et al.*, 1968; Whanger *et al.*, 1968; Shizuta *et al.*, 1969) contains pyridoxal phosphate which, in addition to its catalytic role, contributes to the stability of the enzyme conformation. When crystallized in the presence of AMP, the enzyme has a molecular weight of approximately 150,000 and contains 4 moles of pyridoxal phosphate and 4 moles of AMP. The enzyme was resolved and inactivated by dialysis against a buffer-containing cysteine. AMP prevented both the resolution of pyridoxal phosphate and the loss of activity. On the other hand, addition of pyridoxal phosphate to the resolved inactive protomer, with a molecular weight of approximately 40,000, caused the re-formation of an active protomer of the same molecular weight, for the polymerization of which AMP and certain SH groups are essential.

It was observed that incubation of the two subunits α and β_2 of the tryptophan synthetase of *E. coli* with pyridoxal phosphate markedly increased the association of these subunits (Creighton and Yanofsky, 1966) and thus promoted the formation of the fully associated enzyme.

V. General Summary

This survey of the available data has revealed that the regulation of the activities of pyridoxal phosphate enzymes even in so restricted a field as pyridoxal phosphate and other pyridoxine derivatives, is very complex.

Remarkable differences have been observed, in responses to pyridoxine deficiency, depending on the enzyme under consideration. In general, the enzymes of the cell sap are far more sensitive to pyridoxine deprivation than the enzymes associated with the particulate fractions.

Furthermore, the enzymes whose turnovers are high are more rapidly altered than the enzymes whose turnovers are low.

Injections of large doses of pyridoxine into animals presumably increased the level of pyridoxal phosphate in the tissues. This increase was reflected in a higher percentage of saturation of some pyridoxal phosphate enzymes, which led to an increase in their stability. Unfortunately, until now few experiments have been conducted that were designed to observe changes in the activities of pyridoxine phosphate oxidase (Wada and Snell, 1961) and pyridoxal kinase (McCormick et al., 1961) in response to various treatments or hormonal modifications. Further clarification will not be likely until more is known of the changes in the activities of these enzymes. It is quite possible that most of the effects observed in response to pyridoxine injection only reflect an increased stability of the enzymes against physiological degradation. Indeed, in the case of tyrosine transaminase from rat liver whose endogenous activity was increased in response to pyridoxine injection, it has been postulated, and at least in some instances shown, that hormonal factors may be involved in this phenomenon.

It is now well established that holoenzymes are far more stable than apoenzymes. The claim that pyridoxal phosphate bound to appropriate apoenzymes will produce a profound change of the conformation of these apoenzymes is supported by various experimental data and is currently a topic of increasing interest in relation to the functions of pyridoxal phosphate at the molecular level. It is of interest to recall that several pyridoxal phosphate-dependent enzymes consist of subunits, and that these enzymes have at least as many subunits as pyridoxal phosphate binding sites (Boecker and Snell, 1968).

REFERENCES

Arias, I. M., Doyle, D., and Schimke, R. T. (1969). J. Biol. Chem. 244, 3303.
Ayling, J. E., and Snell, E. E. (1968a). Biochemistry 7, 1616.
Ayling, J. E., and Snell, E. E. (1968b). Biochemistry 7, 1626.
Baranowski, T., Illingworth, B., Brown, D. H., and Cori, C. F. (1957). Biochim. Biophys. Acta 25, 16.
Bergeret, B., Chatagner, F., and Fromageot, C. (1955). Biochim. Biophys. Acta 17, 128.

Bergeret, B., Chatagner, F., and Fromageot, C. (1956). *Biochim. Biophys. Acta* **22**, 329.

Black, I. R., and Axelrod, J. (1969). *J. Biol. Chem.* **244**, 6124.

Boecker, E. A., and Snell, E. E. (1968). *J. Biol. Chem.* **243**, 1678.

Buell, M. V., and Hansen, R. E. (1960). *J. Amer. Chem. Soc.* **82**, 6042.

Cammarata, P. S., and Cohen, P. P. (1950). *J. Biol. Chem.* **187**, 439.

Canham, J. E., Baker, E. M., Harding, R. S., Sauberlich, H. E., and Plough, I. C. (1969). *Ann. N. Y. Acad. Sci.* **166**, Art. 1, 16.

Chatagner, F., and Durieu-Trautmann, O. (1965). *Nature (London)* **207**, 1390.

Chatagner, F., Tabechian, H., and Bergeret, B. (1954). *Biochim. Biophys. Acta* **13**, 313.

Chatagner, F., Durieu-Trautmann, O., and Rain, M. C. (1968a). *In* "Pyridoxal Catalysis, Enzymes and Model Systems" (E. E. Snell *et al.*, eds.), p. 693. Wiley (Interscience), New York.

Chatagner, F., Durieu-Trautmann, O., and Rain, M. C. (1968b). *Bull. Soc. Chim. Biol.* **50**, 129.

Chatagner, F., Van Heijenoort, Y., and Portemer, C. (1968c). *Nature (London)* **218**, 566.

Chatagner, F., Gicquel, Y., Portemer, C., and Tixier, M. (1970). *Experientia* **26**, 602.

Churchich, J. E., and Farrelly, J. G. (1969). *J. Biol. Chem.* **244**, 3685.

Cori, C. F., and Illingworth, B. (1957). *Proc. Nat. Acad. Sci. U.S.* **43**, 547.

Creighton, T. E., and Yanofsky, C. (1966). *J. Biol. Chem.* **241**, 980.

Davis, V. E. (1963). *Endocrinology* **72**, 33.

De Marco, C. (1957). *Biochim. Biophys. Acta* **25**, 634.

Denman, R. F., Hoare, D. S., and Work, E. (1955). *Biochim. Biophys. Acta* **16**, 442.

Dewey, D. E., Hoare, D. S., and Work, E. (1954). *Biochem. J.* **58**, 523.

Durieu-Trautmann, O., Rain, M. C., and Chatagner, F. (1964). *C. R. Acad. Sci.* **259**, 2547.

Eisenstein, A. B. (1962). *Biochim. Biophys. Acta* **58**, 244.

Fellman, J. H., Vanbellinghen, P. J., Jones, R. T., and Koler, D. D. (1969). *Biochemistry* **8**, 615.

Fischer, E. H., Forrey, A. W., Hedrick, J. L., Hughes, R. C., Kent, A. B., and Krebs, E. G. (1963). *In* "Chemical and Biological Aspects of Pyridoxal Catalysis" (E. E. Snell *et al.*, eds.), p. 543. Pergamon Press, Oxford.

Fischer, E. H., Pocker, A., Shaltiel, S., Hedrick, J. L., and Elsom, S. D. (1968). *In* "Symposium on Pyridoxal Enzymes" (K. Yamada, N. Katunuma, and H. Wada, eds.), p. 119. Maruzen, Tokyo.

Fujioka, M., and Snell, E. E. (1965). *J. Biol. Chem.* **240**, 3050.

Furbish, F. S., Fonda, M. L., and Metzler, D. E. (1969). *Biochemistry* **8**, 5169.

Gershoff, S. N. (1968). *In* "Pyridoxal Catalysis, Enzymes and Model Systems" (E. E. Snell *et al.*, eds.), p. 703. Wiley (Interscience), New York.

Greengard, O. (1963). *Advan. Enzyme Regulation* **1**, 161.

Greengard, O. (1964). *Advan. Enzyme Regulation* **2**, 277.

Greengard, O., and Gordon, M. (1963). *J. Biol. Chem.* **238**, 3708.

Gunsalus, I. C., Bellamy, W. D., and Umbreit, W. W. (1944). *J. Biol. Chem.* **155**, 685.

Hedrick, J. L., and Fischer, E. H. (1965). *Biochemistry* **4**, 1337.

Hedrick, J. L., Shaltiel, S., and Fischer, E. H. (1966). *Biochemistry* **5**, 2117.

Hedrick, J. L., Shaltiel, S., and Fischer, E. H. (1969). *Biochemistry* **8**, 2422.

Heyl, D., Harris, S. A., and Folkers, K. (1948). *J. Amer. Chem. Soc.* **70**, 3429.

Holten, D., Wicks, W. D., and Kenney, F. T. (1967). *J. Biol. Chem.* **242**, 1053.

Holzer, H., Boll, M., and Cennamo, C. (1963). *Angew. Chem.* **75**, 894.
Hope, D. B. (1955). *Biochem. J.* **59**, 497.
Hsu, J. M. (1963). *Vitam. Horm.* (*N. Y.*) **21**, 113.
Illingworth, B., Konfeld, R., and Brown, D. H. (1960). *Biochim. Biophys. Acta* **42**, 486.
Kent, A. B., Krebs, E. G., and Fischer, E. H. (1958). *J. Biol. Chem.* **232**, 549.
Khairallah, E. A., and Pitot, H. C. (1968). *In* "Symposium on Pyridoxal Enzymes" (K. Yamada, N. Katunuma, and H. Wada, eds.), p. 159. Maruzen, Tokyo.
Kolb, H., Cole, R. D., and Snell, E. E. (1968). *Biochemistry* **7**, 2946.
Levitan, I. B., and Webb, T. E. (1969). *J. Biol. Chem.* **244**, 4684.
Lin, E. C. C., Civen, M., and Knox, W. E. (1958). *J. Biol. Chem.* **233**, 1183.
Litwack, G., Sears-Gessel, M. L., and Winicov, I. (1966). *Biochim. Biophys. Acta* **118**, 351.
Luque, J., Cascales, M., and Santos-Ruiz, A. (1970). *Rev. Espan. Fisiol.* **26**, 135.
McCormick, D. B., Gregory, M. E., and Snell, E. E. (1961). *J. Biol. Chem.* **236**, 2076.
Meister, A. (1965). "Biochemistry of The Amino Acids," 2nd ed., Vols. 1 and 2, Academic Press, New York.
Morino, Y., and Snell, E. E. (1967a). *J. Biol. Chem.* **242**, 5591.
Morino, Y., and Snell, E. E. (1967b). *J. Biol. Chem.* **242**, 5602.
Novogrodsky, A., and Meister, A. (1964). *Biochim. Biophys. Acta* **85**, 170.
Phillips, A. T., Whanger, P. D., Rabinowitz, K. W., Shada, J. D., and Wood, W. A. (1968). *In* "Pyridoxal Catalysis, Enzymes and Model Systems" (E. E. Snell *et al.*, eds.), p. 549. Wiley (Interscience), New York.
Roberts, E., and Frankel, S. (1951). *J. Biol. Chem.* **188**, 789.
Rosen, F., and Milholland, R. J. (1960). *Fed. Proc., Fed. Amer. Soc. Exp. Biol.* **19**, 414.
Schimke, R. T., Sweeney, E. W., and Berlin, C. M. (1965). *J. Biol. Chem.* **240**, 4609.
Sevilla, C. L., and Fischer, E. H. (1969). *Biochemistry* **8**, 2161.
Shaltiel, S., Hedrick, J. L., and Fischer, E. H. (1966). *Biochemistry* **5**, 2108.
Shaltiel, S., Hedrick, J. L., and Fischer, E. H. (1969). *Biochemistry* **8**, 2429.
Shizuta, Y., Nakazawa, A., Tokushige, M., and Hayaishi, O. (1969). *J. Biol. Chem.* **244**, 1883.
Tate, S. S., and Meister, A. (1969a). *Biochemistry* **8**, 1056.
Tate, S. S., and Meister, A. (1969b). *Biochemistry* **8**, 1660.
Valeriotte, F. A., Aurrichio, F., Tomkins, G. M., and Riley, D. (1969). *J. Biol. Chem.* **244**, 3618.
Wada, H., and Morino, Y. (1964). *Vitam. Horm.* (*N. Y.*) **22**, 411.
Wada, H., and Snell, E. E. (1961). *J. Biol. Chem.* **236**, 2089.
Whanger, P. D., Phillips, A. T., Rabinowitz, K. W., Piperno, J. R., Shada, J. D., and Wood, W. A. (1968). *J. Biol. Chem.* **243**, 167.
Williams, M. A. (1964). *Vitam. Horm.* (*N. Y.*) **22**, 495.
Wilson-Miles, E., Novogrodsky, A., and Meister, A. (1968). *In* "Pyridoxal Catalysis, Enzymes and Model Systems" (E. E. Snell *et al.*, eds.), p. 425. Wiley (Interscience), New York.
Wiss, O., and Weber, F. (1964). *Vitam. Horm.* (*N. Y.*) **22**, 495.
Wooten, E., Nelson, M. M., Simpson, M. E., and Evans. H. M. (1958). *Endocrinology* **63**, 860.

Effect of Conformation on the Binding of Flavins to Flavoenzymes

K. V. RAJAGOPALAN, F. O. BRADY,* AND M. KANDA

*Department of Biochemistry, Duke University Medical Center,
Durham, North Carolina*

I. INTRODUCTION

The interaction of flavin adenine dinucleotide (FAD) and flavin mononucleotide (FMN) with specific proteins confers a great degree of versatility to these coenzymes as evidenced by the wide variety of reactions catalyzed by flavoproteins. An examination of the detailed tabulation of flavoproteins compiled by Palmer and Massey (1968) reveals the diversity of reactions catalyzed by these enzymes. A large number of flavoproteins effect the transfer of electrons between a donor and an acceptor; displaying considerable specificity for the former and much less for the latter. A smaller group of flavoenzymes serve as mixed function oxygenases. In addition, FAD and FMN are also members of multicomponent electron transfer systems such as those present in the metalloflavoproteins (Rajagopalan and Handler, 1968) and respiratory chain-linked dehydrogenases (Singer, 1968). The functional diversity of these enzymes must to a large extent reside in the interactions between the flavocoenzyme and the protein matrices. It may therefore be profitable to focus attention on those aspects of flavoproteins which bear on such interactions.

II. NATURE OF BINDING

The flavin moieties of most flavoproteins are released in solution on denaturation of the proteins by acid or heat. The noncovalent interactions which are involved in linking the flavin to the protein are in many cases strong enough to keep the holoenzymes intact under a variety of moderately harsh treatments. A notable exception is D-amino acid oxidase from pig kidney, which loses its flavin on dilution and requires extraneously added FAD for maintaining linear rates of activity.

Several techniques have been used for the preparation of apoproteins

* Present address: Institute for Cancer Research, Columbia University Medical Center, New York, New York.

TABLE I

PREPARATION AND PROPERTIES OF APOFLAVOPROTEINS

Enzyme	Method of resolution	Extent of reconstitution (%)	Reference
Old yellow enzyme	Acid ammonium sulfate precipitation	70–80	Theorall and Nygaard (1954)
D-Amino acid oxidase	Acid ammonium sulfate precipitation	60–80	Massey and Curti (1966)
D-Amino acid oxidase	Dialysis vs KBr	93–100	Massey and Curti (1966)
NADH-cytochrome b_5 reductase	Acid ammonium sulfate precipitation	75–90	Strittmatter (1961)
NADH-cytochrome b_5 reductase	Acid charcoal treatment	90–97	Strittmatter (1968)
Lipoyl dehydrogenase	Acid ammonium sulfate precipitation	Temperature dependent	Veeger (1968)

from flavoproteins. Results obtained with some of the enzymes are summarized in Table I. The method of choice has been acid ammonium sulfate precipitation of the apoproteins as applied by Strittmatter (1961) for the preparation of apocytochrome b_5 reductase.

III. EFFECT ON FLAVIN ABSORPTION SPECTRUM

The absorption spectrum of flavin is modified to varying degrees in different flavoproteins. Palmer and Massey (1968) have classified two main categories of flavoprotein absorption spectra, as the "resolved" and "unresolved" types. The unresolved spectra are similar in shape to that of the free FAD in water, and the resolved spectra are characterized by pronounced shoulders in the regions of 430 and 470 nm. Figure 1 shows the spectra of D-amino acid oxidase and of NADH-cytochrome b_5 reductase as representative samples of the two classes of spectra. The unresolved type has been characterized as hydrophilic and the resolved type as hydrophobic on the basis of studies with model flavins in different solvents (Harbury et al., 1959).

The addition of benzoate, a competitive inhibitor, to a solution of D-amino acid oxidase transforms the flavin spectrum to the resolved type, suggesting that the binding of benzoate to the enzyme causes a conformational change involving the transfer of the flavin from a polar to a nonpolar region (Yagi and Ozawa, 1962). Palmer and Massey (1968) have interpreted the spectral changes as being the result of the abolition by benzoate of a hydrogen bond between a charged amino group in the pro-

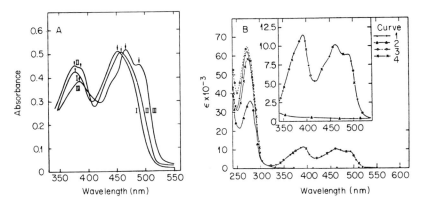

Fɪɢ. 1. (A) Absorption spectra of FAD (I), ᴅ-amino acid oxidase (II); and ᴅ-amino acid oxidase and benzoate (III). (Yagi *et al.*, 1968). (B) Absorption spectra: curve *1*, native NADH-cytochrome b_5 reductase; curve *2*, aporeductase; curve *3*, aporeductase plus 1 equivalent of FAD; curve *4*, aporeductase plus 1 equivalent of FMN (Strittmatter, 1961).

tein and a carbonyl group in the isoalloxazine nucleus of the FAD, followed by the sequestration of the FAD in a nonpolar region.

Similar modifications of flavin spectra, in the presence of substrates or inhibitors, have been observed in other systems, including metalloflavoproteins, such as succinic dehydrogenase (Dervartanian and Veeger, 1964) dihydroorotic dehydrogenase (Aleman and Handler, 1967) and avian xanthine dehydrogenase (Rajagopalan and Handler, 1967).

IV. Pʀᴏᴘᴇʀᴛɪᴇs ᴏꜰ Aᴘᴏꜰʟᴀᴠᴏᴘʀᴏᴛᴇɪɴs

In general it would appear that apoflavoproteins, irrespective of the method of preparation, are less stable than the corresponding holoenzymes. In many cases incomplete reconstitution is observed on addition of flavin to the apoenzyme. In the case of ᴅ-amino acid oxidase (Massey and Curti, 1966) and lipoyl dehydrogenase (Veeger, 1968), formation of catalytically active holoenzyme from apoenzyme and FAD has been reported to require a conformational change of the initially formed apoprotein-FAD complex. Multiple, conformationally distinct species of intermediates have been detected by Strittmatter (1968) in the reconstitution of NADH-cytochrome b_5 reductase from its apoprotein and FAD.

V. Mᴇᴛᴀʟʟᴏꜰʟᴀᴠᴏᴘʀᴏᴛᴇɪɴs

In the case of simple flavoproteins, a functional role for the flavin in catalysis is tacitly assumed and can be substantiated by preparation of inactive apoprotein and subsequent reactivation on adding the coenzyme.

TABLE II

PROPERTIES OF METALLOFLAVOPROTEINS

Enzyme	Source	Molecular weight	Cofactor content	Phyiological electron acceptor
Xanthine oxidase	Milk	280,000	2 Mo, 2 FAD, 8 Fe–S	O_2
Xanthine dehydrogenase	Chicken liver	280,000	2 Mo, 2 FAD, 8 Fe–S	NAD^+
Xanthine dehydrogenase	Micrococcus lactilyticus	280,000	2 Mo, 2 FAD, 8 Fe–S	Ferredoxin
Aldehyde oxidase	Rabbit liver	280,000	2 Mo, 2 FAD, 8 Fe–S	O_2
Dihydroorotic dehydrogenase	Zymobacterium oroticum	120,000	2 FAD, 2 FMN, 4 Fe–S	NAD^+

Metalloflavoproteins of the xanthine oxidase family present complexities of a larger magnitude since they contain multiple electron carriers as shown in Table II. Nonheme iron of the type present in spinach ferredoxin is a component of all the enzymes listed while molybdenum is additionally present in all except dihydroorotic dehydrogenase. All contain FAD, and FMN is also present in dihydroorotic dehydrogenase. It is of interest that the three xanthine-oxidizing enzymes have identical cofactor content but display independent and mutually exclusive electron acceptor specificity in terms of their physiological activity. All the enzymes listed are capable of transferring electrons to a wide variety of artificial electron acceptors.

Studies on the differential inhibition of electron transfer to diverse acceptors by hepatic aldehyde oxidase (Rajagopalan and Handler, 1964b) strongly suggested the presence of a multicomponent internal electron transport chain in the enzyme, and by inference, in related enzymes as well. It is also known that the absorption spectra of these enzymes in the region 400–700 nm is nearly completely due to flavin and nonheme iron (Rajagopalan and Handler, 1964a). While it has not been possible to resolve and reconstitute these enzymes in regard to their metal components, recently reconstitutively active deflavoenzymes have been obtained from them by different techniques (Komai *et al.*, 1969; Brady *et al.*, 1970; Uozumi *et al.*, quoted in Orme-Johnson and Beinert, 1969). These studies have great relevence to the sequence of internal electron transport chains in these enzymes, and at the same time provide strong evidence for the occurrence of conformational changes when they cycle between the oxidized and the reduced states.

In the course of studies on the macromolecular organization of chicken liver xanthine dehydrogenase, it was observed that a number of protein denaturants, especially certain monovalent anions, inactivated the enzyme with respect to its ability to transfer electrons from xanthine to NAD$^+$, while having no effect on the efficiency of electron transfer to DCIP. The results observed with iodide are seen in Fig. 2. The effect of iodide concentration on the inactivation process is shown in Fig. 3. From experiments similar to those in Fig. 3, the time required for 50% inactivation at different concentrations of several protein denaturants was determined and is graphically represented in Fig. 4. These relationships take the shape of "melting" curves, the midpoints of which occur at different concentrations for the diverse salts. The relative efficiencies of the anions in this regard follow the well established Hofmeister series. The enzyme is surprisingly stable in 6.5 M urea for several hours. Quite similar patterns were obtained with milk xanthine oxidase and hepatic aldehyde oxidase.

In all cases thiocyanate and iodide were the most effective of the anions

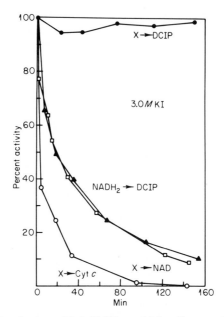

Fig. 2. Effect of incubation with 3 M KI on chicken liver xanthine dehydrogenase. KI concentration in the assay mixture was 0.01 M. Activities are expressed as percentage of control activities measured in the presence of 0.01 M KI. Xanthine → cytochrome c activity represents an increase over control, rather than a decrease.

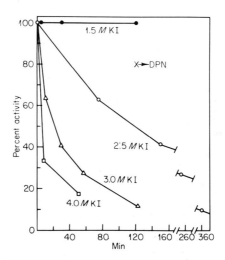

Fig. 3. Effect of KI concentration on the inactivation of xanthine → NAD activity of xanthine dehydrogenase.

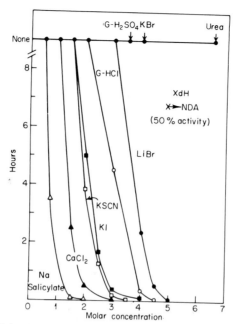

FIG. 4. Relative efficiencies of protein denaturants in effecting 50% inactivation of xanthine → NAD⁺ activity of xanthine dehydrogenase. G·HCl and G·H₂SO₄ are guanidine hydrochloride and guanidine sulfate, respectively.

tried, and were about equally so. These effects were apparently not the result of general protein denaturation, since the ability of xanthine oxidase or xanthine dehydrogenase to transfer electrons to DCIP was not decreased under conditions where the overall activities were completely abolished. Since these treatments did not abolish the visible absorption of the nonheme iron complex, it was considered likely that the flavin moiety of these enzymes was being labilized. Accordingly, xanthine dehydrogenase was incubated with 3 M KI for 16 hours and dialyzed against 0.5 M KI for 3–4 hours. The absorption spectrum of the resultant preparation, shown in Fig. 5, was typical of flavin-free nonheme iron protein (Rajagopalan and Handler, 1964a) and showed that treatment with iodide had indeed resolved the enzyme from its flavin component. Similar flavin-free preparations were also obtained from milk xanthine oxidase and aldehyde oxidase.

The rates of deflavination of milk xanthine oxidase and chicken liver xanthine dehydrogenase by thiocyanate, iodide, and Ca²⁺ at different temperatures was determined, and the results were fitted to an Arrhenius plot, shown in Fig. 6. It is seen that the slopes of the lines for the three

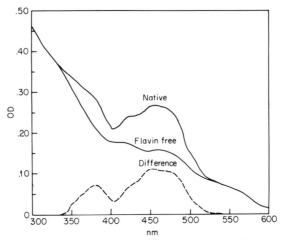

FIG. 5. Absorption spectra of native and flavin-free xanthine dehydrogenase

reagents are quantitatively very similar, indicating that an identical process was involved in all cases. The energy of activation for deflavination can be calculated from these data, and is in the region of 9000–10,000 cal/mole. This is much smaller than the enthalpy of protein denaturation, and is similar in magnitude to the energy of a hydrogen bond in water and in proteins. Thus it would appear that the deflavination process involves rupture of one or two hydrogen bonds between the FAD and the proteins with resultant tendency for the flavin to be completely freed

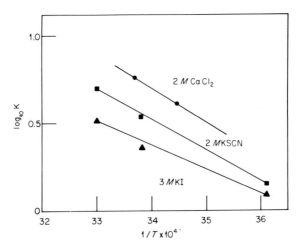

FIG. 6. Arrhenius plots of the temperature dependence of deflavination of xanthine oxidase by KI, KSCN, and CaCl₂.

from its interaction with the protein. It may be mentioned that Theorell and Nygaard (1954) calculated the energy of activation for the deflavination of old yellow enzyme to be about 24,000 cal/mole while Massey and Curti (1966) reported that the deflavination of D-amino acid involves about 20,000 cal/mole. The reconstitution of lipoyl dehydrogenase from apoprotein and FAD has been found to require 8000 cal/mole (Veeger, 1968).

Although the energy of activation for the deflavination process was low, it required prolonged incubation with the denaturating salt, with the result that the final preparation was rather unstable and had a tendency to aggregate and become insoluble. The reconstitution with FAD was never complete, indicating partial denaturation of the protein. In a search for less rigorous conditions of treatment, the effect of iodide on chicken liver xanthine dehydrogenase previously reduced with xanthine was examined. The results, presented in Fig. 7, show that $3\,M$ KI almost instantaneously deflavinates the enzyme, in contrast to 12–16 hours required for complete deflavination of native, oxidized enzyme. The effects of lower concentrations of KI on the reduced enzyme were then examined.

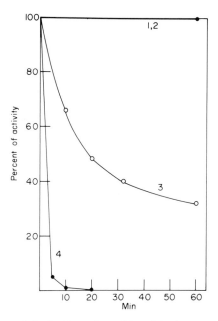

FIG. 7. Effect of KI on deflavination of xanthine dehydrogenase prereduced with xanthine. Curves *1* and *2*, xanthine → DCIP activities of native and reduced XDH respectively; curves *3* and *4*, xanthine → NAD⁺ activities of native and prereduced XDH, respectively.

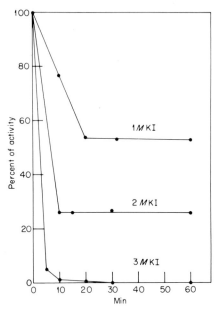

Fɪɢ. 8. Effect of KI concentration on deflavination of XDH prereduced with xanthine.

Figure 8 shows that the deflavination of reduced enzyme by KI is an equilibrium process, in that the final extent of the process was dependent on iodide concentrations and occurred immediately on exposure to the salt and remained constant thereafter. Accordingly, dialysis of xanthine dehydrogenase against 1 M KI in the presence of xanthine resulted in total deflavination in 3 hours. The deflavoenzyme obtained by this treatment was much more stable than the one described earlier, and also yielded considerably higher reconstitution on treatment with FAD. When milk xanthine oxidase was reduced anaerobically with xanthine and then treated with KI anaerobically, it too underwent an enhanced rate of deflavination, again yielding a more stable flavin free product.

These findings suggest that the reduction of metalloflavoproteins by substrate results in a conformational change such that the flavin moiety is less strongly attached to the protein, and is readily removed by treatment with comparatively low concentrations of anions. Similar differences in conformation have been reported for ferri- and ferrocytochrome c (Margoliash and Schejter, 1966). Massey and co-workers (1962) found that while oxidized lipoyl dehydrogenase was stable in 6 M urea for several hours, enzyme reduced with NADH was rapidly inactivated under the same conditions. Thus it would seem that changes in the redox state are associated with changes in conformation in many of the flavo- and metalloflavoproteins.

The catalytic activities of flavin-free xanthine dehydrogenase are compared with those of native enzyme in Table III. Noteworthy is the enhanced ability of the flavin-free enzyme to transfer electrons to nitroblue tetrazolium and cytochrome c. When the holoenzyme is reconstituted from the apoprotein and FAD, these activities return to their normal levels. It would seem that the flavin-free enzyme exists in a conformation in which interaction with nitroblue tetrazolium and cytochrome c is possible and that the addition of FAD alters the conformation wherein there is much less interaction with those acceptors. Exactly similar findings have been made with milk xanthine oxidase.

These results may be considered in the general context of the nature of binding of flavins to flavoproteins. It is reasonable to assume that the flavin moiety is accommodated in a crevice which is largely nonpolar in many instances. Kierkagaard and co-workers (1969) have shown that flavoquinones have a planar configuration while in flavohydroquinones the isoalloxazine ring has a "butterfly" structure. It might then be speculated that conversion of a flavoquinone to flavohydroquinone will force a widening of the crevice, such that the forces of interaction between the protein and the flavin are lessened, with perhaps increased interaction of the flavin with the polar aqueous medium. Under these conditions it is

TABLE III

Ratios of Activity of Flavin-free XdH to Activity of Native XdH, Using Xanthine (0.15 mM) as Substrate and the Indicated Electron Acceptors[a]

Electron acceptor	Activity of deflavoenzyme
	Activity of native enzyme
O$_2$	0
DPN	0
DCIP	1.00
MB	1.18
TNBS	1.02
PMS	1.20
K$_3$Fe(CN)$_6$	40
NBT	40
Cytochrome c	40

[a] Abbreviations: DCIP, dichlorophenolindophenol; MB, methylene blue; TNBS, trinitrobenzene sulfonic acid; PMS, phenazine methosulfate; NBT, nitroblue tetrazolium.

conceivable that the presence of denaturants results in rapid loosening of the flavin from the protein as seen in the experiments described here.

ACKNOWLEDGMENTS

This work was made possible by the kind interest and encouragement of Professor Philip Handler, and was supported by Public Health Service Grant GM-0091. The expert technical assistance of Mr. Ralph Wiley is also acknowledged.

REFERENCES

Aleman, V., and Handler, P. (1967). *J. Biol. Chem.* **242**, 4087.

Brady, F. O., Rajagopalan, K. V., and Handler, P. (1970). *In* "Flavins and Flavoproteins" (H. Kamin, ed.). University Park Press, Baltimore, Maryland (in press).

Dervartanian, D. V., and Veeger, C. (1964). *Biochim. Biophys. Acta* **92**, 233.

Harbury, H. A., LaNoue, K. F., Loach, P. A., and Amick, R. M. (1969). *Proc. Nat. Acad. Sci. U. S.* **45**, 1708.

Kierkagaard, P., Norrestam, R., Werner, P.-E., Csöregh, I., von Glehn, M., Karlsson, R., Leijonmarck, M., Rönnquist, O., Stensland, B., Tillberg, O., and Torbjörnsson, L. (1969). *In* "Flavins and Flavoproteins" (H. Kamin, ed.). University Park Press, Baltimore, Maryland (in press).

Komai, H., Massey, V., and Palmer, G. (1969). *J. Biol. Chem.* **244**, 1692.

Margoliash, E., and Schejter, A. (1966). *Advan. Protein Chem.* **21**, 113.

Massey, V., and Curti, B. (1966). *J. Biol. Chem.* **241**, 3417.

Massey, V., Hofmann, T., and Palmer, G. (1962). *J. Biol. Chem.* **237**, 3820.

Orme-Johnson, W. H., and Beinert, H. (1969). *Biochem. Biophys. Res. Commun.* **36**, 905.

Palmer, G., and Massey, V. (1968). *In* "Biological Oxidations" (T. P. Singer, ed.), p. 263. Wiley (Interscience), New York.

Rajagopalan, K. V., and Handler, P. (1964a). *J. Biol. Chem.* **239**, 1509.

Rajagopalan, K. V., and Handler, P. (1964b). *J. Biol. Chem.* **239**, 2022.

Rajagopalan, K. V., and Handler, P. (1967). *J. Biol. Chem.* **242**, 4097.

Rajagopalan, K. V., and Handler, P. (1968). *In* "Biological Oxidations" (T. P. Singer, ed.), p. 301. Wiley (Interscience), New York.

Singer, T. P. (1968). *In* "Biological Oxidations" (T. P. Singer, ed.), p. 339. Wiley (Interscience), New York.

Strittmatter, P. (1961). *J. Biol. Chem.* **236**, 2329.

Strittmatter, P., (1968). *In* "Flavins and Flavoproteins" (K. Yagi, ed.), p. 85. University Park Press, Baltimore, Maryland.

Theorell, H., and Nygaard, A. P. (1954). *Acta Chem. Scand.* **8**, 1649.

Veeger, C. (1968). *In* "Flavins and Flavoproteins" (K. Yagi, ed.), p. 252. University Park Press, Baltimore, Maryland.

Yagi, K., and Ozawa, T. (1962). *Biochim. Biophys. Acta* **56**, 413.

Yagi, K., Ozawa, T., Naoi, M., and Kotaki, A. (1968). *In* "Flavins and Flavoproteins" (K. Yagi, ed.), p. 237. University Park Press, Baltimore, Maryland.

The Binding of NAD$^+$ and NADH to Glyceraldehydephosphate Dehydrogenase

E. C. SLATER, J. J. M. DE VIJLDER, AND W. BOERS

Laboratory of Biochemistry, B.C.P. Jansen Institute, University of Amsterdam, Amsterdam, The Netherlands

I. Introduction

Glyceraldehydephosphate dehydrogenase [D-glyceraldehyde-3-phosphate:NAD$^+$ oxidoreductase (phosphorylating), EC 1.2.1.12] catalyzes the reaction given in Eq. (1).

$$R \cdot CHO + NAD^+ + P_i \rightleftharpoons R \cdot COO \sim P + NADH + H^+ \tag{1}$$

The physiological substrate is D-glyceraldehyde 3-phosphate, but the enzyme reacts also with other aldehydes (glyceraldehyde, acetaldehyde, and propionaldehyde), although much more slowly. Arsenate can replace phosphate (Needham and Pillai, 1937). In this case the product, an acyl arsenate, hydrolyzes spontaneously so that the sum reaction is

$$R \cdot CHO + NAD^+ + OH^- \rightarrow R \cdot COOH + NADH \tag{2}$$

Early studies of its mechanism of action were carried out with enzyme crystallized from yeast (Warburg and Christian, 1939) and rabbit muscle (Cori *et al.*, 1948). More recently, the enzyme isolated from lobster-tail muscle has been used, since the crystals obtained from this source are more suitable for structure determinations by X-ray analysis (Watson and Banaszak, 1964). Only minor differences in properties between the two muscle enzymes have been observed, but the yeast enzyme differs considerably from these two.

In all three cases, the enzyme is a tetramer (Harris and Perham, 1965; Harrington and Karr, 1965), composed of four identical subunits each containing 331–333 amino acids. The amino acid sequence is known for the lobster-muscle and pig-muscle enzymes (Harris and Perham, 1968).

X-ray analysis has revealed that the lobster-muscle enzyme has at least one 2-fold axis of symmetry (Watson and Banaszak, 1964).

II. Muscle Enzymes

A. Binding of NAD⁺

It was already clear from the early studies that the rabbit-muscle enzyme binds NAD⁺ much more firmly than other dehydrogenases, since the crystalline enzyme contains bound NAD⁺ (Taylor et al., 1948). However, it does not bind NAD⁺ as firmly as activated charcoal, which completely removes NAD⁺ from the enzyme (Velick, 1953).

It was early recognized that glyceraldehydephosphate dehydrogenase is the site of the inhibitory action of iodoacetate on glycolysis (Lundsgaard, 1930), and a cysteine side chain was implicated in this inhibition. Although each subunit contains from 2 (yeast) (Harris and Perham, 1963) to 5 (lobster) (Davidson et al., 1967) cysteine residues, only one of these in the native enzyme reacts with iodoacetate, and the rate of this reaction is increased by NAD⁺ (Racker and Krimsky, 1952a). Interestingly, the addition of one molecule of NAD⁺ per tetramer is sufficient maximally to activate the single cysteine residue in all four subunits (Conway and Koshland, 1968). When the enzyme is denatured by urea, all the thiol groups react with iodoacetic acid (Harris and Perham, 1965).

Binding of NAD⁺ to charcoal-treated enzyme causes the appearance of a broad absorption band with maximum at 360 nm, and the formation of the band is inhibited by iodoacetate or acetyl phosphate (Racker and Krimsky, 1952a,b; Velick, 1953). Since acetyl phosphate acetylates the same thiol group as iodoacetate, it is clear that this group is concerned, either directly or indirectly, with the formation of the 360-nm band. Indeed, it was thought at one time that a covalent bond is formed between a carbon atom in the nicotinamide ring and the sulfur atom (Eq. 3) and that this bond is split by "aldehydolysis" with the formation of a thiol ester (Eq. 4), followed finally by phosphorolysis (or arsenolysis) of the thiol ester (Eq. 5) (Racker and Krimsky, 1952a,b).

$$\text{E—SH} + \text{NAD}^+ \rightleftharpoons \text{E—S—NAD} + \text{H}^+ \tag{3}$$
$$\text{E—S—NAD} + \text{R·CHO} \rightleftharpoons \text{E—S—CO·R} + \text{NADH} \tag{4}$$
$$\text{E—S—CO·R} + \text{P}_i \rightleftharpoons \text{E—SH} + \text{R·COO}P \tag{5}$$

$$\textit{Sum:} \quad \text{R·CHO} + \text{NAD}^+ + \text{P}_i \rightleftharpoons \text{R·COO}P + \text{NADH} \tag{1}$$

The suggestion that an acylated enzyme—a thiol ester—is an intermediate in the enzyme reaction is now well established (Krimsky and Racker, 1955; Koeppe et al., 1956). It appears unlikely, however, that it is formed by "aldehydolysis" of a carbon-sulfur bond. Kosower (1956) pointed out that the 360-nm band has the characteristics of a charge-transfer complex between an electron donor in the enzyme and the pyridine ring. The electron donor is probably the active thiol group, although the indole group of tryptophan has also been suggested (Cilento and Tedeschi, 1961; see also Boross and Cseke, 1966).

The binding constants of NAD⁺ to each of the four subunits in the muscle enzymes have been determined by Conway and Koshland (1968) by equilibrium dialysis, and by De Vijlder and Slater (1968) and De Vijlder *et al.* (1969a), using both ultracentrifugation and equilibrium dialysis to separate free NAD⁺ from that bound to the enzyme. Figure 1 shows the results, given as a Scatchard plot, of the measurements with the lobster enzyme. The curved line, convex to the abscissa, shows that the binding constants become successively less as more NAD⁺ becomes bound to the enzyme, i.e., there is negative cooperativity. The inset shows that a straight-line Scatchard plot is obtained when the binding of the fourth molecule is plotted on the assumption that the first three sites are completely occupied before NAD⁺ is bound to the fourth site. Table I summarizes all the results obtained with the rabbit, lobster, and yeast enzymes. Velick *et al.* (1970) have shown that the binding constants of

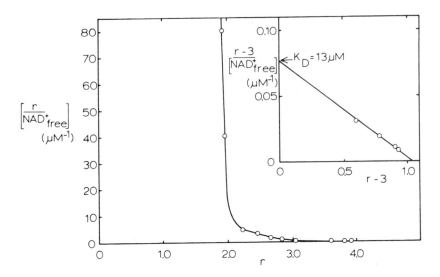

Fig. 1. Scatchard plot of binding of NAD⁺ to lobster-muscle enzyme, measured by equilibrium dialysis at 4°C. *Inset:* Scatchard plot of fourth molecule, calculated on the assumption that the first three sites are completely occupied before NAD⁺ is bound to the fourth site. $r =$ number of molecules NAD⁺ bound per molecule enzyme.

TABLE I

DISSOCIATION CONSTANTS OF NAD[+] BOUND TO GLYCERALDEHYDEPHOSPHATE DEHYDROGENASE

Reaction	Dissociation constants (M)			
	Rabbit		Lobster[d] (dialysis[f])	Yeast[e] (dialysis[f])
	Ultracentrifugation[a,b]	Dialysis[c,f]		
E + NAD[+] ⇌ E-NAD	$<5 \times 10^{-8}$	$<10^{-11}$	$<5 \times 10^{-9}$	5.5×10^{-5}
E-NAD + NAD[+] ⇌ E-(NAD)$_2$	$<5 \times 10^{-8}$	$<10^{-9}$	$<5 \times 10^{-9}$	4.6×10^{-6}
E-(NAD)$_2$ + NAD[+] ⇌ E-(NAD)$_3$	4×10^{-6}	3×10^{-7}	6×10^{-7}	4.2×10^{-5}
E-(NAD)$_3$ + NAD[+] ⇌ E-(NAD)$_4$	3.5×10^{-5}	2.6×10^{-5}	1.3×10^{-5}	1.1×10^{-3}

[a] De Vijlder and Slater (1968).
[b] At 20–25°C.
[c] Conway and Koshland (1968).
[d] De Vijlder et al. (1969a).
[e] Koshland et al. (1970).
[f] At 4°C.

the first two molecules of NAD$^+$ with the rabbit-muscle enzyme, measured by the quenching by added NAD$^+$ of the fluorescence of the apoprotein, decrease with increasing temperature, while that of the third is little temperature dependent. The net result is that the differences between the first three molecules disappear at 36°.

De Vijlder and Slater (1967, 1968) and De Vijlder et al. (1969a) showed that only the first three molecules of NAD$^+$ bound to the enzyme contribute to the 360-nm band. This is illustrated for the lobster-muscle enzyme in Fig. 2. The first two molecules of NAD$^+$ are stoichiometrically bound to the enzyme and bring about an equal increase in $A_{360\ nm}$. The departure from the straight line after 2 molecules of NAD$^+$ are added (Fig. 2A) is due to the fact that the third molecule dissociates from the complex with a significant dissociation constant. When $A_{360\ nm}$ is plotted against enzyme-bound NAD, calculated from that added and the value of $6 \times 10^{-7} M$ for the dissociation constant of the third molecule (see Table I), it may be seen that this molecule of NAD$^+$ contributes to the 360-nm band to the same extent as the first two (Fig. 2B). The fourth molecule, on the other hand, contributes little, if anything, to this band. The slightly higher values of $A_{360\ nm}$ obtained with a large excess of NAD$^+$ is probably due to contact charge-transfer interaction (Kosower, 1960).

The 360-nm band is optically active, giving a very broad positive circular dichroism band, centered at 350 nm, with a molecular elipticity of 18,000 per mole of enzyme (De Vijlder and Harmsen, 1969). When changes in the molecular elipticity at 350 nm of the Moffit-Yang parameter b_0 are plotted against the amount of NAD$^+$ added to the enzyme, curves similar to those of Fig. 2 are obtained (De Vijlder and Harmsen, 1969). Thus, each of the first three molecules of NAD$^+$ bound to the enzyme contribute equally to the circular dichroism, and the fourth molecule does not. All the effects of NAD$^+$ addition on the circular dichroism spectrum occur in the region where NAD$^+$ itself gives positive bands, and no changes are observed on the positive circular dichroism band at 299 nm, given by the apoenzyme. The changes observed may thus be ascribed to extrinsic effects of the NAD$^+$ and do not reflect overall changes in the protein conformation.

The fourth molecule also differs from the other three in having no effect on the fluorescence of the protein (the first three molecules quench the fluorescence of tryptophan in the molecule; Velick, 1958; Velick et al., 1970) and differs from the third in having no effect on the viscosity of a solution of the protein (the third molecule increases the viscosity; Conway and Koshland, 1968). Of particular interest is the finding of Velick et al. (1970) that binding of the first three molecules of NAD$^+$ to the rabbit-muscle enzyme is an exothermic reaction, and that ΔH is the same

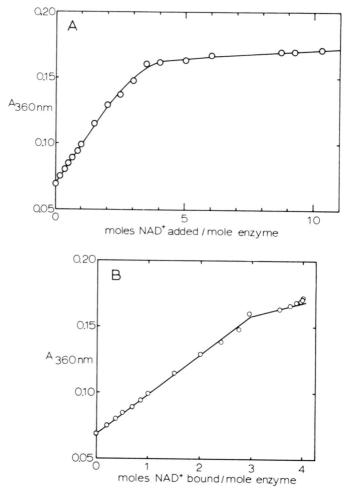

Fig. 2. Titration at 360 nm with NAD⁺ of charcoal-treated glyceraldehydephos-phate dehydrogenase (28.3 μM) isolated from lobster muscle. The enzyme was dis-solved in 100 mM Tris-HCl buffer (pH 8.2) containing 5 mM EDTA. Temperature, 23°C. (A) $A_{360\ nm}$ as a function of added NAD⁺; (B) $A_{360\ nm}$ as a function of bound NAD⁺.

for all three reactions (16 kcal/mole), whereas it is zero for the fourth molecule. From these data and the values for ΔG_0 calculated from the binding of NAD⁺ to the enzyme, the change of entropy may be calculated for each of the four reactions. For this calculation, Velick *et al.* (1970) used binding constants for the first three molecules calculated from the effect of NAD⁺ at 25° on the protein fluorescence, assuming that each molecule of NAD⁺ has the identical effect. These values $(1.7 \times 10^{-7} M,$ $3.4 \times 10^{-7} M$ and $1.9 \times 10^{-6} M)$ differ somewhat from those found by ultracentrifugation or equilibrium dialysis (Table I). The value used for the binding constant for the fourth molecule was that reported by De Vijlder and Slater (1968) by ultracentrifugation.

In several respects, then, the binding of NAD⁺ to the fourth subunit differs from that to the first three. The first molecule also differs in some respects from the second and third. This was shown by De Vijlder and Slater (1967, 1968) with the rabbit enzyme for the rate of reaction between the enzyme and NAD⁺, as followed in the stopped-flow apparatus by the rate of increase of $A_{360\ nm}$. With less than 1 mole of NAD⁺ per mole of enzyme, an almost maximal increase of the absorbance is reached in 3–5 msec, the mixing time of the instrument. On addition of more than 1 mole of NAD⁺, rapid and slow phases are observed. If the enzyme was previously treated with 1 mole of NAD⁺ per mole of enzyme, the slow phase on reaction with an additional 1 mole NAD⁺ was more rapid than when 2 moles of NAD⁺ were added to NAD⁺-free enzyme. This may indicate that the first NAD⁺ molecule prepares the binding site for the second molecule. Similarly, the third molecule was bound more rapidly to enzyme already containing two molecules. Strangely, the lobster enzyme differs in this respect from the rabbit muscle. Even at 10°, with amounts of NAD⁺ between 0.7 and 9.4 moles of NAD⁺ per mole of enzyme, the absorbance change was completed within 3–5 msec of mixing the enzyme with the NAD⁺ (De Vijlder et al., 1969a). This corresponds to a second-order rate constant of more than $10^{10} M^{-1}sec^{-1}$. These experiments give, of course, no information on the rate of binding of the fourth molecule.

The first molecule of NAD⁺ also activates the reactive —SH group in all four subunits (Conway and Koshland, 1968). The activation involves a lowering of the pK so that, at neutral pH, these groups become ionized (Stockell, 1959).

Finally, as already mentioned, the third molecule differs from the first two in having a lower binding constant at lower temperatures (Conway and Koshland, 1968; De Vijlder and Slater, 1968; De Vijlder et al., 1969a) and in the effect of temperature on this binding constant. Thus, differences have been detected at all four binding sites. At physiological temperatures for the rabbit, however, the differences between the fourth site and the other three are quantitatively much more important.

It is clear that binding of NAD⁺ to one subunit invokes asymmetric conformation changes in other subunits. This is not easily explained on the basis of the limiting model for allostery worked out in detail by Monod et al. (1965) and would seem to require a sequential model of the type proposed by Conway and Koshland (1968). Indeed, it seems necessary to invoke four conformations of subunits in order to explain the results, *viz*.

(i) R, in which the —SH group in the active center is not activated (high pK).

(ii) S, in which this —SH group is activated (low pK).

(iii) T, a variant of S in which the conformation is changed in such a way that the subunit can combine with NAD⁺.

(iv) U, a variant of T, induced by combination with NAD⁺, in which the —S⁻ group is favorably placed with respect to the pyridine ring so that a charge-transfer complex may be formed.

The four reactions may then be written, for the rabbit-muscle enzyme

		ΔG_0 (kcal/mole)	ΔH (kcal/mole)	ΔS_0 (entropy unit)
(a)	$R_4 + N \rightleftharpoons S_2 \cdot T \cdot UN$	−9	−16	−23
(b)	$S_2 \cdot T \cdot UN + N \rightleftharpoons S \cdot T \cdot (UN)_2$	−9	−16	−24
(c)	$S \cdot T \cdot (UN)_2 + N \rightleftharpoons T \cdot (UN)_3$	−8	−16	−27
(d)	$T \cdot (UN)_3 + N \rightleftharpoons TN \cdot (UN)_3$	−6	0	+21

On the basis of this formulation we may draw the following conclusions:

1. The binding of NAD⁺ to T, the conformation ready to receive it (Reaction d), is entropy driven, perhaps as the result of hydrophobic interactions between the protein and the NAD⁺ molecule (Velick *et al.*, 1970).

2. The NAD-induced conformation change S → T → U (Reactions b and c) are strongly exothermic.

3. Since, although Reaction a includes the conformation changes 4 R → 4 S and S → T in addition to the S → T → U also involved in Reactions b and c, the thermodynamic parameters are similar to those for Reactions b and c, it may be concluded that the strongly exothermic conformation change is T → U.

In summary, the binding of NAD⁺ to the muscle enzyme is dominated thermodynamically by an entropy-driven binding reaction, followed by a strongly exothermic conformation change in three of the subunits. The formation of the charge-transfer complex can contribute to only a minor extent to this conformation change, since the —ΔG_0 for the formation of such complexes is usually only about 2–3 kcal/mole (Kosower, 1966).

NAD⁺ is also necessary for the reduction of acyl phosphate by NADH, catalyzed by the enzyme (the reverse of Eq. 1) (Hilvers and Weenen, 1962; Hilvers *et al.*, 1964; De Vijlder *et al.*, 1969b). and for transfer reactions catalyzed by the enzyme, such as arsenolysis of acyl phosphate (Harting and Velick, 1954). Maximal activity is found with 3 moles of

NAD$^+$ bound to the enzyme, indicating that the conformation T$\cdot$(UN)$_3$ is the catalytically active form in these reactions. NAD$^+$ in excess of 3 moles per mole of enzyme inhibits the oxidation of NADH by acyl phosphate, competitive with respect to NADH. The inhibition constant, 45 μM, is close to the dissociation constant of the fourth site (35 μM). Thus, we may write

$$T\cdot(UN)_3 + NADH \rightleftharpoons T\text{-}NADH\cdot(UN)_3 \qquad (6)$$
$$T\cdot(UN)_3 + NAD^+ \rightleftharpoons T\text{-}NAD^+\cdot(UN)_3 \qquad (7)$$

where Eq. (6) describes a reaction involved in the oxidation of NADH catalyzed by the enzyme, and Eq. (7) an inhibitory reaction.

B. BINDING OF NADH

The binding of NADH to the enzyme has been studied by determining the quenching of NADH fluorescence on binding to the enzyme (Velick, 1953, 1958) and by ultrafiltration (Boers, 1970). Preliminary measurements by the latter technique indicate that the binding constants of the four molecules of NADH are similar to those of the corresponding molecules of NAD$^+$.

C. MECHANISM OF ACTION

The rate of oxidation of NADH by acetyl phosphate, in the presence of high concentrations of enzyme, is proportional to the concentration of NADH until 1 mole NADH per mole of enzyme is added. In an experiment described by De Vijlder et al., 1969b), the first-order reaction constant with respect to NADH, in the presence of 3 moles of NAD$^+$ per mole of enzyme, was 0.19 min^{-1}. Between 1 and 6 moles NADH per mole of enzyme, the first-order constant declined to 0.05 min^{-1}. A similar result was obtained with 1 mole NAD$^+$ per mole enzyme. Thus, the first molecule of NADH bound to the enzyme is oxidized more rapidly than subsequent molecules.

In contrast, the fourth molecule of NAD$^+$ bound is reduced more than twice as rapidly by glyceraldehyde as the other three (De Vijlder et al., 1969b).* The K_m for this fourth molecule is the same as that for the

---

* The actual values for the catalytic-center activity calculated by De Vijlder et al. (1969b) were 0.014 sec^{-1} for the first three sites and 0.035 sec^{-1} for the fourth. Closely similar results have also been obtained for the lobster enzyme. Teipel and Koshland (1970) have recently calculated a value of 0.78 min^{-1} (i.e., 0.013 sec^{-1}) for the first three sites in the rabbit enzyme, in excellent agreement with the findings of De Vijlder et al. (1969b). The value calculated for the fourth site by Teipel and Koshland (1970) is, however, much less than that of De Vijlder et al. (1969b). The difference appears to lie in the method of calculation, for when the method of De Vijlder et al. was applied to the data of Teipel and Koshland, a value of 0.024 sec^{-1} was obtained. The K_m for the fourth site (33 μM), calculated in this way, was also close to that found by De Vijlder et al. (1969a,b) (17 μM for rabbit, 24 μM for lobster).

overall reaction catalyzed by low concentrations of enzyme, and is also the same as the dissociation constant of the fourth site.

These findings and the fact that NAD^+ and $NADH$ compete for the fourth site (see above) when the amount of NAD^+ exceeds 3 molecules per molecule enzyme suggest that the catalytically most active form of enzyme in both glycolysis (Eq. 1 from left to right) and glucogenesis (Eq. 1 from right to left) is the enzyme with 3 of the 4 subunits occupied by NAD^+, and in the conformation that we have written $T \cdot (UN)_3$. The catalysis takes place on the fourth subunit. In the following mechanism $T \cdot (UN)_3$ is written $E - S^-$ where S^- represents the active thiol group that has formed no charge-transfer complex with NAD^+.

According to this mechanism, the catalytically active enzyme is a

$$
E{-}S^- + NAD^+ \rightleftharpoons E\overset{\textstyle S^-}{\underset{\textstyle NAD^+}{<}} \tag{i}
$$

$$
RCHO + E\overset{\textstyle S^-}{\underset{\textstyle NAD^+}{<}} \rightleftharpoons (RCHO){-}E\overset{\textstyle S^-}{\underset{\textstyle NAD^+}{<}} \tag{ii}
$$

$$
(RCHO){-}E\overset{\textstyle S^-}{\underset{\textstyle NAD^+}{<}} \rightleftharpoons E\overset{\textstyle S{\cdot}COR}{\underset{\textstyle NADH}{<}} + H^+ \tag{iii}
$$

$$
E\overset{\textstyle S{\cdot}COR}{\underset{\textstyle NADH}{<}} \rightleftharpoons E{-}S{-}COR + NADH \tag{iv}
$$

$$
or \qquad E\overset{\textstyle S{\cdot}COR}{\underset{\textstyle NADH}{<}} + P_i \rightleftharpoons E\overset{\textstyle S^-}{\underset{\textstyle NADH}{<}} + R{\cdot}COOP \tag{iv'}
$$

$$
E{-}S{-}COR + P_i \rightleftharpoons E{-}S^- + R{\cdot}COOP \tag{v}
$$

$$
or \qquad E\overset{\textstyle S^-}{\underset{\textstyle NADH}{<}} \rightleftharpoons E{-}S^- + NADH \tag{v'}
$$

$$
Sum: \quad R{\cdot}CHO + NAD^+ + P_i \rightleftharpoons R{\cdot}COOP + NADH + H^+ \tag{1}
$$

conjugated protein with 3 firmly bound prosthetic groups per tetramer. The charge-transfer complex plays no direct role in the enzyme-catalyzed reaction. The fourth NAD$^+$ molecule, which does not form a charge-transfer complex, is a substrate.

It cannot be excluded, however, that enzyme molecules containing fewer than 3 molecules of bound NAD$^+$ also play a minor role in the catalysis.

The hydride transfer (Eq. iii) may be visualized as in Fig. 3. Experiments with [1-^{3}H]glyceraldehyde phosphate have shown that, with this enzyme, a direct hydrogen transfer from the aldehyde to the nicotinamide takes place (Allison *et al.*, 1969), in contrast to alcohol, lactate, and malate dehydrogenases, where hydrogen transfer between substrate and nicotinamide occurs via a tryptophan in the protein (Chan and Schellenberg, 1968).

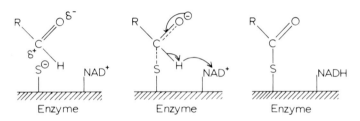

Fig. 3. Proposed mechanism of hydride transfer to NAD bound to fourth site of glyceraldehydephosphate dehydrogenase.

III. YEAST ENZYME

Remarkable differences between the behavior of the muscle and yeast enzymes have been reported despite the fact that the primary structures are sufficiently similar to allow the formation of hybrid tetramers (Kirschner and Schuster, 1970). These differences are:

1. The binding constants are so much less (Table I) that the yeast enzyme as usually prepared contains little NAD$^+$ (Warburg and Christian, 1939).

2. A positive cooperativity is observed in the binding of successive molecules of NAD$^+$, especially at higher temperatures. There is a difference of opinion between Koshland *et al.*, (1970) (see Table I), who has reported a mixture of positive cooperativity (between first and second sites) and negative cooperativity (between second and third, and third and fourth) and Kirschner and co-workers (1966; Kirschner, 1968; Kirschner and Schuster, 1970), who consider that only positive cooperativity is present.

3. According to Kirschner and Schuster (1970) and Chance and Harting Park (1967), all four NAD^+ molecules contribute equally to the 360-nm band. However, if the low value of Koshland et al. (1970) for the binding constant of the fourth site is correct, the fourth site could scarcely have been occupied in the experiments of Kirschner and Schuster (1970) and Chance and Harting Park (1967).

Kirschner and co-workers interpret the results in terms of the allosteric model of Monod et al. (1965), which may be written

$$R_4 \underset{k_{-0}}{\overset{k_0}{\rightleftharpoons}} T_4 \qquad\qquad L_0 = \frac{[T_4]}{[R_4]}$$

$$R_4 + N \underset{k_D}{\overset{k_A}{\rightleftharpoons}} R_3 \cdot RN \qquad\qquad T_4 + N \underset{k'_D}{\overset{k'_A}{\rightleftharpoons}} T_3 \cdot TN$$

$$R_3 \cdot RN + N \rightleftharpoons R_2 \cdot (RN)_2 \qquad\qquad T_3 \cdot TN + N \rightleftharpoons T_2 \cdot (TN)_2$$
$$R_2 \cdot (RN)_2 + N \rightleftharpoons R \cdot (RN)_3 \qquad\qquad T_2 \cdot (TN)_2 + N \rightleftharpoons T \cdot (TN)_3$$
$$R \cdot (RN)_3 + N \rightleftharpoons (RN)_4 \qquad\qquad T \cdot (TN)_3 + N \rightleftharpoons (TN)_4$$

Kinetic studies by rapid-mixing and temperature-jump techniques yielded the following values at pH 9.0 and 20° (Kirschner and Schuster, 1970):

k_0	1.2 sec^{-1}		
k_{-0}	0.05 sec^{-1}	$L_0 = 24$	
k_A	$5.3 \times 10^5 \, M^{-1} \text{ sec}^{-1}$	$K_R = 3.0 \times 10^{-5} \, M$	
k_D	16 sec^{-1}		
$k_{A'}$	$4.2 \times 10^6 \, M^{-1} \text{ sec}^{-1}$	$K_T = 3.0 \times 10^{-4} \, M$	$c = \dfrac{K_R}{K_T} = 0.1$
$k_{D'}$	$1.25 \times 10^3 \text{ sec}^{-1}$		

$K_R =$ intrinsic dissociation constant of R form with NAD^+; $K_T =$ intrinsic dissociation constant of T form with NAD^+.

The T state is enzymatically inactive. The transition from the R to the T state is accompanied by an increase in anisotropy and a volume contraction of 7%. Indeed the T state can be regarded as a reversible denatured state of the enzyme.

REFERENCES

Allison, W. S., Connors, M. J., and Parker, D. J. (1969). *Biochem. Biophys. Res. Commun.* **34**, 503.

Boers, W. (1970). Unpublished data.

Boross, L., and Cseke, E. (1966). *Acta Biochim. Biophys.* **2**, 47.

Chan, T. L., and Schellenberg, K. A. (1968). *J. Biol. Chem.* **243**, 6284.

Chance, B., and Harting Park, J. (1967). *J. Biol. Chem.* **242**, 5093.

Cilento, G., and Tedeschi, P. (1961). *J. Biol. Chem.* **236**, 907.

Conway, A., and Koshland, D. E., Jr., (1968). *Biochemistry* **7**, 4011.

Cori, G. T., Slein, M. W., and Cori, C. F. (1948). *J. Biol. Chem.* **173**, 605.

Davidson, B. E., Sajgò, M., Noller, H. F., and Harris, J. I. (1967). *Nature (London)* **216**, 1181.

De Vijlder, J. J. M., and Harmsen, B. J. M. (1969). *Biochim. Biophys. Acta* **178**, 434.

De Vijlder, J. J. M., and Slater, E. C. (1967). *Biochim. Biophys. Acta* **132**, 207.

De Vijlder, J. J. M., and Slater, E. C. (1968). *Biochim. Biophys. Acta* **167**, 23.

De Vijlder, J. J. M., Boers, W., and Slater, E. C. (1969a). *Biochim. Biophys. Acta* **191**, 214.

De Vijlder, J. J. M., Hilvers, A. G., Van Lis, J. M. J., and Slater, E. C. (1969b). *Biochim. Biophys. Acta* **191**, 221.

Harrington, W. F., and Karr, G. M. (1965). *J. Mol. Biol.* **13**, 885.

Harris, J. I., and Perham, R. N. (1963). *Biochem. J.* **89**, 60P.

Harris, J. I., and Perham, R. N. (1965). *J. Mol. Biol.* **13**, 876.

Harris, J. I., and Perham, R. N. (1968). *Nature (London)* **219**, 1025.

Harting, J., and Velick, S. F. (1954). *J. Biol. Chem.* **207**, 857.

Hilvers, A. G., and Weenen, J. H. M. (1962). *Biochim. Biophys. Acta* **58**, 380.

Hilvers, A. G., Van Dam, K., and Slater, E. C. (1964). *Biochim. Biophys. Acta* **85**, 206.

Kirschner, K. (1968). *In* "Regulation of Enzyme Activity and Allosteric Interactions" (E. Kvamme and A. Pihl, eds.), p. 39. Academic Press, New York.

Kirschner, K., and Schuster, I. (1970). *In* "Pyridine Nucleotide-Dependent Dehydrogenases" (H. Sund, ed.), p. 217. Springer, Berlin.

Kirschner, K., Eigen, M., Bittman, R., and Voigt, B. (1966). *Proc. Nat. Acad. Sci. U. S.* **56**, 1661.

Koeppe, O. J., Boyer, P. D., and Stulberg, M. P. (1956). *J. Biol. Chem.* **219**, 569.

Koshland, D. E., Jr., Cook, R. A., and Cornish-Bowden, A. (1970). *In* "Pyridine Nucleotide-Dependent Dehydrogenases" (H. Sund, ed.), p. 199. Springer, Berlin.

Kosower, E. M. (1956). *J. Amer. Chem. Soc.* **78**, 3497.

Kosower, E. M. (1960). *In* "The Enzymes" (P. D. Boyer, H. Lardy, and K. Myrbäck, eds.), 2nd rev. ed., Vol. 3, p. 171. Academic Press, New York.

Kosower, E. M. (1966). *In* "Flavins and Flavoproteins" (E. C. Slater, ed.), B.B.A. Library, Vol. 8, p. 1. Elsevier, Amsterdam.

Krimsky, I., and Racker, E. (1955). *Science* **122**, 319.

Lundsgaard, E. (1930). *Biochem. Z.* **227**, 51.

Monod, J., Wyman, J., and Changeux, J. P. (1965). *J. Mol. Biol.* **12**, 88.

Needham, D. M., and Pillai, R. K. (1937). *Biochem. J.* **31**, 1837.

Racker, E., and Krimsky, I. (1952a). *Nature (London)* **169**, 1043.

Racker, E., and Krimsky, I. (1952b). *J. Biol. Chem.* **198**, 731.

Stockell, A. (1959). *J. Biol. Chem.* **234**, 1286.

Taylor, J. F., Velick, S. F., Cori, G. T., Cori, C. F., and Slein, M. W. (1948). *J. Biol. Chem.* **173**, 619.

Teipel, J., and Koshland, D. E., Jr. (1970). *Biochim. Biophys. Acta* **198**, 183.

Velick, S. F. (1953). *J. Biol. Chem.* **203**, 563.

Velick, S. F. (1958). *J. Biol. Chem.* **233**, 1455.

Velick, S. F., Baggott, J. P., and Sturtevant, J. M. (1970). *In* "Pyridine Nucleotide-Dependent Dehydrogenases" (H. Sund, ed.), p. 229. Springer, Berlin.

Warburg, O., and Christian, W. (1939). *Biochem. Z.* **303**, 40.

Watson, H. C., and Banaszak, L. J. (1964). *Nature (London)* **204**, 918.

The Role of Phosphopantetheine in the Yeast Fatty Acid Synthetase Complex

E. SCHWEIZER,* K. WILLECKE, W. WINNEWISSER,
AND F. LYNEN

*Max-Planck-Institut für Zellchemie und Chemisches Laboratorium der Universität,
Institut für Biochemie, Munich, Germany*

I. Introduction

Since the original definition of the term "vitamin" as "an organic base essential for life," as given by Funk in 1912 during his work on thiamine (Funk, 1912), our knowledge of the number, chemical nature, and physiological role of these substances has considerably increased. Today, we know that despite rather specific pathological manifestations of various vitamin deficiencies in higher organisms, the role of vitamins in cellular metabolism is quite basic: they represent in the form of coenzymes and prosthetic groups an indispensable part of the cellular capacity for enzymatic catalysis. The elucidation of a great number of coenzyme-involved reaction mechanisms in detail during the past two decades has revealed that the function of many of these cofactors consists in their ability to transfer substrates or intermediates in an activated and reactive form from one catalytic site to another.

Whereas freely diffusible coenzymes like the pyridine nucleotides or coenzyme A represent carriers between independent and spatially separated enzymes, some of the so-called prosthetic groups which are tightly or even covalently linked to some enzymes, fulfill, in a more elaborate system, a very similar function. It may be worthwhile in this context to point to the distinct selective advantage which the "concentration" of

* Present address: Institut für Biochemie der Universität Würzburg, 87 Würzburg, Germany.

functionally related enzymes in close spatial proximity and ultimately within a multifunctional enzyme or enzyme complex has for the cell. Kinetically, this advantage becomes most evident by the consideration that a reaction sequence which is catalyzed by separate enzymes, and where the intermediates have to migrate, by diffusion, from one enzyme to another, is severely hampered by high transient times and the hazards of unwanted side reactions. On the other hand, even in a complex it may be an exceptional situation when all catalytic sites are located so close together that a rigidly bound substrate is exposed to all of them at the same time. More often, a substance may have to move from one catalytic site to another, either by diffusion or, in a more directed, and therefore more efficient way, by its binding to a suitable prosthetic group. Such a group should, by its chemical structure, be flexible enough to contact the different catalytic sites by a simple rotatory movement around its point of fixation. As an example, this type of function has been attributed to the enzyme-bound biotin (Lane and Lynen, 1963) and lipoic acid (Reed and Cox, 1966), the prosthetic groups of carboxylases and α-ketoacid dehydrogenases, respectively. Their own carbon side chain together with that of lysine, to which they are fixed, should provide their functional groups with the necessary flexibility mentioned.

Ever since the discovery of coenzyme A by Lipmann (1948–1949) and the identification of its acetyl thioester as the metabolically active form of acetate by Lynen (Lynen et al., 1951), the significance of the vitamin pantothenic acid has been solely viewed in terms of a constituent of this principal cellular carrier substance. While the unique aptness of the thioester bond for the enzymatic catalysis of transacylations and of condensation reactions was evident very early, there was no indication, however, which pointed to the significance of the rest of this complicated molecule, especially to that of its rather curious chemical constituent pantothenic acid. Since few enzymes only were strictly dependent on the intact molecule of coenzyme A, many of them working also, at a reduced rate, with simpler model substrates like N-acetylcysteamine derivatives, one was led to the conclusion that the occurrence of pantothenic acid in the cell was of not more than fortuitous significance.

It was only recently, however, that the study of fatty acid biosynthesis in various organisms disclosed a completely new role of pantothenic acid in cellular metabolism. Working with the soluble enzyme system from bacteria, Vagelos et al. (1966) as well as Pugh and Wakil (1965) discovered the involvement of a new cofactor, protein-bound 4'-phosphopantetheine, in bacterial fatty acid synthesis. Subsequently, fatty acid synthetases from plants (Simoni et al., 1967), mammals (Larrabee et al., 1965), and birds (Butterworth et al., 1967) as well as from yeast (Lynen, 1967) could equally be shown to contain this component. In

Escherichia coli, 4'-phosphopantetheine is bound to a heat-stable acidic protein which has a molecular weight of **8847** and contains **77** amino acid residues (Vanaman *et al.,* 1968). The results of studies relating to the isolation, structure and function of this cofactor in the yeast fatty acid synthetase complex will be presented in the following sections.

II. REACTION SCHEME OF FATTY ACID BIOSYNTHESIS

The first step in fatty acid biosynthesis consists of the carboxylation of acetyl-CoA to malonyl-CoA with ATP as an energy source, as indicated in Eq. (1):

$$\text{Acetyl-CoA} + \text{ATP} + \text{CO}_2 \rightarrow \text{malonyl-CoA} + \text{ADP} + \text{P}_i \qquad (1)$$

This reaction is catalyzed by a distinct acetyl-CoA carboxylase, an enzyme which is independent from the fatty acid synthetase complex and which shall not be considered further in this context. The following steps which lead from acetyl-CoA and malonyl-CoA as starting materials to the final production of palmityl-CoA and stearyl-CoA are catalyzed by the multienzyme complex of fatty acid synthetase according to the following overall equation:

$$\text{Acetyl-CoA} + 7 \text{ malonyl-CoA} + 14 \text{ NADPH} + 14\text{H}^+ \rightarrow$$
$$\text{palmityl-CoA} + 7\text{CoASH} + 14 \text{ NADP}^+ + 7\text{CO}_2 + 7\text{H}_2\text{O} \qquad (2)$$

The study of this enzyme system from yeast in the Munich laboratory during the past several years has provided us with a refined knowledge of the details of this synthetic process as well as of the structure of the enzyme system involved (Lynen, 1967). In yeast, this system represents a very stable aggregate of at least seven different enzymatic activities. It may be isolated as a single protein of a molecular weight of **2.3** millions which appears to be free of contaminations according to the criteria of ultracentrifugation, electrophoresis, and electron microscopy (Schweizer *et al.,* 1966). Although no intermediates are released from the complex during fatty acid synthesis, the use of appropriate model substrates as well as the isolation of the enzyme-bound intermediates has led to a detailed scheme of the reaction sequence (Fig. 1). In this scheme, the two substrates acetate and malonate are covalently bound by the complex at two different SH groups, designated as "peripheral" ($-\text{SH}_p$) and "central" ($-\text{SH}_c$) SH-groups, respectively. In these positions, both acyl groups condense to form enzyme-bound acetoacetate with concomitant release of CO_2. The next steps consist of the reduction of enzyme-bound acetoacetate to β-hydroxybutyrate, which is dehydrated to crotonyl enzyme and in turn gets reduced to butyryl enzyme. The butyrate is not released but enters, instead of acetate, a corresponding reaction sequence. This cycle is repeated until finally a carbon chain of **16–18** C atoms has been

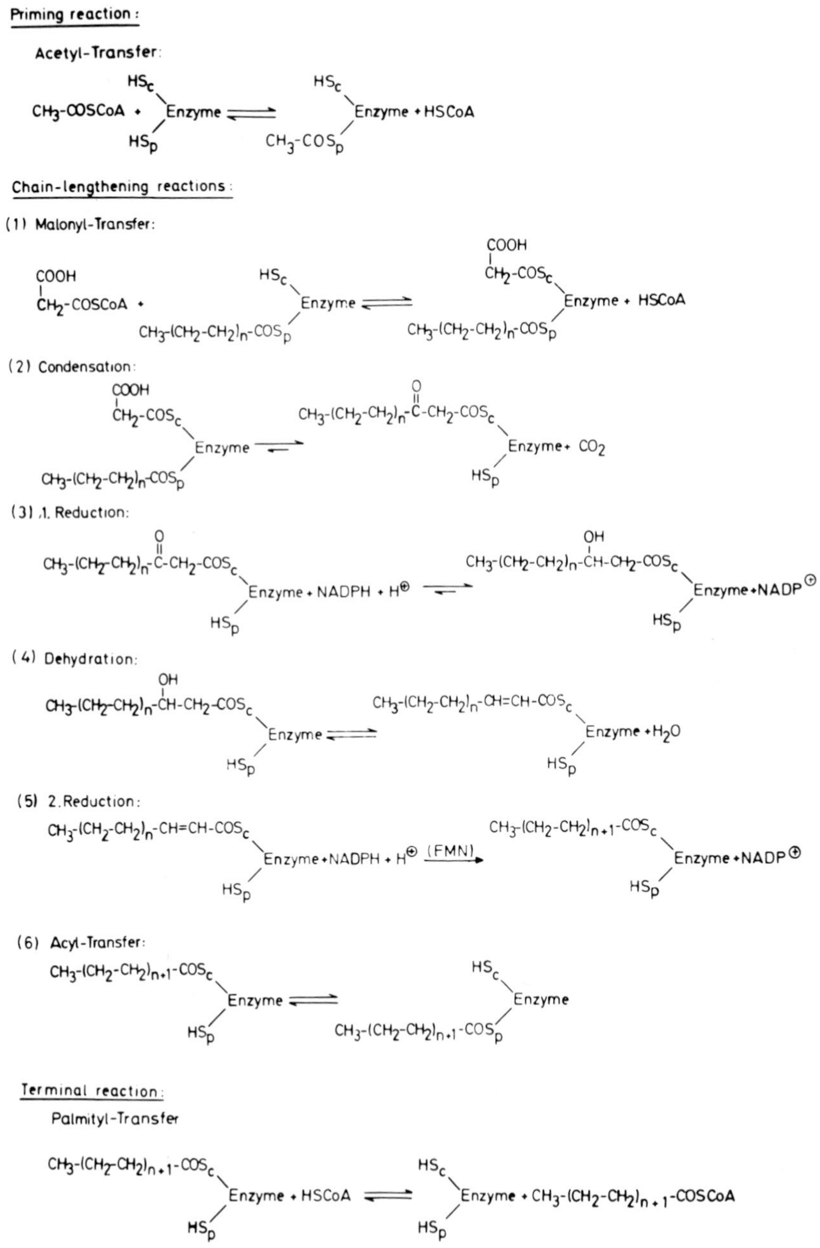

FIG. 1. Reaction scheme of fatty acid biosynthesis.

synthesized, which then gets transferred in a final reaction step from the enzyme to free coenzyme A.

III. Substrate Binding Sites of the Multienzyme Complex

When purified yeast fatty acid synthetase was incubated with ^{14}C-labeled acetyl-CoA or malonyl-CoA, radioactively labeled acetyl-enzyme or malonyl-enzyme compounds were formed and could be isolated by Sephadex filtration or trichloroacetic acid precipitation. The treatment of both compounds with performic acid revealed that in both cases only a minor portion of the enzyme-substrate bonds were thioester linkages, since an appreciable amount of the substrate was not released from the enzyme by oxidation (Schweizer et al., 1966). Further insight as to the chemical nature of the different substrate binding sites came from protein structural studies, the results of which are summarized briefly below.

A. Malonyltransferase Binding Site

When malonyl-^{14}C-enzyme was subjected to pepsin digestion and the digest was subsequently chromatographed on DEAE-Sephadex, three radioactive peptide fragments were eluted from the column (Fig. 2). Two of these, the malonyl peptides B and C, proved to be stable against performic acid oxidation and therefore represented the non-thiol binding sites of malonate. Two further purification steps, a Dowex 50 chromatography and a paper chromatography yielded both peptides in analytically pure form so that their amino acid composition could be determined. Malonyl peptide B proved to be a heptapeptide containing the amino acids His, Ser, Glu, Gly, Gly, Ala, Leu. Malonyl peptide C was apparently derived from peptide B by further digestion, since it contained two amino acid residues (Glu and Gly) less than peptide B. A detailed study of these two peptides made it most likely that malonate is bound to the hydroxyl group of serine (Schweizer et al., 1970). Since in earlier studies with the thiol inhibitors N-ethylmaleimide and iodoacetamide we had found that total fatty acid synthesis was completely inhibited while the malonyl-, acetyl-, and palmityl transfer reactions of the complex were not affected (Schweizer et al., 1966), we had assumed that these transferase binding sites were non-thiol binding sites. In the light of these experiments the isolation of the serine containing malonyl peptide suggested that it represents the active center of the malonyltransferase enzyme of the complex.

B. Acetyltransferase Binding Site

An analogous study of the non-thiol acetate binding site of the complex led Ziegenhorn (1970), after trypsin digestion of acetyl-^{14}C enzyme at pH 6.9, gel filtration, ion exchange chromatography, and paper electrophoresis, to the isolation of a performic acid stable acetyl-^{14}C peptide. By stepwise degradation with carboxypeptidase A the following amino acid sequence was established (Ziegenhorn, 1970): ^{14}C labeled N-acetyl-Ser-Gln-Gly-Leu-Thr-Val-Ala-Val. Since, by model experiments, it could be shown that acetate bound to the hydroxyl group of aminoterminal serine very easily moves to the serine amino group, it is conceivable that also in the acetyl peptide isolated the acyl residue originally was bound to the hydroxyl group of serine. Since we assume that, by analogy with malonyltransferase, this peptide represents the active site of acetyltransferase, it is evident from the amino acid sequences of both peptides isolated that the two transferases, although both have serine at their active sites, are not identical.

C. The Peripheral SH Group

According to our concept of the yeast fatty acid synthetase reaction mechanism (see Fig. 1) the so-called peripheral SH group is the acetate-binding thiol group which probably belongs to the condensing enzyme component of the complex. Attempts to isolate pure acetyl peptides derived from this binding site have not been successful so far because of the enormous amount of contaminating peptides. In spite of that, Oesterhelt (1967) has purified the peripheral acetyl peptide to such a degree that he was able to demonstrate that cysteine was the thiol group involved.

D. The Central SH Group

Since the extraordinarily stable structure of the yeast fatty acid synthetase made it impossible to isolate in a way, analogous to the bacterial system, a heat-stable acyl carrier protein component from this complex, the starting material for our investigation of the "central" SH-group in the yeast enzyme was the malonyl-thioester-peptide obtained after pepsin digestion of malonyl-^{14}C enzyme and subsequent DEAE-Sephadex chromatography, the malonyl peptide A in Fig. 2. Although we did not succeed in a complete purification of this peptide, 4′-phosphopantetheine as a constituent of it was made very likely after the analytical demonstration of the presence of equimolar amounts of organic phosphate, β-alanine, cysteamine, and malonic acid in this fraction (Table I). This was the first experimental hint for the occurrence of 4′-phosphopantetheine as a prosthetic group also in the yeast fatty acid synthesizing system. Further support came from the experiments of Wells in our laboratory (Wells et al., 1967), who was able to demonstrate the incorporation of ^{14}C-labeled pantothenic acid into the yeast fatty acid synthetase complex, after this vitamin had been fed to a pantothenate heterotrophic strain of yeast.

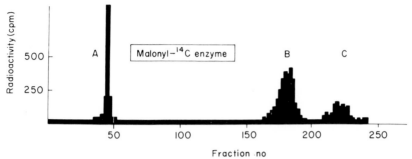

Fraction no

FIG. 2. Chromatography of the peptic hydrolyzate of malonyl-¹⁴C-enzyme on DEAE-Sephadex. Preparation of malonyl-¹⁴C-enzyme: 1.6 g synthetase, 28 μmoles of malonyl-3-¹⁴C-CoA (1.2 × 10⁶ cpm/μmole), 120 ml 0.05 M K-phosphate buffer, pH 6.5, were incubated for 2 min at 22°C. Pepsin digestion: precipitation of malonyl-¹⁴C-enzyme with 6 ml 3 M trichloroacetic acid, 3 careful washings of the precipitate, then suspension in 2 liters of 0.01 M HCl, digestion with 160 mg of pepsin for 12 hours at room temperature. Then evaporation to dryness, solution in 7 ml of pyridine acetate, pH 6.25. Insoluble material is removed by centrifugation. Chromatography on DEAE-Sephadex (2.1 × 150 cm): After application of the sample elution with 0.05 M pyridine acetate, pH 6.25, until fraction 70 (fraction volume, 6 ml); thereafter a continuous gradient with 0.2 M acetic acid in the reservoir and 200 ml of 0.05 M pyridine acetate, pH 6.25, in the constant-volume mixing chamber was applied.

The unequivocal identification of enzyme-bound 4'-phosphopantetheine was possible after the hydrolytic cleavage of the phosphodiester bond, the subsequent purification of freed 4'-phosphopantetheine as a S-benzoyl-ester by ion exchange and paper chromatography, which then was characterized by chemical analysis and comparison with an authentic reference substance (Schweizer et al., 1970). In Figure 3 the complete identity between the UV spectra of authentic S-benzoyl-4'-phosphopantetheine

TABLE I

ANALYSIS OF MALONYL-3-¹⁴C PEPTIDE A[a]

Constituent	Content (μmoles)
Organic phosphate	0.080
β-Alanine	0.068
Cysteamine (as taurine)	0.061
Malonic acid	0.063

[a] The four constituents were separately determined in aliquots of the malonyl-3-¹⁴C peptide fraction eluted from DEAE-Sephadex. β-Alanine and cysteamine were determined in the amino acid analyzer, the latter after performic acid oxidation. The amount of malonic acid was calculated from its known specific activity.

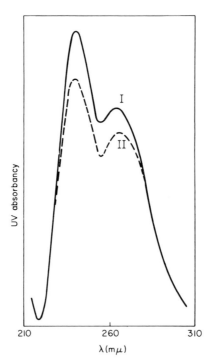

Fig. 3. UV spectrum of *S*-benzoyl-4'-phosphopantetheine isolated from fatty acid synthetase (I) and authentic reference (II).

and the compound isolated from the fatty acid synthetase is evident. The cleavage of the phosphodiester bond was effected in this experiment according to a method indicated by Vagelos (see Larrabee *et al.*, 1965) by alkali treatment at pH 12 and 70°C for 1 hour.

The quantitative determination of 4'-phosphopantetheine in yeast fatty acid synthetase has been performed in two different ways: (1) 4'-phosphopantetheine released from the complex by alkaline hydrolysis was treated according to Novelli *et al.* (1949) with liver peptidase and alkaline phosphatase to yield free pantothenic acid, which then was determined microbiologically with *Lactobacillus plantarum* (ATCC 8014) as a test organism; (2) the 4'-phosphopantetheine released was freed from the apoenzyme by trichloroacetic acid precipitation and subsequent passage of the supernatant through a Dowex 50 (H⁺) column. Then it was hydrolyzed in a sealed and evacuated glass tube for 20 hours at 110°C in 6 *N* HCl, and subsequently the *β*-alanine was determined in an amino acid analyzer. In both cases the time-dependent destruction of pantothenic acid in alkaline solution has to be corrected for. This was

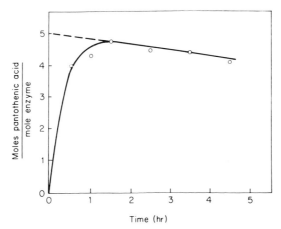

FIG. 4. Kinetics of 4'-phosphopantetheine release from fatty acid synthetase by alkali treatment. After incubation of 14.7 mg of enzyme and 0.4 mmole of KOH 40°C, hydrolysis is stopped at various times by addition of 0.1 mmole of Tris pH 8.3 and 0.1 mmole of H_2SO_4. Incubation is carried out with 15 μg alkaline phosphatase and crude liver extract (2.5 mg protein) for 12 hours at 37°C. Released pantothenate was subjected to microbiological testing.

done either by following the kinetics of 4'-phosphopantetheine release and extrapolation to zero time (Fig. 4) or by the establishment of standard conditions and the introduction of an appropriate correction factor. Using the microbiological pantothenate assay, Winnewisser (1969) obtained for two different preparations of fatty acid synthetase values of 5.0 ± 0.35 and 4.93 ± 0.35 moles of pantetheine per mole of enzyme. The specific activities of the two enzyme preparations were 2400 and 1800 mU/mg, respectively. The values were averaged from 8 individual determinations. Similar results were obtained by the β-alanine assay method mentioned: the average β-alanine content of five different synthetase preparations was 4.9 ± 0.6 moles per mole enzyme (Schweizer et al., 1970).

IV. ISOLATION OF THE ACYL CARRIER PROTEIN

After attempts to isolate the acyl carrier protein (ACP) from native yeast fatty acid synthetase were not successful because of the very stable quarternary structure of the complex, Willecke in our laboratory has devised a procedure for the isolation of ACP from the denatured complex (Willecke et al., 1969). Pantothenate-^{14}C labeled synthetase was denatured in 6 M guanidine hydrochloride and subjected to Sephadex G-200 chromatography. As indicated in Fig. 5, the radioactive ACP is eluted slightly behind the nonradioactive bulk proteins. The radioactive

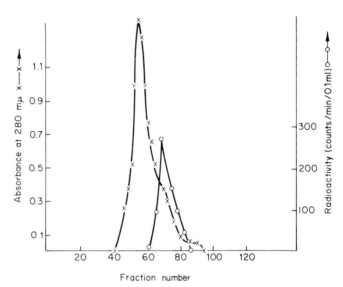

Fɪɢ. 5. Purification of the yeast acyl carrier protein on Sephadex G-200. Thirty milligrams of pantetheine-^{14}C synthetase (1×10^5 cpm) was subsequently treated, in saturated guanidine HCl, with $0.25\,M$ dithiothreitol and $0.6\,M$ iodoacetamide at pH 8.6, then dialyzed against $6\,M$ guanidine HCl $0.1\,M$ potassium citrate pH 3.5 for 12 hours. Chromatography was on Sephadex G-200 (81×2 cm) with the same buffer. ×—×, Absorbancy at 280 mμ, ○—○, radioactivity.

fractions were pooled, concentrated and, to check their purity, subjected to analytical polyacrylamide gel electrophoresis. The gel was then stained with Amido Black 10B. Its densitometer tracing at 546 mμ is shown in Fig. 6. The position of radioactive fractions, as determined in thin slices of the block, is indicated by the dotted line. Apparently, there are two radioactive peaks A and B which, by rechromatography, could be shown to reproducibly migrate at the two different positions indicated in Fig. 6b. So, we are left with the rather unexpected observation of two different pantothenate containing proteins in yeast fatty acid synthetase. The question has to remain open so far, if these two fractions really represent two different types of ACP, or if the splitting into two peaks was an artificial process. In this context a report of Matsumura and Stumpf (1968) is noteworthy; these workers during their study of the soluble spinach ACP observed that in starch gel electrophoresis also this ACP separated into two different bands with slightly different amino acid compositions.

V. Concluding Remarks

The apparent presence of ACP or at least 4′-phosphopantetheine in all fatty acid synthesizing systems so far investigated, clearly points to a

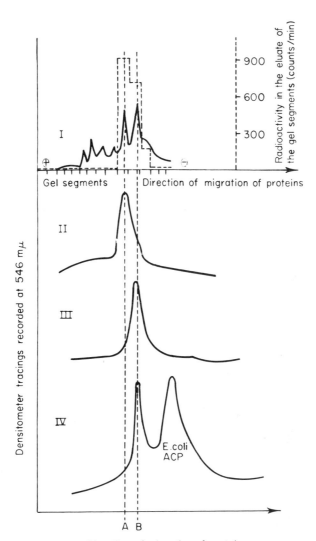

Fig. 6. Analytic electrophoretic runs of yeast ACP and *Escherichia coli* ACP in polyacrylamide gel. Panel I: pantetheine-^{14}C yeast ACP after Sephadex G-200 filtration (—, densitometer tracing after Amido Black 10 B staining; - - -, radioactivity). Panels II and III: reelectrophoresis of bands A and B from panel I. Panel IV: reelectrophoresis of band B together with *E. coli* ACP.

central role of this prosthetic group within the mechanism of this process. In bacteria, fatty acid synthetase may also exist as a complex within the intact cell, but the quarternary structure of this complex must be very weak since after cell breakage the individual component enzymes including ACP are independent and may be separately purified. Therefore, the role of ACP could be most easily, and has been most extensively studied in this system. As could be shown by the laboratories of Vagelos (Vagelos *et al.*, 1969) and of Wakil (Williamson and Wakil, 1966) the ACP derivatives of acetate, malonate, and the intermediates act as substrates for all the individual enzymes, some of them being absolutely specific for ACP. Although the rigid structure of the yeast fatty acid synthetase, which so far has prevented the isolation and study of the individual enzymes separately, makes an experimental approach to this question very difficult, it seems feasible to assume that ACP in yeast fatty acid synthetase exhibits a quite similar function. Thus, the ACP is not a diffusible carrier like coenzyme A, but a carrier fixed at a certain position within the network of the multienzyme complex. Assuming an aggregate structure of the intact *E. coli* system, the ACP may be located at a fixed position, or positions, within this complex, too. To fulfill this carrier function without any diffusion being possible, the distinct structural features of this prosthetic group may be of importance. As demonstrated in Fig. 7, the 4′-phosphopantetheine moiety of ACP may be considered as a long flexible arm about 20 Å in length when fully extended, which, when placed in an appropriate central position of the complex, could "reach" an intermediate from one enzyme to another. This would, other than in coenzyme A, point to an important function of pantothenic acid as a constituent of this prosthetic group.

As a recent study of Majerus (1968) using *E. coli* ACP suggests, the protein part of ACP may have the function of ensuring the proper incorporation of the prosthetic group into the quaternary structure of the complex. Majerus showed that all but the three last amino acids of the polypeptide chain were necessary for the affinity, i.e., the proper combination of ACP and the individual enzymes. It remains to demonstrate, however, that ACP has distinct sites to combine with more than one component enzyme at the same time.

Since five molecules of 4′-phosphopantetheine have been found per molecule of yeast fatty acid synthetase, one may ask whether all five prosthetic groups are involved in the same function or whether there is a functional differentiation between them. In other words, either the synthetase as a whole or its ACP-containing portion could be a pentamer, or there are five ACP residues placed at different locations within the complex. The finding of two different types of ACP in yeast may hint at the latter possibility. On the other hand, *E. coli* pyruvate dehydrogenase, another intensively studied multienzyme system, which comprises three different enzyme components, contains these enzymes in widely differing molecular amounts (Reed and Cox, 1966). One molecule of this complex

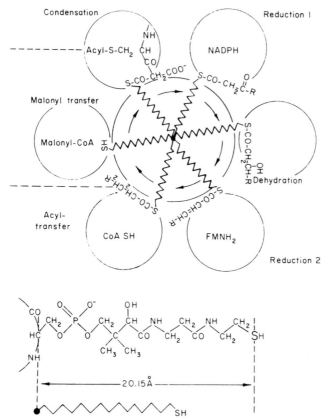

Fig. 7. Structure and function of 4′-phosphopantetheine in the yeast fatty acid synthetase complex.

even contains 48 molecules of covalently bound lipoic acid as prosthetic groups. It has been suggested that eventually major gaps between the active sites may be bridged by the interaction of several of these flexible groups. To answer this question for the yeast fatty acid synthetase complex, one has to await further technical advances in the dissociation of the complex.

After Oesterhelt found that, besides malonate, acetate is also bound to the 4′-phosphopantetheine.of yeast fatty acid synthetase (Oesterhelt, 1967)—an observation supported by ·competition experiments between acetate and malonate for the "central" SH group (Schweizer et al., 1970) —the following model was developed for substrate binding sites and their respective functions (Fig. 8). The two substrates acetate and malonate

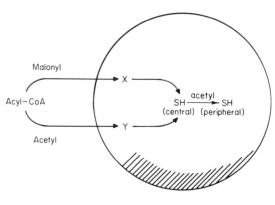

Multienzyme complex

Fig. 8. Specificity of acyl transfer to the different acceptor groups on the multi-enzyme complex.

enter the synthetase complex by a transfer reaction from coenzyme A to their respective transferase non-thiol binding sites. From here, both move to the central SH-group (4'-phosphopantetheine), from which acetate finally gets transferred to the peripheral SH group, while malonate remains to undergo the condensation with peripherally bound acetate. All intermediates up to palmitate remain bound to the central SH group, thereby preventing another acetate molecule from priming a new synthetic sequence. This takes place only after palmitate has finally been transferred to coenzyme A. This model also accounts for the observation that preincubation of fatty acid synthetase with acetyl-CoA yields higher initial rates of synthesis than preincubation with malonyl-CoA, since in the latter case malonate blocks the accessibility of the peripheral SH group for acetate.

Another interesting question represents the problem of ACP biosynthesis. Very recently, Elovson and Vagelos (1966) reported that in extracts of *E. coli* an enzyme is found which catalyzes the transfer of 4'-phosphopantetheine from coenzyme A to ACP-apoprotein, according to the following equation:

$$\text{Coenzyme A} + \begin{array}{c} -\text{CO} \\ \diagdown \\ \text{CH—CH}_2\text{OH} \\ \diagup \\ -\text{NH} \end{array} \rightarrow \begin{array}{c} -\text{CO} \\ \diagdown \\ \text{CH—CH}_2\text{O—P-pantetheine} \\ \diagup \\ -\text{NH} \end{array}$$

$$+\ 3',5'\text{-adenosine diphosphate} \quad (3)$$

In this reaction, the equilibrium should be shifted far to the side of ACP formation because of the higher energy content of a pyrophosphate bond compared to the phosphodiester bond. In agreement with this consideration are results of Alberts and Vagelos (1966) with a pantothenate heterotrophic strain of *E. coli*. When grown under increasing pantothenate limitations, the ratio of cellular coenzyme A to ACP concentrations was increasingly shifted in favor of the ACP content. Apparently, the synthesis of ACP proceeds at the expense of coenzyme A. This means that coenzyme A, besides its widespread carrier function in cellular metabolism, also plays an important role as the precursor of ACP.

REFERENCES

Alberts, A. W., and Vagelos, P. R. (1966). *J. Biol. Chem.* **241**, 5201.

Butterworth, P. H. W., Jacob, E. J., Dorsey, J. A., and Porter, J. W. (1967). *Fed. Proc., Fed. Amer. Soc. Exp. Biol.* **26**, 671.

Elovson, J., and Vagelos, P. R. (1966). *J. Biol. Chem.* **243**, 3603.

Funk, C. (1912). *J. State Med.* **20**, 341.

Lane, M. D., and Lynen, F. (1963). *Proc. Nat. Acad. Sci. U. S.* **49**, 397.

Larrabee, A. R., McDaniel, E. G., Bakerman, H. A., and Vagelos, P. R. (1965). *Proc. Nat. Acad. Sci. U. S.* **54**, 267.

Lipmann, F. (1948–1949). *Harvey Lect.* **44**, 99.

Lynen, F. (1967). *Biochem. J.* **102**, 381.

Lynen, F., Reichert, E., and Rueff, L. (1951). *Justus Liebigs Ann. Chem.* **578**, 1.

Majerus, P. W. (1968). *Science* **159**, 428.

Matsumura, S., and Stumpf, P. K. (1968). *Arch. Biochem. Biophys.* **125**, 932.

Novelli, G. D., Kaplan, N. O., and Lipmann, F. (1949). *J. Biol. Chem.* **177**, 97.

Oesterhelt, D. (1967). Ph.D. Thesis, University of Munich.

Pugh, E. L., and Wakil, S. J. (1965). *J. Biol. Chem.* **240**, 4727.

Reed, L. J., and Cox, D. J. (1966). *Annu. Rev. Biochem.* **35**, 57.

Schweizer, E., Oesterhelt, D., Chan, W., Duba, C., and Lynen, F. (1966). *Colloq. Ges. Physiol. Chem.* **16**, 49.

Schweizer, E., Piccinini, F., Duba, C., Günther, S., Ritter, E., and Lynen, F. (1970). *Eur. J. Biochem.* (submitted for publication).

Simoni, R. D., Criddle, R. S., and Stumpf, P. K. (1967). *J. Biol. Chem.* **242**, 573.

Vagelos, P. R., Majerus, P. W., Alberts, A. W., Larrabee, A. R., and Ailhaud, G. P. (1966). *Fed. Proc., Fed. Amer. Soc. Exp. Biol.* **25**, 1485.

Vagelos, P. R., Alberts, A. W., and Majerus, P. W. (1969). *Methods Enzymol.* **14**, 39.

Vanaman, T. C., Wakil, S. J., and Hill, R. L. (1968). *J. Biol. Chem.* **243**, 6420.

Wells, W. W., Schultz, J., and Lynen, F. (1967). *Biochem. Z.* **346**, 474.

Willecke, K., Ritter, E., and Lynen, F. (1969). *Eur. J. Biochem.* **8**, 503.

Williamson, I. P., and Wakil, S. J. (1966). *J. Biol. Chem.* **241**, 2326.

Winnewisser, W. (1969). Diplomarbeit, University of Munich.

Ziegenhorn, J. (1970). Ph.D. Thesis, University of Munich.

Tricarboxylic Acid Activator-Induced Changes at the Active Site of Acetyl-CoA Carboxylase

M. DANIEL LANE, JOHN EDWARDS, ERWIN STOLL,
AND JOEL MOSS

*Department of Physiological Chemistry, The Johns Hopkins University
School of Medicine, Baltimore, Maryland*
and
*Department of Biochemistry, New York University School of Medicine,
New York, New York*

I. INTRODUCTION

Acetyl-CoA carboxylase catalyzes the first committed step of extra-mitochondrial fatty acid synthesis in animal tissues and appears to be an important control point in this biosynthetic pathway (Vagelos, 1964; Lowenstein, 1968; Lane and Moss, 1970). The carboxylase appears to be regulated both by alterations of its level in tissues (Majerus and Kilburn, 1969) and by modification of its catalytic efficiency with allosteric effectors (Vagelos, 1964; Numa et al., 1965; Gregolin et al., 1966a; Miller and Levy, 1969). Certain tricarboxylic acids, notably citrate and isocitrate, markedly activate the carboxylase-catalyzed reaction (Martin and Vagelos, 1962; Waite and Wakil, 1962; Matsuhashi et al., 1962; Kallen and Lowenstein, 1962; Gregolin et al., 1966a,b, 1968a,b). Activation by these acids is rather specific in that tricarballylate, a close structural analog, is completely inactive (Ryder et al., 1967; Gregolin et al., 1968a). Citrate appears to serve the dual role in fatty acid synthesis of precursor of extramitochondrial acetyl-CoA via the citrate-cleavage reaction (Lowenstein, 1968) and of "feed-forward" activator of acetyl-CoA carboxylase. As demonstrated in this laboratory (Gregolin et al., 1966a,b, 1968b; Kleinschmidt et al., 1969; Moss et al., 1969), activation by tricarboxylic acids is accomplished by the rapid polymerization of carboxylase protomers to give rise to polymeric filaments. Electron micrographs of the catalytically active filamentous forms of the avian liver and bovine adipose tissue acetyl-CoA carboxylases in the presence of citrate are shown in Fig. 1. Investigations with both carboxylases show that these filamentous forms are catalytically active; however, dissociation into protomers occurs under assay conditions when tricarboxylic acid activator

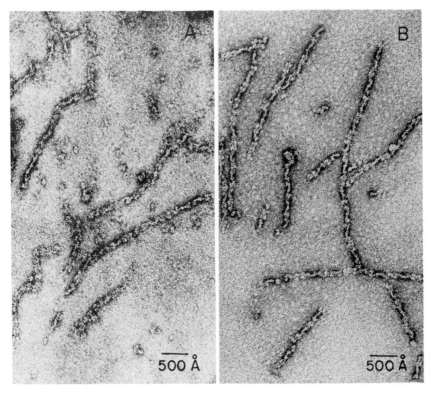

FIG. 1. Filamentous forms of avian liver (A) and bovine adipose tissue (B) acetyl-CoA carboxylases in the presence of citrate. Dilute solutions (20 μg/ml) of avian liver (Gregolin et al., 1968a) or bovine perirenal adipose tissue (Kleinschmidt et al., 1969; Moss et al., 1970) carboxylase in 50 mM Tris (Cl⁻) buffer containing 10 mM potassium citrate, 5 mM 2-mercaptoethanol and 0.1 M EDTA at pH 7.5 were applied to carbon support films. After staining with 4% aqueous uranyl acetate, the preparations were examined in the electron microscope. From Kleinschmidt et al. (1969).

TABLE I

MOLECULAR PROPERTIES OF AVIAN LIVER ACETYL-CoA CARBOXYLASE[a]

Form of carboxylase	Conditions	$s_{20,w}$	Molecular weight (by sedimentation equilibrium)
Polymeric	i-citrate, citrate, or P_i	55–59S	4,000,000–8,000,000
"Protomeric"	0.5 M NaCl	13.1S	410,000
Subunit	0.1–1.0% SDS	4S	110,000

Biotin prosthetic group	0.93 ⎫	
Acetyl-CoA binding sites[b]	1.0 ⎬	per protomeric unit (410,000 molecular weight)
Citrate binding sites[b]	1.16 ⎭	

[a] Adapted from Gregolin et al. (1968b).

[b] At 4°, pH 7.5, and 2 mg carboxylase protein per ml; K_D (acetyl CoA) = 5 × 10⁻⁶ M; K_D (citrate) = 2 × 10⁻⁶ M.

is not present (Gregolin et al., 1966a,b, 1968b; Kleinschmidt et al., 1969). Some of the molecular characteristics of the polymeric and protomeric forms of the avian liver carboxylase are summarized in Table I. The polymeric filamentous species are composed of a linear assemblage of 10–20 protomers of 410,000 daltons and each protomer in turn consists of 4 subunits of approximately 110,000 daltons.

The fundamental question to be considered in this paper is how conformational changes at the active site, induced by the remote binding of the allosteric activator, result in increased catalytic efficiency. Two types of activator effects are anticipated in allosteric systems (Monod et al., 1963, 1965), namely V_{max} and K_m effects, which are associated either with an increase in catalytic capacity or an increase in the affinity of the enzyme for substrate or cofactor, respectively. It is generally agreed on the basis of investigations with the rat liver (Numa et al., 1965), avian liver (Ryder et al., 1967; Gregolin et al., 1968a), and bovine adipose tissue (Moss et al., 1969) acetyl-CoA carboxylases that the primary kinetic effect of tricarboxylic acid activator is on the maximal velocity, not on the K_m's for substrates. It will be demonstrated that tricarboxylic acid activators promote specific changes at the active site which accompany activation and account for the observed increase in V_{max}.

II. EFFECT OF ACTIVATOR ON THE PARTIAL REACTIONS OF ACETYL-CoA CARBOXYLATION

The carboxylation of acetyl-CoA catalyzed by acetyl-CoA carboxylases from animal tissues involves the following minimal partial reaction sequence (Eqs. 1 and 2) (Matsuhashi et al., 1964; Numa et al., 1964):

$$\text{Enz} + \text{HCO}_3^- + \text{ATP} \overset{\text{Mg}^{2+}}{\rightleftharpoons} \text{Enz-CO}_2^- + \text{ADP} + \text{P}_i \qquad (1)$$

$$\text{Enz-CO}_2^- + \text{acetyl-CoA} \rightleftharpoons \text{Enz} + \text{malonyl-CoA} \qquad (2)$$

$$\textit{Overall:} \quad \text{HCO}_3^- + \text{ATP} + \text{acetyl-CoA} \overset{\text{Mg}^{2+}}{\rightleftharpoons} \text{malonyl-CoA} + \text{ADP} + \text{P}_i \qquad (3)$$

The occurrence of these reactions has been demonstrated by appropriate exchange reactions, by the formation and isolation of enzyme-CO_2^-, and by carboxyl transfer from enzyme-CO_2^- to acetyl-CoA to form malonyl-CoA. Both half-reactions (Eqs. 1 and 2), as well as the overall carboxylation and decarboxylation reactions (Eq. 3), appear to be activated by citrate or isocitrate. The rates of ATP-^{32}P$_i$-and ATP-^{14}C-ADP-exchange, which involve the first half-reaction (Eq. 1), and of malonyl-CoA-^{14}C-acetyl-CoA exchange, which involves the carboxyl transfer step (Eq. 2), are all markedly increased by tricarboxylic acid activator (Matsuhashi *et al.*, 1964; Gregolin *et al.*, 1966b, 1968a; Ryder *et al.*, 1967). Attempts to measure the kinetics of enzyme-CO_2^- formation or subsequent carboxyl transfer from enzyme-CO_2^- to acetyl-CoA by conventional techniques have been unsuccessful because of the rapidity of these stoichiometric processes (Stoll *et al.*, 1968). It was possible to circumvent this problem, however (Stoll *et al.*, 1968), by use of enzymatic models for each of the forward half-reactions, namely (1) the carboxylation of free (+)-biotin to form free 1'-*N*-carboxybiotin, and (2) carboxyl transfer from enzyme-CO_2^- to acetyl pantetheine to form malonyl pantetheine. The effect of tricarboxylic acid activator on both of these reactions is discussed below (Sections I,A and II,B).

A. EFFECT ON THE CARBOXYLATION OF FREE BIOTIN

It was commonly believed (Ochoa and Kaziro, 1965) that the ability to carboxylate free biotin was a unique property of the bacterial β-methylcrotonyl-CoA carboxylase studied extensively in Lynen's laboratory (Knappe *et al.*, 1961a,b; Lynen *et al.*, 1961). This view became untenable when it was found by Stoll *et al.* (1968) that the avian liver acetyl-CoA carboxylase also catalyzes the carboxylation of free biotin (see Fig. 2). The carboxylation product was identified as 1'-*N*-carboxybiotin by methylation with diazomethane and by comparison of the chromatographic behavior of the methylated product with authentic 1'-*N*-methoxycarbonyl biotin methyl ester (Stoll *et al.*, 1968) as described by Knappe *et al.* (1961b). It was demonstrated that citrate (see Fig. 2) and isocitrate markedly activate this carboxylation, whereas tricarballylate has no effect. The fact that the reaction is a model for the initial step in the carboxylation of acetyl-CoA indicates that this half-reaction (Eq. 1) is also stimulated by tricarboxylic acid activator.

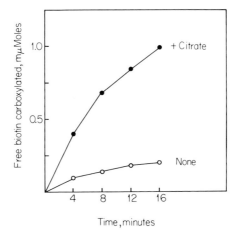

Fig. 2. Kinetics of carboxylation of free biotin. The reaction mixture contained the following components (in micromoles per milliliter, unless specified): Tris (Cl⁻) buffer, pH 7.5, 60; (+)-biotin, 20; ATP, 2; MgCl₂, 8; KH¹¹CO₃ (specific radioactivity, 5 to 7 × 10⁶ cpm/μmole), 10; dithiothreitol, 2; bovine serum albumin, 0.6 mg/ml; and acetyl-CoA carboxylase (8–9 units per milligram of refractometrically determined protein), 0.8 mg/ml. Potassium citrate was added at a level of 10 mM as indicated. After incubation at 37°C, the reaction was terminated by rapidly transferring 0.1-ml aliquots to 0.8 ml of water (0–2°C) containing 1 drop of n-octanol and bubbling CO₂ through the solution for 40 minutes at 0–2°C to remove excess H¹¹CO₃⁻. The gassed solution was made alkaline and residual ¹¹C-activity (1'-N-carboxybiotin) determined using a liquid scintillation spectrometer. From Stoll *et al.* (1968).

Since the functional ureido group of the bicyclic biotin ring resides at the distal end of a flexible 14 Å side chain* which anchors it to the apoprotein, some means must exist for precisely orienting this group with respect to bound substrate. The existence of secondary binding sites on the enzyme for interaction with the bicyclic ring and its side-chain amide group is suggested by the pattern of specificity exhibited by the carboxylase for (+)-biotin and biocytin relative to that of certain biotin analogs. The effects of structural and stereochemical modifications of the (+)-biotin molecule on carboxylation rate are shown in Table II. Biocytin (ϵ-N-(+)-biotinyl-L-lysine), which has a side-chain amide group in the same position as the biotin prosthetic group of the enzyme, is a somewhat

* Although the biotinyl prosthetic group is covalently linked in amide linkage to lysyl ϵ-amino groups in biotin enzymes, it is evident that its functional bicyclic ring must be bound at a secondary site on the enzyme for the carboxylation to take place. Measurements made with Corey-Pauling models (Koltun connectors) of ϵ-N-(+)-biotinyllysine reveal that the maximum distance from the α-carbon to the juncture of the side chain with the thiophane ring is about 14 Å.

TABLE II

THE SPECIFICITY OF THE CARBOXYLATION OF FREE BIOTIN[a]

Derivative	Concentration (mM)	Carboxylation rate relative to (+)-biotin[b] (%)
(+)-Biotin	20	100
(−)-Biotin	20	0
Biocytin	20	122
(+)-Homobiotin	20	31
(+)-Norbiotin	20	28
d,l-O-Heterobiotin	40	27
d,l-Dethiobiotin	40	0
2-Imidazolidone (ethyleneurea)	20–100	0

[a] From Stoll et al. (1968).

[b] Carboxylation rates were determined as described in the legend for Fig. 2; biotin derivatives were substituted for (+)-biotin in the reaction mixture.

better substrate than free biotin. On the other hand, the biotin side-chain homologs, norbiotin (C_4), and homobiotin (C_6), are much less reactive biotin (C_5). This suggests that the distance from the carboxyl group to the thiophane ring is critical, and in the case of biotin, optimal. The inactivity of dethiobiotin and 2-imidazolidone (ethyleneurea), as well as the reduction in activity caused by the substitution of O for S in the thiophane ring, as with oxybiotin (O-heterobiotin), emphasizes the importance of the thiophane ring in binding. It is evident from Table II that a change in configuration about the 2-position (the point of juncture of the side chain with the thiophane ring), i.e., from (+)- to (−)-biotin, completely abolishes activity. These observations suggest that a specific enzyme site hydrogen bonds the side-chain amide of the prosthetic group or, alternatively, the carboxyl or amide of free biotin or its analogs.

An investigation of the kinetic parameters for the carboxylation of (+)-biotin, (+)-homobiotin, and biocytin (see Table III) showed that citrate causes a 5- to 10-fold increase in the K_m values for these biotin derivatives (Stoll et al., 1968). The relevance of these effects in terms of a conformational change in the vicinity of the active site is considered later (see Section V). The V_{max} for the carboxylation of free (+)-biotin in the presence of citrate is about 5 mμmoles per minute per milligram of protein, which is about 1/2000 that for the carboxylation of acetyl-CoA. The K_m for citrate in this reaction is about 5 mM which is in good agreement with those for the overall carboxylation and ATP-$^{32}P_i$ exchange reactions (Gregolin et al., 1966a,b, 1968a).

The high degree of specificity, as well as the high concentration of

TABLE III

THE EFFECT OF CITRATE ON KINETIC PARAMETERS OF THE CARBOXYLATION
OF "FREE" BIOTIN DERIVATIVES

Derivative	Side-chain length	K_m (mM) No citrate	K_m (mM) + citrate	V_{max} (relative, %)[a] No citrate	V_{max} (relative, %)[a] + citrate
(+)-Biotin	C_5	10	45	11	100
(+)-Homobiotin	C_6	19	200	10	100
(+)-Biocytin	$\cong C_{11}$	12	50	17	151

[a] V_{max} is expressed as percent relative to that for free (+)-biotin in the presence of citrate, 5 mμmoles per minute per milligram of protein at 37°C. The method for determining carboxylation rate is given in the legend for Fig. 2.

(+)-biotin required to saturate the enzyme, supports the view that free biotin and certain of its derivatives bind and are carboxylated at the enzyme site normally occupied by the bicyclic ring of the biotin prosthetic group. The resolution of a biotin-free subunit from the acetyl-CoA carboxylase system of *E. coli* which catalyzes the carboxylation of free (+)-biotin provides a precedent for a site of this type on biotin enzymes (Alberts *et al.*, 1969; Lane *et al.*, 1970).

B. EFFECT ON CARBOXYL TRANSFER FROM ENZYME-CO$_2^-$
TO ACETYL-PANTETHEINE

Stoichiometric carboxyl transfer from enzyme-CO$_2^-$ to acetyl-CoA is too rapid to follow by conventional methods even at low temperatures and nonoptimal pH's. Therefore, a valid test of the effect of tricarboxylic acid activator on the rate of transcarboxylation to acetyl-CoA was not feasible. On the other hand, carboxyl transfer to acetylpantetheine, an analog of acetyl-CoA and a poorer acceptor, was sufficiently slow to permit a valid kinetic test (Stoll *et al.*, 1968). The maximal velocity for *S*-acetyl-D-pantetheine in the overall carboxylation reaction is at least two orders of magnitude slower than that for acetyl-CoA. As illustrated in Fig. 3, carboxyl transfer from enzyme-CO$_2^-$ to *S*-acetyl-D-pantetheine to form malonyl-pantetheine exhibits an almost absolute requirement for tricarboxylic acid activator even at an essentially saturating concentration of acetyl-pantetheine (20 mM). It is evident from Fig. 3 that the K_m for acetylpantetheine in the carboxyl transfer reaction is about 5 mM, which is similar to that ($K_m = 6$ mM) for the overall carboxylation reaction (Stoll *et al.*, 1968). The fact that the K_m values for acetyl-CoA (Gregolin *et al.*, 1968a) and acetylpantetheine in the overall carboxylation reaction are not altered by tricarboxylic acid activator suggests that

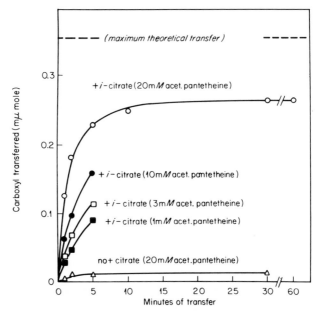

FIG. 3. Kinetics of carboxyl transfer from enzyme-CO$_2^-$ to acetyl-pantetheine to form malonyl pantetheine. Enzyme-^{14}CO$_2^-$ (0.35 mμmole; specific radioactivity 2.5 $\times$ 10^4 cpm/mμmole) was incubated at 25° in a reaction mixture (1 ml total volume and final pH, 7.5) which contained 60 μmoles of Tris (Cl$^-$) buffer, 3 μmoles of GSH, 0.1 μmole of EDTA, and the levels of S-acetyl-D-pantetheine and potassium DL-isocitrate indicated. Aliquots were withdrawn at various times, acidified with HCl, and acid-stable radioactivity (^{14}C-malonyl pantetheine) determined. From Stoll et al. (1968).

binding of the acceptor is not affected by activation. Similarly, the affinity of the carboxylase for acetyl-CoA as determined in direct binding experiments is also not affected by the activator (Gregolin et al., 1968b).

These findings, along with the results of the isotopic exchange experiments, show that both half-reactions (Eqs. 1 and 2), i.e., the carboxylation of the biotin prosthetic group and subsequent transcarboxylation to thioester acceptor, are activated by citrate or isocitrate. This suggests that a substituent at the active site of the carboxylase common to both half-reactions (Eqs. 1 and 2) is the focal point of the citrate-induced conformational change. The fact that citrate is an activator of the V_{max} type and that the isotopic exchange reactions which characterize each half-reaction involve different substrates indicates that this common participant is not a substrate. The most obvious substituent common to both partial reactions is the covalently bound biotin prosthetic group. Further investigation revealed that citrate-induced conformational changes in the vicinity of the prosthetic group could be detected and that these changes were correlated with an enhanced reactivity of the carboxylated biotin prosthetic group.

III. Effect of Activator on the Environment of the Prosthetic Group

In order to evaluate any citrate-induced changes which might be found in the vicinity of the biotinyl group, it was important to have more complete information concerning the number and arrangement of catalytic sites on the carboxylase protomers. As pointed out earlier, the protomer has a molecular weight of 410,000 and is composed of four subunits of about 100,000 daltons each. Furthermore, the enzyme contains 1 mole of covalently bound biotin and binds tightly 1 mole of citrate and 1 mole of acetyl-CoA per 410,000 gm of protein (Gregolin *et al.*, 1966b, 1968b). This is insufficient information to decide whether each protomer has 1 biotin prosthetic group, 1 citrate site, and 1 acetyl-CoA site as visualized in panel B of Fig. 4 or whether these sites are nonuniformly distributed among protomers, e.g., as in panel A of Fig. 4. In the latter case the protomers would be nonidentical. Experiments were undertaken to determine how biotin prosthetic groups are distributed among the protomers within the polymeric form of the carboxylase.

A. Distribution of Biotin Prosthetic Groups within the Polymeric Form of the Carboxylase

To label the biotin-containing protomers, avidin–protomer complexes were formed by reacting the polymeric form of the carboxylase with a stoichiometric excess of avidin for several hours at 0°. Avidin has 4

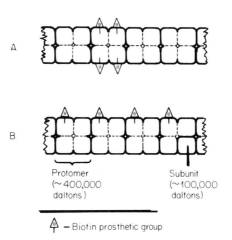

FIG. 4. Distribution of biotin prosthetic groups on carboxylase protomers within the polymeric filamentous form.

biotin-binding sites per molecule and binds either free biotin or the biotinyl group of enzymes almost irreversibly, the K_D for free biotin being
about $10^{-15} M$ (Green, 1963a,b, 1964). An attempt was made to resolve
any avidin–protomer complex which contains biotin from protomers not
containing biotin on biocytin-Sepharose columns as illustrated diagrammatically in Fig. 5. Biocytin-Sepharose was prepared by coupling biocytin (ϵ-N-($+$)-biotinyl-L-lysine) to cyanogen bromide-activated
Sepharose 4B as described by Cuatrecasas and Wilchek (1968). Interaction with avidin depolymerizes the polymeric form of the enzyme, and
the avidin-protomer complex reaggregates and precipitates. Since the
polymer-to-protomer transition involves a conformational change in the
protomer (Gregolin et al., 1968b), this is illustrated diagrammatically in
Fig. 5 by a change in shape of the protomer. The precipitated avidin-
protomer complex was solubilized in $1 M$ guanidine·HCl and applied to
a column of biocytin-Sepharose; the column was eluted with $1 M$
guanidine·HCl. Since each avidin–protomer complex has 3 biotin-binding
sites remaining, on the average, the avidin-bearing protomers, as well
as excess free avidin, should be retained by the column as a result of

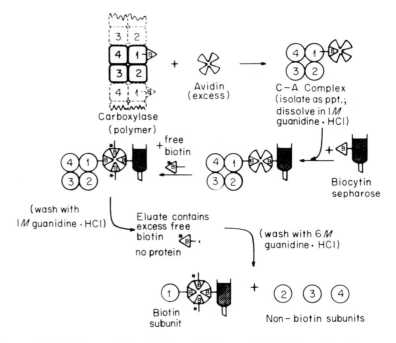

FIG. 5. Method for resolving biotin-containing and biotin-free subunits or protomers.

interaction with biotinyl groups of biocytin-Sepharose. More than 90% of the carboxylase protein applied to the column was retained even after extensive washing with 1 M guanidine·HCl (Fig. 6). The small amount of protein that was eluted from the column at this point was shown to be a minor protein contaminant of the avidin preparation. These results coupled with the biotin content of the carboxylase (1 mole per 410,000 gm of protein) indicate that each protomer contains a single biotin prosthetic group. Thus, it appears that the protomers are identical in this respect and probably monovalent both with respect to carboxylation and activator sites.

It was also possible by this technique to resolve biotin-containing subunits from those not containing biotin by further elution of the biocytin-Sepharose column with higher concentrations of guanidine·HCl. However, it was necessary to protect the "avidin link" from the dissociating effect of guanidine·HCl by loading its remaining sites with free ^{14}C-biotin. It has been demonstrated by Green (1963c), that only when all 4 binding sites are occupied by biotin is avidin resistant to dissociation with 6 M guanidine·HCl. To accomplish this an excess of ^{14}C-biotin was passed

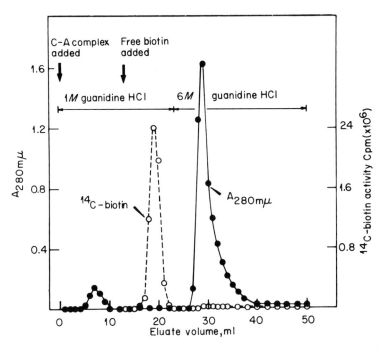

Fig. 6. Resolution of biotin-containing and biotin-free subunits by affinity chromatography on biocytin-Sepharose.

through the column (see Figs. 5 and 6). The amount of ^{14}C-biotin retained by the column could be accounted for by the number of sites theoretically available in the avidin-protomer complex and avidin applied to the column. The carboxylase subunits not containing biotin, i.e., about 75% of the carboxylase protein applied to the column, were eluted from the column with the $6\,M$ guanidine·HCl. Since no biotin-^{14}C appeared in the eluate at this point and since 25% of the carboxylase protein originally applied to the column remained bound, it is evident that the biotin-containing subunits were not eluted from the column by this treatment. These data are consistent with our earlier proposal (Gregolin *et al.*, 1968b) that one of the four 110,000-molecular weight subunits that comprise the protomer contains a biotin prosthetic group.

B. EFFECT ON THE ACCESSIBILITY OF THE BIOTIN PROSTHETIC GROUP TO AVIDIN

To test the hypothesis that activation of acetyl-CoA carboxylase by citrate induces conformational changes at the active site in the vicinity of the biotin prosthetic group, the accessibility of this group to avidin was investigated (Ryder *et al.*, 1967). Avidin inactivates biotin enzymes by binding irreversibly to the bicyclic ring system of biotin, thereby blocking its functional ureido group (Green, 1963a,b). The kinetics of inactivation of acetyl-CoA carboxylase by avidin would be expected to be influenced by changes in the environment of the prosthetic group. As illustrated in Fig. 7, in the presence of citrate the carboxylase is completely resistant to inactivation by avidin, whereas in the absence of activator it is nearly completely inactivated by avidin within 2 minutes. Similar kinetic inactivation patterns were obtained under carboxylase assay conditions in the presence or absence of citrate (Moss and Lane, 1970) indicating that the catalytically active species is not susceptible to avidin while the catalytically inactive species is almost instantly inactivated. It was also observed (Fig. 7) that acetyl-CoA partially protects the carboxylase from avidin. In other experiments, in which the rates of inactivation were increased by raising the avidin to carboxylase ratio, the protection afforded by citrate and acetyl-CoA was synergistic. As will be discussed later (Section IV) tricarboxylic acid and acetyl-CoA also act synergistically in the activation of the decarboxylation of carboxybiotin enzyme. The specificity pattern for the activation of the carboxylase and protection from inactivation by avidin are similar; citrate and isocitrate, which are activators, protect the enzyme from avidin, whereas tricarballylate, neither activates nor protects. Apparently, the biotin prosthetic group becomes shielded by neighboring groups as a result of activator-induced conformational changes at the active site. These results

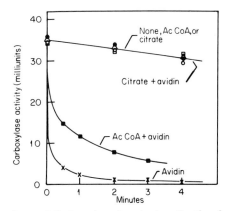

FIG. 7. Susceptibility of acetyl-CoA carboxylase to inactivation by avidin. Avian liver acetyl-CoA carboxylase (4.2 μg) was incubated at 25° in a total volume of 0.5 ml in the presence of 50 μmoles of Tris (Cl⁻), pH 7.5; 5 μmoles of GSH; and 0.1 μmole of EDTA, with the following variable additions: 10 μg of avidin, 5 μmoles of citrate, and 0.1 μmole of acetyl-CoA. Aliquots were withdrawn and assayed by the standard carboxylation assay procedure (Gregolin et al., 1968a) except that 25 μg of (+)-biotin were added to the reaction mixture.

are consistent with the hypothesis that the biotin prosthetic group is the focal point of citrate-induced conformational changes.

IV. EFFECT OF ACTIVATOR ON THE REACTIVITY OF THE CARBOXYLATED BIOTIN PROSTHETIC GROUP

In view of the apparent changes in conformation near the biotin prosthetic group which accompany citrate activation, the possibility was considered that the reactivity of the biotinyl- or N-carboxybiotinyl group might also be altered. Studies on the effect of tricarboxylic acid activator on malonyl-CoA and enzyme-CO_2^- decarboxylation, both of which involve decarboxylation of the N-carboxybiotinyl prosthetic group as the rate-limiting step, indicate that the activator greatly enhances the reactivity of this group.

A. EFFECT ON THE RATE OF MALONYL-CoA DECARBOXYLATION

In the course of investigations on the ¹⁴C-labeled acetyl-CoA–malonyl-CoA exchange, it was observed that acetyl-CoA carboxylase catalyzes an isocitrate- and acetyl-CoA-dependent decarboxylation of malonyl-CoA (Ryder et al., 1967). The rate of this reaction is about 2.5% and 10% that of the overall carboxylation (Eq. 3) and malonyl-CoA-¹⁴C–acetyl-CoA exchange reactions, respectively. As shown in Fig. 8, carboxylase alone supports only a slow rate of malonyl-CoA decarboxylation,

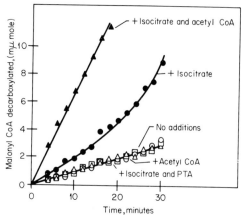

Fig. 8. Kinetics of malonyl-CoA decarboxylation. The rate of malonyl-CoA decarboxylation was determined using a reaction mixture which contained the following components (in μmoles, unless specified): Tris (Cl⁻) buffer, pH 7.5, 30; malonyl-3-¹⁴C-CoA (specific activity, 6.4 × 10⁶ cpm per μmole), 0.02; glutathione (GSH), 1.5; ethylenediaminetetraacetate, 0.1; K·arsenate, 2.5; and acetyl-CoA carboxylase, 8.8 μg, in a total volume of 0.5 ml. Variable additions were: potassium DL-isocitrate, 5 μmoles; acetyl-CoA, 0.03 μmoles; crystalline phosphotransacetylase (PTA), 5 μg (specific activity, 1200 units/mg). The reaction was initiated by the addition of enzyme, allowed to proceed at 25°C, and was terminated by addition of 0.1 ml of 6 N HCl. An aliquot was taken to dryness in a scintillation counting vial at 85°C, water and scintillator were added, and residual acid-stable ¹⁴C-activity was determined using a liquid scintillation spectrometer. From Ryder *et al.* (1967).

which is essentially unaffected by acetyl-CoA, but is increased somewhat by addition of isocitrate. A marked activation of the carboxylase-catalyzed decarboxylation results when both isocitrate (or citrate) and acetyl-CoA are present simultaneously. A synergism between isocitrate and acetyl-CoA is evident from the autocatalytic character of the kinetics of decarboxylation in the presence of isocitrate (Fig. 8). That this is due to the generation of acetyl-CoA from the decarboxylation reaction per se is demonstrated by the reversion from autocatalytic kinetics to zero-order kinetics when an acetyl-CoA trapping system (arsenate and phosphotransacetylase or oxaloacetate and citrate synthase) is added. Like all the other acetyl-CoA carboxylase-catalyzed reactions studied in our laboratory (Gregolin *et al.*, 1968a), malonyl-CoA decarboxylation is avidin-sensitive and is not activated by tricarballylate.

The isocitrate- and acetyl-CoA-activated decarboxylation of malonyl-CoA can be described by the following minimal reaction sequence which is consistent with experimental findings:

$$
\begin{array}{c}
\phantom{E + M\text{-}CoA}\quad \overset{\text{CO}_2^-}{|}\qquad \overset{\text{CO}_2^-}{|} \\
\overset{1'}{E + M\text{-}CoA} \rightleftharpoons \overset{2'}{E(M\text{-}CoA)} \rightleftharpoons \overset{3'}{E(A\text{-}CoA)} \rightleftharpoons E + A\text{-}CoA \\
\qquad\qquad\qquad\downarrow 4' \qquad \downarrow 5' \\
E(A\text{-}CoA) + CO_2 \quad E + CO_2
\end{array}
$$

E represents the enzyme; M-CoA, malonyl CoA; and A-CoA, acetyl CoA. Malonyl-CoA-^{14}C-acetyl-CoA exchange, which involves only the reversible Reactions 1′, 2′, and 3′, is considerably faster than the decarboxylation of malonyl-CoA under comparable conditions either in the presence or the absence of isocitrate. Therefore, either Reaction 4′ or 5′, both of which involve the decarboxylation of a "carboxylated" enzyme species, must be rate-limiting in malonyl-CoA decarboxylation. Since removal of acetyl-CoA by a trapping system (e.g., arsenate and phosphotransacetylase or oxaloacetate and citrate synthase) drastically reduces the rate of malonyl-CoA decarboxylation, it is apparent that

$$
\begin{array}{c}
\text{CO}_2^- \\
| \\
E(A\text{-}CoA)
\end{array}
$$

undergoes decarboxylation (Reaction 4′) more rapidly than

$$
\begin{array}{c}
\text{CO}_2^- \\
| \\
E \;(\text{Reaction } 5')
\end{array}
$$

More direct evidence from studies on the decarboxylation of enzyme-CO_2^- per se supports the idea that both isocitrate and acetyl-CoA affect the reactivity of the carboxy group of enzyme-CO_2^-, hence its susceptibility to decarboxylation.

B. Effect on the Rate of Enzyme-CO_2^- Decarboxylation

The investigations on the decarboxylation of malonyl-CoA indicated that tricarboxylic acid activator and acetyl-CoA activate the rate-limiting step, i.e., the decarboxylation of enzyme-CO_2^-. These findings were corroborated in a more direct manner by following the rate of decarboxylation of enzyme-$^{14}CO_2^-$ (1′-N-^{14}C-carboxybiotinyl enzyme) per se in the presence and absence of isocitrate and/or acetyl-CoA (Ryder $et\ al.$, 1967). As shown in Fig. 9, citrate markedly activates the decarboxylation of enzyme-CO_2^- at pH 7.5 and 25°. This is reflected in the shortening of the half-life of enzyme-CO_2^- from 17–20 minutes to 4–5 minutes and corresponds to a 4- to 5-fold increase in the first-order decarboxylation rate. The effect of citrate is greatly enhanced by the presence of less than saturating concentrations of acetyl-CoA as shown in Table IV. At an acetyl-CoA concentration of 0.5 μM, the addition of citrate activates

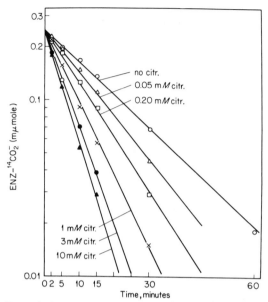

FIG. 9. The effect of citrate on the kinetics of "enzyme-$^{14}CO_2^-$" decarboxylation. Enzyme-$^{14}CO_2^-$, prepared as described by Ryder *et al.* (1967), was warmed to 25°C for 2 minutes and then incubated at 25°C in a reaction mixture containing (in μmoles): Tris (Cl$^-$), pH 7.5, 84; GSH, 4; and EDTA, 0.13 in a total volume of 1.4 ml. Potassium citrate was added as shown in the figure. At each time indicated, a 0.2-ml aliquot was withdrawn and added to 0.2 ml of "transfer" reaction mixture containing 4 μmoles of potassium citrate and 0.075 μmole of acetyl-CoA. One minute at room temperature was allowed for "-$^{14}CO_2^-$" transfer to acetyl-CoA, after which 0.1 ml of 6 N HCl was added. Acid-stable ^{14}C-activity (as malonyl-3-^{14}C-CoA) was then determined. The ordinate in the figure, i.e., mμmoles of "Enz-$^{14}CO_2^-$," represents acid-stable ^{14}C-activity as malonyl-CoA after the transfer reaction. From Ryder *et al.* (1967).

enzyme-CO_2^- decarboxylation at least 10-fold. Since this concentration of acetyl-CoA is 5% of the K_m value (10 μM) and equal to the K_D for acetyl-CoA (Gregolin *et al.*, 1968b), the enzyme is probably far less than half-saturated with acetyl-CoA under these conditions. It would be anticipated, therefore, that at saturating concentrations of acetyl-CoA, activation by citrate would be much greater. However, this cannot be tested by the present method since at higher acetyl-CoA concentrations the decarboxylation rate exceeds the upper reliability limit of measurement. It should also be noted that in the experiments in which acetyl-CoA is added (0.5 μM), the equilibrium described by Reactions 1′, 2′, and 3′ in the preceding section is rapidly established. Since the method used to

TABLE IV

The Effect of Citrate and Acetyl-CoA on the Rate of
Decarboxylation of "Enzyme-CO₂⁻"

Additions	Rate of enzyme-CO_2^- decarboxylation[a] (min^{-1})
None	0.034
+Citrate (10 mM)	0.110 (0.086)
+Acetyl-CoA (0.5 μM)	0.063 (0.029)
+Citrate + acetyl-CoA (0.5 μM)	0.635 (0.601)

[a] Determined at pH 7.5 and 25° as described in legend for Fig. 9 with the avian liver carboxylase (Gregolin et al., 1968a). Values in parentheses are increments above control value.

follow the decay of "-$^{14}CO_2^-$" measures the sum of the rates of decay of enzyme-$^{14}CO_2^-$ and malonyl-3-^{14}C-CoA, the rate of decarboxylation of enzyme-$^{14}CO_2^-$ is slightly underestimated because the concentration of the rate-determining species, i.e., enzyme-CO_2^-, is lower by about 10% in the presence of acetyl-CoA (see Ryder et al., 1967). It is evident that the simultaneous presence of citrate and acetyl-CoA renders enzyme-CO_2^- more susceptible to decarboxylation, presumably because of conformational changes at the active site which enhance the reactivity of the carboxy group of carboxybiotinyl enzyme.

V. Discussion and Summation

Extensive earlier investigations have shown that acetyl-CoA carboxylases from animal tissues are capable of oscillating between catalytically inactive protomeric and catalytically active polymeric states, the level of carboxylase activity being determined by the position of the protomer-polymer equilibrium (Gregolin et al., 1966a,b, 1968a,b; Numa et al., 1966; Kleinschmidt et al., 1969). Citrate and isocitrate are capable of shifting this equilibrium in favor of the catalytically active form presumably by binding preferentially to the polymeric species. As demonstrated above, activation is also accompanied by a conformational change at the active site in the vicinity of the biotin prosthetic group as evidenced by the decreased accessibility of the prosthetic group to avidin in the presence of tricarboxylic acid activator. This and several other lines of evidence are consistent with the hypothesis that the biotin prosthetic group is the focal point of citrate-induced conformational changes. The observations, that citrate is an allosteric activator of the V_{max} type and that the half-reactions (Eqs. 1 and 2), both of which involve the biotinyl group as a common participant, are citrate activated, support this view. Furthermore, it is evident that the reactivity of the carboxy group of carboxy-biotinyl enzyme is greatly enhanced by tricarboxylic acid activator, particularly in the presence of acetyl-CoA.

Further insight into the effect of citrate on the biotinyl prosthetic group was gained in experiments on the carboxylation of free biotin. The high degree of specificity for (+)-biotin or closely related derivatives in this reaction indicates that binding and carboxylation of the free species occurs at the same specific site normally occupied by the bicyclic ring of the biotinyl prosthetic group. Since the functional bicyclic ring resides at the distal end of a flexible 14 Å side chain (Stoll *et al.*, 1968) which anchors it to the apoprotein, secondary binding sites must be required to precisely orient the ureido ring system with respect to the substrates with which it must react. One possible mechanism for the citrate effect on transcarboxylation rate is that the carboxybiotin prosthetic group may be brought into closer proximity to substrate binding sites by activator-induced conformational changes as illustrated diagrammatically in Fig. 10. Citrate may enhance the affinity of a binding site in the

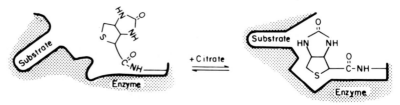

Fig. 10. Hypothetical scheme depicting the effect of tricarboxylic acid activator on the biotin prosthetic group of acetyl-CoA carboxylase.

vicinity of the substrate site for the bicyclic ring of the prosthetic group and thereby facilitate reaction. This would account for the V_{max} effect of the activator and would be consistent with the observation (Table III) that the K_m values for free (+)-biotin, (+)-homobiotin, and biocytin are increased by citrate. If citrate increases the affinity of an enzyme site for the bicyclic ring of the biotinyl prosthetic group, higher concentrations of the free biotin analogs would be required to displace this group. This interpretation is also supported by the fact that the biotinyl prosthetic group is less accessible to avidin in the citrate-activated enzyme.

ACKNOWLEDGMENTS

Many of the investigations reported in this paper were supported by research grants from the National Institutes of Health, USPHS (AM14574 and AM14575) and the American Heart Association, Inc. and a USPHS Research Career Program Award (K3-AM-18487).

REFERENCES

Alberts, A. W., Nervi, A. M., and Vagelos, P. R. (1969). *Proc. Nat. Acad. Sci. U. S.* **63**, 1319.

Cuatrecasas, P., and Wilchek, M. (1968). *Biochem. Biophys. Res. Commun.* **33**, 235.

Green, N. M. (1963a). *Biochem. J.* **89**, 585.

Green, N. M. (1963b). *Biochem. J.* **89**, 599.

Green, N. M. (1963c). *Biochem. J.* **89**, 609.

Green, N. M. (1964). *Biochem. J.* **90**, 564.

Gregolin, C., Ryder, E., Kleinschmidt, A. K., Warner, R. C., and Lane, M. D. (1966a). *Proc. Nat. Acad. Sci. U. S.* **56**, 148.

Gregolin, C., Ryder, E., Warner, R. C., Kleinschmidt, A. K., and Lane, M. D. (1966b). *Proc. Nat. Acad. Sci. U. S.* **56**, 1751.

Gregolin, C., Ryder, E., and Lane, M. D. (1968a). *J. Biol. Chem.* **243**, 4227.

Gregolin, C., Ryder, E., Warner, R. C., Kleinschmidt, A. K., Chang, H. C., and Lane, M. D. (1968b). *J. Biol. Chem.* **243**, 4236.

Kallen, R. G., and Lowenstein, J. (1962). *Arch. Biochem. Biophys.* **96**, 188.

Kleinschmidt, A. K., Moss, J., and Lane, M. D. (1969). *Science* **166**, 1276.

Knappe, J., Schlegal, H. G., and Lynen, F. (1961a). *Biochem. Z.* **335**, 101.

Knappe, J., Ringelmann, E., and Lynen, F. (1961b). *Biochem. Z.* **335**, 168.

Lane, M. D., and Moss, J. (1971). *In* "Metabolic Pathways" (D. M. Greenberg, ed.), 3rd ed., Vol. V. Academic Press, New York (in preparation).

Lane, M. D., Moss, J., Dimroth, P., Guchhait, R. B., Stoll, E., Edwards, J. B., and Kleinschmidt, A. K. (1970). *Abstr. 8th Int. Congr. Biochem., 1969* (in press).

Lowenstein, J. (1968). *Biochem. Soc. Symp.* **27**, 61–86.

Lynen, F., Knappe, J., Lorch, E., Jütting, G., Ringelmann, E., and LaChance, J. P. (1961). *Biochem. Z.* **335**, 123.

Majerus, P. W., and Kilburn, E. (1969). *J. Biol. Chem.* **244**, 6254.

Martin, D. B., and Vagelos, P. R. (1962). *J. Biol. Chem.* **237**, 1787.

Matsuhashi, M., Matsuhashi, S., Numa, S., and Lynen, F. (1962). *Fed. Proc., Fed. Amer. Soc. Exp. Biol.* **21**, 288.

Matsuhashi, M., Matsuhashi, S., and Lynen, F. (1964). *Biochem. Z.* **340**, 263.

Miller, A. L., and Levy, H. R. (1969). *J. Biol. Chem.* **244**, 2334.

Monod, J., Changeux, J. P., and Jacob, F. (1963). *J. Mol. Biol.* **6**, 306.

Monod, J., Wyman, J., and Changeux, J. P. (1965). *J. Mol. Biol.* **12**, 88.

Moss, J., and Lane, M. D. (1970). Unpublished observations.

Moss, J., Kleinschmidt, A. K., Yamagishi, M., and Lane, M. D. (1969). *Fed. Proc., Fed. Amer. Soc. Exp. Biol.* **28**, 1548.

Moss, J., Yamagishi, M., and Lane, M. D. (1970). Unpublished observations (manuscript in preparation).

Numa, S., Ringelmann, E., and Lynen, F. (1964). *Biochem. Z.* **340**, 228.

Numa, S., Ringelmann, E., and Lynen, F. (1965). *Biochem. Z.* **343**, 243.

Numa, S., Ringelmann, E., and Riedel, B. (1966). *Biochem. Biophys. Res. Commun.* **24**, 750.

Ochoa, S., and Kaziro, Y. (1965). *Comp. Biochem.* **16**, 244–378.

Ryder, E., Gregolin, C., Chang, H. C., and Lane, M. D. (1967). *Proc. Nat. Acad. Sci. U. S.* **57**, 1455.

Stoll, E., Ryder, E., Edwards, J., and Lane, M. D. (1968). *Proc. Nat. Acad. Sci. U. S.* **60**, 986.

Vagelos, P. R. (1964). *Annu. Rev. Biochem.* **33**, 139.

Waite, M., and Wakil, S. J. (1962). *J. Biol. Chem.* **237**, 2750.

Thiamine Pyrophosphate-Catalyzed Enzymatic Decarboxylation of α-Oxo Acids

JOHANNES ULLRICH, YURI M. OSTROVSKY,*
JAIME EYZAGUIRRE,† AND HELMUT HOLZER

Biochemisches Institut der Universität, Freiburg im Breisgau, Germany

I. Introduction

The first enzymatic decarboxylation of an α-oxo acid was described by Neuberg and Karczag (1911): a fermenting extract from brewer's yeast cleaves pyruvate into acetaldehyde and carbon dioxide. Auhagen (1932) found that, besides the protein of the enzyme, a thermostable cofactor ("cocarboxylase") is necessary for this enzymatic cleavage of pyruvate. Five years later, Lohmann and Schuster (1937) established the identity of cocarboxylase with thiamine pyrophosphate (Fig. 1). For decarboxylation of other α-oxo acids to the corresponding aldehydes, for their oxidative decarboxylation leading to acyl coenzyme A derivatives, and for a number of other enzymatic reactions (Table I), the same coenzyme was found to be necessary (summary by Metzler, 1960).

Theories on the mechanism of thiamine pyrophosphate-catalyzed α-oxo acid decarboxylation were developed by Langenbeck (1933), Karrer and Viscontini (1946), Reed (1953), Wiesner and Valenta (1956), Breslow (1956), and others (see review by Metzler, 1960), until Breslow (1957a,b) formulated the concept that is now generally accepted (Fig. 2a–c).

* Present address: Department of Biochemistry, State Medical Institute, Grodno, Bielorussian SSR, USSR.

† Present address: Department of Biochemistry, Catholic University, Santiago, Chile.

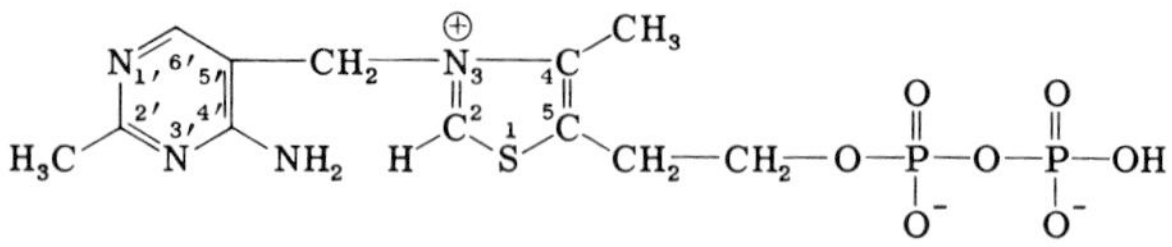

FIG. 1. Formula of thiamine pyrophosphate with conventional numbering.

Experimental data that could have led to at least partial elucidation of Breslow's mechanism had been collected since 1937: when measuring H-D exchange of thiaminium dichloride in D_2O, Hamill (1937) found a single exchangeable C-bound hydrogen with comparably slow exchange rate in addition to the expected four N- and O-bound hydrogens, which exchange very rapidly. Todd and Bergel (1937), Bergel and Todd (1937), and Schultz (1940), after screening the vitamin B_1 efficiency of numerous homologs and analogs of thiamine, stated total and persistent failure of 2-alkylated thiamine derivatives to show B_1 activity, whereas thiamines with altered substituents at other C atoms exhibited only gradual and nonsystematic differences in their vitamin B_1 effect (summary by Rogers, 1962). Ugai et al. (1943), Mizuhara et al. (1951), Mizuhara and Handler (1954), and Downes and Sykes (1957) found the same situation to apply to nonenzymatic "model" reactions catalyzed by thiazolium salts, e.g., acyloin condensations from a variety of aldehydes in slightly alkaline solution.

Finally, Breslow (1957a,b) succeeded in directly localizing the catalytic site of thiamine and of model thiazolium compounds by infrared and

TABLE I

THIAMINE PYROPHOSPHATE DEPENDENT ENZYMATIC REACTIONS

Pyruvate → acetaldehyde + CO_2
Pyruvate → acetyl-CoA + CO_2 + 2H
Glyoxylate → formyl-CoA(δ) + CO_2 + 2H
α-Oxobutyrate → propionyl-CoA + CO_2 + 2H
α-Oxoisovalerate → isobutyryl-CoA + CO_2 + 2H
α-Oxoisocaproate → isovaleryl-CoA + CO_2 + 2H
α-Oxo-β-methylvalerate → α-methylbutyryl-CoA + CO_2 + 2H
Hydroxypyruvate → glycolyl-CoA + CO_2 + 2H
α-Oxoglutarate → succinyl-CoA + CO_2 + 2H
α-Oxoadipate → glutarate (δ) + CO_2 + 2H
Pyruvate + acetaldehyde → acetoin + CO_2
Pyruvate + pyruvate → α-acetolactate + CO_2
Pyruvate + α-oxobutyrate → α-aceto-α-hydroxybutyrate + CO_2
Glyoxylate + glyoxylate → tartronic semialdehyde + CO_2
α-Oxoglutarate + glyoxylate → γ-oxo-δ-hydroxyhexanoate + CO_2
Transketolase reactions
Phosphoketolase reactions

nuclear magnetic resonance spectrometry of their proton-deuterium exchange in D_2O. From these experiments he developed the scheme for the reaction mechanism shown in Fig. 2, which in the following years became generally accepted and, in its main parts, is still valid today. It is the basis of all subsequent work in the field of thiamine catalysis and is thus discussed in detail in the next section.

II. Mechanism of Nonenzymatic Thiamine (Thiazolium) Catalysis

By comparison of thiamine catalysis with that of cyanide in the acyloin condensation, Breslow (1957a,b, 1958; reviews, 1961, 1962) came to the following conclusions (Fig. 2a): thiamine (I) forms a 2-carbanion (II) with a pK comparable to that of HCN (pK ~9); the upper limit found for the pK was 20 (McNelis, 1960). The exclusively kinetic measurements could not account for activation energy, and therefore the pK of thiamine is expected to be several units lower. The 2-carbanion (II) has the character of an ylid (zwitterion with adjacent charges). By its addition to the polarized oxo group of the substrate, an intermediate (III) is formed which decarboxylates rapidly to the α-carbanion (IV) of a 2-α-hydroxy-alkylthiamine (V). This α-carbanion is aliphatic and thus must be a very strong nucleophile. In Breslow's scheme it is stabilized by resonance with the species (VI). Pullman and Spanjaard (1961) arrived at the same conclusions in their calculations of energy levels and electron distribution in the thiamine molecule. A protonation equilibrium is assumed to exist between (IV) and (V), their relative concentrations depending on the pH of the solution.

For the liberation of aldehyde, the final step of the decarboxylation reaction, Breslow could not decide whether (IV) or (V) or even a third species (VII) is the most likely starting molecule; he used all three of them in his various formulations of the mechanism.

For the enzymatic decarboxylation, Schellenberger (1967) assumed a base catalysis by the 4'-NH_2 group, resulting in the release of the aldehyde moiety, as an addition to Breslow's concept of the mechanism.

For the acyloin condensation (Fig. 2b), the α-carbanion (IV) is the only possible candidate[*] for the addition to the polarized oxo group of an acceptor aldehyde (or α-oxo acid), leading to thiamine-bound acyloin (VIII) or 2-acyl-2-hydroxycarboxylic acid). For the formulation of the liberation of these species from the thiamine residue, the same difficulties arise as for simple aldehydes.

The oxidative transfer of the aldehyde group from thiamine pyrophos-

---

[*] From electron paramagnetic resonance measurements, Babitcheva et al. (1968) assumed a mixed-type mechanism for the acyloin condensation, partly ionic and partly radicalic, due to the ability of the thiazolium ring to hide single electrons in its π-electron system.

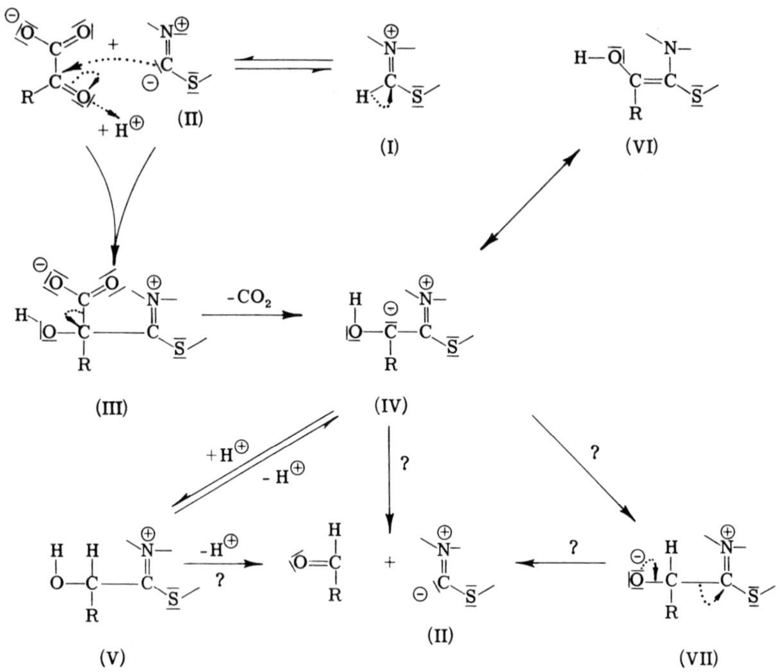

Fig. 2a.

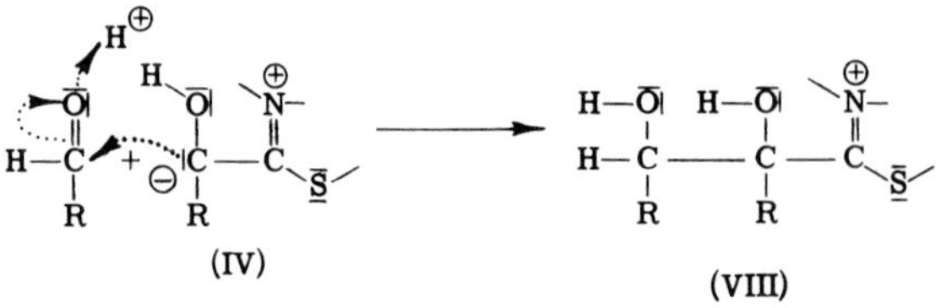

Fig. 2b.

phate to lipoic acid, occurring exclusively in enzymatic reactions catalyzed by α-oxo acid dehydrogenase complexes (review by Reed and Cox, 1966), with the aid of several coenzymes, again can be best formulated with the α-carbanion (IV) as starting species (Fig. 2c). In a concerted multicenter mechanism oxidized lipoic acid and the α-carbanion of 2-α-hydroxyalkyl-thiamine pyrophosphate (IV) are converted to 6-S-acylated dihydrolipoic acid and free thiamine pyrophosphate as 2-carbanion (II). The subsequent and last step of the enzymatic reaction sequence catalyzed by the complex is a transfer of the acyl group from lipoic acid to coenzyme A without changing the thioester-type bonding and the oxidation state of the residue.

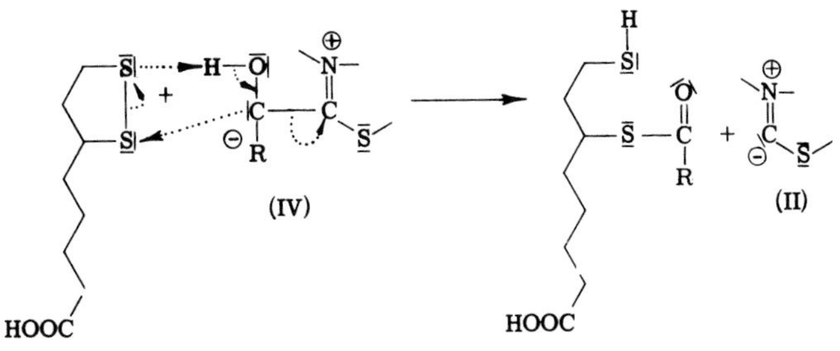

Fig. 2c.

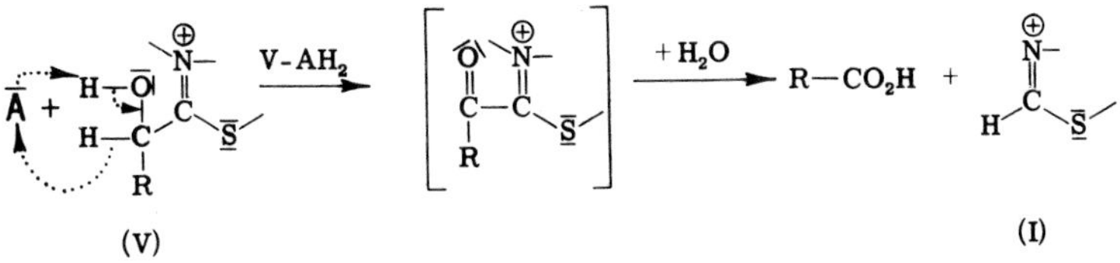

Fig. 2d.

Fig. 2. Breslow's mechanism of thiazolium catalysis and related reactions. (a) Full sequence with liberation of aldehyde. (b) Acyloin condensation. (c) Oxidative transfer of the aldehyde residue from thiamine pyrophosphate (TPP) to lipoic acid. (d) Nonenzymatic oxidation of 2-α-hydroxyalkyl-TPP by an artificial hydrogen acceptor (A) to 2-acyl-TPP, which is rapidly hydrolyzed to carboxylic acid and TPP.

Schellenberger (summary, 1967) emphasized that the above-mentioned resonance stabilization of the α-carbanion (IV), which plays a key role at least in the latter two reactions, must depend on parallel orientation of the two α-substituents (alkyl and OH) to the thiazolium ring. This conformation, however, is prevented by steric hindrance (Fig. 3) at least for 2-α-hydroxyalkylthiamine pyrophosphates bound to the active site of pyruvate decarboxylase. Thus a ready re-formation of the α-carbanion (IV) from the protonated species (V) appears doubtful, at least in the enzymatic process.

2-α-Hydroxyethylthiamine has been synthesized by Krampitz et al. (1958) and Miller et al. (1962) in the protonated form. Upon treatment with an ATP-regenerating system and alkali-washed yeast containing thiamine pyrophosphokinase this product is converted to a substance which can substitute for thiamine pyrophosphate as coenzyme in the decarboxylation of pyruvate. These experiments first indicated a biological significance of Breslow's theory (for further references, see the review by Krampitz, 1969). Definite evidence that Breslow's model functions in the enzymatic catalysis was obtained by the isolation of 2-α-hydroxyethylthiamine pyrophosphate from enzymatic reaction mixtures, as described in the following section.

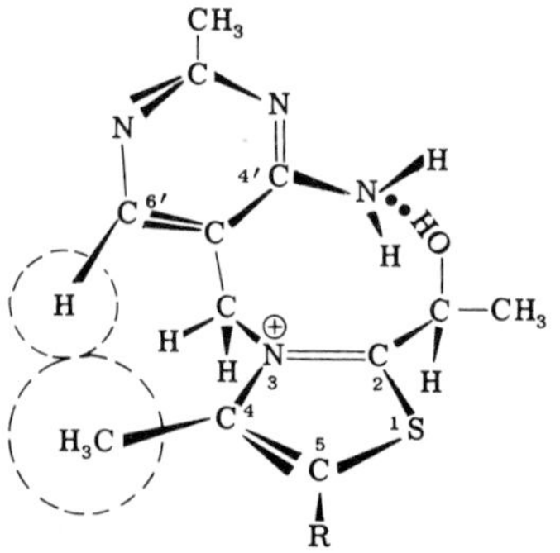

$$R = -(CH_2)_2-O-P_2O_6H_3$$

FIG. 3. Space formula of 2-α-hydroxyethyl thiamine pyrophosphate in the conformation of most intense interaction of α-hydroxy and 4'-amino groups (Schellenberger, 1967).

III. ISOLATION OF 2-α-HYDROXYALKYL DERIVATIVES OF THIAMINE PYROPHOSPHATE FROM ENZYMATIC INCUBATION MIXTURES

Direct proof that 2-α-hydroxyalkyl derivatives of thiamine pyrophosphate are intermediates in an enzyme-catalyzed reaction was presented by Holzer and Beaucamp (1959, 1961), working with purified pyruvate decarboxylase from brewer's yeast. From enzymatic incubations with 2- or 3-^{14}C-labeled pyruvate, small quantities of ^{14}C-labeled "active pyruvate" and "active acetaldehyde" could be isolated by paper chromatography. By enzymatic conversion of these intermediates to acetaldehyde and CO_2, or to acetoin, and particularly by sulfite cleavage (Williams et al., 1935) and identification of the cleavage products, the structures of these intermediates were proved to be 2-α-hydroxy-α-carboxyethyl-TPP* for "active pyruvate" and 2-α-hydroxyethyl-TPP for "active acetaldehyde." From incubation mixtures of wheat germ pyruvate decarboxylase with pyruvate or acetaldehyde, Carlson and Brown (1960) isolated compounds which, after dephosphorylation, were compared with synthetic 2-α-hydroxyethylthiamine by paper chromatography. One spot exhibiting the R_f value of 2-α-hydroxyethylthiamine could be identified by bioautography as thiamine derivative and found to contain ^{14}C from pyruvate-^{14}C applied to the mixture. Larger quantities of 2-α-hydroxyalkyl derivatives of TPP could be prepared using a crude preparation of α-oxo acid dehydrogenase complexes from pig heart. This was incubated

---

* TPP: nonstandard abbreviation for thiamine pyrophosphate.

with an excess of α-oxo acid and TPP, but without NAD and coenzyme A (summary by Deus et al., 1970). Using pyruvate, 2-α-hydroxyethyl-TPP ("active acetaldehyde") was isolated (Scriba and Holzer, 1961; Ullrich and Holzer, 1963) and shown to be the levorotatory enantiomer (Ullrich and Mannschreck, 1967); from glyoxylate, 2-hydroxymethyl-TPP ("active formaldehyde") was formed (Kohlhaw et al., 1965); hydroxypyruvate gave 2-α,β-dihydroxyethyl-TPP ("active glycolaldehyde") (H. Holzer et al., 1962; Da Fonseca-Wollheim et al., 1962; Pohlandt et al., 1967). All three "active aldehydes" were obtained in good yields. α-Oxoglutarate could be converted to 2-α-hydroxy-γ-carboxypropyl-TPP ("active succinic semialdehyde") only with poor yield (Deus et al., 1970). The structures of the compounds were shown, by a variety of methods, to agree with those proposed by Breslow (1957a,b, 1958, 1961, 1962) (see Fig. 2).

2-α-Hydroxyethyl-TPP is oxidized by dichlorophenolindophenol, ferricyanide, or several other electron acceptors to acetic acid and TPP. The same artificial oxidants had been shown to cause acetate production by yeast pyruvate decarboxylase (Holzer and Goedde, 1957b; Holzer and Crawford, 1960). Very probably this oxidation proceeds via 2-acetyl-TPP. In this derivative the acetyl residue is attached to the C-2 of TPP by a very high-energy bond (Breslow and McNelis, 1960; Nash et al., 1961; White and Ingraham, 1962; Lienhard, 1966) and is released very rapidly in aqueous solution by hydrolysis (Fig. 2d).

IV. Enzymatic Conversions of 2-α-Hydroxyalkyl Derivatives of Thiamine Pyrophosphate

Figure 4 demonstrates the reactions of 2-α-hydroxyethyl-TPP which could be anticipated from earlier knowledge of pyruvate metabolism. "Active acetaldehyde," isolated from incubations with α-oxo acid dehydrogenase complex, could be demonstrated to undergo all the formulated enzymatic reactions (summaries, Holzer, 1961; H. Holzer et al., 1962; Goedde, 1963; Ullrich et al., 1968). 2-α,β-Dihydroxyethyl-TPP ("active glycolaldehyde") was shown to be used by transketolase for the formation of sedoheptulose 7-phosphate (Prochoroff et al., 1962) and of erythrulose (Holzer, 1961). By phosphoketolase it was converted to acetylphosphate (Schröter and Holzer, 1963).

In contrast to the normal behavior of intermediates in enzymatic reactions, the conversions of the "active aldehydes," fed into the appropriate enzyme systems, are considerably slower than the complete reaction sequences of the same enzyme systems, starting from the α-oxo acids. This problem deserves detailed treatment.

Figure 5 shows the single reaction steps of the conversion of pyruvate

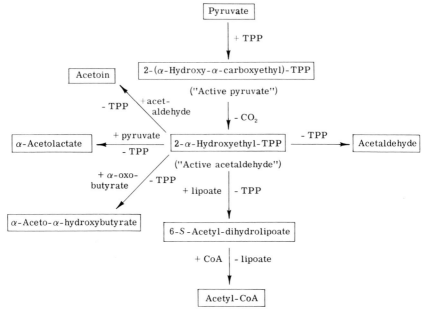

Fig. 4. Enzymatic reactions of 2-α-hydroxyethyl thiamine pyrophoshate.

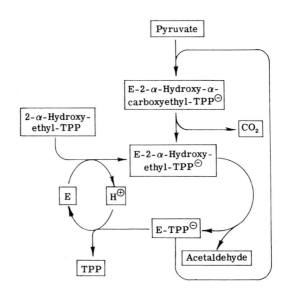

Fig. 5. Liberation of acetaldehyde from pyruvate and from 2-α-hydroxyethyl-TPP. Scheme of single reaction steps.

to acetaldehyde (top to bottom, right side) and of 2-α-hydroxyethyl-TPP to acetaldehyde (from left to right side, bottom). That the conversion rate of 2-α-hydroxyethyl-TPP is 3–4 orders of magnitude lower than that of pyruvate (Goedde, 1963; Goedde et al., 1965) was first thought to be due to a rate-limiting exchange of the enzyme-bound TPP against 2-α-hydroxyethyl-TPP (Holzer, 1961; Goedde, 1963; Krampitz et al., 1961, 1963). If this were true, the rate-limiting step could be avoided by incubation of 2-α-hydroxyethyl-TPP with stoichiometric quantities of apopyruvate decarboxylase and Mg^{2+}. An initial rapid reaction was found in qualitative experiments with wheat germ pyruvate decarboxylase by Krampitz et al. (1961). More detailed experiments with yeast pyruvate decarboxylase (Table II), however, failed to show any initial rapid conversion of 2-α-hydroxyethyl-TPP to acetaldehyde in amounts stoichiometric to the added enzyme. In these experiments, a burst of acetaldehyde equal to 10% of the amount of active apoenzyme present in the mixture would have been detected with certainty, based on the assumptions of 2 TPP-binding sites of pyruvate decarboxylase and of only 50% of the enzyme surviving the coenzyme resolution treatment (Ullrich et al., 1966). Therefore slow dissociation of TPP was ruled out as a possible explanation for the low conversion rate of "active acetaldehyde." Another possibility, a slow and thus rate-limiting recombination of 2-α-hydroxyethyl-TPP with apopyruvate decarboxylase, was checked by Schellenberger and his group (summary, Schellenberger, 1967), who found indeed no enzyme-binding of any 2-substituted TPP derivative because of steric hindrance (Fig. 3). Since Schellenberger got "all-or-nothing" effects, no calculation of the ratio of the conversion rate of 2-α-hydroxyethyl-TPP to that of pyruvate could be based on his data. Measurements of the concentration for half-maximal rate of 2-α-hydroxyethyl-TPP conversion

TABLE II

CHECK FOR STOICHIOMETRIC CONVERSION OF 2-α-HYDROXYETHYL
THIAMINE PYROPHOSPHATE BY APOPYRUVATE DECARBOXYLASE[a]

Apo-PDC[b] (nmoles)	1.2	2.3	6.5	11.5
$\Delta A_{366\,nm}$ observed[c]	+0.002	0.000	+0.002	0.000
$\Delta A_{366\,nm}$ calculated[d]	−0.004	−0.008	−0.021	−0.038

[a] Each sample contained in a total volume of 2 ml: 230 μmoles of citrate, 30 μmoles of phosphate, 10 μmoles of $MgSO_4$, ca. 0.5 μmole of NADH, 1 mg of alcohol dehydrogenase, 1 μmole of 2-α-hydroxyethyl-TPP (in 0.1 ml used for starting). Light path, 1 cm; final pH = 6.2; temperature 25°C. Readings were taken before and 1 minute after start.

[b] Active enzyme in the preparation which after the experiment had a specific activity of 31 units/mg (30°, TPP and Mg^{2+} saturated) (Ullrich et al., 1966).

[c] Corrected with the absorption difference of a blank without enzyme.

[d] Assuming 2 binding sites for TPP per enzyme molecule.

TABLE III

LIBERATION OF ACETALDEHYDE FROM 2-α-HYDROXYETHYL-TPP AND FROM
PYRUVATE BY CYTOPLASMIC APO- AND HOLOPYRUVATE DECARBOXYLASE
FROM BREWER'S YEAST[a]

Substrate	K_M	Turnover number per second (moles of substrate per mole of enzyme)
2-α-Hydroxyethyl-TPP	$4.8 \times 10^{-4} M$[b]	0.013
Pyruvate	$1.3 \times 10^{-3} M$[c]	42.5[d]

[a] Goedde *et al.* (1965). Conditions: pH = 6.0, 25°, Mg^{2+}-saturation; NADH consumption by the liberated acetaldehyde with alcohol dehydrogenase was measured.
[b] For TPP was found $K_M = 2.4 \times 10^{-5} M$. Later measurements of the authors gave $6 \times 10^{-6} M$.
[c] Values of several earlier authors for this reaction.
[d] The enzyme was only partially purified. With pure enzyme the highest turnover number per second and mole of enzyme obtained thus far was 220.

to acetaldehyde by apopyruvate decarboxylase (Table III) gave a value of $4.8 \times 10^{-4} M$ (Goedde *et al.*, 1965). Even at full saturation with 2-α-hydroxyethyl-TPP, the rate of its conversion to acetaldehyde is 3–4 orders of magnitude slower than that of pyruvate. Thus lower affinity of 2-α-hydroxyethyl-TPP to the enzyme cannot explain the low reaction rate of this substance.

Therefore a third possibility is worth considering: 2-α-hydroxyethyl-TPP, as isolated in the proton-saturated form (V), may not be the real intermediate, but requires previous activation by removal of a proton, i.e., conversion to its α-carbanion (IV). Breslow (1962) had postulated ready re-formation of this α-carbanion. Nuclear magnetic resonance measurements (Ullrich and Mannschreck, 1967; Mieyal *et al.*, 1967) revealed, however, that the re-formation of the α-carbanion can proceed at a detectable rate only at pH values above 8 and must be very slow at the pH optimum (6–7) of pyruvate decarboxylase activity. Therefore the dissociation of the α-proton from 2-α-hydroxyethyl-TPP might well be the rate-limiting step for its conversion to free acetaldehyde and enzyme-bound TPP.

This last possibility is supported by an isotope effect on the production of free acetaldehyde and of acetoin (Table IV) when D_2O was used as solvent for the enzymatic decarboxylation of pyruvate. Acetoin is a side product which is always formed in relatively small quantities (Neuberg and Hirsch, 1921; Neuberg and Ohle, 1922; Juni, 1961) in addition to acetaldehyde, which is a potent uncompetitive inhibitor of the overall reaction (Gruber and Wesselius, 1962). While the overall reaction rate,

TABLE IV

PYRUVATE DECARBOXYLATION AND ACETOIN FORMATION BY
YEAST PYRUVATE DECARBOXYLASE IN H_2O AND D_2O[a]

Solvent	H_2O	D_2O	H_2O	D_2O	H_2O	D_2O
Holopyruvate Decarboxylase[b] (μg)	2		2		4	
Reaction time (min)	60		30		60	
CO_2 evolved[b] (μmoles)	6.14	3.79	3.33	2.22	9.07	5.50
Acetoin formed[c] (μmoles)	0.125	0.145	0.073	0.090	0.251	0.297
Acetoin/CO_2[d]	0.02	0.04	0.02	0.04	0.03	0.06

[a] Each sample contained 40 μmoles of pyruvate in 1.00 ml of 0.1 M citrate pH = 6.0 at 25°C.

[b] Prepared by the method of Ullrich et al. (1966).

[c] Determined manometrically (Umbreit et al., 1964).

[d] Determined by the method of Westerfeld (1945) after distillation.

measured by CO_2 liberation, was approximately halved by use of D_2O as solvent instead of H_2O, the yield of acetoin was found to be slightly increased. As in earlier experiments by Juni (1961), acetaldehyde added to the reaction mixture reduced the overall rate of pyruvate decarboxylation, but had no effect on the yield of acetoin. This indicates that acetoin condensation involves only acetaldehyde molecules just formed and probably still attached to the enzyme in appropriate position.

Based on Schellenberger's concept (1967) of product release being the rate-limiting step of the overall reaction, the following interpretation of the experimental observations can be given.

The "active intermediate" for acetoin condensation is the α-carbanion (IV). Since acetoin formation is not subjected to a deuterium effect, reformation of the α-carbanion from the protonated molecule appears to be ruled out. Acetoin thus originates from the primary α-carbanion which is left after the decarboxylation step.

Acetaldehyde liberation, on the other hand, is affected by deuterium. Therefore protons or a proton-carrying group should be involved in this process. In this context several possibilities have to be considered, namely, the protonation of the α-carbanion [(IV) → (V)], the proton transfer from the α-OH to the α-C [(IV) → (VII)], and the base catalysis by the 4'-NH_2 group assumed by Schellenberger (1967).

V. EFFECTS OF SUBSTITUENTS AT THE THIAZOLIUM RING

A strong dependence of C-2 reactivity on the nature of the substituent at N-3⊕ was found already in model experiments by Mizuhara et al.

(1951), Mizuhara and Handler (1954), Downes and Sykes (1957), Breslow (1958), and Breslow and McNelis (1959). The most efficient group turned out to be a 5-(4-aminopyrimidine)methyl residue which is most strongly electron-withdrawing. This is followed by a benzyl group and, at great distance, by simple alkyl groups.

The 4-methyl group appears to have no significant influence on C-2 reactivity. Its enlargement, however, gives rise (see Fig. 3) to some steric hindrance of protein-binding (Schellenbereger, 1967). On the other hand, the 5-β-hydroxyethyl group has pronounced influence on the electronic state at C-2 (Risinger and Dove, 1965; Ostrovsky, 1967, 1968). Changes in its chain length, phosphorylation, or replacement of the β-hydroxy group in thiamine or oxythiamine by chlorine or hydrogen produce striking differences in the ninhydrin and formalin-azo reactions of the homologs or analogs (Table V) and in their catalytic activity for the forma-

TABLE V

NINHYDRIN AND FORMALIN-AZO REACTIONS OF THIAMINE ANALOGS AND
HOMOLOGS WITH ALTERED 5-SUBSTITUENT[a]

Compound	Ninhydrin reaction[a] ($A_{430 nm}$)	Formalin-Azo reaction[b]
Thiamine	0.30	0.30
Thiamine monophosphate	0.15	0.22
Thiamine pyrophosphate	0.09	0.14
Thiamine triphosphate	0.03	0.10
5-Ethylthiamine	0.27	0.27
5-Methylthiamine	0.10	0.22
5-Hydroxymethylthiamine	0.27	0.01
5-γ-Hydroxypropylthiamine	0.24	0.01
5-β-Chloroethylthiamine	0.01	0.06
Tetrahydrothiamine	0.00	0.00

[a] Ostrovsky and Gvozdeva (1959, 1960).
[b] Conditions as described by Kinnersley and Peters (1934).

tion of acetoin (Risinger and Dove, 1965). The pK's, the rates of pseudobase formation, and the Hammett-Taft induction constants are changed as well (Table VI, Figs. 6 and 7). As a general rule, increased electrophilicity of the 5-substituent weakens the binding of the 2-proton and lowers the pK of pseudobase formation. The main mechanism for such action of substituents may be σ-σ-interaction and σ-π-hyperconjugation (Palm, 1968). The effects depend on the functioning of an intact thiazolium π-electron system. Even the imidazolium analog of TPP is catalytically inactive (Schellenberger et al., 1969). Decrease of reactivity at C-2 by phosphorylation of the OH group is probably more than overcome

TABLE VI

C-2-Reactivities and Hammett-Taft Constants of Thiamine Analogs and Homologs with Altered 5-Substituent[a]

Compound	pK	$k \times 10^{2b}$			Hammett-Taft constant σ*			
		pH 10.2	pH 10.8	pH 11.2	pH 7.4	pH 10.2	pH 10.8	pH 11.2
Thiamine	9.20	3.37	3.59	4.80	+0.59	−0.14	−0.33	−0.47
5-Ethylthiamine	9.60	2.66	3.81	7.45	−0.11	−0.25	−0.30	−0.28
5-Methylthiamine	9.50	4.70	7.60	14.3	—	—	—	—
5-Hydroxymethylthiamine	7.60	31.0	37.0	43.8	+2.23	+0.82	+0.68	+0.49
5-γ-Hydroxypropylthiamine	9.45	2.60	2.90	3.10	+0.56	−0.26	−0.42	−0.56
5-β-Chloroethylthiamine	7.05	1140	1800	—	+1.75	+2.38	+2.55	—

[a] Ostrovsky (1967) and Ostrovsky et al. (1970).

[b] $k = \frac{1}{t} \ln \frac{a}{a - x}$ (h^{-1}).

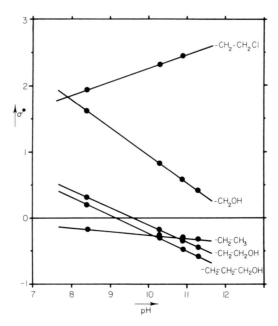

FIG. 6. pH dependence of the Hammett-Taft constants σ^* of thiamine homologs and analogs with altered 5-substituent (Ostrovsky *et al.*, 1970). Note the different behavior of 5-ethyl- and particularly 5-chloroethylthiamine.

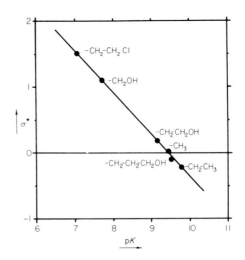

FIG. 7. Interdependence of Hammett-Taft constants σ^* and pK values of thiamine homologs and analogs with altered 5-substituent (Ostrovsky *et al.*, 1970).

by secondary inductive effects of the protein in the enzymatic reactions. Similar effects of the 5-substituent are detectable in the basicity of N-1'. They must cross the whole molecule via the methylene bridge or the hydrogen bond between C-2 and the 4'-amino group.

VI. Effects of Substituents at the Pyrimidine Ring

On the other hand, altered substituents at the pyrimidine ring have distinct effects on the pK (Fig. 8) and on the rate of pseudobase formation at the thiazole ring (Fig. 9) (Ostrovsky et al., 1970).

Although not necessary in the nonenzymatic model reactions, the intact 4'-amino group is a prerequisite for coenzymatic activity which is destroyed even by monomethylation (Schellenberger, 1967). It is thought to be hydrogen-bonded to an unknown group of the protein, which, by this hydrogen bond, may regulate the activity of the 4'-amino group. In protein-free solution this amino group is hydrogen-bonded to the C-2 of the thiazolium ring (Metzler, 1960; Ullrich and Mannschreck, 1966; Pletcher and Sax, 1966). The most basic site in the whole molecule is N-1' (Metzler, 1960), which in acidic solutions is protonated with a pK of ~5.0. In the TPP crystal, this nitrogen is found protonated as well (Pletcher and Sax, 1966). Replacement of this N by CH results in complete loss of coenzymatic activity (Schellenberger, 1967), whereas the other N in position 3' seems to be of much less importance. Incorporation of an additional CH_2 into the substituents at 2' and 6' gives only a gradual decrease of coenzymatic activity. A methyl group at 6' can be partially compensated for by removal of the 4-methyl group, which clearly indicates that these substituents act only by sterically hindering proper positioning of the coenzyme (see Fig. 3) in the active site of the protein (Schellenberger, 1967). Elongation of the methylene bridge by an additional CH_2 group completely destroys the coenzymatic activity because of heavily altered geometry of the molecule (Schellenberger et al., 1968), and also reduces the catalytic activity in the nonenzymatic model reactions to that of a thiazolium salt with simple 3-alkyl group. Most of the effects, touched here only very shortly, are summarized in Table VII. For further details see the reviews by Schellenberger (1967, 1969).

VII. Groups Involved in Protein-Binding of Thiamine Pyrophosphate

Morey and Juni (1968) as well as Schellenberger (1967) developed a simple protein-binding test for thiamine pyrophosphate homologs or analogs and for metals. Apopyruvate decarboxylase is treated with the TPP derivative and metal under investigation and run through a Sephadex G-25 column. Strongly bound cofactors run with the protein

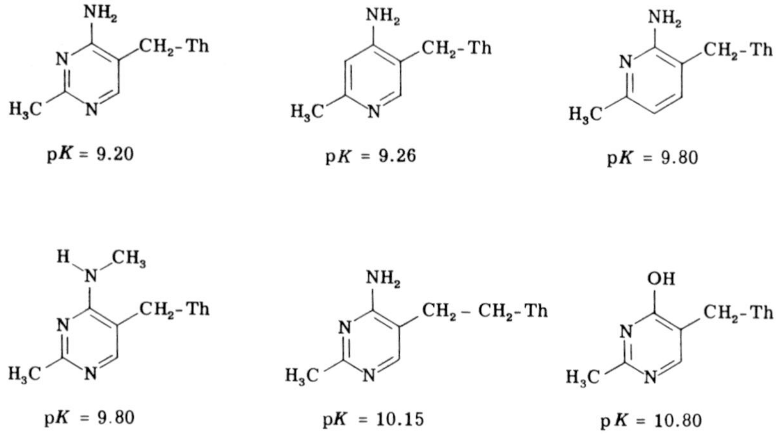

R	p*K*
$-O-C_6H_5$	9.40
$-C_6H_5$	9.50
$-CH_2-C_6H_5$	9.60
$-CH_2-CH_3$	9.26
$-O-CH_3$	9.75

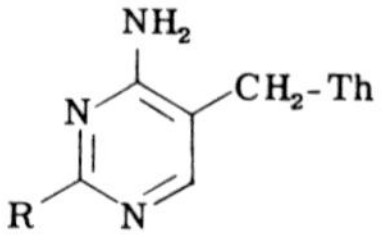

FIG. 8. p*K* values of thiamine homologs and analogs with altered substituents at the pyrimidine ring (Ostrovsky *et al.*, 1970). Th = thiazolium residue.

front; others are subjected to retardation by the molecular sieve, proportional to their tendency to dissociate from the protein. This test was supported by enzymatic inhibition experiments with derivative and unaltered TPP present in equal amounts and competing with each other for the binding sites on the apoenzymes (Schellenberger, 1967).

A number of groups were found in these experiments to be necessary in an unaltered state for proper protein binding: pyrophosphate, N-′, N-3$^{\oplus}$,4′-NH_2 (may be replaced by 4′-OH), and the methylene bridge. There may be other groups involved in additional weaker bonds between the coenzyme and the protein. Of the possible divalent metals, Mg^{2+} and Mn^{2+} give the strongest binding, followed by Co^{2+}, Ni^{2+}, Ca^{2+}, and Zn^{2+} (Schellenberger *et al.*, 1966).

VIII. Properties and Effects of the Pyruvate Decarboxylase Protein

Following recognition of yeast pyruvate decarboxylase as a magnesium protein (Green *et al.*, 1941; Kubowitz and Lüttgens, 1941), methods were

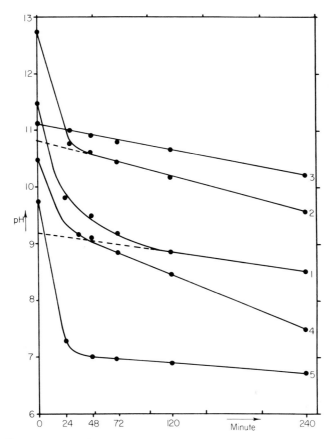

Fig. 9. Kinetics of pseudobase formation from thiamine and several analogs, demonstrated by pH measurements (Ostrovsky *et al.*, 1970). Curves; *1*, thiamine; *2*, 4'-hydroxythiamine; *3*, 3-benzyl-4-methyl-5-β-hydroxyethyl thiazolium chloride; *4*, 2'-phenoxythiamine; *5*, 5-β-chloroethylthiamine.

developed for resolution for cofactors at pH 8.5–9 (Kubowitz and Lüttgens, 1941; Holzer *et al.*, 1956) and for recombination with an excess of these in neutral solution (Steyn-Parvé and Westenbrink, 1944). In the native or fully reconstituted enzyme, TPP and Mg^{2+} were found to be almost undissociable at pH 6–7 (Steyn-Parvé and Westenbrink, 1944; Schellenberger *et al.*, 1966). The kinetics of the formation of the ternary complex between apopyruvate decarboxylase, TPP, and Mg^{2+} has been studied in detail by Schellenberger and his group (summary, Schellenberger, 1967) : TPP or Mg^{2+} alone are reversibly bound to the protein at different sites and show regular Michaelis-Menten behavior. Protein molecules which have bound both undergo a conformational change and

TABLE VII

PROTEIN BINDING, COENZYMATIC ACTIVITY, COMPETITION WITH THIAMINE PYROPHOSPHATE (TPP), AND NONENZYMATIC CATALYTIC ACTIVITY OF HOMOLOGS AND ANALOGS OF TPP AND THIAMINE[a]

Compound	Protein binding of pyrophosphate (TPP = 100)	Coenzymatic activity of pyrophosphate (TPP = 100)	Inhibition of TPP activity by pyrophosphate	Catalytic activity in Mizuhara model reaction for acetoin formation (thiamine = 100)[b]	
				Acetaldehyde	Pyruvate
Thiamine	100	100	—	100	100
4'-Hydroxythiamine	100	0	52 ± 7	65	15
Deaminothiamine	—	—	30 ± 5	—	—
N-Methylthiamine	1	0	25 ± 3	165	96
N,N-Dimethylthiamine	—	0	22 ± 3	281	74
2-Methylthiamine	1	0	0	0	0
2-α-Hydroxyethylthiamine	16	0	0	—	—
6'-Methylthiamine	44	0	10 ± 3	—	18
6'-Methyl-4'-hydroxythiamine	26	0	2 ± 1	—	—
6'-Methyl-4'-northiamine	100	22	—	—	—
4-Northiamine	4	24	25 ± 4	—	—
4'-Ethylthiamine	>90	32	4 ± 1	—	—
2-Methyl-4-northiamine	—	0	18 ± 5	—	—
2'-Ethylthiamine	>90	48	11 ± 2	—	—
5-γ-Hydroxypropylthiamine	—	0	22 ± 3	—	—
N-1-Pyridine analog	6	13	11 ± 2	—	—
N-3-Pyridine analog	0	0	0	—	—
Pyrithiamine	3	0	0	—	—
Imidazole analog[c]	~100	0	—	0	—
Ethylene-bridged thiamine homolog[d]	—	0	0	66	—

[a] Schellenberger (1967, 1969).
[b] Biggs and Sykes (1961).
[c] Schellenberger et al. (1969).
[d] Schellenberger et al. (1968).

thus form the stable ternary complex at a rather slow but well-defined reaction rate, which is increased by the presence of substrate (pyruvate). There is no agreement on the role of the metal: several authors tend to assign its position between the pyrophosphate group of TPP and a group of the protein, while Schellenberger (1967) assumes it forms a complex bond between the N-1' of TPP and some unknown residue of the protein. Additional Mg^{2+} was once thought to be necessary for maintaining the conformation of the whole protein, but no evidence for this has been found as yet. Whether the Mg^{2+}, besides its importance for coenzyme binding, participates somehow in the enzymatic thiamine catalysis is still unknown. Perhaps its replacement by Mn^{2+}, leading to a completely intact and active enzyme, would make these problems accessible to electron paramagnetic resonance studies.

While the first studies on the behavior and function of pyruvate decarboxylase were undertaken with crude or little-fractionated yeast extracts (review, Vennesland, 1951), more detailed investigations required purified pyruvate decarboxylase. An efficient partial purification by a series of fractional precipitations is described by H. Holzer et al. (1956,

TABLE VIII

AMINO ACID COMPOSITION OF CYTOPLASMIC YEAST PYRUVATE DECARBOXYLASE[a,b]

	Mole %		Mole %
Lys	6.18	Ala	9.74
His	2.12	Val	7.85
Arg	2.49	Leu	9.63
		Ile	6.39
(Basic:	10.79)		
		(Alkyl chain:	33.61)
Asp (+ASN)	10.36		
Glu (+GLN)	9.48	Phe	4.09
		Tyr	2.85
(Acidic:	19.84)	Try	1.42
Ser	4.81	(Aromatic:	8.36)
Thr	7.22		
Pro	4.75	Pro	4.75
		Met	2.02
(Antihelical:	16.78)		
		(Lipophilic:	48.74)
Gly	7.75		
Cys (+half-cystine)	0.85		

[a] Ullrich et al. (1969).
[b] Molecular weight: 170.000; 2 subunits.

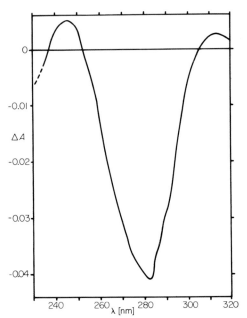

Fɪɢ. 10. Absorption difference spectrum of ternary complex formation between apopyruvate decarboxylase in the first chambers and thiamine pyrophosphate + Mg^{2+} in the second chambers of a pair of tandem cuvettes 15 minutes after mixing of the solutions in the sample beam against the unmixed reference (Ullrich and Wollmer, 1971). pH = 6.8, 25°C.

1962). Pure enzyme was obtained by subsequent Sephadex gel filtration (Ullrich et al., 1966; Ullrich, 1970). Its molecular weight was determined by sucrose density gradient centrifugation with reference proteins (Ullrich et al., 1966) to be 175,000. By analytical ultracentrifugation a value of 170,000 was obtained, and upon denaturation with 6 M guanidine hydrochloride and 0.1 M 2-mercaptoethanol two subunits of molecular weight 85,000–90,000 were found (Ullrich and Kempfle, 1969). The isolated enzyme was found to contain a little less than 3 TPP per molecule and could be enhanced in activity by about one-third when saturated with TPP and Mg^{2+} (Ullrich et al., 1966). Thus 4 binding sites for TPP were assumed. Kinetic measurements including extreme substrate concentrations, however, indicated only two substrate-binding sites at the intact enzyme (Hill slope $n = 1.8$) (Ullrich and Donner, 1970). This is in agreement with the two subunits, but in contrast to the apparently 4 TPP-binding sites mentioned above.

The amino acid composition of yeast pyruvate decarboxylase (Table VIII) has been determined by Ullrich et al. (1969). Lipophilic amino acid

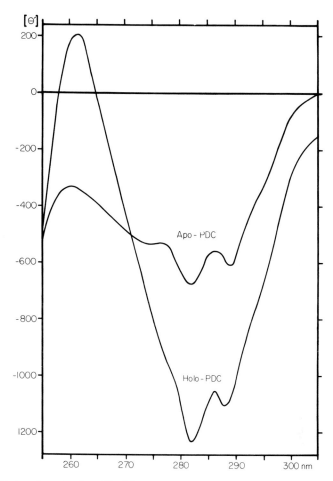

Fig. 11. Reduced molecular ellipticity spectrum of holo- and apopyruvate decar-boxylase at 27° and pH = 6.8. By addition of saturating concentrations of TPP and Mg^{2+} to the apopyruvate decarboxylase solution, the spectrum is changed back almost to that of the holoenzyme (Ullrich and Wollmer, 1971).

residues amount to almost 50% of the total, although the protein has a good solubility in water. Measurements of the radius of gyration of the protein by small-angle X-ray scattering (Dibble et al., 1970) gave 35.5 Å. From this value the longest diameter of the molecule was calculated to be 92 Å, which is not much above the value of 75 Å calculated for a spherical protein of 175,000 molecular weight (Reed et al., 1964). There-fore the shape of the molecule must be quite compact and not far from spherical.

The α-helix content of yeast pyruvate decarboxylase was estimated by a number of methods to be near 25% (Ullrich and Wollmer, 1971), a value allowed by the 17% of antihelix amino acids (Havsteen, 1966).

In the Moffitt plots and the far-UV circular dichroism spectra, only small differences were found between holo- and apopyruvate decarboxylase (Ullrich and Wollmer, 1971). From these results it may be concluded that the conformational changes, postulated by Schellenberger (1967) for the formation of the ternary complex from protein, TPP, and Mg^{2+}, do not appreciably involve the secondary structure of the protein.

Changes in the absorption of aromatic side chains upon coenzyme binding (Fig. 10) indicate alterations of aromatic interactions involving mainly tryptophan (Ullrich and Wollmer, 1971). Evidence for such alterations comes also from circular dichroism measurements in the same spectral range (Fig. 11), where very strong differences between holo- and apopyruvate decarboxylase were found (Ullrich and Wollmer, 1971). Further evidence was contributed by Wittorf and Gubler (1970) from fluorescence studies. The fluorescence of apopyruvate decarboxylase, due mainly to tryptophan (excitation maximum 280–290 nm, emission maximum 340 nm), is drastically quenched by the binding of TPP. Using thiochrome pyrophosphate instead of TPP, the same quenching of tryptophan fluorescence is observed, but a considerable part of the excitation energy is reemitted at longer wavelength of about 440 nm as thiochrome fluorescence (Wittorf and Gubler, 1970). This energy transfer indicates that certain tryptophan residues and the bound coenzyme analog are located near each other.

An attractive possibility for the type of binding between TPP and a tryptophan located in the active site of the protein has been shown by Mieyal et al. (1969) in model experiments: thiamine and indole-β-acetic acid in aqueous solution form molecular complexes which were detected by difference spectrometry (Biaglow et al., 1969). Their geometry, shown in Fig. 12, could be calculated from the chemical shifts of the involved protons in the nuclear magnetic resonance spectra of the single compounds and the mixture. The complexes are not formed with thiamine-like compounds containing nonquaternized N-3. Thus the predominant type of interaction between the indole ring of tryptophan and the thiazolium ring of TPP seems to be a π-electron transfer.

Another fluorescence indicator, 2-p-toluidinonaphthalene-6-sulfonate, is preferentially bound to the lipophilic areas on the surface of proteins or other biological structures (McClure and Edelman, 1966; Edelman and McClure, 1968). While almost nonfluorescent in aqueous solution, the dye shows strong fluorescence in a lipophilic environment. Its excitation maximum is 360–370 nm; its emission maximum, between 410 and

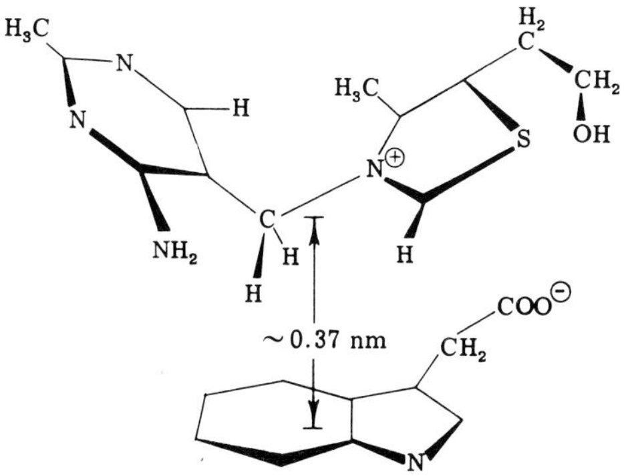

FIG. 12. Space formula of the complex of β-indoleacetic acid with thiamine (Mieyal et al., 1969).

490 nm, decreases with enhanced lipophilicity of the environment. Apopyruvate decarboxylase was found to be able to bind about twice the amount of dye as the holoenzyme (Fig. 13) (Ullrich and Donner, 1970b). By recombination with TPP and Mg^{2+}, half of the dye is removed from the protein, as measured by the disappearance of ca. 50% of the fluorescence (Table IX). The residual dye was found to act as a competitive inhibitor for pyruvate decarboxylation catalyzed by the enzyme.

Half of the dye may be bound directly to the TPP-binding site, but

TABLE IX

RELATIVE FLUORESCENCE INTENSITY OF 2-p-TOLUIDINONAPHTHALENE-6-SULFONATE BOUND TO YEAST PYRUVATE DECARBOXYLASE[a]

Sample	Fluorescence[b] (arbitrary units)
Complete[c]	19.7
Complete without TPP and Mg^{2+}	41.8
Complete without Mg^{2+}	42.2
Complete without TPP	41.5
Complete without enzyme	1.3
Complete without dye	0.5
Native holopyruvate decarboxylase + dye[d]	18.8
Native holopyruvate decarboxylase without dye[d]	0.9

[a] Ullrich and Donner (1970b).

[b] Excitation at 365–366 nm (Hg lamp), emission measured in 45° remission with secondary filter 400–3000 nm.

[c] 6 μM Apopyruvate decarboxylase (Ullrich et al., 1966) of specific activity 50 units/mg, 1 mM TPP and $MgSO_4$, 0.1 mM dye, 50 mM phosphate pH = 6.8; 25°, 3-ml cuvettes 1 × 1 cm².

[d] In the same buffer as that described in footnote c.

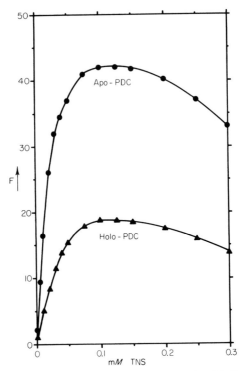

Fɪɢ. 13. Apparent fluorescence saturation curves for binding of 2-*p*-toluidino-naphthalene-6-sulfonate (TNS) to holo- and apopyruvate decarboxylase from brewer's yeast (Ullrich and Donner, 1970b). pH = 6.8, 25°C. Excitation at 365 nm.

less strongly than TPP. Another explanation would be that a coenzyme-induced conformational change distant from the TPP-binding site blocks a dye-binding site previously available to the dye. By analogy with a better investigated example, the binding of a similar dye to apohemoglobin (Stryer, 1968), the first version seems to be more likely.

Kinetic studies of the complicated interaction between pyruvate decarboxylase and 2-*p*-toluidinonaphthalene-6-sulfonate (Ostrovsky and Ullrich, 1970) further support the concept of dye binding at the TPP-binding site. In apopyruvate decarboxylase three different types of binding sites are indicated by 3 different rates of appearance of fluorescence after addition of the dye (Fig. 14). The first type is very rapid and saturated already before the fluorescence measurements start (the curves start well above zero). The second one shows a kinetics comparable to that of TPP-binding (see Schellenberger, 1967). The third one is much slower and probably represents an active denaturation of the protein by the dye. For holopyruvate decarboxylase, only the rate types 1 and 3

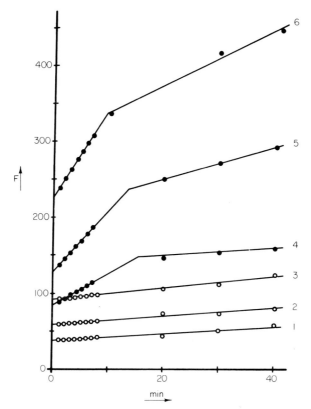

Fig. 14. Kinetics of binding of 0.33 mM 2-p-toluidinonaphthalene-6-sulfonate to pyruvate decarboxylase, measured by relative fluorescence intensity (Ostrovsky and Ullrich, 1970). ○ = Holopyruvate decarboxylase (curves: *1*, 0.17 mg/ml; *2*, 0.34 mg/ml; *3*, 0.67 mg/ml). ● = Apopyruvate decarboxylase (curves: *4*, 0.2 mg/ml; *5*, 0.4 mg/ml; *6*, 0.8 mg/ml).

can be observed (Fig. 14). This can be taken as an indication, that rate type 2 represents the binding of dye at the TPP-binding sites, whereas type 1 is probably due to occupation of the substrate-binding sites.

The experiments with the fluorescent dye show both the TPP-binding sites and the substrate-binding sites to be strongly lipophilic, whereas the rest of the surface of the protein appears to be in general hydrophilic, despite the high percentage of lipophilic amino acids, the bulk of which are obviously located in the interior of the compact protein molecule and probably serve to maintain the tertiary structure. These conclusions are supported by many earlier observations from comparative measurements on decarboxylation rates of various α-oxo acids (summaries, Vennesland, 1951; Schellenberger, 1967). α-Oxo acids with larger alkyl groups than

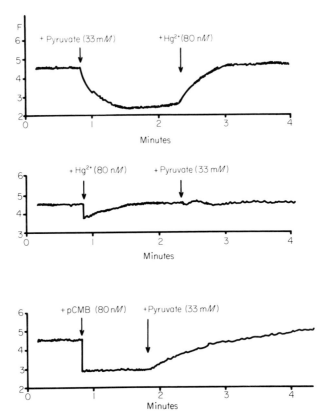

FIG. 15. Effect of pyruvate on the fluorescence intensity of 2-p-toluidinonaphtha-lene-6-sulfonate bound to holopyruvate decarboxylase; influence of Hg^{2+} on this effect; reversal of the effect of p-chloromercuribenzoate (pCMB) by pyruvate (Ostrovsky and Ullrich, 1970).

methyl—if not highly branched—are decarboxylated by pyruvate de-carboxylase with Michaelis constants lower than that for pyruvate, al-though at a lower rate; they are potent competitive inhibitors of pyruvate. The larger alkyl groups have greater lipophilicity and thus are better bound to the lipophilic substrate-binding sites of the enzyme. Glyoxylate, the smallest and simplest α-oxo acid molecule, represents a unique excep-tion: one molecule of it is decarboxylated per active site, but the reaction stops at the 2-hydroxymethyl-TPP stage, because the liberation mecha-nism for the aldehyde residue fails to work in this case (Schellenberger, 1967). Schellenberger explains this phenomenon by lack of inductive in-fluence of the alkyl group which is also responsible for the very stable hydration of formaldehyde.

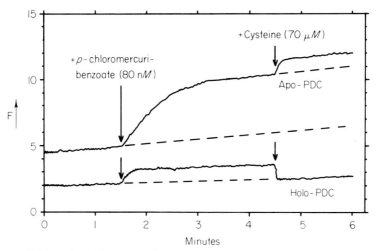

Fɪɢ. 16. Effect of p-chloromercuribenzoate and of cysteine on the fluorescence intensity of 2-p-toluidinonaphthalene-6-sulfonate bound to apo- and holopyruvate decarboxylase (Ostrovsky and Ullrich, 1970).

Figure 15 demonstrates that pyruvate diminishes the fluorescence of 2-p-toluidinonaphthalene-6-sulfonate bound to pyruvate decarboxylase. Hg^{2+} reverses or prevents this effect. On the other hand, pyruvate reverses the effect of p-chloromercuribenzoate, which, under certain conditions, strongly reduces the fluorescence of the dye. Organic mercurial and pyruvate together may induce a conformational change which opens additional lipophilic sites otherwise inaccessible to the dye. These sites must be different from the ones influenced by TPP, as demonstrated by a difference in their half-saturation concentrations (Ostrovsky and Ullrich, 1970). In the presence of TPP and Mg^{2+} the effect of the mercurial can be counteracted by excess cysteine (Fig. 16), whereas without TPP and Mg^{2+} cysteine enhances the fluorescence.

These experiments indicate that sulfhydryl groups are involved in substrate binding. They agree with earlier findings of Stoppani *et al.* (1952), Kanopkaite (1956), and Schellenberger and Hübner (1968), who could inactivate pyruvate decarboxylase by treatment with mercurials or *N*-ethyl maleimide.

IX. Sᴛʀᴜᴄᴛᴜʀᴇ ᴀɴᴅ Fᴜɴᴄᴛɪᴏɴ ᴏꜰ α-Oxᴏ Aᴄɪᴅ Dᴇʜʏᴅʀᴏɢᴇɴᴀꜱᴇ Cᴏᴍᴘʟᴇxᴇꜱ

α-Oxo acid dehydrogenase complexes have been isolated from *Escherichia coli* (Koike *et al.*, 1960; Dennert and Höglund, 1970, obtained greatly improved activity) and from mitochondria of several vertebrate tissues (Jagannathan and Schweet, 1952; Schweet et al., 1952; Sanadi et al., 1952; Hayakawa et al., 1964); they have been also described in yeast mitochondria (Holzer and Goedde, 1957a; Holzer et al., 1963). Two types of such multienzyme complexes have been thoroughly investigated: pyruvate dehydrogenase and α-ketoglutarate dehydrogenase (reviews by Reed and Cox, 1966 and Reed and Oliver, 1968). Furthermore, there is evidence for the existence of at least one additional complex of this type which catalyzes the oxidative decarboxylation of α-oxoisovalerate, α-oxo-isocaproate, and α-oxo-β methylvalerate, the deamination products of valine, leucine, and isoleucine, respectively (Goedde et al., 1967; Goedde and Keller, 1967; Connelly et al., 1968; Bowden and Connelly, 1968; Namba et al., 1969; Wohlhueter and Harper, 1970). Its nonfunctioning in human infants is known as inherited "maple syrup urine" disease.

All the α-oxo acid dehydrogenase complexes consist of 3 different types of enzymes: α-oxo acid decarboxylase (TPP-dependent), lipoyl reductase-transacylase (containing lipoic acid), and dihydrolipoyl dehydrogenase (containing FAD and NAD-dependent). These complexes can be dissociated into their constitutive enzymes and reassembled with almost complete restoration of activity (reviews by Reed and Cox, 1966 and Reed and Oliver, 1968).

The E. coli pyruvate dehydrogenase complex has been found to contain 12 molecules of pyruvate decarboxylase of molecular weight 183,000, 6 molecules of dihydrolipoyl dehydrogenase (molecular weight 112,000), and an aggregate of 48 subunits of lipoyl reductase-transacetylase (molecular weight 35,000). One molecule of the decarboxylase consists of 2 pairs of peptide chains (Henning et al., 1966) of similar molecular weight with alanine and leucine as N-terminal amino acids (Reed, 1968b). It binds TPP and Mg^{2+} at different binding sites and finally forms a ternary complex similar to that of yeast pyruvate decarboxylase (Schwartz and Reed, 1970); it was found to have 2 substrate-binding sites.

Organic mercurials inactivate apopyruvate decarboxylase by modifying two sulfhydryl groups per molecule of enzyme (Schwartz and Reed, 1970). TPP and Mg^{2+} were found to protect against this inactivation; pyruvate, on the other hand, has no such effect. In the presence of TPP and Mg^{2+}, however, two other SH groups are modified, which are otherwise inaccessible for the mercurial and which seem to be nonessential for enzyme activity. The sites involved in binding the pyruvate decarboxylase unit to lipoyl reductase-transacetylase remain intact. From these results it was concluded that coenzyme binding of pyruvate decarboxylase contained in the multienzyme complex is of a type similar to that in the cytoplasmic pyruvate decarboxylase, but that substrate binding is different. The catalytic sites and the protein-binding sites are assumed to be independent of each other. The pyruvate dehydrogenase complexes from mammalian sources have been investigated to a similar extent during recent years and seem to be similar in macromolecular organization, but different in size (Ishikawa *et al.*, 1966; Hayakawa *et al.*, 1966, 1969; Hirashima *et al.*, 1967; Kanzaki *et al.*, 1969; Bremer, 1969).

The α-oxoglutarate dehydrogenase complex of *E. coli* has a molecular weight of 2.4 million, which is only half that of the pyruvate dehydrogenase complex. It contains fewer decarboxylase units and probably less dihydrolipoyl dehydrogenase. The latter enzyme is interchangeable and probably identical with that of the pyruvate dehydrogenase complex (Pettit and Reed, 1967). The lipoyl reductase-transsuccinylase contained in the α-oxoglutarate dehydrogenase complex has been shown to be different from lipoyl reductase-transacetylase of the pyruvate dehydrogenase complex in molecular weight and in the amino acid sequence around the ε-*N*-lipoyllysine (Daigo and Reed, 1962). Despite its smaller size, the α-oxoglutarate dehydrogenase complex exhibits about ten times the substrate turnover rate of the pyruvate dehydrogenase complex (for further details, see the reviews by Reed and Cox, 1966 and Reed and Oliver, 1968).

X. Conclusions

As has been stated for a number of other enzymes, the active site of cytoplasmic yeast pyruvate decarboxylase seems to be partially buried in a sort of pocket. TPP is bound in this pocket from different sides by various residues of the protein chain. One of these is probably tryptophan, forming a charge transfer complex with the thiazolium part of TPP. Another bond is mediated by Mg^{2+}; the nature of the rest of the binding residues is still unknown.

The pocket is certainly much more open or may not even exist in the apoenzyme. It is formed when TPP and Mg^{2+} are properly bound to different lobes of the protein, in reversible equilibria independent of one another by a change in tertiary structure which brings together the two lobes of the protein. The ternary complex between protein, TPP, and Mg^{2+} thus formed has a much higher structural stability than the apoenzyme, even when this is saturated with one of the ligands, TPP or Mg^{2+} alone. The shape of the pocket apparently does not allow much alteration of the TPP molecule, for steric as well as for electronic reasons. The substrate specificity of pyruvate decarboxylase is, presumably, determined by the size of the entrance to the catalytic site which lies within the pocket; highly branched α-oxo acids are excluded.

Incorporated in this lipophilic environment must be a pattern of specific binding sites for the different parts of the TPP molecule. The lipophilicity of the whole structure appears to be sufficient to exclude during the enzymatic reaction solvent molecules bearing protons or hydroxyl groups. Thus "micro pH values" can be sustained, as has been shown for other enzymes, and the lifetimes of very active intermediates, e.g., the α-carbanion of 2-α-hydroxyethyl-TPP, can be prolonged "kinetically," allowing them to undergo reactions that would be prevented if accessible to protons or other particles of the solvent.

Particular attention should be drawn to the exceptional case of the decarboxylation of glyoxylate, leading not to free formaldehyde, but only to terminal stoichiometric formation of 2-hydroxymethyl-TPP. The alkyl group of the substrate may well be necessary for completion of the lipophilic envelope around the α-carbanion during the reaction. If it is missing, protons may be better able to penetrate into this zone and saturate the reactive species, diverting it from the normal path of conversion.

In the α-oxo acid dehydrogenase complexes a similar lipophilic zone may be built up by the array of different proteins forming the complex. Binding of TPP in the decarboxylase of the pyruvate dehydrogenase complex is probably of the same type as in cytoplasmic pyruvate decarboxylase, but less firm. In the α-oxoglutarate dehydrogenase complex TPP seems to be more firmly bound. The decarboxylase part of all of these complexes must have a more open structure, allowing the lipoic acid, attached to another protein of the complex, to enter the decarboxylation site and effect transfer of the residue. A plausible concept of the details of this transfer has been developed by Reed and Cox (1966) and Reed (1968a).

ACKNOWLEDGMENTS

For information very valuable in the preparation of this manuscript we thank Professor Gubler, Professor Reed, and Professor Schellenberger. Many of the experimental data were obtained with skillful technical assistance of Frl. Ingrid Donner. Financial support for our investigations came from the Deutsche Forschungsgemeinschaft and from the Bundesministerium für Bildung und Wissenschaft, Bonn. J. E. received a fellowship from the Humboldt-Stiftung.

REFERENCES

Auhagen, E. (1932). Z. Physiol. Chem. 204, 149; 209, 20.
Babitcheva, A. F., Polumbrik, O. M., and Yasnikov, A. A. (1968). Org. Reactiv. (USSR) 5, 802.
Bergel, F., and Todd, A. R. (1937). J. Chem. Soc. (London) p. 1504.
Biaglow, J. E., Mieyal, J. J., Suchy, J., and Sable, H. Z. (1969). J. Biol. Chem. 244, 4054.
Biggs, J., and Sykes, P. (1961). J. Chem. Soc. London 1961, 2595.
Bowden, J. A., and Connelly, J. L. (1968). J. Biol. Chem. 243, 3526.
Bremer, J. (1969). Eur. J. Biochem. 8, 535.

Breslow, R. (1956). *Chem. Ind. (London)* p. R28.
Breslow, R. (1957a). *Chem. Ind. (London)* p. 893.
Breslow, R. (1957b). *J. Amer. Chem. Soc.* 79, 1762.
Breslow, R. (1958). *J. Amer. Chem. Soc.* 80, 3719.
Breslow, R. (1961). *Ciba Found. Study Group* No. 11, 65–73.
Breslow, R. (1962). *Ann. N. Y. Acad. Sci.* 98, 445.
Breslow, R., and McNelis, E. (1959). *J. Amer. Chem. Soc.* 81, 3080.
Breslow, R., and McNelis, E. (1960). *J. Amer. Chem. Soc.* 82, 2394.
Carlson, G. L., and Brown, G. M. (1960). *J. Biol. Chem.* 235, PC3.
Connelly, J. L., Danner, D. J., and Bowden, J. A. (1968). *J. Biol. Chem.* 243, 1198.
Da Fonseca-Wollheim, F., Bock, K. W., and Holzer, H. (1962). *Biochem. Biophys. Res. Commun.* 9, 466.
Daigo, K., and Reed, L. J. (1962). *J. Amer. Chem. Soc.* 84, 666.
Dennert, G., and Höglund, S. (1970). *Eur. J. Biochem.* 12, 502.
Deus, B., Ullrich, J., and Holzer, H. (1970). *Methods Enzymol.* 18, 259.
Dibble, W. E., Benson, A. K., and Wittorf, J. H. (1970). In press.
Downes, J., and Sykes, P. (1957). *Chem. Ind. (London)* p. 1095.
Edelman, G. M., and McClure, W. O. (1968). *Accounts Chem. Res.* 1, 65.
Goedde, H. W. (1963). *Int. Z. Vitaminforsch.* 33, 18.
Goedde, H. W., and Keller, W. (1967). In "Amino Acid Metabolism and Genetic Variation" (W. L. Nyhan, ed.), pp. 191–215. McGraw-Hill, New York.
Goedde, H. W., Ulrich, B., Stahlmann, C., and Holzer, H. (1965). *Biochem. Z.* 343, 204.
Goedde, H. W., Hüfner, M., Möhlenbeck, F., and Blume, K. G. (1967). *Biochim. Biophys. Acta* 132, 524.
Green, D. E., Herbert, D., and Subrahmanyan, V. (1941). *J. Biol. Chem.* 138, 327.
Gruber, M., and Wesselius, J. C. (1962). *Biochim. Biophys. Acta* 57, 171.
Hamill, W. H. (1937). *J. Amer. Chem. Soc.* 59, 1152.
Havsteen, B. H. (1966). *J. Theor. Biol.* 10, 1.
Hayakawa, T., and Koike, M. (1969). *J. Biochem. (Tokyo)* 65, 645.
Hayakawa, T., Muta, H., Hirashima, M., Ide, S., Okabe, K., and Koike, M. (1964). *Biochem. Biophys. Res. Commun.* 17, 51.
Hayakawa, T., Hirashima, M., Ide, S., Hamada, M., Okabe, K., and Koike, M. (1966). *J. Biol. Chem.* 241, 4694.
Hayakawa, T., Kanzaki, T., Kitamura, T., Fukuyoshi, Y., Sakurai, Y., Koike, K., Suematsu, T., and Koike, M. (1969). *J. Biol. Chem.* 244, 3660.
Henning, U., Dennert, G., Hertel, R., and Shipp, W. S. (1966). *Cold Spring Harbor Symp. Quant. Biol.* 31, 227.
Hirashima, M., Hayakawa, T., and Koike, M. (1967). *J. Biol. Chem.* 242, 902.
Holzer, E., Söling, H. D., Goedde, H. W., and Holzer, H. (1962). In "Methoden der enzymatischen Analyse" (H. U. Bergmeyer, ed.), pp. 602–605. Verlag Chemie, Weinheim.
Holzer, H. (1961). *Angew. Chem.* 73, 721.
Holzer, H., and Beaucamp, K. (1959). *Angew. Chem.* 71, 776.
Holzer, H., and Beaucamp, K. (1961). *Biochim. Biophys. Acta* 46, 225.
Holzer, H., and Crawford, R. M. M. (1960). *Nature (London)* 188, 410.
Holzer, H., and Goedde, H. W. (1957a). *Biochem. Z.* 329, 175.
Holzer, H., and Goedde, H. W. (1957b). *Biochem. Z.* 329, 192.
Holzer, H., Schultz, G., Villar-Palasi, C., and Jüntgen-Sell, J. (1956). *Biochem. Z.* 327, 331.

Holzer, H., Da Fonseca-Wollheim, F., Kohlhaw, G., and Woenckhaus, C. W. (1962). *Ann. N. Y. Acad. Sci.* **98**, 453.

Holzer, H., Hierholzer, G., and Witt, I. (1963). *Biochem. Z.* **337**, 115.

Ishikawa, E., Oliver, R. M., and Reed, L. J. (1966). *Proc. Nat. Acad. Sci. U. S.* **56**, 534.

Jagannathan, V, and Schweet, R. S. (1952). *J. Biol. Chem.* **196**, 551.

Juni, E. (1961). *J. Biol. Chem.* **238**, 2302.

Kanopkaite, S. I. (1956). *Biokhimiya* **21**, 834.

Kanzaki, T., Hayakawa, T., Hamada, M., Fukuyoshi, Y., and Koike, M. (1969). *J. Biol. Chem.* **244**, 1183.

Karrer, P., and Viscontini, M. (1946). *Helv. Chim. Acta* **29**, 711.

Kinnersley, H. W., and Peters, R. A. (1934). *Biochem. J.* **28**, 667.

Kohlhaw, G., Deus, B., and Holzer, H. (1965). *J. Biol. Chem.* **240**, 2135.

Koike, M., Reed, L. J., and Caroll, W. R. (1960). *J. Biol. Chem.* **235**, 1924.

Krampitz, L. O. (1969). *Annu. Rev. Biochem.* **38**, 213.

Krampitz, L. O., Greull, G., Miller, C. S., Bicking, J. B., Skeggs, H. R., and Sprague, J. M. (1958). *J. Amer. Chem. Soc.* **80**, 5893.

Krampitz, L. O., Suzuki, I., and Greull, G. (1961). *Fed. Proc., Fed. Amer. Soc. Exp. Biol.* **20**, 971.

Krampitz, L. O., Suzuki, I., and Greull, G. (1963). *Proc. 5th. Int. Congr. Biochem., 1961* Vol. 4, p. 321.

Kubowitz, F., and Lüttgens, W. (1941). *Biochem. Z.* **307**, 170.

Langenbeck, W. (1933). *Ergeb. Enzymforsch.* **2**, 314.

Lienhard, G. E. (1966). *J. Amer. Chem. Soc.* **88**, 5642.

Lohmann, K., and Schuster, P. (1937). *Biochem. Z.* **294**, 188.

McClure, W. O., and Edelman, G. M. (1966). *Biochemistry* **5**, 1908.

McNelis, E. (1960). Ph.D. Thesis, Columbia University, New York.

Metzler, D. E. (1960). *In* "The Enzymes" (P. D. Boyer, H. Lardy, and K. Myrbäck, eds.), 2nd rev. ed., Vol. 2, Part A, pp. 295–337. Academic Press, New York.

Mieyal, J. J., Votaw, R. G., Krampitz, L. O., and Sable, H. Z. (1967). *Biochim. Biophys. Acta* **141**, 205.

Mieyal, J. J., Suchy, J., Biaglow, J. E., and Sable, H. Z. (1969). *J. Biol. Chem.* **244**, 4063.

Miller, C. S., Sprague, J. M., and Krampitz, L. O. (1962). *Ann. N. Y. Acad. Sci.* **98**, 401.

Mizuhara, S. M., and Handler, P. (1954). *J. Amer. Chem. Soc.* **76**, 571.

Mizuhara, S. M., Tamura, R., and Arata, H. (1951). *Proc. Jap. Acad.* **27**, 302, 700, and 705.

Morey, A. V., and Juni, E. (1968). *J. Biol. Chem.* **243**, 3009.

Namba, Y., Yoshizawa, K., Ejima, A., Hayashi, T., and Kaneda, T. (1969). *J. Biol. Chem.* **244**, 4437.

Nash, C. P., Olsen, C. W., White, F. G., and Ingraham, L. L. (1961). *J. Amer. Chem. Soc.* **83**, 4106.

Neuberg, C., and Hirsch, J. (1921). *Biochem. Z.* **115**, 282.

Neuberg, C., and Karczag, L. (1911). *Biochem. Z.* **37**, 170.

Neuberg, C., and Ohle, H. (1922). *Biochem. Z.* **127**, 327; **128**, 610.

Ostrovsky, Yu. M. (1967). *Biokhimiya* **32**, 933.

Ostrovsky, Yu. M. (1968). *J. Vitaminol. (Kyoto)* **14**, 98.

Ostrovsky, Yu. M., and Gvozdeva, M. (1959). *Bull. Exp. Biol. Med. (USSR)* **11**, 120.

Ostrovsky, Yu. M., and Gvozdeva, M. (1960). *Aptech. Delo* **2**, 52.

Ostrovsky, Yu. M., and Ullrich, J. (1970). *Biokhimiya* (in press).

Ostrovsky, Yu. M., Sadovnik, M., Masolov, N., and Gritzenko, E. (1970). *Biokhimiya* (in press).

Palm, V. (1968). *Org. Reactiv. (USSR)* **5**, XXX.

Pettit, F., and Reed, L. J. (1967). *Proc. Nat. Acad. Sci. U. S.* **58**, 1126.

Pletcher, J., and Sax, M. (1966). *Science* **154**, 1331.

Pohlandt, F., Kohlhaw, G., and Holzer, H. (1967). *Z. Naturforsch.* **B22**, 407.

Prochoroff, N. N., Kattermann, R., and Holzer, H. (1962). *Biochem. Biophys. Res. Commun.* **9**, 477.

Pullman, B., and Spanjaard, C. (1961). *Biochim. Biophys. Acta* **46**, 576.

Reed, L. J. (1953). *Physiol. Rev.* **33**, 544.

Reed, L. J. (1968a). *J. Vitaminol. (Kyoto)* **14**, 77.

Reed, L. J. (1968b). Personal communication.

Reed, L. J., and Cox, D. J. (1966). *Annu. Rev. Biochem.* **35**, 57.

Reed, L. J., Koike, M., and Willms, C. R. (1964). *Science* **145**, 930.

Reed, L. J., and Oliver, R. M. (1968). *Brookhaven Symp. Biol.* **21**, 397.

Risinger, G. E., and Dove, M. F. (1965). *Chem. Ind. (London)* p. 510.

Rogers, E. F. (1962). *Ann. N. Y. Acad. Sci.* **98**, 412.

Sanadi, D. R., Littlefield, J. W., and Bock, R. M. (1952). *J. Biol. Chem.* **197**, 851.

Schellenberger, A. (1967). *Angew. Chem.* **79**, 1050; *Angew. Chem., Int. Ed. Engl.* **6**, 1024.

Schellenberger, A. (1969). *Wiss. Z. Univ. Halle* **18**, 319.

Schellenberger, A., and Hübner, G. (1968). *Angew. Chem.* **80**, 41; *Angew. Chem., Int. Ed. Engl.* **7**, 68.

Schellenberger, A., Winter, K., Hübner, G., Schwaiberger, R., Helbig, D., Schumacher, S., Thieme, R., Bouillon, G., and Rädler, K. P. (1966). *Z. Physiol. Chem.* **346**, 123.

Schellenberger, A., Hanke, H., and Hübner, G. (1968). *Z. Physiol. Chem.* **349**, 517.

Schellenberger, A., Thieme, H., and Hübner, G. (1969). *Z. Chem.* **9**, 62.

Schröter, W., and Holzer, H. (1963). *Biochim. Biophys. Acta* **77**, 474.

Schultz, F. (1940). *Z. Physiol. Chem.* **265**, 113.

Schwartz, E. R., and Reed, L. J. (1970). *J. Biol. Chem.* **245**, 182.

Schweet, R. S., Katchman, B., Bock, R. M., and Jagannathan, V. (1952). *J. Biol. Chem.* **196**, 563.

Scriba, P., and Holzer, H. (1961). *Biochem. Z.* **334**, 473.

Steyn-Parvé, E. P., and Westenbrink, H. G. K. (1944). *Int. Z. Vitaminforsch.* **15**, 1.

Stoppani, A. O. M., Actis, A. S., Deferrari, J. O., and Gonzalez, E. L. (1952). *Nature (London)* **170**, 812.

Stryer, L. (1968). *Science* **162**, 526.

Todd, A. R., and Bergel, F. (1937). *J. Chem. Soc.* p. 364.

Ugai, T., Tanaka, S., and Dokawa, S. (1943). *J. Pharm. Soc. Jap.* **63**, 269.

Ullrich, J. (1970). *Methods Enzymol.* **18**, 109.

Ullrich, J., Deus, B., and Holzer, H. (1968). *Int. Z. Vitaminforsch.* **38**, 273.

Ullrich, J., and Donner, I. (1970a). *Z. Physiol. Chem.* **351**, 1026.

Ullrich, J., and Donner, I. (1970b). *Z. Physiol. Chem.* **351**, 1030.

Ullrich, J., and Holzer, H. (1963). *Biochem. Z.* **337**, 345.

Ullrich, J., and Kempfle, M. (1969). *FEBS Letters* **4**, 273.

Ullrich, J., and Mannschreck, A. (1966). *Biochim. Biophys. Acta* **115**, 46.

Ullrich, J., and Mannschreck, A. (1967). *Eur. J. Biochem.* **1**, 110.

Ullrich, J., and Wollmer, A. (1971). Manuscript in preparation.

Ullrich, J., Wittorf, J. H., and Gubler, C. J. (1966). *Biochim. Biophys. Acta* **113**, 595.

Ullrich, J., Wittorf, J. H., and Gubler, C. J. (1969). *FEBS Letters* **4**, 275.

Umbreit, W. W., Burris, R. H., and Stauffer, J. F. (1964). "Manometric Techniques," 4th ed. Burgess, Minneapolis, Minnesota.

Vennesland, B. (1951). *In* "The Enzymes" (J. B. Sumner and K. Myrbäck, eds.), Vol. 2, Part 1, pp. 183–215. Academic Press, New York.

Westerfeld, W. W. (1945). *J. Biol. Chem.* **161**, 495.

White, F. G., and Ingraham, L. L. (1962). *J. Amer. Chem. Soc.* **84**, 3109.

Wiesner, K., and Valenta, Z. (1956). *Experientia* **12**, 190.

Williams, R. R., Waterman, R. E., Keresztesy, J. C., and Buchman, E. R. (1935). *J. Amer. Chem. Soc.* **57**, 536.

Wittorf, J. H., and Gubler, C. J. (1970). *Eur. J. Biochem.* **14**, 53.

Wohlhueter, R. M., and Harper, A. E. (1970). *J. Biol. Chem.* **245**, 2391.

Mechanism and Stereochemistry of Transamination[*]

HARMON C. DUNATHAN

Haverford College, Haverford, Pennsylvania

I. Introduction

In a recently published book on catalysis (Jencks, 1969), pyridoxal phosphate is described as God's gift to those enzymologists and chemists who enjoy "pushing electrons." Their satisfaction is derived from the tremendous variety of reactions catalyzed by enzymes dependent on this cofactor and from the existence of broad mechanistic concepts, first stated by Snell (Metzler *et al.*, 1954) and by Braunstein and Shemyakin, 1953), which encompass all these reactions. These concepts, supported and elaborated by extensive model studies, allow enzymologists to approach these reactions knowing the probable sequence of chemical events leading to products. These enzymes are then ideally suited for investigating the basic question of how the apoenzyme impresses reaction specificity, stereospecificity and catalytic efficiency on a sequence of known chemical steps between cofactor and substrate. In these investigations stereochemistry plays a large role since both cofactor and amino acid substrates offer many possibilities for observing stereospecific steps.

II. Stereospecificity[†]

The aldimine complex between pyridoxal phosphate and an amino acid shown in Fig. 1 can react to cleave reversibly many of the bonds shown. In most cases this bond making or breaking is completely stereospecific.

[*] New results reported here were supported by a grant (AM 09309) from the National Institutes of Health, U. S. Public Health Service.
[†] The notation of Fig. 1 (C_p, C_a, C_β, etc.) will be used throughout this paper.

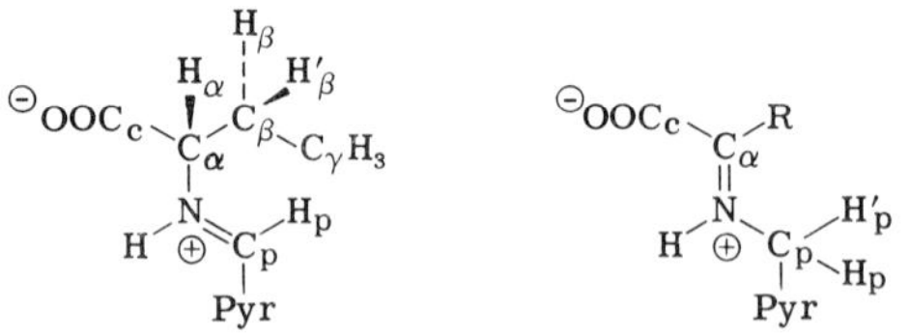

FIG. 1. A generalized structure of the pyridoxal phosphate–amino acid Schiff base complex. Most enzyme-catalyzed reactions at C_p, C_α, and C_β have been shown to be stereospecific. Pyr = 2-methyl-3-hydroxy-5-hydroxymethyl-4-pyridyl.

C_p. This carbon is protonated stereospecifically in the course of enzymatic transamination. The proton H'_p is exchanged while the original pyridoxal proton H_p is conserved (Dunathan et al., 1968a,b; Ayling et al., 1968).

$C_\alpha - H$. When this bond is broken and re-formed as in transamination, α-decarboxylation, α-β elimination-addition, or β-γ isomerizations and additions, the C_α always preserves its original configuration. Furthermore, the amino acids which serve as substrates for a common transaminase are always of the same symmetry, be it L or D (Martinez-Carrion and Jenkins, 1965).

On the other hand, pyridoxal phosphate-dependent racemases are able to labilize $C_\alpha - H$ bonds of either D or L configuration (Rosso et al., 1969).

$C_\alpha - C_c$. Decarboxylation replaces the $C_\alpha - C_c$ bond with $C_\alpha - H$. It has been shown for tyrosine decarboxylase that the entering solvent proton occupies the same stereochemical position as the C_c which is lost (Belleau and Burba, 1960).

$C_\alpha - C_\beta$. Serine transhydroxymethylase, now known to be identical with threonine and allothreonine aldolases, catalyzes the formation and cleavage of the $C_\alpha - C_\beta$ bond (Schirch and Gross, 1968). It has been known for some time that this enzyme will interconvert (+)-S-methyl-serine (Takamura et al., 1967) and D-alanine (Wilson and Snell, 1962). In this reaction the entering formaldehyde moiety occupies the same position as did the H_α of D-alanine. More recently, Jordan and Akhtar (1970) have shown that the glycine-L-serine interconversion follows the same stereochemical pattern, the pro S proton (Hanson, 1966) of glycine being replaced by the hydroxymethyl group of L-serine (Fig. 3). It is notable that with acetaldehyde as substrate, the new asymmetric center at C_β is formed in both configurations (threonine and allothreonine) at about the same rate (Schirch and Gross, 1968).

$C_\beta - H_\beta(X)$. A number of pyridoxal phosphate enzymes catalyze elimination, isomerization, and replacement reactions which involve

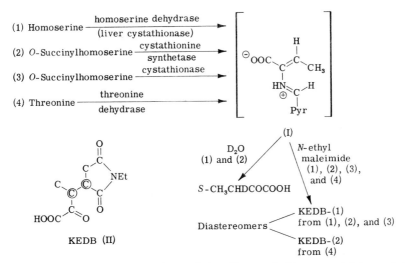

FIG. 2. Stereospecific reactions of an enimine (I), a probable common intermediate for each of the reactions shown.

breaking the C_β—H or C_β—X bond (X = —COOH, —OPO H⁻, —SH, 3-indoyl). Many of these reactions proceed via the intermediate enimine shown in Fig. 2 (I). Subsequent reactions at C_β are stereospecific. Thus the substrates homoserine and succinylhomoserine both yield in D_2O solvent, S-3-deutero-2-ketobutyrate in reactions catalyzed by homoserine dehydrase* (Krongelb et al., 1968) and cystathionine synthetase (Guggenheim and Flavin, 1969). In four of these enzyme systems, this same intermediate has been trapped by the electrophilic reagent N-ethyl maleimide (Flavin and Slaughter, 1969). In all cases the trapped product [Fig. 2 (II)] is optically active; however, the product from the threonine dehydrase reaction differs at one of the asymmetric centers from the product produced in the cystathionine synthetase and the two cystathionase catalyzed reactions.

Finally, in the γ replacement reactions catalyzed by cystathionine γ-synthase, only a single H_β is labilized, showing that here too the bond breaking at C_β is stereospecific (Guggenheim and Flavin, 1969).

Complete stereospecificity at C_p, C_α, and C_β has so far been observed in all but two systems. In one of these, pyridoxal phosphate-dependent racemases, enzyme function itself depends on a lack of complete stereospecificity. In the other, threonine aldolase does not discriminate between threonine and allothreonine in breaking or forming the C_α—C_β bond. That is, the enzyme does not distinguish between the si and re faces (Han-

* This enzyme is in fact the cystathionase of rat liver.

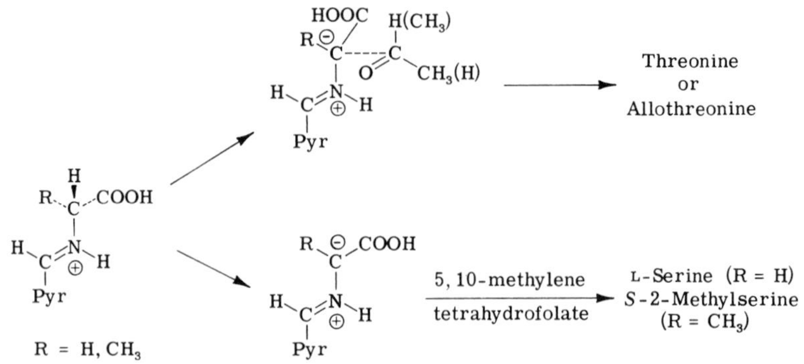

Fig. 3. The stereochemistry of C_α—C_β bond formation in threonine-allothreonine aldolase or serine hydroxymethylase.

son, 1966) of the acetaldehyde carbonyl group as it approaches the open face of the ionized glycine-pyridoxal phosphate imine (Fig. 3). This is understandable since the approaching acetaldehyde is not covalently bound to the cofactor. In all other cases, stereospecificity can be viewed as a natural consequence of strictly defined relationships between C_p, C_α, and C_β and the cofactor ring. That the cofactor chromophore is in an asymmetric environment is clearly seen in optical rotatory dispersion (ORD) measurements of various pyridoxal phosphate holoenzymes. In many cases a Cotton effect can be observed, centered about the λ_{max} of the cofactor imine. Jenkins has pointed out that the sign of this Cotton effect is positive for a number of L-amino acid specific enzymes but is negative for the single D specific enzyme so far examined (Schirch and Slotter, 1966).

III. REACTION SPECIFICITY

The specific binding of the cofactor substrate complex to the apoenzyme which yields stereospecificity must also be a primary factor in determining the chemical fate of that complex. In terms of the Braunstein-Snell concept, apoenzyme interactions control which of the three bonds to C_α is labilized. Some years ago we suggested that this appears specifically in apoenzyme control of the C_α—N bond conformation in complex (I) (Dunathan, 1966). The bond to C_α which is to be broken should lie in a plane (defined by N—C_α—X) which is perpendicular to the plane of the cofactor π-electron system. This conformation achieves maximum electronic interaction between the cofactor π system and the breaking sigma bond as well as minimizing the movement of the other groups on C_α as the bond breaks. Figure 4 shows C_α—N conformations appropriate to C_α—H, C_α—C_c, and C_α—C_β bond breaking. This view is consistent with and would predict many of the results presented in the discussion of

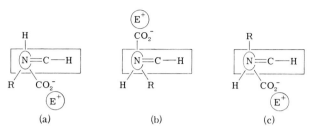

(a) (b) (c)

FIG. 4. Various conformations of a pyridoxal-amino acid Schiff base as viewed along the C_a-N bond. The atoms of the pyridine ring lie in a plane shown by the box. C_a-N bond conformation is controlled by the position of the enzyme binding site for the carboxylase anion E^+.

stereochemistry. Here too, the existence of pyridoxal phosphate-dependent racemases must be viewed as an exception to the tight control of C_α—N conformation.

A decarboxylase-transaminase described by Bailey and Dempsey (1967) would also seem to violate this tight control of C_α—N conformation. This enzyme catalyzes the decarboxylation-transamination of D-isovaline and other α-dialkyl amino acids (Eq. 1a). The enzyme is returned to its aldehyde form by transamination with pyruvate yielding L-alanine (Eq. 1b). Reaction (1b) can be demonstrated in the absence of (1a). Together, Eq. (1c), they define a transamination-dependent decarboxylase that is capable of labilizing the C_α—C_c or a C_α—H_α bond.

$$\text{DL-Isovaline + PLP enzyme} \rightleftarrows \text{2-butanone} + CO_2 + \text{PMP enzyme} \quad (1a)$$

$$\text{PMP enzyme + pyruvate} \rightleftarrows \text{PLP enzyme + L-alanine} \quad (1b)$$

$$\text{DL-Isovaline + pyruvate} \rightleftarrows \text{2-butanone} + CO_2 + \text{L-alanine} \quad (1c)$$

This implies either unexpected conformational freedom about C_α—N or alternate binding sites for the carboxylate group (Fig. 5). The latter interpretation is supported by the fact that this enzyme decarboxylates α-methyl-α-aminomalonate (Bailey et al., 1969) presumably binding this substrate as in Fig. 5 (III).

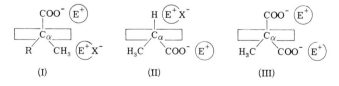

(I) (II) (III)

FIG. 5. Conformations which may be available to substrates of a decarboxylase-transaminase. The view is of the substrate α-carbon distant from the amino nitrogen. Cofactor atoms lie in a plane represented by the box.

IV. TRANSAMINATION

A. THE MECHANISTIC UNKNOWNS IN TRANSAMINATION

Transamination is the most common reactivity dependent on pyridoxal phosphate. Figure 6 shows the key steps of transamination. This sequence is supported by a wealth of data, most recently by quantitative conversion of glutamic aspartic transaminase (GAT) from its aldehyde to amino forms (Jenkins and D'Ari, 1966). For transaminases to show high turnover numbers, they must achieve a remarkable balance between the relative rates of these steps. Both C_α—H and C_p—H bond breaking must be rapid, and rates of reprotonation of the anion [Fig. 6 (II)] at C_α and C_p must be comparable. Both the ketimine [Fig. 6 (III)] and aldimine [Fig. 6 (I)] must be susceptible to rapid hydrolysis. This is in marked contrast to other systems. For example, in the α-decarboxylases and aldolases addition of the proton after loss of CO_2 or C_β must always be on C_α (if C_p is protonated reversibly, the resulting ketimine must be protected from hydrolysis).

Using the concepts of Section III, we became convinced that it should be possible to determine the detailed mechanism of the key reaction of transamination [Fig. 6, reactions (2) and (3)] including the configuration and conformation of all bonds and asymmetric centers involved (Dunathan et al., 1968a,b).

Figure 7 shows how the configuration of the proton removed at C_α is related to the configuration of the proton added to C_p by three variables: the conformation of C_α—N, and of C_p=N and the stereochemistry of the transfer reaction. This can be described as *cis* if proton addition and ab-

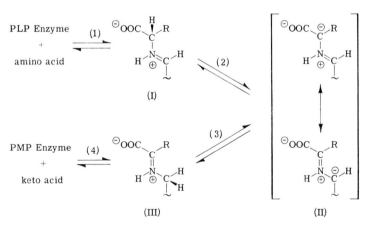

FIG. 6. The key chemical steps of enzymatic transamination.

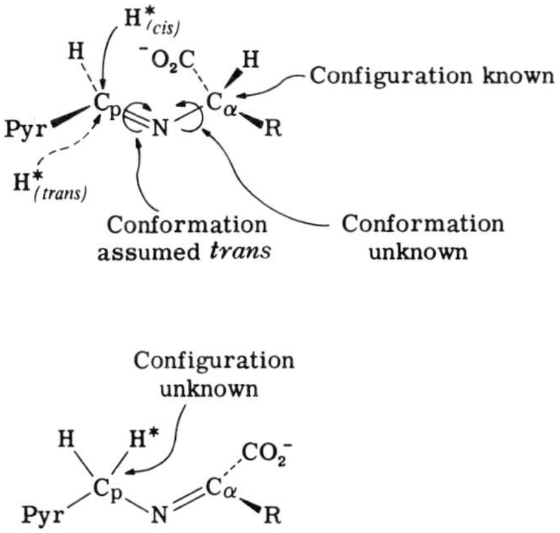

Fig. 7. Stereochemical variables in transamination.

straction occur on the same side of the cofactor π system and *trans* if on opposite sides.

Viewed as a problem in chemical algebra there are five unknowns in the equation of this tautomerism, each with only two possible values; R or S configurations, conformations differing by 180°, and a mechanism which is *cis* or *trans*. Changing the sign of any one of these variables must change the sign of one of the others. It also follows that knowledge of four of the variables will allow definition of the fifth.

B. STEREOSPECIFICITY AT THE COFACTOR 4′ CARBON (C_p)

An experimental definition of these variables depended on a method for isotopically labeling the cofactor molecule and an enzyme capable of a rapid turnover of cofactor molecules. It was found that a mixture of pyridoxal and pyridoxamine at slightly acid pH underwent self-trans-amination incorporating solvent protons in the 4′-methylene position of pyridoxamine and the aldehyde position of pyridoxal (Dunathan *et al.,* 1968a,b). These nonphosphorylated cofactor molecules act as freely diffus-ible substrates for the apoenzyme of glutamic aspartic transaminase (Wada and Snell, 1962a). These reactions (reaction 2) show the same substrate and stereospecificity as the holoenzyme reaction. We believe that the apoenzyme catalyzed reactions proceed by the same mechanism as the holoenzyme half reactions and that our stereochemical results apply to both.

$$\text{Pam} + \text{2-ketoglutarate} \underset{}{\overset{\text{apoGAT}}{\rightleftharpoons}} \text{Pal} + \text{L-glutamate}$$

$$\text{Pam} + \text{oxaloacetate} \underset{}{\overset{\text{apoGAT}}{\rightleftharpoons}} \text{Pal} + \text{L-aspartate}$$

(2)

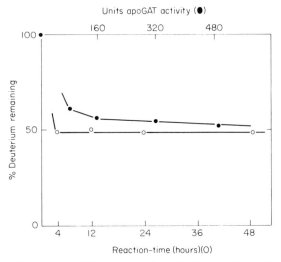

FIG. 8. Loss of deuterium label from the 4'-methylene position of pyridoxamine in transamination with ketoglutarate catalyzed by apo-glutamic-aspartic transaminase.

When pyridoxamine dideuterated in the 4-methylene position was incubated with apo-glutamic-aspartic transaminase in H_2O, only one deuteron exchanged with solvent protons independent of time or quantity of enzyme (Fig. 8). As expected, the enzyme in D_2O catalyzed the incorporation of only one deuteron into the 4-methylene groups of pyridoxamine. The enantiomeric relationship between the two monodeuteropyridoxamines so produced was confirmed by measurements of the kinetic isotope effect in the forward reaction.

C. The Relative Stereospecificity of Different Transaminases at the Cofactor Carbon (C_p)

The above results, first reported in 1966 and in more detail in 1968 (Dunathan et al., 1968a,b) established the stereospecificity of protonation at the cofactor carbon C_p. This raised the interesting question of the relative symmetry of the proton added to C_p in the course of other enzymatic transaminations. Unfortunately the very small K_m values for binding of the phosphorylated cofactor of most of these enzymes makes the symmetry comparison dependent on isolation of very large quantities of enzyme. The single comparison that has been possible involves an enzyme which, like apo-glutamic-aspartic transaminase, catalyzes the transamination of the nonphosphorylated cofactor molecules.*

* Recently, Bailey has shown that the decarboxylase-transaminase described in Section III shows the same absolute stereospecificity in protonating C_p as does apoGAT and PPT (Bailey et al., 1970).

This enzyme, pyridoxamine-pyruvate transaminase (PPT) (Wada and Snell, 1962b) is L-alanine specific and can be used to prepare samples of enantiomeric monodeuteropyridoxamines. When these were used as substrates in the apo-GAT reaction, the observed kinetic isotope effects proved that PPT was labilizing the same cofactor proton as apo-GAT (Ayling et al., 1968). One is tempted to predict a one-to-one relationship between amino acid symmetry and the symmetry of the labilized cofactor proton. This is not likely to be established in the near future as the single D-specific transaminase which has been highly purified would be very difficult to prepare in quantity (Martinez-Carrion and Jenkins, 1965).

D. The Absolute Symmetry of the Labile Cofactor Proton

The absolute symmetry of the labilized proton at C_p might be established by an independent asymmetric synthesis of monodeuteropyridoxamine of predictable symmetry or by degradation of an enzymatically produced monodeuteropyridoxamine to a known asymmetric compound.

Both paths have now been followed. An asymmetric synthesis led to the assignment of pro S symmetry to the labilized pyridoxamine proton (Dunathan et al., 1968b). This tentative assignment was confirmed by Besmer and Arigoni (1969), who prepared pyridoxamine specifically tritiated in the 4-methylene position via the apo-GAT-catalyzed transamination of pyridoxal and aspartate in tritiated water. Degradation of the labeled pyridoxamine to glycine and thence to tritiated glycolate allowed assignment of S symmetry to the original pyridoxamine.

With the configuration of the labile proton on C_p established as pro S, and the C_α configuration defined by the absolute symmetry of the amino acid substrate, only the mechanism of transfer and the two bond conformations remain unknown. Of the two bond conformations, one, the $C_p{=}N$ double bond, can be defined by inspection. A cis conformation of this bond would require the amino acid residue to lie so close to the cofactor ring that the coplanarity of $C_p{=}N$ and the pyridine ring would be destroyed and the geometry available to the anion [Fig. 6 (II)] correspondingly unfavorable. Only the trans geometry at this bond is consistent with the cofactor's action in labilizing C_α bonds. We are then left with an unknown conformation at C_α—N and a choice of two mechanisms for the transfer.

E. The Mechanism of the Prototropic Shift

Isomerizations involving 1,3 proton shifts have been studied for more than 75 years in a variety of organic systems (Ingold, 1969). Various mechanisms have been proposed for 1,3 prototropy as shown in Fig. 9. These are characterized by the cis or trans nature of the transfer, concerted or stepwise bond breaking and making, and the involvement of a

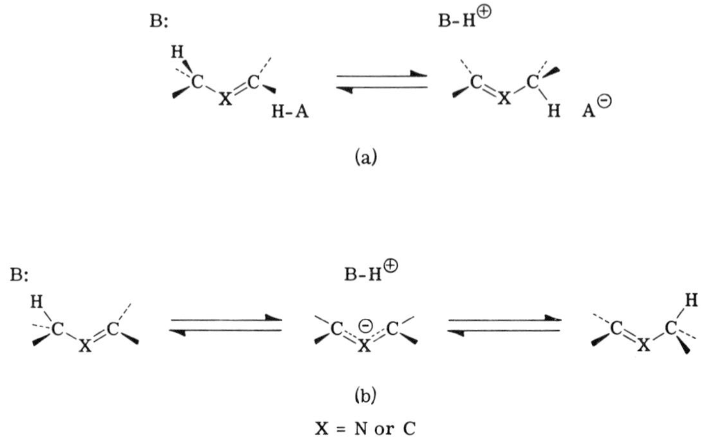

FIG. 9. Proposed paths for 1,3-prototropic isomerization.

single or two acid-base groups. The existence of a bimolecular mechanism (Fig. 9a) in a methylene azomethine isomerization was claimed by Ossario and Hughes (1952). Recent work by Cram and his co-workers (Cram and Guthrie, 1965) has provided strong evidence that such isomerisms proceed via an anionic intermediate (Fig. 9b). Other work from this group has revealed a wealth of mechanistic detail about these simple prototropic shifts. Most important from our viewpoint were the results with an imine system shown in Fig. 10 (Guthrie et al., 1967). These results are remarkable for the high degree of asymmetric induction observed in this acyclic system. For steric reasons there is a great preference for the conformation (III) as opposed to (IV) for the anion in the path leading to isomerization.

At about the same time, Auld and Bruice (1967) provided compelling evidence that the nonenzymatic transamination of a simple pyridoxal analog with alanine proceeded with intermediate formation of an anion.

These results suggested that enzymatic transamination might proceed via an intermediate anion with a single apoenzyme group acting as general acid-base catalyst. If this was so, one might hope to observe an intramolecular proton shift in the cofactor amino acid complex. An intramolecular proton shift would effectively define the *cis* mechanism for this transfer.

Early experiments with apo-GAT were frustrated by traces of remaining holoenzyme activity which catalyzed rapid exchange of the amino acid alpha proton or deuteron with solvent. This problem is avoided with pyridoxamine-pyruvate transaminase. Results from several experiments are given in Table I. Using that enzyme, 4–5 atom % deuterium was

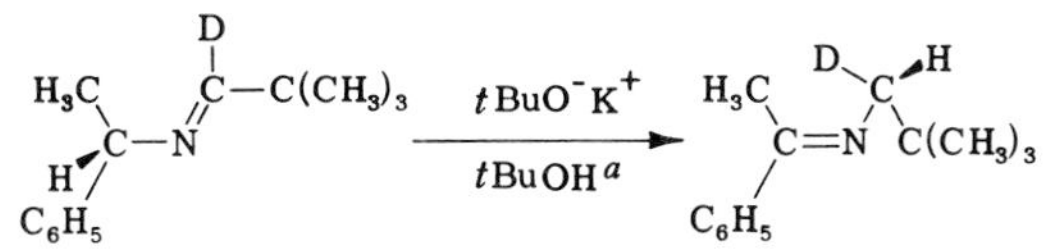

FIG. 10. Asymmetric induction in an imine prototropic isomerization (Guthrie et al., 1967). [a]When carried out in tBuOD, the proton is transferred intramolecularly to the extent of 13%.

transferred intramolecularly from the α position of L-alanine to the C_p of pyridoxamine (Ayling et al., 1968). The unreacted α-deutero-L-alanine suffered very little loss of label. Deuterium analyses were carried out by mass spectrometry on the pyridoxamine molecule in the first experiments and later by the more accurate method of Graff and Rittenberg (1952) (combustion, conversion of labeled water to H_2—HD mixtures, and analysis by mass spectrometer).

TABLE I

INTRAMOLECULAR TRANSFER OF DEUTERIUM IN PYRIDOXAMINE
PYRUVATE TRANSAMINASE CATALYZED REACTIONS

Reaction[a]	Solvent	% Conversion	% Intramolecular transfer
2-²H-L-Ala + Pal	H_2O	2	4.0[b]
2-²H-L-Ala + Pal	H_2O	5	2.0[b]
2-²H-L-Ala + Pal	H_2O	10	4.5[c]
2-¹H-L-Ala + Pal	D_2O	10	50[c]
Pam(¹H) + Pyr	D_2O	22	38[d]
Pam(²H) + Pyr	H_2O	17	<5[d]

[a] Ala = alanine, Pal = pyridoxal, Pam = pyridoxamine, Pyr = pyruvate.

[b] Mass spectrometer analysis of intact pyridoxamine. We are grateful to Dr. Thomas Kinstle of the Department of Chemistry, Iowa State University for supervising the mass spectral analyses.

[c] Analysis by the combustion method of Graff and Rittenberg (1952).

[d] Analysis by 220 mc NMR. Supervised by Dr. J. Leogh, University of Pennsylvania.

When the same reaction was carried out in 99% D_2O with proton substrates, the α-hydrogen of L-alanine was conserved by intramolecular transfer to the extent of 50 atom %.

Followed in the reverse direction, the intramolecular transfer of deuterium from dideuteropyridoxamine to alanine in H_2O amounted to <5 atom %. In D_2O solution the pyridoxamine proton is transferred intramolecularly to alanine to the extent of 38%.

A 10-fold difference in intramolecular transfer is observed when proton transfer in D_2O is compared to deuteron transfer in H_2O. This is compelling evidence that the proton or deuteron which is transferred becomes equivalent to other deuterons or protons respectively during the transfer.

Figure 11 shows a possible scheme to account for the results of Table I. An active site lysine amino group acts as a general base in removing H_α to form the ion pair. This might be the same lysine that binds the cofactor in the absence of substrate, as was suggested by Snell (1962). As the result of rapid rotation, the $-NH_2D^+$ of this ion pair can transfer H or D at relative rates dependent only on the kinetic isotope effect and a statistical factor of 2, favoring proton transfer. If we assume that the Schiff base species [Fig. 11 (I), (III), (IV), (V)] are in rapid equilibrium with substrate molecules in solution, the concentration of (IV) will always be small under conditions of low percentage of conversion. Under these conditions, the ratio of proton transfer to deuteron transfer is simply $2k_{4(H)}/k_{4(D)}$ or 2 times the kinetic isotope effect for reaction (4). The percentage of deuteron transfer from C_α to C_p is then only 9% when the

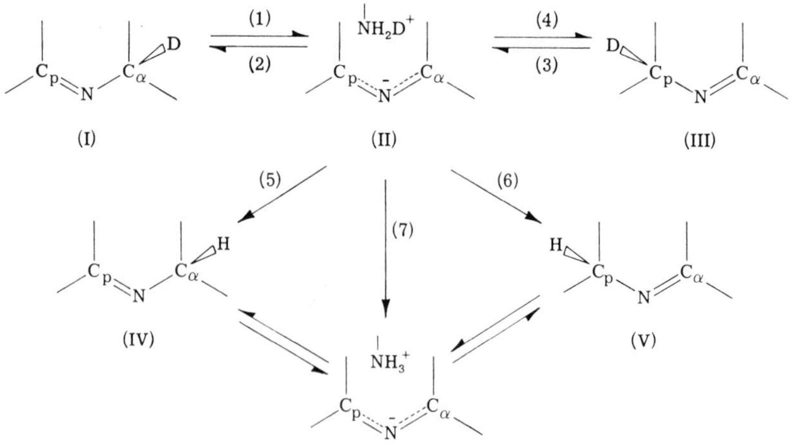

FIG. 11. A possible pathway for intramolecular transfer of deuterium label in transamination.

kinetic isotope effect is $k_{4(H)}/k_{4(D)} = 5$. However, transfer of a proton from C_α to C_p in D_2O is favored by a rate ratio of $k_{4(H)}/2k_{4(D)}$ or $\frac{1}{2}$ times the kinetic isotope effect. This is equal to an observed percentage transfer of 71% when $k_{4(H)}/k_{4(D)}$ is 5. Both of these numbers are higher than the 4% and 50% observed. The efficiency of transfer is undoubtedly reduced by exchange of the ion pair [Fig. 11, reaction (7)] or more likely, by reaction through species (I), (II), (IV). The results of Table I can be reconciled with catalysis by a histidine residue's imidazole ring only if rather unusual kinetic and solvent isotope effects are postulated. For example, postulating much larger kinetic isotope effect for transfer of H or D to C_p compared to the isotope effect in the transfer to solvent.

Other transaminases may in fact utilize a different basic residue to catalyze this reaction. Bailey *et al.* (1970) has observed transfer of tritium from C_α to C_p catalyzed by the decarboxylase-transaminase discussed in Section III. The high efficiency of this transfer makes it unlikely that the tritium is carried by an amino group. Recent experiments on the photooxidation of GAT suggest that a histidine imidazole group may be responsible for proton transfer in that enzyme (Peterson and Martinez-Carrion, 1970). However, photosensitized oxidation of alanine aminotransferase does not destroy an active site imidazole side chain (Beis and Swoboda, 1970).

Quite aside from the question of the nature of the enzyme basic group, there is mounting evidence that conservation of the mobile proton and thus a *cis* transfer will be a general phenomenon. Guggenheim and Flavin (1968) have observed 80% conservation of a substrate proton in the enzymatic conversion of succinyl homoserine to 2-ketobutyrate. The conserved proton must come from the α or β carbon of the succinylhomoserine. Figure 12 shows a possible sequence involving proton conservation in 1-3 and 1-5 prototropic shifts. The intramolecular transfer of a deuteron in these same shifts is apparently much less efficient (Flavin, 1970).

More recent work indicates that the conserved proton added at C_γ comes from both C_α and C_β with nearly equal efficiency (Posner and Flavin, 1970). Figure 12 is then at best an incomplete description of the reaction path.

Finally, Besmer *et al.* (1970) have been able to show that both the aldimine and ketimine [Fig. 6, (I) and (III)] are reduced by borodeuteride from the same side (si and re, respectively) from which they are protonated during transamination. This is strong evidence of a different kind that the *cis* mechanism operates and that all bond making and breaking takes place on the same side of the cofactor π system.

With the establishment of the *cis* mechanism of transfer and the determination of the absolute symmetry of the proton added to C_p, the stereo-

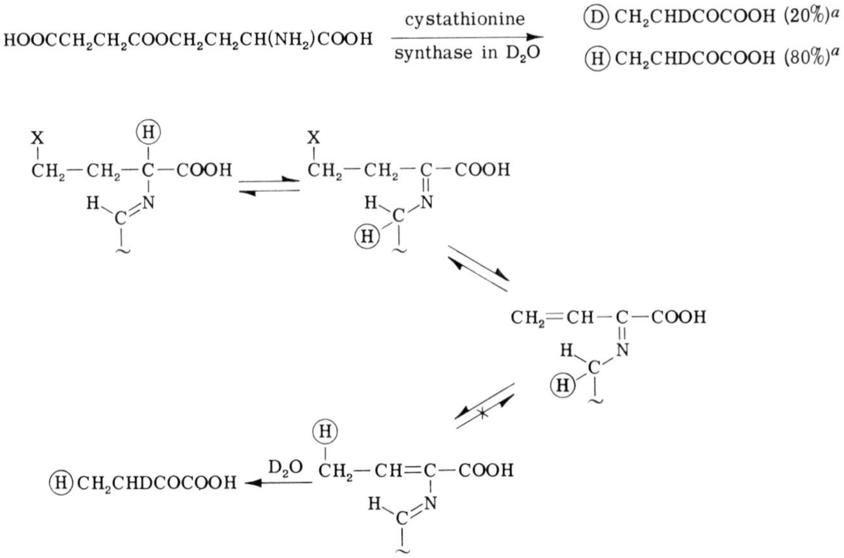

$$HOOCCH_2CH_2COOCH_2CH_2CH(NH_2)COOH \xrightarrow[\text{synthase in } D_2O]{\text{cystathionine}}$$

(D) $CH_2CHDCOCOOH$ (20%)[a]

(H) $CH_2CHDCOCOOH$ (80%)[a]

FIG. 12. A reaction sequence leading to conservation of a substrate proton in a β-γ elimination reaction. [a] Results of Guggenheim and Flavin (1968).

chemical picture of transamination is complete. The conformationally and configurationally correct structures are shown in Fig. 13.

If the *cis* mechanism of transfer is general and if all L-amino acid specific transaminases add and remove the pro *S* proton of pyridoxamine, we must conclude that the C_α—N conformation shown in Fig. 13 (1) has always been favored in the evolution of the active site geometry of these enzymes. This conformation places the amino acid α-carboxylate ion at a maximum distance from the phosphate ester group of the cofactor. This fact alone may account for the apparent favoring of this conformation.

Satisfying as it may be to define so precisely the stereochemistry of this

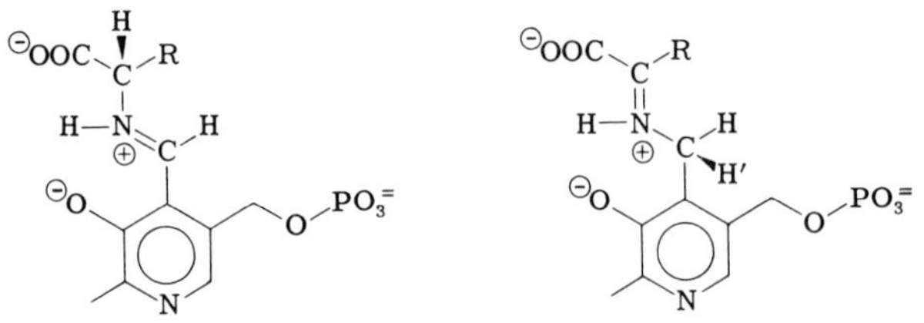

(I)   (II)

FIG. 13. The aldimine and ketimine complexes of pyridoxamine pyruvate transaminase-catalyzed reactions shown in their correct conformation and configuration.

reaction, this knowledge does not necessarily help us understand the basis for the catalytic efficiency of the holoenzyme.

The thermodynamic acidity of the C_α—H or C_p—H protons in the enzymatic reaction is hard to estimate but is probably much greater than in model systems (Schirch and Slotter, 1966). On the other hand, the rate of imidazole-catalyzed C_α—H bond breaking in a model transamination studied by Auld and Bruice (1967) is remarkably high even when compared to the rapid first-order constants obtained by Fasella and Hammes (1967) from temperature-jump studies of glutamic aspartic transaminase. How these rates are achieved can only be guessed at. Is the pyridinium-positive charge buried in an apolar region, thus raising the energy of the aldimine and ketimine relative to the quininoid anion [Fig. 6 (II)]? Does the enzyme bind this planar anion more tightly than either of the imines? Does the phosphate group in a holotransaminase play a catalytic role beyond its binding properties? Recent evidence (Furbish *et al.*, 1969) supports this conclusion. Once produced, what subtle steric and electronic factors control the position of reprotonation of the anion and what factors determine the relative rates of hydrolysis of aldimine and ketimine?

In the end one cannot help but be impressed by the finesse with which nature uses this cofactor's ability to support a negative charge on the α carbon of an amino acid.

REFERENCES

Auld, D. S., and Bruice, T. C. (1967). *J. Amer. Chem. Soc.* **89**, 2098.

Ayling, J. E., Dunathan, H. C., and Snell, E. E. (1968). *Biochemistry* **7**, 4537.

Bailey, G. B., and Dempsey, W. B. (1967). *Biochemistry* **6**, 1526.

Bailey, G. B., Chotamangsa, O., and Vuttivej, K. (1969). *Fed. Proc., Fed. Amer. Soc. Exp. Biol.* **28**, 351.

Bailey, G. B., Kusamrarn, T., and Vuttivej, K. (1970). *Fed. Proc., Fed. Amer. Soc. Exp. Biol.* **29**, 857.

Beis, I., and Swoboda, B. E. P. (1970). Unpublished results.

Belleau, B., and Burba, J. (1960). *J. Amer. Chem. Soc.* **82**, 5751.

Besmer, P., and Arigoni, D. (1968). *Chimia* **22**, 494.

Besmer, P., and Arigoni, D. (1969). *Chimia* **23**, 190.

Besmer, P., Bertola, E., and Arigoni, D. (1970). Personal communication.

Braunstein, A. E., and Shemyakin, M. M. (1953). *Biokhimiya* **18**, 393.

Cram, D. J., and Guthrie, R. D. (1965). *J. Amer. Chem. Soc.* **87**, 397.

Dunathan, H. C. (1966). *Proc. Nat. Acad. Sci. U. S.* **55**, 712.

Dunathan, H. C., Davis, L., and Kaplan, M. (1968a). *In* "Pyridoxal Catalysis: Enzymes and Model Systems" (E. E. Snell *et al.*, eds.), pp. 325–337. Wiley (Interscience), New York.

Dunathan, H. C., Davis, L., Kury, P. G., and Kaplan, M. (1968b). *Biochemistry* **7**, 4532.

Fasella, P., and Hammes, G. G. (1967). *Biochemistry* **6**, 1798.

Flavin, M. (1970). Personal communication.

Flavin, M., and Slaughter, C. (1969). *J. Biol. Chem.* **244**, 1434.

Furbish, F. S., Fonda, M. L., and Metzler, D. E. (1969). *Biochemistry* **8**, 5169.

Graff, J., and Rittenberg, D. (1952). *Anal. Chem.* **24**, 878.

Guggenheim, S., and Flavin, M. (1968). *Biochim. Biophys. Acta* **151**, 664.

Guggenheim, S., and Flavin, M. (1969). *J. Biol. Chem.* **244**, 6217.

Guthrie, R. D., Meister, W., and Cram, D. J. (1967). *J. Amer. Chem. Soc.* **89**, 5288.

Hanson, K. R. (1966). *J. Amer. Chem. Soc.* **88**, 2731.

Ingold, C. K. (1969). "Structure and Mechanism in Organic Chemistry," 2nd ed., p. 806. Cornell Univ. Press, Ithaca, New York.

Jencks, W. (1969). "Catalysis in Chemistry and Enzymology," p. 136. McGraw-Hill, New York.

Jenkins, W. T., and D'Ari, L. (1966). *Biochem. Biophys. Res. Commun.* **22**, 376.

Jordan, P. M., and Akhtar, M. (1970). *Biochem. J.* **116**, 277.

Krongelb, M., Smith, T. A., and Abeles, R. H. (1968). *Biochim. Biophys. Acta* **167**, 473.

Martinez-Carrion, M., and Jenkins, W. T. (1965). *J. Biol. Chem.* **240**, 3538.

Metzler, D. E., Ikawa, M., and Snell, E. E. (1954). *J. Amer. Chem. Soc.* **76**, 648.

Ossario, R. P., and Hughes, E. D. (1952). *J. Chem. Soc.* p. 426.

Peterson, D. L., and Martinez-Carrion, M. (1970). *J. Biol. Chem.* **245**, 806.

Posner, B., and Flavin, M. (1970). Unpublished results.

Rosso, G., Takashima, K., and Adams, E. (1969). *Biochem. Biophys. Res. Commun.* **34**, 134.

Schirch, L., and Gross, T. (1968). *J. Biol. Chem.* **243**, 5651.

Schirch, L., and Slotter, R. A. (1966). *Biochemistry* **5**, 3175.

Snell, E. E. (1962). *Brookhaven Symp. Biol.* **15**, 39.

Takamura, N., Terashima, S., Achiwa, K., and Yamada, S. (1967). *Chem. Pharm. Bull.* **15**, 1776.

Wada, H., and Snell, E. E. (1962a). *J. Biol. Chem.* **237**, 127.

Wada, H., and Snell, E. E. (1962b). *J. Biol. Chem.* **237**, 133.

Wilson, E. M., and Snell, E. E. (1962). *J. Biol. Chem.* **237**, 3180.

Roles of Vitamin B_{12} and Folic Acid in Methionine Synthesis*

HERBERT WEISSBACH AND ROBERT T. TAYLOR

Roche Institute of Molecular Biology, Nutley, New Jersey, and Bio-Medical Division, Lawrence Radiation Laboratory, University of California, Livermore, California

I. BACKGROUND

It is well established that in *Escherichia coli* there are two types of enzymes capable of catalyzing methyl group transfer from N^5-methyltetrahydrofolic acid (N^5-methyl-H_4-folate) to homocysteine. One of these enzymes is a cobamide-containing protein (Guest *et al.*, 1960, 1964a; Hatch *et al.*, 1961; Larrabee *et al.*, 1961; Takeyama *et al.*, 1961) which requires catalytic levels of S-adenosylmethionine (AMe) (Foster *et al.*, 1964; Rosenthal and Buchanan, 1963; Weissbach *et al.*, 1963), and a reducing system (Hatch *et al.*, 1961; Larrabee *et al.*, 1961; Takeyama *et al.*, 1961). N^5-Methyl-H_4-folates containing one or more L-glutamate moieties can function as methyl group substrates for the B_{12} enzyme (Reaction 1).

$$N^5\text{-Methyl-H}_4\text{-folate (Glu}_1\text{, Glu}_3\text{, etc.)} + \text{homocysteine} \xrightarrow[\substack{\text{AMe} \\ \text{reducing system}}]{\text{B}_{12}\text{ protein}}$$
$$\text{methionine} + \text{H}_4\text{-folate} \quad (1)$$

Unlike the B_{12} protein, the bacterial noncobamide enzyme requires Mg^{2+}, is stimulated by inorganic phosphate, and utilizes only poly-L-glutamate forms of N^5-methyl-H_4-folate to synthesize methionine (Reaction 2)

---

* In 1966 we reviewed the role of vitamin B_{12} in methionine synthesis (Weissbach and Taylor, 1966). The reader should refer to that article for the historical development of the problem and studies prior to that time. The present report will emphasize studies performed since 1966.

(Buchanan *et al.*, 1964; Burton *et al.*, 1969; Guest *et al.*, 1964b; Jones *et al.*, 1961; Whitfield *et al.*, 1970).

$$N^5\text{-Methyl-H}_4\text{-folate (Glu}_2,\ \text{Glu}_3,\ \text{etc.)} + \text{homocysteine} \xrightarrow[\text{Pi}]{\text{Mg}^{2+}}$$
$$\text{methionine} + \text{H}_4\text{-folate} \quad (2)$$

Another distinguishing feature between these two bacterial methyltransferases is the influence of oxygen which causes marked inhibition of the cobamide-containing enzyme but has no effect on catalysis by the noncobamide protein (Buchanan *et al.*, 1964).

It is of interest to note the species distribution of the two types of enzymes. In addition to various strains of *E. coli*, both methyltransferases have been reported in *Aerobacter aerogenes* (Morningstar and Kisliuk, 1965) and *Salmonella typhimurium* (Cauthen *et al.*, 1966); whereas only the B_{12}-dependent enzyme has been observed in *Rhodopseudomonas spheroides* (Cauthen *et al.*, 1967), *Ochromonas malhamensis* (Griffiths and Daniel, 1969), mammalian liver (Dickerman *et al.*, 1964; Loughlin *et al.*, 1964), and several lines of mammalian cells grown in tissue culture (Mangum *et al.*, 1969). Thus far, however, yeast and higher plants have been found to contain only noncobamide, N^5-methyl-H_4-folate methyltransferases (Botsford and Parks, 1967; Burton and Sakami, 1967; Guest *et al.*, 1964a). The absence of the B_{12} enzyme in higher plants is consistent with the fact that corrinoids are not constituents of their tissues except in the root nodules of species that carry out symbiotic nitrogen fixation (Evans and Kliewer, 1964).

Until this past year, it was generally considered that the inability to use N^5-methyl-H_4-folate (Glu$_1$) was a distinguishing feature of all the non-B_{12} folate methyltransferases. In fact, Burton *et al.* (1969) suggested that their homogeneous enzyme preparation from *Saccharomyces cerevisiae* (Burton and Sakami, 1970), as well as the non-B_{12} enzymes in *E. coli* and *Neurospora crassa*, should be called N^5-methyl-H_4-folate (polyglutamate)-homocysteine transmethylases. The non-B_{12} enzymes from all three of the sources are totally inactive with N^5-methyl-H_4-folate (Glu$_1$). Very recently, though, extracts of pea seeds (Dodd, 1969), green beans, spinach, and barley sprouts (Burton and Sakami, 1969) were found to catalyze the transmethylation of homocysteine with N^5-methyl-H_4-folate (Glu$_1$) in the presence of Mg^{2+} and phosphate buffer. In both of these reports the possible participation of some contaminating B_{12} enzyme was rigorously excluded. Moreover, with an extract of green beans the transmethylase activities for N^5-methyl-H_4-folate (Glu$_1$) and N^5-methyl-H_4-folate (Glu$_3$) were eluted in the exact same fractions from a Sephadex G-100 column. The rate of catalysis with the monoglutamate substrate was about one-seventh of that with the triglutamate folate (Burton and Sakami, 1969). These observations clearly indicate the occurrence in higher plants of a second type of non-B_{12} methyltransferase that resembles the bacterial non-B_{12} enzyme in its requirement for only Mg^{2+}, but resembles the E. coli B_{12} enzyme in its ability to utilize N^5-methyl-H_4-folate (Glu_1). The existence of this type of non-B_{12} enzyme also suggests that extra glutamate groups are only involved in the binding or positioning of the N^5-methyl-H_4-folate to the active sites of the microbial enzymes (Burton and Sakami, 1969; Whitfield and Weissbach, 1970). It argues against a direct involvement of the α-carboxyl group, on the second glutamate residue, in the catalysis of Reaction (2). At this date it would appear that the crucial point to be determined concerning the non-B_{12} methyltransferases is the function of the Mg^{2+}.

The B_{12}-dependent methyltransferase in mammalian liver appears to be quite analogous to the corresponding enzyme in E. coli insofar as it requires both AMe and a reducing system in order to catalyze Reaction (1) (Mangum and Scrimgeour, 1962; Loughlin et al., 1964; Dickerman et al., 1964). The most active mammalian enzyme B_{12} preparation described thus far is that of Loughlin et al. (1964); yet, even their isolation procedure from pig liver did not yield the B_{12} protein in a sufficient quantity or purity to permit any mechanistic studies with substrate levels of the enzyme. Consequently, practically all the work concerning the mechanism of Reaction (1) has been carried out with B_{12} enzyme preparations purified from various strains of E. coli that were cultured in the presence of vitamin B_{12}. E. coli cells are a much richer source of the B_{12} enzyme than animal liver, and the bacterial B_{12} protein is more stable than the mammalian enzyme. Therefore, this review deals primarily with the role of the vitamin in the catalysis of methionine synthesis (Reaction 1) by a B_{12} protein derived from extracts of E. coli B.

II. N^5-METHYLTETRAHYDROFOLATE-HOMOCYSTEINE COBALAMIN METHYLTRANSFERASE (B_{12} TRANSMETHYLASE)

A. CHARACTERISTICS OF THE ENZYME

The cobamide-containing enzyme has been extensively purified from E. coli B (Taylor and Weissbach, 1967a) and an unspecified strain of E. coli (Stravrianopoulos and Jaenicke, 1967). Both B_{12}-protein preparations sedimented with $s_{20,w}$ values of approximately 7.0 S and, assuming a partial specific volume of 0.728, were calculated to have molecular weights of about 140,000. The best preparation (not homogeneous) from E. coli B contained 0.35 mole of bound cobamide per mole of protein, and the preparation obtained by Stravrianopoulos and Jaenicke (1967) (shown to be homogeneous with respect to its sedimentation behavior) contained 0.51–0.59 mole of bound cobamide per mole of protein. Enzyme preparations isolated from *E. coli* B are salmon-colored and display a prominent absorption maximum in the visible region at 475 nm (Taylor and Weissbach, 1967a). This absorption maximum at 475 nm is due to the cobamide chromophore since it shifts to yield double maxima at 540 nm and 580 nm upon the addition of alkaline cyanide. While the shape of the absorption spectrum, especially the 475 nm peak, closely resembles the spectrum of a one-electron reduced derivative of the vitamin (i.e., B_{12r}), the salmon-colored B_{12}-protein did not yield the electron spin resonance spectrum (Taylor and Weissbach, 1967a) that is characteristic of B_{12r} (Hogenkamp *et al.*, 1963). Furthermore, the bound-B_{12} chromophore is stable to oxygen in contrast to B_{12r}. An absorption maximum at 470 nm is not unique for B_{12r}; it is also given by a variety of corrinoid compounds in acidic media (Hill *et al.*, 1962). Conclusive evidence has been obtained, however, that the salmon-colored enzyme does contain a complete corrinoid, i.e., a 5,6-dimethylbenzimidazolylcobamide (Ertel *et al.*, 1968) ; hence, it is appropriate to refer to it as a cobalamin enzyme. Throughout the remainder of this review, therefore, the symbol B_{12} is used to denote a cobalamin, e.g., methyl-B_{12}, methylcobalamin, etc. (Fig. 1).

In addition to Reaction (1), purified preparations of the *E. coli* B_{12} enzyme also catalyze Reaction (3) and (4).

$$S\text{-Adenosyl-L-methionine} + \text{homocysteine} \xrightarrow{\text{reducing system}}$$
$$\text{methionine} + S\text{-adenosyl-L-homocysteine} \quad (3)$$

$$\text{Methyl-}B_{12} + \text{homocysteine} \xrightarrow{\text{aerobic}}$$
$$\text{methionine} + \text{hydroxy-}B_{12} \quad (4)$$

Reaction (3) is catalyzed by the enzyme at $<1\%$ the rate of Reaction (1) (Taylor and Weissbach, 1967a; Rosenthal *et al.*, 1965) but is absolutely dependent on the presence of a reducing system. An $FMNH_2$ + 1,4-dithiothreitol (DTT) reducing system (Taylor and Weissbach, 1967a) has been employed routinely to provide the optimal catalysis of Reactions (1) and (3). Moreover, as will be seen later, this potent artificial reducing system was used exclusively in the experiments utilizing substrate amounts of enzymes. Despite its extremely slow rate relative to Reaction (1), the synthesis of methyl-^{14}C-methionine from methyl-^{14}C-AMe is not inhibited by unlabeled N^5-methyl-H_4-folate (Taylor and Weissbach, 1967a; Rosenthal *et al.*, 1965). In contrast to Reactions (1) and (3), Reaction (4) requires no reducing system. Also, unlabeled methyl-B_{12} does not inhibit the synthesis of methyl-^{14}C-methionine from N^5-methyl-^{14}C-H_4-folate (Taylor and Weissbach,

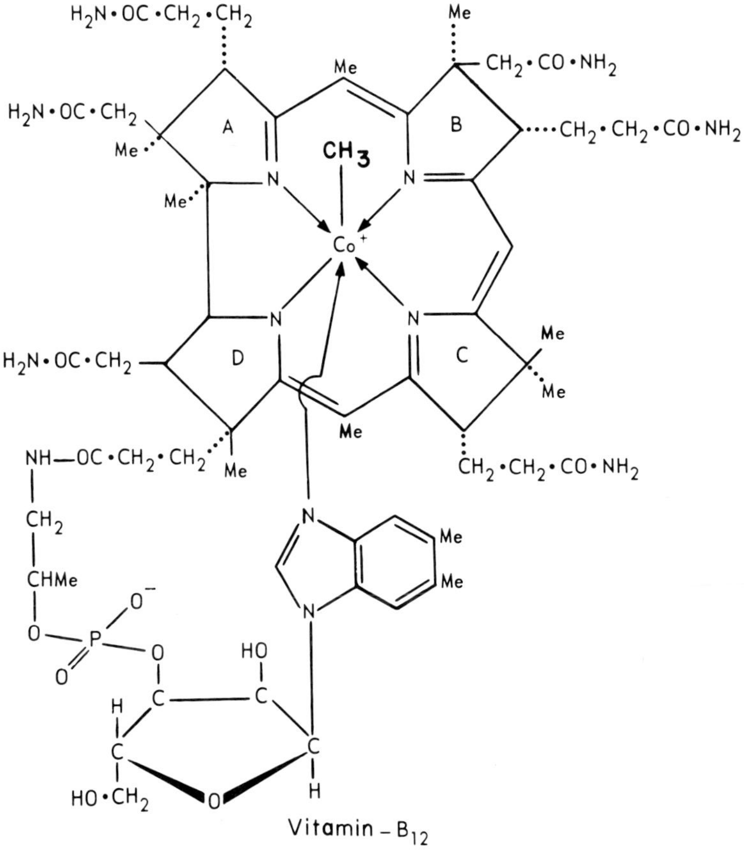

$H_2N \cdot OC \cdot CH_2 \cdot CH_2$

Me

$CH_2 \cdot CO \cdot NH_2$

Me

$H_2N \cdot OC \cdot CH_2$

Me

A

CH_3

B

$\cdots CH_2 \cdot CH_2 \cdot CO \cdot NH_2$

Me

N

N

Co^+

N

N

Me

Me

$H_2N \cdot OC \cdot CH_2$

D

C

$CH_2 \cdot CH_2 \cdot CO \cdot NH_2$

Me

$NH-OC \cdot CH_2 \cdot CH_2$

Me

CH_2

N

Me

$CHMe$

Me

N

O^-

HO

$O-P-O$

C

C

H

O

C

C

$HO \cdot CH_2$

O

H

Vitamin $-B_{12}$

FIG. 1. Structure of methyl-B₁₂ (5,6-dimethylbenzimidazolylcobamide methyl). For structures of various other cobamide compounds the reader should refer to Bonnett (1963).

1967a). Reaction (4) now appears to be a side reaction that is catalyzed by the B₁₂ enzyme (Taylor and Weissbach, 1967b; Brot et al., 1966). Yet, in retrospect, it was the observation made initially by Guest et al. (1962) that the B₁₂ transmethylase also catalyzed a methyl group transfer from methyl-B₁₂ to homocysteine (Reaction 4) which stimulated much of the interest in B₁₂-dependent methionine synthesis. This observation focused attention on the possibility that a cobalamin on the enzyme was functioning as a methyl group carrier, i.e., accepting a methyl group from N^5-methyl-H₄-folate to form a methyl-B₁₂-enzyme which could transfer its methyl group to homocysteine to form methionine. The availability of millimicromole amounts of purified B₁₂ enzyme (Taylor and Weissbach, 1967a) made it possible to investigate whether the enzyme-bound cobalamin is methylated during the reaction, and how AMe functions catalytically in methyl group transfer.

B. STUDIES WITH RADIOACTIVE N^5-METHYLTETRAHYDROFOLATE

In the initial experiments, methyl-^{14}C labeled N^5-methyl-H$_4$-folate was used in an attempt to see whether a stable methylated enzyme could be detected (Taylor and Weissbach, 1967c,d, 1968). As seen in Table I, incubation of the radioactive folate substrate with the purified B$_{12}$ enzyme yields a radioactive enzyme. Radioactivity on the protein was assayed by precipitating the enzyme with cold 10% TCA, and collecting the precipitate on a nitrocellulose (Millipore) filter. The radioactivity on the filter was then determined. The dependencies for the formation of a radioactive protein, namely AMe and a reducing system, and the inability to accumulate any ^{14}C-protein in the presence of homocysteine, suggested that the B$_{12}$ protein had reacted with radioactive N^5-^{14}C-methyl-H$_4$-folate. Figure 2 shows the effects of the N^5-methyl-^{14}C-H$_4$-folate and the protein concentrations on the formation of a radioactive enzyme. A folate (active stereoisomer) to B$_{12}$ protein ratio of 5:1 gave maximal TCA precipitable counts per minute, and based on the B$_{12}$ content of the

TABLE I

REQUIREMENTS FOR THE FORMATION OF ^{14}C-B$_{12}$-TRANSMETHYLASE WITH N^5-METHYL-^{14}C-H$_4$-FOLATE

Reaction mixture	Trichloroacetic acid precipitate (cpm)	^{14}C bound (mμmoles)
Complete system, $0°^a$	187	<0.01
Complete system, 37°	6219	0.51
−Enzyme[b]	147	—
−FMNH$_2$ and platinum oxide	1278	0.09
−Dithiothreitol	2369	0.18
−FMNH$_2$, platinum oxide, and dithiothreitol	147	—
−AMe	276	0.01
+Homocysteine	180	<0.01

[a] Complete system (0.2 ml) contained potassium phosphate, pH 7.4, 20 μmoles; ±N^5-methyl-^{14}C-H$_4$-folate (12,300 cpm/mμmole), 3 mμmoles; AMe, 10 mμmoles; dithiothreitol, 5 μmoles; FMNH$_2$, 50 mμmoles; platinum oxide, 0.1 mg; and B$_{12}$ transmethylase, 0.6 mg. Homocysteine, 0.1 μmole, was added to the complete system as indicated. Incubations were for 10 minutes at 37° under continuous H$_2$ gassing.

[b] The amount of B$_{12}$-enzyme added was estimated spectrophotometrically to contain about 1.4 mμmoles of bound B$_{12}$-chromophore. From Taylor and Weissbach (1967c).

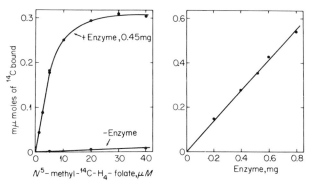

FIG. 2. Effect of N^5-methyl-H$_4$-folate and enzyme concentration on the formation of trichloroacetic acid-precipitable counts per minutes from N^5-methyl-^{14}C-H$_4$-folate. Reaction mixtures (0.2 ml) contained potassium phosphate, pH 7.4, 20 μmoles; AMe, 10 mμmoles; dithiothreitol, 5 μmoles; FMNH$_2$, 50 mμmoles; platinum oxide, 0.1 mg; enzyme, 0.45 mg; and the indicated concentrations of N^5-methyl-^{14}C-H$_4$-folate active stereoisomer (16,500 cpm/mμmole) (left). Reaction mixtures (right) were the same as on the left except that the concentration of N^5-methyl-^{14}C-H$_4$-folate active stereoisomer was 40 μM while the amounts of enzyme were varied. Incubations were for 15 minutes at 37° in the dark. From Taylor and Weissbach (1968).

enzyme determined spectrophotometrically it was concluded that under the conditions used, 0.5 equivalent of ^{14}C was bound per equivalent of B$_{12}$ enzyme.

The results in Table I and Fig. 2 gave no indication, however, as to whether the intact N^5-methyl-^{14}C-H$_4$-folate molecule was bound to the enzyme, or if a methylated enzyme had been formed. By employing differently labeled N^5-methyl-H$_4$-folates, it was possible to show that only the methyl group of N^5-methyl-H$_4$-folate is transferred to the enzyme (Taylor and Weissbach, 1968). As seen in Table II, pteridine labeled N^5-methyl-H$_4$-folate (either with ^{14}C or ^{3}H) did not react with the B$_{12}$ enzyme under conditions in which the methyl-^{14}C labeled substrate formed a radioactive enzyme.

In order to examine the various characteristics of an enzyme methylated with N^5-methyl-^{14}C-H$_4$-folate, Sephadex G-25 chromatography was used to isolate a methylated enzyme which still retained catalytic activity (Taylor and Weissbach, 1967c). After incubation of the B$_{12}$ enzyme with N^5-methyl-^{14}C-H$_4$-folate as described in Table I, the reaction mixtures were filtered through Sephadex G-25 columns. As seen in Fig. 3, radioactivity is associated with the protein component (fractions 13 to 16) and, similar to the results in Table I, a dependency on AMe was again observed. Peaks II and III in Fig. 3 represent an oxidized degradation product of the labeled methyl-folate and the unreacted N^5-methyl-^{14}C-

TABLE II

FORMATION OF TRICHLOROACETIC ACID-PRECIPITABLE COUNTS PER MINUTE
WITH THREE DIFFERENTLY LABELED N^5-METHYL-H$_4$-FOLATES[a]

Folate in complete system	Trichloroacetic acid precipitate (cpm)	Isotope bound (mμmoles)
(1) N^5-Methyl-^{14}C-H$_4$-folate, 16,500 cpm/mμmole	6222	0.37
−Enzyme	128	0
(2) N^5-Methyl-H$_4$-folate-2-^{14}C, 9300 cpm/mμmole	374	<0.01
−Enzyme	352	0
(3) N^5-Methyl-^{3}H$_4$-folate, 22,000 cpm/mμmole	235	<0.01
−Enzyme	179	0

[a] Incubation conditions were the same as in Table I except that all the systems contained 10 mμmoles of labeled N^5-methyl-H$_4$-folate and 0.52 mg of enzyme. From Taylor and Weissbach (1968).

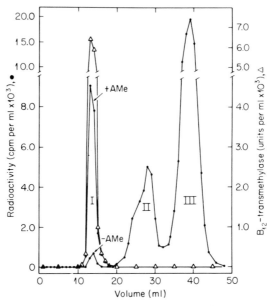

FIG. 3. Isolation of ^{14}C-B$_{12}$-transmethylase by Sephadex filtration. A reaction mixture (0.28 ml) containing 2.0 mg of B$_{12}$-enzyme, 6 μmoles of dithiothreitol, 10 mμmoles of ±N^5-methyl-^{14}C-H$_4$-folate (12,300 cpm/mμmole), and all the other components of the complete system in Table I were incubated 10 minutes at 37°C under H$_2$. Then 0.3 ml of water was added and the entire mixture was applied to a Sephadex G-25 column (for details, see Taylor and Weissbach, 1967c). A second identical reaction mixture minus AMe was treated in the same manner.

H_4-folate, respectively. The Sephadex G-25 procedure made it possible to separate a catalytically active methylated enzyme from the other components in the preliminary incubation mixture and to answer the following questions: (1) Can the methylated enzyme transfer its methyl group to homocysteine? and (2) Is the methylated enzyme a methyl-B_{12} enzyme?

A methylated enzyme, isolated by Sephadex G-25 chromatography almost quantitatively transferred its methyl group to homocysteine to form methionine (Taylor and Weissbach, 1967c). As seen in Table III, 80% of the radioactivity associated with the enzyme could be recovered as the methyl group of methionine, and the transfer was not dependent on AMe or a reducing system. It should also be noted that methyl group transfer from the methylated enzyme to homocysteine occurred in the dark under anerobic conditions (Table III, experiment 1) or in the light in an aerobic environment (Table III, experiment 2). Although a 15-minute incubation was used initially in Table III, this transfer actually occurs at a rate that is too rapid to measure (Taylor and Weissbach, 1969b).

At first, the light stability of the methylated enzyme argued against it being a methyl-B_{12}-enzyme. After exposure to visible light, the radioactivity on the methylated enzyme could not be recovered as formaldehyde, the major product obtained after light decomposition of methyl-B_{12}

TABLE III
REQUIREMENT FOR METHYL-^{14}C-METHIONINE FORMATION
FROM ^{14}C-B_{12}-TRANSMETHYLASE

Experiment	Reaction mixture[a]	Cpm	Methionine formed (mμmoles)
1, Dark (anaerobic)	Complete system (^{14}C-enzyme + homocysteine)	2000	0.16
	−Homocysteine	160	0.01
	Complete system + AMe + reducing system	1900	0.15
2, Light (aerobic)	Complete system (^{14}C-enzyme + homocysteine)	2650	0.21
	−Homocysteine	230	0.02

[a] Complete systems (0.3 ml) contained ^{14}C-enzyme, 2600 cpm (experiment 1) or 2730 cpm (experiment 2) and homocysteine, 0.2 μmole. In experiment 1 AMe 10 mμmoles, and a reducing system were included in the reaction mixture as indicated. The reducing system consisted of $FMNH_2$, 50 mμmoles; platinum oxide, 0.1 mg; and dithiothreitol, 5 μmoles. Incubations were for 15 minutes at 37° under H_2 gas in the dark (experiment 1) or aerobic for 15 minutes at 37°C in room light (experiment 2). From Taylor and Weissbach (1967c).

(Hogenkamp, 1966). In addition, as seen in Table III, the methyl group on the enzyme was readily transferred to homocysteine after exposure of the enzyme to light. There was also no reason to believe that a protein-bound methyl-B_{12} would be light stable since previous studies (Brot and Weissbach, 1965; Taylor and Weissbach, 1967b) on the chemical alkylation of the B_{12} enzyme has shown that a propyl-B_{12} enzyme was inactive but could be reactivated by exposure to light (Reaction 5).

$$
\begin{array}{ccc}
\underset{\substack{\diagdown\, |\, \diagup \\ \text{Co} \\ \diagup\, |\, \diagdown \\ \text{Enz}}}{\text{C—C—C}} & \xrightarrow{\text{light}} & \underset{\substack{\diagdown\, |\, \diagup \\ \text{Co} \\ \diagup\, |\, \diagdown \\ \text{Enz}}}{} + [\text{C—C—C}]
\end{array}
\qquad (5)
$$

$$
\begin{array}{cc}
\text{Inactive} & \text{Active} \\
\text{propyl-}B_{12} & \text{holoenzyme} \\
\text{enzyme} &
\end{array}
$$

However, despite the light stability of the methylated enzyme, other

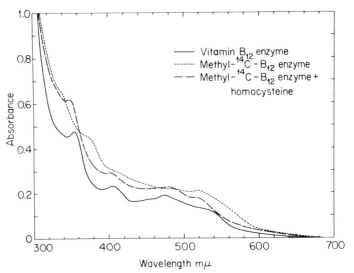

FIG. 4. Effect of methylation with N^5-methyl-^{14}C-H_4-folate on the absorption spectrum of vitamin-B_{12} transmethylase. Vitamin-B_{12} enzyme: initial enzyme, 22 mg/ml, in 0.05 M potassium phosphate, pH 7.4; methyl-^{14}C-B_{12} enzyme: same concentration of enzyme in phosphate buffer after methylation with N^5-methyl-^{14}C-H_4-folate (plus unlabeled AMe) followed by Sephadex G-25 filtration and lyophilization in the dark; same tracing was obtained in the dark and after illumination for 20 minutes with a 100-W tungsten lamp at 10 cm and 0°; methyl-^{14}C-B_{12} enzyme + homocysteine: spectrum immediately after the addition of 0.2 μmole of homocysteine at 22°C; same tracing was obtained after an additional 30 minutes aerobic incubation at 37°. From Taylor and Weissbach (1968).

experiments demonstrated conclusively that methylation of the enzyme with N^5-methyl-^{14}C-H$_4$-folate did, in fact, yield a methyl-^{14}C-B$_{12}$ enzyme. As seen in Fig. 4, methylation of the enzyme resulted in a shift of the absorption peak in the visible region of the spectrum from 475 nm to 520 nm. Such a change would be expected if a methyl-B$_{12}$ chromophore had been formed. Exposure of the methylated enzyme to homocysteine resulted in a new absorption spectrum similar to that of the original nonmethylated B$_{12}$ enzyme. In addition to the spectral data, it was possible to obtain more direct evidence for the presence of a methyl-

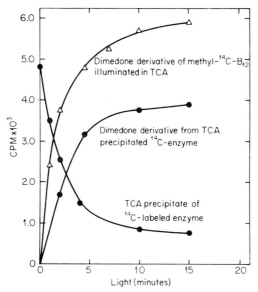

FIG. 5. Dependence of loss of radioactivity from ^{14}C-labeled enzyme on time of illumination in trichloroacetic acid. Lower curve: Vitamin-B$_{12}$ enzyme (11.5 mg) was incubated with N^5-methyl-^{14}C-H$_4$-folate and isolated by Sephadex chromatography as described in Fig. 3. Then separate samples of ^{14}C-labeled enzyme (0.12 ml containing 6000 cpm each) were precipitated with cold 10% trichloroacetic acid and exposed to a 100-W tungsten lamp at 0° at a distance of 10–15 cm for the times indicated. Middle curve: Other samples of ^{14}C-labeled enzyme (0.2 ml containing 10,000 cpm each) were mixed with 0.2 ml of 0.1 M formaldehyde, precipitated with 0.1 ml of cold 25% trichloroacetic acid, and then exposed to light for varying times. After centrifugation at 20,000g and 0°, the supernatant liquids were removed in the dark and the amount of dimedone-^{14}C-reactive material was determined in the dark (Taylor and Weissbach, 1965). Upper curve: Samples of authentic methyl-^{14}C-B$_{12}$ (6 mμmoles containing 15,000 cpm) were mixed with formaldehyde and trichloroacetic acid and then photolyzed for varying times. Release of dimedone-^{14}C reactive formaldehyde-^{14}C was then determined as for the trichloroacetic acid precipitated enzyme above. From Taylor and Weissbach (1968).

B_{12} enzyme. After methylation of the enzyme with N^5-methyl-^{14}C-H$_4$-folate, the isolated methylated enzyme was extracted in the dark with hot 80% ethanol to remove the protein-bound cobalamin. After concentration of the alcohol extract, a single radioactive component which behaved like methyl-^{14}C-B$_{12}$ could be separated by paper chromatography and paper electrophoresis (Taylor and Weissbach, 1968). Thus, despite the light stability of the methylated enzyme, it was clear from the spectral and chromatographic results that N^5-methyl-^{14}C-H$_4$-folate reacted with the B$_{12}$ protein in the presence of a reducing system and AMe to yield a methyl-^{14}C-B$_{12}$ enzyme.

A more detailed investigation of the light stability of the methylated enzyme indicated that the native enzyme protects the bound methyl-B$_{12}$ from photolytic decomposition. It was noted that acidification of the methyl-^{14}C-B$_{12}$ enzyme (isolated by Sephadex chromatography) rendered the radioactivity on the enzyme light-sensitive (Taylor and Weissbach, 1968). As seen in Fig. 5 light treatment of a TCA-precipitated methylated enzyme yielded the formation of ^{14}C-formaldehyde which was assayed as the dimedone derivative. The release of ^{14}C-formaldehyde upon light exposure paralleled the loss of radioactivity from the enzyme, and the rate of ^{14}C-formaldehyde released from the enzyme in TCA was the same as that observed with chemically synthesized methyl-^{14}C-B$_{12}$ (Fig. 5). A variety of treatments of the methylated enzyme were examined to determine what conditions were needed to make the carbon to cobalt bond of the enzyme bound methyl-B$_{12}$ light sensitive. As seen in Table IV, acidification of the enzyme with HCl to below pH 2.5 resulted in almost complete photolysis of the enzyme-bound methyl-^{14}C group; whereas, exposure of the methylated enzyme at 0° to alkaline cyanide, urea, etc., did not convert the methylated enzyme to a photolabile enzyme.

The foregoing results gave support for the two partial reactions depicted below (Reactions 6 and 7).

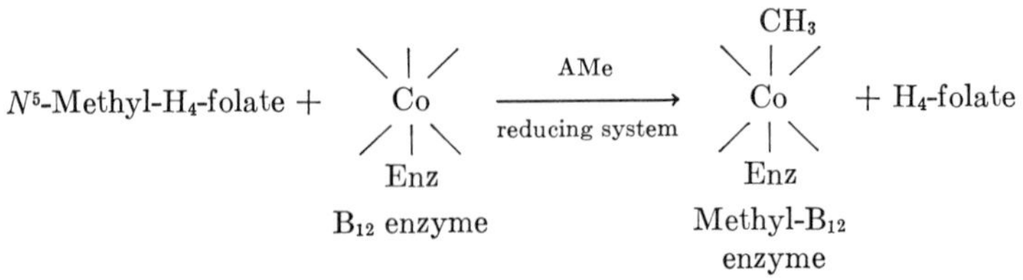

$$N^5\text{-Methyl-H}_4\text{-folate} + \underset{\substack{\diagdown \mid \diagup \\ \diagup \mid \diagdown \\ \text{Enz} \\ \text{B}_{12}\text{ enzyme}}}{\text{Co}} \xrightarrow[\text{reducing system}]{\text{AMe}} \underset{\substack{\diagdown \mid \diagup \\ \diagup \mid \diagdown \\ \text{Enz} \\ \text{Methyl-B}_{12} \\ \text{enzyme}}}{\overset{\text{CH}_3}{\text{Co}}} + \text{H}_4\text{-folate} \qquad (6)$$

$$\underset{\substack{\diagdown \mid \diagup \\ \diagup \mid \diagdown \\ \text{Enz}}}{\overset{\text{CH}_3}{\text{Co}}} + \text{homocysteine} \longrightarrow \text{methionine} + \underset{\substack{\diagdown \mid \diagup \\ \diagup \mid \diagdown \\ \text{Enz}}}{\text{Co}} \qquad (7)$$

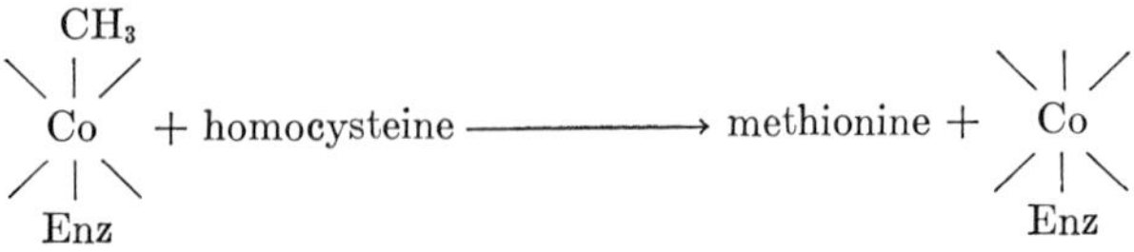

TABLE IV

PHOTOLABILITY OF TRICHLOROACETIC ACID-PRECIPITABLE ^{14}C
UNDER VARIOUS CONDITIONS[a]

Condition	Trichloroacetic acid precipitate (cpm light/cpm dark)
Distilled water	0.98
Distilled water; 37°C	0.80
0.1 M Potassium cyanide	1.0
1.0 M Potassium phosphate, pH 7.4	1.0
2.0 M Urea, pH 7.4	0.95
1 mM Mercuric acetate	1.0
0.1 M Imidazole phosphate, pH 7.4	0.92
0.1 M Sodium acetate, pH 4.4	0.97
0.1 M Acetic acid, pH 2.5	0.80
3 mM HCl, pH 2.5	0.75
10% Trichloroacetic acid (0.6 M)	0.24
20 mM HCl, pH 2	0.03

[a] To duplicate 0.1-ml aliquots of ^{14}C-enzyme (0.85 mg containing 6000 cpm each) which had been labeled with $\pm N^5$-methyl-^{14}C-H$_4$-folate and passed through a Sephadex G-25 column, 2 ml of the indicated solutions were added. One mixture of each pair was exposed to a 100-W tungsten lamp at 10–15 cm for 15 minutes at 0° (with one exception at 27°C), and the other was kept at 0° in the dark. Subsequently, 1 ml of 40% trichloroacetic acid was added to each mixture and the protein precipitates were collected and washed with 10% trichloroacetic acid in the dark. From Taylor and Weissbach (1968).

Reaction (6) requires AMe plus a reducing system and involves methylation of the enzyme by N^5-methyl-H$_4$-folate to form a methyl-B$_{12}$ enzyme. Reaction (7) is simply a transfer of the methyl group from the methyl-B$_{12}$ enzyme to homocysteine to form methionine.

C. STUDIES ON THE ROLE OF S-ADENOSYL-L-METHIONINE (AMe)

Mangum and Scrimgeour (1962) first directed attention to AMe by reporting that catalytic amounts of AMe were required by a crude pig liver enzyme preparation in order to observe methyl transfer from N^5-methyl-H$_4$-folate to homocysteine. Similarly, as mentioned in Section I, AMe is also needed in catalytic amounts by the E. coli B$_{12}$ enzyme. Consequently, over the years various postulates have been put forth to explain the requirement of this metabolite of methionine in cobalamin-dependent methionine synthesis. A priori, AMe could be functioning as an allosteric effector or could be donating an essential methyl group or a 5'-deoxyadenosyl moiety to the enzyme. The first clue to the function of AMe came from the finding that methyl iodide, a chemical methylating agent, could partially satisfy the requirement for AMe in Reaction (1) (Taylor and Weissbach, 1966). It was further shown (Taylor and Weissbach, 1967e) that methyl iodide could promote the synthesis of 7–8 equivalents of methyl-^{14}C-methionine and hence was functioning catalytically like AMe. The key technical aspect of these experiments (Taylor and Weissbach, 1966, 1967e) was the use of a labeled folate substrate (N^5-methyl-^{14}C-H$_4$-folate) so that any nonenzymatic reaction between the nonradioactive methyl iodide and homocysteine would not influence the results. These observations suggested that AMe could only be serving as a methyl group donor.

Using methyl-^{14}C labeled AMe, it was then demonstrated that this compound could also transfer its methyl group to the B$_{12}$ enzyme to yield a methyl-B$_{12}$ enzyme (Table V). As expected, a reducing system was required for this reaction, and the properties of the methyl-^{14}C-B$_{12}$ enzyme (light stability, etc.) formed from methyl-^{14}C AMe were similar to those found earlier with a methyl-B$_{12}$ enzyme formed from N^5-methyl-^{14}C-H$_4$-folate (Taylor and Weissbach, 1969a). It is also seen in Table V that after a 15-minute incubation, both homocysteine and unlabeled N^5-methyl-H$_4$-folate prevented the accumulation of a methyl-^{14}C-B$_{12}$ enzyme from methyl-^{14}C-AMe. Homocysteine was obviously acting as a methyl group acceptor and demethylating the methyl-B$_{12}$ enzyme. But the affect of N^5-methyl-H$_4$-folate on methyl-^{14}C-B$_{12}$ enzyme formation from methyl-^{14}C-AMe (Table V) suggested initially that AMe did not methylate the bound-B$_{12}$ in the presence of the normal methyl donor, N^5-methyl-H$_4$-folate. However, kinetic studies (Fig. 6) on the rate of methyl-^{14}C-B$_{12}$ enzyme formation showed that methylation of the enzyme by methyl-^{14}C-AMe occurred very rapidly even in the presence of N^5-methyl-H$_4$-folate. As seen in Fig. 6, methylation of the enzyme with

TABLE V

REQUIREMENTS FOR THE FORMATION OF TRICHLOROACETIC ACID-PRECIPITABLE ^{14}C WITH METHYL-^{14}C-AMe

Reaction mixture	Trichloroacetic acid precipitate (cpm)	^{14}C Bound (mμmoles)
Complete (37°)[a]	12,800	0.61
−B$_{12}$ Enzyme	1,480	0
−FMNH$_2$ and platinum	2,074	0.03
+N^5-Methyl-H$_4$-folate	2,600	0.06
+Homocysteine	2,470	0.05

[a] Complete systems (0.2 ml) contained potassium phosphate buffer, pH 7.4, 20 μmoles; methyl-^{14}C-AMe (18,500 cpm per mμmole), 10 mμmoles; dithiothreitol, 5 μmoles; B$_{12}$ enzyme, 0.54 mμmole; FMNH$_2$, 50 mμmoles; and platinum, 0.1 mg. Where indicated N^5-methyl-H$_4$-folate, 30 mμmoles, or homocysteine 0.2 μmole, was added to the complete system. Incubations were for 15 minutes in the dark under H$_2$ gas. From Taylor and Weissbach (1969a).

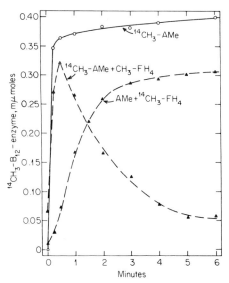

FIG. 6. Time dependence of methyl-^{14}C-B$_{12}$ enzyme formation with methyl-^{14}C-AMe and N^5-methyl-^{14}C-H$_4$-folate. All reaction mixtures (0.2 ml) contained 0.46 mμmole of B$_{12}$ enzyme; 10 mμmoles of AMe either unlabeled or methyl-^{14}C (18,000 cpm per mμmole); and, where indicated, 10 mμmoles of N^5-methyl-H$_4$-folate either unlabeled or methyl-^{14}C (73,000 cpm per mμmole). Incubations were under H$_2$ gas at 37° for the times indicated. They were initiated within 3 minutes after the injection at 0° of reduced flavin. From Taylor and Weissbach (1969a).

methyl-^{14}C-AMe occurred within 30 seconds and in the absence of non-radioactive N^5-methyl-H$_4$-folate, the methyl group on the enzyme from AMe was stable. Yet, in the presence of N^5-methyl-H$_4$-folate, a loss of the radioactive methyl group on the enzyme occurred over a period of 30 sec to 6 minutes. In analogous experiments with N^5-methyl-^{14}C-H$_4$-folate, methylation of the enzyme to form a methyl-^{14}C-B$_{12}$ enzyme occurred over a period of 5–6 minutes. This reaction was dependent on AMe (not shown in Fig. 6) and the time kinetics showed a discernible lag during the first 30–60 seconds.

The data in Fig. 6 indicated that the methyl group of N^5-methyl-H$_4$-folate was exchanging with the methyl group on the bound-cobalamin (derived from AMe). This was borne out by experiments in which a methyl-^{14}C-B$_{12}$ enzyme was preformed with methyl-^{14}C-AMe and then subjected to Sephadex G-25 column filtration. Upon a subsequent aerobic incubation of this methyl-^{14}C-B$_{12}$ enzyme with racemic, unlabeled N^5-methyl-H$_4$-folate, N^5-methyl-^{14}C-H$_4$-folate (active isomer) was formed (Taylor and Weissbach, 1969a). A plausible mechanism for this exchange (Fig. 7) was realized when it was found (Taylor and Weissbach, 1969a)

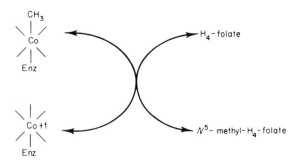

FIG. 7. Role of H_4-folate in methyl group exchange between N^5-methyl-H_4-folate and the methyl-B_{12} enzyme. From Taylor and Weissbach (1969b).

(1) that H_4-folate can accept directly the methyl group from a methyl-^{14}C-B_{12} enzyme yielding active N^5-methyl-^{14}C-H_4-folate and (2) that racemic N^5-methyl-H_4-folate prepared as described by Keresztesy and Donaldson (1961) contained traces of contaminating H_4-folate. In this scheme (Fig. 7), H_4-folate accepts a methyl group from the methyl-B_{12} enzyme to form N^5-methyl-H_4-folate and a postulated Co^{+1} enzyme species (B_{12s} enzyme) which can cyclically react with N^5-methyl-H_4-folate to re-form the methyl-B_{12} enzyme (Taylor and Weissbach, 1969b). Confirmation of such an exchange reaction was obtained by showing that the B_{12} enzyme could catalyze an AMe-dependent exchange reaction between pteridine ring labeled N^5-methyl-H_4-folate and H_4-folate, yielding pteridine ring labeled H_4-folate (Taylor and Weissbach, 1969b).

These results on the exchange of the methyl group of a methyl-B_{12} enzyme with the methyl group of N^5-methyl-H_4-folate suggested a mechanism for the role of AMe in methionine formation (Reaction 1) catalyzed by the B_{12} enzyme. This scheme involved the initial priming or activation of the enzyme by methylation of the enzyme-bound cobalamin. This priming reaction could be accomplished by AMe, methyl iodide and very likely other methylating or ethylating agents (Taylor and Weissbach, 1967e). Once activated (methylated) the enzyme could catalyze methyl transfer from N^5-methyl-H_4-folate to homocysteine.

The experiments described in Table VI support the view that a methyl-B_{12} enzyme is an activated enzyme capable of catalyzing methionine formation from N^5-methyl-H_4-folate. The B_{12} enzyme was preincubated under conditions in which the enzyme-bound cobalamin was methylated by either AMe or methyl iodide in the presence of an $FMNH_2$ reducing system. Each incubation system was then shaken to oxidize the $FMNH_2$ to FMN, and was then incubated aerobically with N^5-methyl-^{14}C-H_4-folate plus homocysteine. As seen in Table VI, the methylated enzyme

TABLE VI

REQUIREMENTS FOR AEROBIC METHYL-^{14}C GROUP TRANSFER FROM
N^5-METHYL-^{14}C-H$_4$-FOLATE TO HOMOCYSTEINE

First incubation reaction mixture	15 min, 37°C[a] Gas phase	Methyl-^{14}C-methionine formed after a second aerobic incubation, 5 min, 37°C[c] (mμmoles)
Complete	H$_2$	3.4–3.8
Complete (FMN)	Air	0.07
−FMNH$_2$ and platinum	H$_2$	0.01
−AMe	H$_2$	0.10
−AMe	H$_2$	0.13 (+AMe)[d]
−AMe + CH$_3$I[b]	H$_2$	3.40
−B$_{12}$ enzyme	H$_2$	0
Complete	H$_2$	0.09 (−homocysteine)[e]

[a] Complete systems (0.2 ml) for the first incubation contained B$_{12}$ enzyme, 0.39 mμmole; potassium phosphate buffer, pH 7.4, 20 μmoles; AMe, 10 mμmoles; FMNH$_2$, 50 mμmoles; and platinum 0.1 mg.

[b] Methyl iodide (0.15 μmole in 2 μl of ethanol) was substituted for AMe and the complete system (0.2 ml) also contained dithiothreitol (5 μmoles) during the first incubation.

[c] At the end of the first incubation the reaction mixtures were chilled to 0° in the dark and shaken for several minutes to oxidize the FMNH$_2$. They were then equilibrated at 37° for 5 minutes and tested for their transmethylase activity by the addition of 0.06 ml of a pH 7.4 substrate solution containing 0.5 mM N^5-methyl-^{14}C-H$_4$-folate (14,400 cpm/mμmole), 2.5 mM homocysteine, 0.05 M dithiothreitol, and 0.05 M potassium phosphate buffer, pH 7.4. Methyl-^{14}C-methionine synthesis was determined at the end of a 5-minute incubation by means of a Dowex 1-Cl column procedure.

[d] AMe (10 mμmoles) was added at the end of the first incubation after the FMNH$_2$ had been oxidized.

[e] Homocysteine was omitted from the second incubation system. From Taylor and Weissbach (1969b).

was able to catalyze the aerobic synthesis of about 10 equivalents of methyl-^{14}C-methionine from N^5-methyl-^{14}C-H$_4$-folate depending on the previous conditions used. This catalytic reaction lasted only about 30 seconds, then the enzyme was again inactivated. Exactly the same dependencies on AMe and reduced flavin were also observed when the preformed methyl-B$_{12}$ enzyme was separated from the components in the first incubation mixture by Sephadex G-25 filtration or charcoal column filtration (Taylor and Weissbach, 1969b). The significant observation was that this limited turnover of the enzyme occurred only when the enzyme had been methylated during the preliminary incubation. Thus, AMe (or methyl iodide) as well as a reducing system were required in order to preform a catalytically active B$_{12}$ protein. It was also observed in other experiments (Taylor and Weissbach, 1969b) that the amount of methionine formed with a given amount of activated enzyme could be increased 10-fold by carrying out the transmethylation reaction in an anaerobic environment.

More recently, conclusive evidence has been obtained that a methyl-B_{12} protein is a fully active enzyme molecule. By a selective treatment of the salmon-colored B_{12} protein (initial B_{12} holoenzyme) with 6 M urea at 37°C, it was resolved into a colorless apoprotein (apoenzyme) plus free B_{12r} (Fig. 8). Release of the bound-cobalamin as B_{12r} is due to the presence of dithiothreitol (DTT) in the resolution mixture (Taylor, 1970) which apparently helps to stabilize the much more labile apoenzyme. By this procedure about 95% of the original (nonmethylated) bound B_{12} was released and was readily separated from the apoenzyme upon Sephadex G-25 column filtration. The resulting apoenzyme was then shown to bind methyl-^{14}C-B_{12} very tightly and specifically at its active site. As seen in Fig. 8, the process of resolution and reconstitution was accompanied by a reversible change in the sedimentation coefficient ($s_{20,w}$). It is clearly indicative of a gross conformational change in the protein, mediated by the B_{12} chromophore. When apoenzyme was incubated with methyl-^{14}C-B_{12} and then freed of unbound methyl-^{14}C-B_{12} by charcoal treatment, a light-stable but homocysteine reactive methyl-^{14}C-B_{12} complex was obtained. The obvious advantage in testing the catalytic activity of a reconstituted methyl-B_{12} enzyme was the fact that it had not been subjected to a preliminary incubation with AMe and FMNH$_2$.

As seen in Table VII, the reconstituted methyl-^{14}C-B_{12} enzyme synthesized about 18 equivalents of methyl-^{14}C-methionine under aerobic conditions, but catalyzed negligible transmethylation if it was first demethylated by a short exposure to homocysteine prior to adding N^5-methyl-H$_4$-folate. These findings are comparable to what was found earlier with enzyme premethylated with AMe (Taylor and Weissbach, 1969b). By carefully pregassing the enzyme and the substrate mixture separately with H$_2$, however, it was possible to increase the catalytic

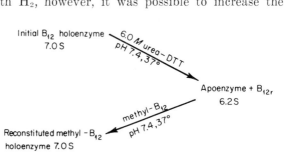

FIG. 8. Schematic summary of the resolution and reconstitution of B_{12} transmethylase. From Taylor (1970).

TABLE VII

EFFECT OF ORDER OF SUBSTRATE ADDITION ON THE AEROBIC CATALYSIS BY A
RECONSTITUTED METHYL-^{14}C-B₁₂ ENZYME[a]

Order of addition	Methyl-^{14}C-methionine formed (mμmoles)
N^5-Methyl-^{14}C-H₄-folate + homocysteine (5 min)	4.5
N^5-Methyl-^{14}C-H₄-folate (15 sec), then homocysteine (5 min)	4.0
Homocysteine (15 sec), then N^5-methyl-^{14}C-H₄-folate (5 min)	0.4

[a] Methyl-^{14}C-B₁₂ enzyme, 0.92 mg (0.25 mμmole) in 0.2 ml of 0.1 M potassium phosphate buffer, pH 7.4, was equilibrated at 37° for 5 minutes. A 1.0 mM solution of N^5-methyl-^{14}C-H₄-folate (29,000 cpm/mμmole), a 5.0 mM solution of homocysteine, and a 1:1 mixture of the substrate solutions were also equilibrated separately at 37° for 5 minutes. Then 0.06 ml of the 1:1 mixture or 0.03 ml of each substrate solution was added and incubated at 37° as shown. From Taylor and Hanna (1970a).

life of the reconstituted methyl-^{14}C-B₁₂ enzyme to several minutes (Fig. 9). Figure 9 also shows the inactivity of the original, nonmethylated B₁₂ enzyme in the presence of only the two substrates. Like an AMe-methylated B₁₂ enzyme (Taylor and Weissbach, 1969b), the reconstituted enzyme in Fig. 9 could not maintain a steady state of catalysis unless both AMe and FMNH₂ were added to the system. Nevertheless, it was possible to calculate that the minimum turnover number after 5 seconds was 910 moles of methionine formed per minute per mole of added methyl-^{14}C-B₁₂ enzyme. The total turnover at the end of 5 minutes was 530-fold. A turnover number of 910 is commensurate with the steady-state turnover rate of 860 which was obtained with this same reconstituted enzyme in the presence of AMe plus FMNH₂ (Taylor and Hanna, 1970a).

D. MECHANISM OF THE B₁₂-DEPENDENT TRANSMETHYLASE REACTION

The combined results discussed in Sections II,B and C suggest a reaction mechanism which is summarized in Fig. 10. The cobalt atom in the routinely isolated salmon-colored enzyme is thought to be linked to a sulfur atom, the source of which has not been determined. The only basis for this view is the independent isolation of sulfito-B₁₂ from two different purified B₁₂ enzyme preparations (Ertel *et al.*, 1968; Takeyama and Buchanan, 1961). In Fig. 10, the symbol

is used to represent collectively all the nonmethylated (inactive) forms

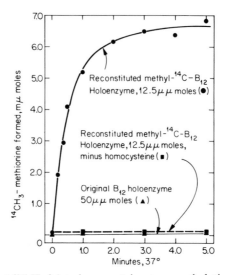

Fig. 9. N^5-Methyl-^{14}C-H$_4$-folate-homocysteine transmethylation under H$_2$ gas by a reconstituted methyl-^{14}C-B$_{12}$ holoenzyme. Final reaction mixtures (0.26 ml) contained potassium phosphate buffer, pH 7.4, 20 μmoles; N^5-methyl-^{14}C-H$_4$-folate (29,000 cpm/mμmole), 30 mμmoles; homocysteine, 50 mμmoles; and enzyme, either 46 μg of reconstituted methyl-^{14}C-B$_{12}$ enzyme (12.5 $\mu\mu$moles of bound methyl-^{14}C-B$_{12}$) or 50 μg of the original B$_{12}$ holoenzyme (50 $\mu\mu$moles of bound B$_{12}$). Enzyme in 0.1 M phosphate buffer (0.2 ml) and a pH 7.4 substrate solution containing 0.5 mM N^5-methyl-^{14}C-H$_4$-folate plus 2.5 mM homocysteine were pregassed separately with H$_2$ for 5 minutes at 0° and with constant agitation. Then the buffered enzyme and substrate mixture were equilibrated separately at 37°C for 5 minutes. Reactions were initiated by the injection of 0.06 ml of substrate mixture and were terminated at the times indicated with 0.8 ml of ice-cold water. From Taylor and Hanna (1970a).

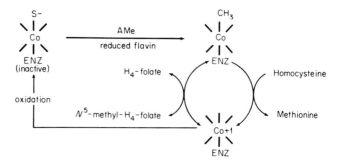

Fig. 10. Schematic reaction mechanism for AMe-dependent methionine synthesis catalyzed by *E. coli* B cobalamin transmethylase. From Taylor and Weissbach (1969b).

of the B$_{12}$ enzyme that may exist, including the salmon-colored enzyme that has been purified from *E. coli* B cells. The initial priming or activation of the enzyme is accomplished by methylation of the bound cobalamin with AMe (or methyl iodide) in the presence of a reducing system. The functional methyl-B$_{12}$ enzyme thus formed can then transfer its methyl group as a carbonium ion to homocysteine to form methionine and a second functional form of the B$_{12}$ enzyme which is pictured as containing a two-electron reduced form of the vitamin (B$_{12s}$),

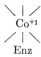

The formation of a

species is an essential feature of the scheme in Fig. 10. In this regard, direct spectral evidence for this type of reduced B$_{12}$ enzyme has recently been obtained in experiments on methyl transfer from AMe to homocysteine (Reaction 3) (Taylor and Hanna, 1970b). During this reaction absorption maxima appear at 385 nm and 460 nm, consistent with the formation of B$_{12s}$. These maxima are transient since the absorption spectrum reverts to a B$_{12r}$ spectrum when the AMe has been consumed. The

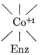

presumably accepts a methyl group preferentially from N^5-methyl-H$_4$-folate to reform the methyl-B$_{12}$ enzyme. Transfer of the methyl group from the methyl-B$_{12}$ enzyme to homocysteine and remethylation of the

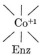

by N^5-methyl-H$_4$-folate would result in the continued formation of methionine selectively from folate. Thus, in this cycle only the first methyl group incorporated into methionine arises from AMe, whereas subsequent methyl groups come from N^5-methyl-H$_4$-folate. In agreement with this picture is the fact that a reconstituted methyl-B$_{12}$ enzyme could form 530–650 equivalents of methyl-^{14}C-methionine from N^5-

methyl-^{14}C-H$_4$-folate in the absence of AMe and FMNH$_2$ (Taylor and Hanna, 1970a).

The observations (Taylor and Weissbach, 1969b; Taylor and Hanna, 1970a) that both AMe and a reducing system are necessary to maintain a constant rate of methionine synthesis, even though one starts the reaction with a functional methyl-B$_{12}$ protein, indicate that an oxygen-labile

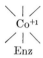

form of the enzyme is being generated during the catalytic cycle. This view is supported by the finding that a methylated enzyme has an extremely short catalytic life in air, but under anaerobic conditions there is a marked increase in the total amount of methionine that it can synthesize (Taylor and Weissbach, 1969b; Taylor and Hanna, 1970a). In addition, the apparent K_m for AMe in Reaction (1), under otherwise identical conditions, increases from $5 \times 10^{-8}\,M$ to $5 \times 10^{-7}\,M$ upon changing from an FMNH$_2$ + DTT reducing system to a 2–2.5-fold less active reducing system (Taylor and Hanna, 1970a). Thus, the

in Fig. 10 can be pictured as continually oxidizing even in a highly anaerobic system to an inactive form which must again be primed (methylated) to utilize N^5-methyl-H$_4$-folate as a substrate. One can, consequently, regard the slow catalysis of AMe-homocysteine transmethylation (Reaction 3) via a methyl-B$_{12}$ enzyme intermediate (Taylor and Weissbach, 1967b, 1969a; Taylor and Hanna, 1970b) as a manifestation of the rate of oxidative inactivation in a given reducing system (Taylor and Hanna, 1970a). Vitamin B$_{12s}$ is perhaps the most powerful nucleophile that has been studied to date (Schrauzer et al., 1968); yet, it is so oxygen-labile that it has been prepared only in solutions containing potent reducing agents, such as sodium borohydride, chromous chloride, or zinc plus NH$_4$Cl, or else by electrolysis (Boos et al., 1953; Hill et al., 1962; Tackett et al., 1963).

E. Additional Remarks

The foregoing results provide strong evidence that in methionine synthesis the enzyme-bound cobalamin functions as a methyl group carrier. Similar conclusions have also been reached by Jaenicke and co-workers

(Rudiger and Jaenicke, 1969; Stravrianopoulos and Jaenicke, 1967) using a purified enzyme preparation from *E. coli*. In contrast, the *E. coli* non-B_{12} transmethylase (Reaction 2) does not form a stable methylated enzyme but reacts with a racemic mixture of the folate substrate to yield a complex containing stoichiometric amounts of enzyme and the active stereoisomer of N^5-methyl-H_4-folate (Glu_3) (Whitfield and Weissbach, 1968, 1970). Unfortunately, for both the B_{12}-dependent and the B_{12}-independent reactions there is still no information as to how the methyl group on the N^5 position of the folate substrate is activated for transfer. It is important to stress that N^5-methyl-H_4-folate is not an onium compound, and therefore, a means must exist so that the nitrogen-carbon bond is labilized. Since labilization of the N^5-methyl group is probably the rate-limiting step in both Reactions (1) and (2), a methyl-B_{12} enzyme intermediate appears to be a much more efficient mechanism of catalysis. The conclusion is drawn from the fact that the turnover number for the *E. coli* non-B_{12} transmethylase is only 14 moles of N^5-methyl groups transferred per minute per mole of enzyme (Whitfield and Weissbach, 1970), while a turnover number (steady-state conditions) of ca. 800/min per mole of bound B_{12} was obtained with a preparation of the *E. coli* B_{12} enzyme (Taylor and Hanna, 1970a).

While this review was being prepared, Galivan and Huennekens (1970) reported that an uncharacterized but low molecular weight protein (M.W. 3000), stimulates the activity of the *E. coli* B_{12} containing protein. The low molecular weight S protein precipitates between 60 and 90% saturation with $(NH_4)_2SO_4$. They conclude that the B_{12}-transmethylase from *E. coli* K-12 is composed of two protein components, an M or B_{12}-protein (M.W. ca. 125,000) plus the S protein. No attempt was reported, however, to stimulate the activity of their M protein with reduced flavin or other reducing systems. Unless it can be shown that highly purified preparations of B_{12} enzyme obtained in other laboratories (Taylor and Weissbach, 1967a; Stravrianopoulos and Jaenicke, 1967) contain firmly attached S protein, the conclusion that the S protein is an integral part of the transmethylase system is not valid. Consequently, at present, it seems more plausible to assume that they have isolated a small thiol protein which behaves like $FMNH_2$, 2-mercaptoethanol + vitamin B_{12} (Taylor and Weissbach, 1967a), H_4-folate (Taylor and Weissbach, 1969b), or lipoyl dehydrogenase (Taylor and Hanna, 1970c), and serves as a reductant for the bound cobalamin.

Finally it should be noted at this point that the B_{12} transmethylase system, per se, does not satisfactorily explain at the enzymatic level the well-documented interrelationship among folic acid, vitamin B_{12}, and one-carbon metabolism in mammalian tissues (Bennett *et al.*, 1951; Machlin *et al.*, 1952; Sunde *et al.*, 1951; Fox *et al.*, 1956, 1961; Silverman and Pitney, 1958). Although a detailed discussion of the folate-B_{12} relationship is beyond the scope of this review, the key points in this controversy appear to be as follows: the major form of tissue and serum folic acid is N^5-methyl-H_4-folate (Herbert *et al.*, 1962), which must transfer its methyl group to homocysteine in order to regenerate H_4-folate for one-carbon unit metabolism (Vitale, 1966). Consequently, when Herbert and Zalusky (1962) observed that the parenteral administration of folic acid to a small number of patients with untreated pernicious anemia appeared to increase the serum level of N^5-methyl-H_4-folate, they proposed a "methylfolate block" hypothesis. According to this proposal a deficiency of vitamin B_{12} yields a pile-up of N^5-methyl-H_4-folate due to the inability to catalyze Reaction (1). This pile-up, in turn, causes a secondary shortage of H_4-folate. Although a very attractive hypothesis, recent studies do not support this viewpoint of Herbert and Zalusky. The increased folate in the serum and urine of pernicious anemia subjects, following an injected dose of tritiated folic acid, was shown to be derived by a displacement of unlabeled tissue folate into the plasma (Chanarin and McLean, 1967), and was not derived from the parenteral dose. In addition, the amount of N^5-methyl-H_4-folate displaced into the urine after a parenteral folic acid injection was less in pernicious anemia patients than in healthy subjects. Equally important was the finding that the plasma clearance of parenteral N^5-methyl-H_4-folate was the same in pernicious anemia patients as it was in control patients (Chanarin and Perry, 1968). Particularly germane is the recent report involving rats fed diets that were deficient in methionine and vitamin B_{12} (Vitale and Hegsted, 1969). Supplementation of their diet with either vitamin B_{12} or methionine resulted in an increase in liver and little or no change in the serum N^5-methyl-H_4-folate levels. Associated with the increase in liver folate there was a decrease in serum H_4-folate, a decrease in urinary formiminoglutamate excretion, and an increase in liver formiminotransferase activity. These findings indicate that the effect of vitamn B_{12} on folate metabolism may be mediated only indirectly via the vitamin B_{12}-dependent transmethylase.

REFERENCES

Bennett, M. A., Joralemon, J., and Halpern, P. E. (1951). *J. Biol. Chem.* **193**, 285.
Bonnett, R. (1963). *Chem. Rev.* **63**, 573.
Boos, R. N., Carr, J. E., and Conn, J. B. (1953). *Science* **117**, 603.
Botsford, J. D., and Parks, L. W. (1967). *J. Bacteriol.* **94**, 966.
Brot, N., and Weissbach, H. (1965). *J. Biol. Chem.* **240**, 3064.
Brot, N., Taylor, R. T., and Weissbach, H. (1966). *Arch. Biochem. Biophys.* **114**, 256.

Buchanan, J. M., Elford, H. L., Loughlin, R. E., McDougall, B. N., and Rosenthal, S. (1964). *Ann. N. Y. Acad. Sci.* **112**, 756.

Burton, E. G., and Sakami, W. (1967). *Fed. Proc., Fed. Amer. Soc. Exp. Biol.* **26**, 387.

Burton, E. G., and Sakami, W. (1969). *Biochem. Biophys. Res. Commun.* **36**, 228.

Burton, E. G., and Sakami, W. (1970). *Methods Enzymol.* **17B** (in press).

Burton, E., Selhub, J., and Sakami, W. (1969). *Biochem. J.* **111**, 793.

Cauthen, S. E., Foster, M. A., and Woods, D. D. (1966). *Biochem. J.* **98**, 630.

Cauthen, S. E., Pattison, J. R., and Lascelles, J. (1967). *Biochem. J.* **102**, 774.

Chanarin, I., and McLean, A. (1967). *Clin. Sci.* **32**, 57.

Chanarin, I., and Perry, J. (1968). *Brit. J. Haematol.* **14**, 297.

Dickerman, H., Redfield, B. G., Bieri, J., and Weissbach, H. (1964). *J. Biol. Chem.* **239**, 2545.

Dodd, W. A. (1969). *Arch. Biochem. Biophys.* **133**, 216.

Ertel, R., Brot, N., Taylor, R. T., and Weissbach, H. (1968). *Arch. Biochem. Biophys.* **126**, 353.

Evans, H. J., and Kliewer, M. (1964). *Ann. N. Y. Acad. Sci.* **112**, 735.

Foster, M. A., Dilworth, M. J., and Woods, D. D. (1964). *Nature (London)* **201**, 39.

Fox, M. R., Ortiz, L. O., and Briggs, G. M. (1956). *Proc. Soc. Exp. Biol. Med.* **93**, 501.

Fox, M. R., Ludwig, W. J., and Baroody, M. D. (1961). *Proc. Soc. Exp. Biol. Med.* **107**, 723.

Galivan, J., and Huennekens, F. M. (1970). *Biochem. Biophys. Res. Commun.* **58**, 46.

Griffiths, J. M., and Daniel, L. J. (1969). *Arch. Biochem. Biophys.* **134**, 463.

Guest, J. R., Helleiner, C. W., Cross, M. J., and Woods, D. D. (1960). *Biochem. J.* **76**, 396.

Guest, J. R., Friedman, S., and Woods, D. D. (1962). *Nature (London)* **195**, 340.

Guest, J. R., Friedman, S., and Woods, D. D., and Smith, E. L. (1964a). *Ann. N. Y. Acad. Sci.* **112**, 774.

Guest, J. R., Friedman, S., Foster, M. A., Tejerina, G., and Woods, D. D. (1964b). *Biochem. J.* **92**, 497.

Hatch, F. T., Larrabee, A. R., Cathou, R. E., and Buchanan, J. M. (1961). *J. Amer. Chem. Soc.* **83**, 4094.

Herbert, V., and Zalusky, R. (1962). *J. Clin. Invest.* **41**, 1263.

Herbert, V., Larrabee, A. R., and Buchanan, J. M. (1962). *J. Clin. Invest.* **41**, 1134.

Hill, J. A., Pratt, J. M., and Williams, R. J. P. (1962). *J. Theor. Biol.* **3**, 423.

Hogenkamp, H. P. C. (1966). *Biochemistry* **5**, 417.

Hogenkamp, H. P. C., Barker, H. A., and Mason, H. S. (1963). *Arch. Biochem. Biophys.* **100**, 353.

Jones, K. M., Guest, J. R., and Woods, D. D. (1961). *Biochem. J.* **79**, 566.

Keresztesy, J. C., and Donaldson, K. O. (1961). *Biochem. Biophys. Res. Commun.* **5**, 281.

Larrabee, A. R., Rosenthal, S., Cathou, R. E., and Buchanan, J. M. (1961). *J. Amer. Chem. Soc.* **83**, 5094.

Loughlin, R. E., Elford, H. L., and Buchanan, J. M. (1964). *J. Biol. Chem.* **239**, 2888.

Machlin, L. J., Denton, C. A., and Bird, H. R. (1952). *Poultry Sci.* **31**, 110.

Mangum, J. H., and Scrimgeour, K. G. (1962). *Fed. Proc., Fed. Amer. Soc. Exp. Biol.* **21**, 242.

Mangum, J. H., Murray, B. K., and North, J. A. (1969). *Biochemistry* **8**, 3496.

Morningstar, J. F., and Kisliuk, R. L. (1965). *J. Gen. Microbiol.* **39**, 43.

Rosenthal, S., and Buchanan, J. M. (1963). *Acta Chem. Scand.* **17**, Suppl. 1, 288.

Rosenthal, S., Smith, L. C., and Buchanan, J. M. (1965). *J. Biol. Chem.* **240**, 836.

Rudiger, H., and Jaenicke, L. (1969). *Euro. J. Biochem.* **10**, 557.

Schrauzer, G. N., Deutsch, E., and Windgassen, R. J. (1968). *J. Amer. Chem. Soc.* **90**, 2441.

Silverman, M., and Pitney, A. J. (1958). *J. Biol. Chem.* **233**, 1179.

Stravrianopoulos, J., and Jaenicke, L. (1967). *Eur. J. Biochem.* **3**, 95.

Sunde, M. L., Waibel, P. E., Cravens, W. W., and Elvehjem, C. A. (1951). *Poultry Sci.* **30**, 668.

Tackett, S. L., Collat, J. W., and Abbott, J. C. (1963). *Biochemistry* **2**, 919.

Takeyama, S., and Buchanan, J. M. (1961). *J. Biochem. (Tokyo)* **49**, 578.

Takeyama, S., Hatch, F. T., and Buchanan, J. M. (1961). *J. Biol. Chem.* **236**, 1102.

Taylor, R. T. (1970). *Arch. Biochem. Biophys.* **137**, 529.

Taylor, R. T., and Hanna, M. L. (1970a). *Arch. Biochem. Biophys.* **137**, 453.

Taylor, R. T., and Hanna, M. L. (1970b). *Biochem. Biophys. Res. Commun.* **38**, 578.

Taylor, R. T., and Hanna, M. L. (1970c). *Arch. Biochem. Biophys.* (manuscript submitted for publication).

Taylor, R. T., and Weissbach, H. (1965). *Anal. Biochem.* **13**, 80.

Taylor, R. T., and Weissbach, H. (1966). *J. Biol. Chem.* **241**, 3641.

Taylor, R. T., and Weissbach, H. (1967a). *J. Biol. Chem.* **242**, 1502.

Taylor, R. T., and Weissbach, H. (1967b). *J. Biol. Chem.* **242**, 1509.

Taylor, R. T., and Weissbach, H. (1967c). *Arch. Biochem. Biophys.* **119**, 572.

Taylor, R. T., and Weissbach, H. (1967d). *Biochem. Biophys. Res. Commun.* **27**, 398.

Taylor, R. T., and Weissbach, H. (1967e). *J. Biol. Chem.* **242**, 1517.

Taylor, R. T., and Weissbach, H. (1968). *Arch. Biochem. Biophys.* **123**, 109.

Taylor, R. T., and Weissbach, H. (1969a). *Arch. Biochem. Biophys.* **129**, 728.

Taylor, R. T., and Weissbach, H. (1969b). *Arch. Biochem. Biophys.* **129**, 745.

Vitale, J. J. (1966). *Nutr. Rev.* **24**, 289.

Vitale, J. J., and Hegsted, D. M. (1969). *Brit. J. Haematol.* **17**, 467.

Weissbach, H., and Taylor, R. T. (1966). *Fed. Proc., Fed. Amer. Soc. Exp. Biol.* **25**, 1649.

Weissbach, H., Peterkofsky, A., Redfield, B. G., and Dickerman, H. (1963). *J. Biol. Chem.* **238**, 3318.

Whitfield, C. D., and Weissbach, H. (1968). *Biochem. Biophys. Res. Commun.* **33**, 6.

Whitfield, C. D., and Weissbach, H. (1970). *J. Biol. Chem.* **245**, 402.

Whitfield, C. D., Steers, E. J., and Weissbach, H. (1970). *J. Biol. Chem.* **245**, 390.

Chemical Properties of Flavins in Relation to Flavoprotein Catalysis*

G. R. PENZER,† G. K. RADDA, J. A. TAYLOR, AND M. B. TAYLOR

Department of Biochemistry, University of Oxford, Oxford, England

I. Introduction

The understanding of the chemistry of flavin excited states contributes in two ways to the interpretation of flavoprotein catalysis.

First, the spectral properties of the flavin chromophore (absorption, fluorescence, phosphorescence) provide an intrinsic probe for the microenvironment of the flavin. Knowing the factors that govern spectral shifts in flavins, the nature of the coenzyme-enzyme interaction can in principle be understood.

Second, flavin photoreactions are models for many reactions catalyzed by flavoenzymes. Among the compounds that can be directly oxidized by a flavin excited state or a flavoprotein are NADH (Radda and Calvin, 1964), amino acids (Byrom and Turnbull, 1968; Penzer and Radda, 1968), hydroxy acids, ketoacids (Brüstlein and Hemmerich, 1968), and dicarboxylic acids (Weatherby and Carr, 1970). Flavin excited states can also sensitize oxidations, e.g., oxidation of purines by oxygen (Sussenbach and Berends, 1963), and hydroxylation of aromatic compounds by hydrogen peroxide (Steele, 1963).

* This work was supported by the Science and Medical Research Councils.
† Present address: Department of Chemistry, University of York, England.

II. Photophysical Properties of the Excited States

A. Absorption Spectra

The absorption spectra of flavins have been studied by a number of other workers both experimentally (Dudley *et al.*, 1964; Müller and Hemmerich, 1966; Müller *et al.*, 1966; Gordon-Walker *et al.*, 1970) and theoretically (Fox *et al.*, 1967; Kurtin and Song, 1968; Tollin, 1968). Of the four absorption bands in flavin mononucleotide (FMN), at 220, 265, 375, and 447 nm, the two long-wavelength bands have been most extensively used in studies of flavoproteins and flavoprotein inhibitor complexes (Massey and Ganther, 1965). The high extinction coefficients of these two transitions (Beinert, 1960), and the fact that the polarization of fluorescence is constant across both bands (Weber, 1966), suggests that these are π-π^* transitions. Any fine structure observed is associated with vibrational bands.

Here we shall review some of our own observations and present some speculations about the nature of the electronic transitions involved. Our starting point is the observation that in many flavoproteins both long-wavelength bands shift on binding to the apoenzyme. In addition, this interaction is often accompanied by the appearance of distinct shoulders in the 447 nm band (Massey and Ganther, 1965). An understanding of these shifts and inflections is essential to any interpretation of flavin binding.

1. Solvent Effects

The 370 nm band in general is blue shifted in nonpolar solvents while the position of the 447 nm band is relatively insensitive to solvent polarity (Harbury *et al.*, 1959; Koziol and Knobloch, 1965). Vibrational fine structure in the latter band is clearly observable in nonpolar solvents. The solvent shifts in the 370 nm band imply that it contains a charge-transfer contribution, perhaps tending to donate electrons to the pyrimidine ring. The sensitivity of this absorption band to solvent is further dependent on the nature of the substituents in the isoalloxazine ring. The correlation between an empirically derived solvent parameter (Z value, Kosower, 1958) and the position of the near-ultraviolet band for a number of flavins is shown in Fig. 1 and Table I. Clearly, substituents that decrease the energy of this electronic transition also lead to an increased charge separation on excitation, as the sensitivity of the band to solvent increases. These correlations suggest that a possible method for measuring the "polarity" of the flavin binding site is a comparison of the shifts with different flavins, as this should eliminate contributions to the shift from specific interactions.

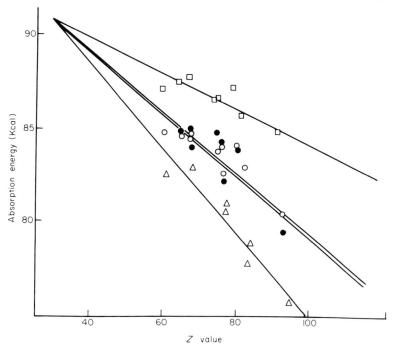

FIG. 1. The variation of the near-ultraviolet band energy of several flavins with solvent polarity. Flavin 1 ●; flavin 2 △; flavin 3 □; flavin 4 ○. The flavins are those listed in Table I.

2. *Dichroic Bleaching*

We have measured the angle between the two long-wavelength oscillators by a novel technique.

When flavins are trapped in a heavily cross-linked polyacrylamide film and are bleached by linearly polarized light consisting only of wavelengths absorbed by the 447 nm band, a partially ordered film of unreacted chromophores is obtained. This is because the probability of bleaching by polarized light is proportional to $\cos^2\alpha$, where α is the angle between an absorption oscillator and the direction of polarization of the exciting light. After bleaching, the dichroic ratio (OD parallel to bleaching/OD perpendicular to bleaching) is constant across a particular absorption band, but is different for the two bands (Fig. 2). This observation confirms that there are two separate electronic transitions involved. In addition, since the extent of orientation can be calculated after the photoselection experiment, the angle between the two long wavelength oscillators may be derived using an extension (Gordon-Walker *et al.*, 1970)

TABLE I

Absorption Maxima for Flavins in Different Solvents

Solvent	Flavin[a]					Z value[b]
	1	2	3	4	5	
Water	338 446	356 447	361 431	375 445		94.6
Methanol	328 440	340 444	341 427		344	83.6
Ethanol	330 448 (476)	340 449	339 436 (464)	353 448 (473)	387	79.6
n-Propanol	330 450 (480)	341 445	337 440 (465)			78.3
t-Butanol		338 452 (472; 430)	340 437 (470; 415)			71.3
Ethylene glycol	334 444	345 448 (470)	345 432 (455)	363 446	352 370	85.1

Solvent	Flavin 1	Flavin 2	Flavin 3	Flavin 4	Flavin 5	Z
Acetic acid		346, 445 (470)	348, 430 (450)	355, 445 (465)		79.2
N,N-Dimethyl formamide	326, 446 (474)	337, 452 (485)	336, 437 (465) (420)		334, 385 (404)	68.5
Chloroform		350 (366), 449 (425; 480)	349 (370), 438 (415; 465)		350, 387	63.2
Pyridine	327, 452 (430) (480)	336, 453 (435; 480)	336, 440	345, 460 (430; 475)		64.0
Acetonitrile	325, 442 (410; 470)	337, 451 (472; 427)	336, 446	344, 445 (468; 421)		71.3
Dimethyl sulfoxide		346, 447 (475)				71.1

a Flavin 1 is 6-chloro-9-(N,N-dimethylaminopropyl)isoalloxazine, flavin 2 is 6-methyl-9-(N,N-diethylaminoethyl)isoalloxazine; flavin 3 is 7-chloro-9-(N,N-dimethylaminopropyl)isoalloxazine; flavin 4 is lumiflavin or riboflavin; flavin 5 is lumichrome. Numbers in parentheses indicate shoulders. Positions of flavin substituents are numbered as in Penzer and Radda (1967b).
b Taken from Kosower (1958).

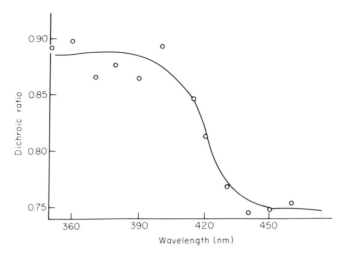

Fig. 2. The dichroic ratio spectrum of flavin mononucleotide in a polyacrylamide film after polarized bleaching. Taken from Gordon-Walker *et al.* (1970).

of Albrecht's work on photoselectivity (Albrecht, 1961). The results for a number of flavins are summarized in Table II. It is not possible to deduce the absolute direction of absorption oscillators simply from their relative orientations. Some theoretical work suggests that the long-wavelength transition is almost parallel to the long axis of the molecule (Kurtin and Song, 1968) with the near-ultraviolet band as shown in Fig. 3.

Now as a general and rough guide, one might expect that specific interactions along either of these axes will predominantly influence the transition with its moment oriented along the particular axis. This effect can be illustrated to a limited extent by examining the effect of substituents on flavin absorption.

TABLE II

ANGLE BETWEEN THE TWO LONG-WAVELENGTH ABSORPTION
OSCILLATORS (θ) FOR SEVERAL FLAVINS

Flavin	$\theta^{\circ a}$
Lumiflavin	37
3-Methyllumiflavin	38
Riboflavin	41
FMN	36
6-Chloro-9-(N,N-dimethylaminoethyl)isoalloxazine	52

[a] From dichroic ratio.

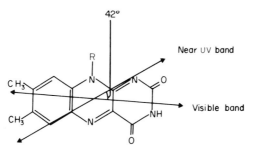

FIG. 3. The directions of the two long-wavelength absorption oscillators of iso-alloxazine. The direction of the longer-wavelength oscillator is taken from Kurtin and Song (1968).

3. *Substituent Effects*

The way substituents affect an absorption spectrum is usually dominated by mesomeric effects as inductive effects often change the energies of the ground and excited states similarly (Jaffé and Orchin, 1962). Some useful deductions can be made about flavin spectra from comparison of flavin spectra with those of similar chromophores for which electronic assignments have already been made, and comparison of the spectra of flavin derivatives with different substituents. It is reasonable to compare the spectra of flavins with those of tricyclic hydrocarbons and other heterocyclic molecules, in view of their planar structure (Kierkegaard *et al.*, 1967).

The spectra of anthracene and acridine at neutral pH are similar. The bands around 350 nm are assigned to the $^1L_a \leftarrow {}^1A$ transition, and the 254 nm band to $^1B_b \leftarrow {}^1A$. For anthracene these have transverse and longitudinal polarizations, respectively (Jones, 1945). Substituents around the ring may change the position of one or both of the bands, and they may effect the extinction by altering the symmetry of the chromophores (Jaffé and Orchin, 1962).

Consider now some aminoacridines (Table III). Most of them have a new absorption around 400 nm. This could be either of the $^1L \leftarrow {}^1A$ transitions shifted from its position in acridine. It is possible that in the 1-, 2-, 3-, and 4-aminoacridines the 400 nm band is $^1L_b \leftarrow {}^1A$, but in 9-aminoacridine it is $^1L_a \leftarrow {}^1A$. This is suggested because increasing the conjugation in the end rings usually favors longitudinally polarized transitions, while a conjugative substituent in the 9- position directly aids a transversely polarized transition across the center ring (Jaffé and Orchin, 1962). The different assignment in 9-aminoacridine is supported by the spectral changes that ocur on protonation of the ring nitrogen.

TABLE III

ABSORPTION MAXIMA OF ANTHRACENE, ACRIDINE, AND SOME ACRIDINE DERIVATIVES[a]

Compound	Long-wavelength absorption maxima (nm)
Anthracene	252 (339, 356, 374)[b]
Acridine	249, 351
Acridinium cation	254, 353
1-Aminoacridine	263 (341, 358), 414
1-Aminoacridinium cation	290, 357, 529
2-Aminoacridine	259 (338, 355), 404
2-Aminoacridinium cation	273, 371, 461
3-Aminoacridine	262 (336, 353), 410
3-Aminoacridinium cation	272 (350, 365), 454
4-Aminoacridine	262 (343, 360), 407
4-Aminoacridinium cation	250, 275, 362, 446
9-Aminoacridine	260, 389 (407, 430)
9-Aminoacridinium cation	259, 326 (400, 422)
1-Hydroxyacridinium cation	272, 355, 454
9-Hydroxyacridine anion	267, 340 (411, 435)
9-Hydroxyacridine zwitterion	254, 294 (380, 398)
2,7-Diaminoacridine	263, 293, 391
3,6-Diaminoacridine	262, 284, 395
4,5-Diaminoacridine	269, 447
2,6-Diaminoacridine	272, 350, 439

[a] All the values are taken from DMS, U.V. Atlas of Organic Compounds, Butterworths and Verlag Chemie, 1966.

[b] Figures in parentheses are maxima of vibrational bands apparently associated with the same electronic transition.

The 400 nm bands of 1-, 2-, 3-, and 4-aminoacridines shift about 50 nm to the red on protonation, but with 9-aminoacridine there is a blue shift of about 10 nm. In diaminoacridines the $^1L_a \leftarrow {}^1A$ band is shifted further to the red because of the increased conjugation of the chromophore.

The extrapolation from acridine spectra of flavin spectra is a big one, and it is not possible to deduce spectral assignments with complete certainty. If the flavin chromophore is considered as a tricyclic nucleus with two strongly conjugating substituents in the 2 and 4 positions, it can be predicted that the $^1L_b \leftarrow {}^1A$ band is red-shifted from its position in acridine and enhanced in intensity, as in the 2- and 4-aminoacridines. Thus it is likely that the 450 nm band of a flavin is the $^1L_b \leftarrow {}^1A$ transition, and hence is polarized longitudinally. The 370 nm band is $^1L_a \leftarrow$ ^1A, and is polarized transversely. These polarizations are not accurately in the directions suggested both because of the dysymmetry of the molecule, and because of the directing effects of the various substituents and heteroatoms.

Any substituent that extends the conjugation of the ring system should cause bathochromic shifts in the π-π^* absorptions. Substituting methyl groups in the benzene ring of an isoalloxazine causes a red shift of the long wavelength absorption band (Penzer and Radda, 1967b). The near-ultraviolet band has a larger shift in the same direction, with 5- and 8-methyl groups being more effective than 6- and 7-ones. This supports the tentative assignments made. The effects of substituting chlorine in the benzene ring are mostly similar to those found for methyl substitution, but the absence of a bathochromatic shift in the visible band of the 7-chloro derivative is inconsistent. Most of the 9-substituents do not conjugate with the ring system, and it is not surprising that they produce insignificant spectral shifts. Apart from substituting in the 3-position, changes in the groups round the pyrimidine ring cause reorganization of the conjugation of the chromophore. It still seems, however, that bathochromic shifts of the visible band are largest when the longitudinal conjugation is increased, while similar shifts for the near-ultraviolet band are greatest for increases in transverse conjugation.

B. Physical Deactivation of Flavin Excited States

1. *Fluorescence*

The possible routes for deactivation of excited singlets are outlined in Fig. 4. The deactivation of higher excited singlets to the first excited singlet (k_1) is very efficient since the quantum yield of flavin fluorescence

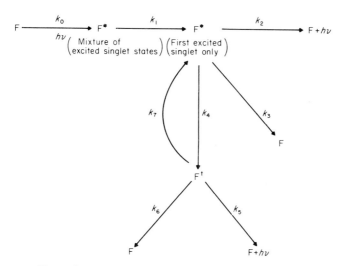

Fig. 4. Routes for deactivation of flavin excited states.

is independent of the exciting wavelength. The quantum yield of fluorescence (k_2) for riboflavin in water is 0.26 (Weber and Teale, 1957), but yields of other derivatives vary from 0.01 to 0.5 so that the processes k_3 and k_4 must account for about three-quarters of the excited singlets. k_4 depends on the magnetic perturbations which reduce the forbiddenness of the singlet to triplet intersystem crossing (see below). k_3 has been measured in some cases, with the conclusion that deactivation to the ground state is relatively unimportant (Brocklehurst, 1970, and references therein). The same conclusion is drawn from the observation that the quantum yields of fluorescence and phosphorescence of 9-phenylanthracene add up to one (Horrocks *et al.*, 1967). Also for flavins, Nathanson *et al.* (1967) have shown that a photochemical reaction involving flavin triplets has a quantum yield of 0.7 under the conditions where the fluorescence yield is 0.25. The positions of fluorescence maxima also vary for flavin derivatives. Generally they shift in the same direction as the visible absorption maximum but by a smaller amount of energy (Fig. 5). The difference between the absorption and fluorescence maxima is a measure of the solvation changes which follow excitation into the Franck-Condon state, and it indicates the extent to which electron distribution and geometry of the first excited singlet differ from those of the ground state. These effects are thus smaller for those flavin derivatives which are excited at lower energies.

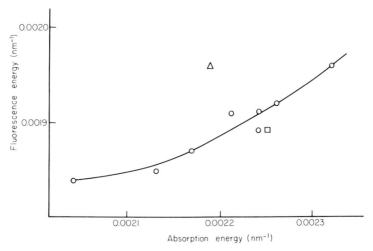

Fig. 5. The relationship between absorption and fluorescence energies of various flavins. Various flavins in water ◯; lumiflavin in acetone ◻; lipoamide dehydrogenase in phosphate buffer, pH 7.0 △.

It should be noted that this correlation holds for a given flavin in different solvents. Interestingly, for the one flavoprotein for which we have data under comparable conditions, the relationship breaks down. One interpretation of this is that the flavin is in some way distorted on binding, but other explanations are possible.

2. Energy Transfer

One general deactivation mechanism which falls into the general class of k_3, which may be very efficient under favorable conditions, is energy transfer by resonance coupling (Förster, 1959). Energy transfer in flavins can readily be demonstrated by trapping the chromophore in a methyl cellulose film (Penzer and Radda, 1967a). In such films one observes low polarizations of fluorescence and arguments have been presented (Penzer and Radda, 1967a) that the flavin is trapped in aqueous "cages" within the film where the microscopic viscosities are significantly lower than the macroscopic viscosity of the methyl cellulose solution. One of the requirements of efficient energy transfer is that the fluorescence emission spectrum of the donor should overlap with the absorption band of the acceptor. Two flavin derivatives which fulfill this condition are 6-chloro-7-methoxy-9-ethyl-2-N-pyrrolidinoisoalloxazine (D) and 4-morpholinolumiflavin (A). Their relevant spectral properties are shown in Table IV. When the two flavins are mixed in a methyl cellulose film, their absorption spectra are additive, but the fluorescence emissions are not (Fig. 6). A little of A (20% or more of total flavin) completely quenches the fluorescence emission of D. We have already shown how this may be accounted for by singlet-singlet transfer (Penzer and Radda, 1967a), where R_0 (the mean intermolecular distance at which energy transfer is as likely as other deactivation processes) can be calculated

TABLE IV

SPECTRAL PROPERTIES OF THE DERIVATIVES CHOSEN FOR MIXED FILM EXPERIMENTS

Flavin	D[a] (nm)	A[a] (nm)
Visible absorption maximum		
In aqueous solution	445	470
In a methyl cellulose film	445	475
Fluorescence maximum		
In aqueous solution	510	540
In a methyl cellulose film	530	570

[a] D is 6-chloro-7-methoxy-9-(ethyl-2'-N-pyrrolidino)isoalloxazine; A is 4-morpholinolumiflavin.

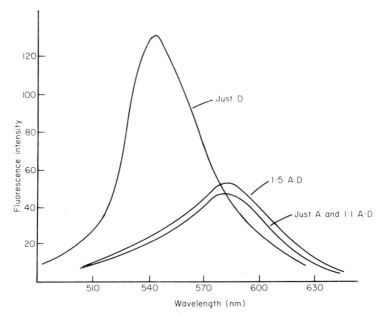

FIG. 6. Fluorescence emission spectra of flavins used in energy transfer experiments.

(Förster, 1959). This is 21 Å for a mixture of the two flavins above. Similarly, R_0 is 14 Å for FMN alone, so that singlet energy transfer between identical molecule can also occur. This can be demonstrated by observing the decrease in fluorescence polarization of FMN in methyl cellulose films as the concentration of the dye is increased (Table V).

TABLE V
FLUORESCENCE POLARIZATIONS OF FMN IN AQUEOUS
METHYL CELLULOSE SOLUTIONS[a]

Methyl cellulose concentration (g/l)	Fluorescence polarization
0	0.014
3.26	0.017
6.41	0.015
9.68	0.020
12.83	0.022
17.66	0.025
22.50	0.029

[a] All measurements were made at room temperature. Fluorescence was excited at 447 nm and measured at 520 nm.

3. Delayed Light Emission

A flavin dispersed in a rigid polyacrylamide matrix has a delayed light emission at room temperature with the following characteristics. The emission maximum is the same as that for fluorescence in solution. The lifetimes of the emissions are in the range 20–100 msec. The decay curves are exponential. The intensity of the delayed emission is proportional to the intensity of excitation, and not to its square. The lifetime of the delayed emission falls but its intensity increases as the temperature is raised. Below room temperature a new delayed emission is also observed, which is the only emission at 77°K, and corresponds in wavelength to phosphorescence (Dhère and Castelli, 1938; Shiga and Piette, 1964; Lhoste et al., 1966; Bowd et al., 1968). The intensities of the two maxima (Fig. 7) always move in opposite directions when the temperature is changed. The delayed fluorescence can be identified as E-type delayed fluorescence (Parker, 1968). The mechanism of this process is thermal reexcitation of a triplet state to the first excited singlet (k_7 in Fig. 4), which subsequently fluoresces.

The lifetimes of delayed fluorescence depend on the rate constants for

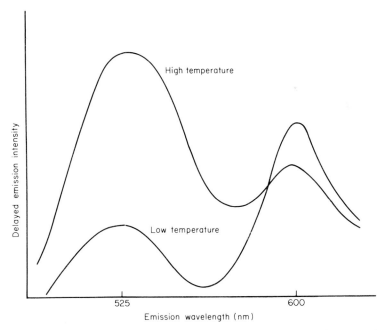

FIG. 7. Change in delayed emission spectrum of flavin mononucleotide in a polyacrylamide film on changing the temperature. Excitation wavelength, 447 nm.

all triplet deactivation routes. Thus the rate constant obtained (k_c) from the reciprocal of delayed lifetime is $k_c = k_5 + k_6 + k_7$ (cf. Fig. 4).

The intensity of delayed emission (I), however, is proportional to k_7 $[F_t]$. From a steady-state treatment then:

$$ I \approx \frac{k_0 k_4 k_7 [F]}{(k_2 + k_3 + k_4)(k_5 + k_6 + k_7)} $$

If we now measure the apparent activation energies from a study of the temperature dependence of lifetimes and intensities, they will be different. This is because of the different way in which the individual rate constants are combined (see Table VI). Thus while the activation energy from the half-life plots is that for the processes described by k_c, the activation energy obtained from intensities is related to k_7/k_c. [The assumptions made in arriving at the latter conclusion have been discussed in detail elsewhere (Gordon-Walker *et al.*, 1970).] Adding the two activation energies therefore gives the true activation energy for k_7. This can be compared with the spectroscopically measured energy separation

TABLE VI

DELAYED EMISSION PARAMETERS FOR DIFFERENT FLAVINS

Substituents in isoalloxazine	Lifetime of delayed fluorescence at 20°C (msec)	E_T (kcal mole^{-1})	E_I (kcal mole^{-1})	A (kcal mole^{-1})	B (kcal mole^{-1})
6,7-Dimethyl-9-D-ribityl	58	1.2	4.4	6.7	5.6
6,7-Dimethyl-9-D-ribityl phosphate	72	2.5	6.0	6.6	8.5
6,7,9-Trimethyl	80	1.8	6.5	6.8	8.3
3,6,7,9-Tetramethyl	80	2.0	5.7	6.4	7.7
9-(N,N-Dimethylaminoethyl)	58	2.3	2.8	6.4	5.1
6-Chloro-7-methoxy-9-(ethyl-2'-N-pyrrolidino)	109	0.9	5.0	8.4	5.9
2-Morpholino-6,7,9-trimethyl	61	3.5	5.1	6.7	8.6
4-Morpholino-6,7,9-trimethyl	26	1.3	4.1	5.7	5.4
5,6-Dimethyl-9-D-ribityl	35	2.7	2.8	5.8	5.5
5,6-Dimethyl-9-peracetyl-D-ribityl	43	2.4	3.4	5.4	5.8
6-Chloro-9-(N,N-dimethylaminopropyl)	30	1.4	3.5	7.0	4.9
6-Methyl-9-(N,N-diethylaminoethyl)	48	2.4	3.9	7.0	6.3

^{a} E_T and E_I are the Arrhenius activation energies calculated from delayed fluorescence lifetimes and intensities, respectively. A is the energy separation between the emission maxima of fluorescence and phosphorescence. B is $(E_T + E_I)$ for delayed fluorescence.

between the fluorescence and phosphorescence maxima (Table VI). Using similar considerations for the temperature dependence of phosphorescence, the activation energies derived from half-life and intensity measurements are due to the rate processes $(k_5 + k_6)$ and $1/(k_5 + k_6)$, respectively. The activation energies which can be deduced from the various rate processes, although only semiquantitative, are of considerable interest as indications of the relative magnitudes of the energies required in the various mechanisms of triplet deactivation. The results for 3-methyllumiflavin are summarized in Fig. 8.

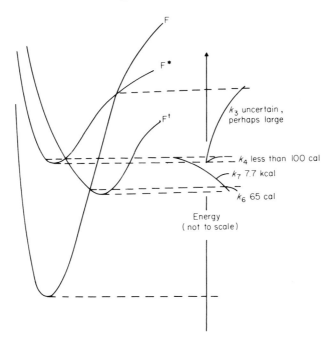

Fig. 8. Morse curves for the electronic states of 3-methyllumiflavin. After Gordon-Walker *et al.* (1970).

III. Photochemical Properties of Flavin Excited States

A. Photoreduction

Under anaerobic conditions, flavins may be photoreduced to dihydroflavins by a variety of electron donors, e.g., the ribityl side chain (Holmström and Oster, 1961), amines (Penzer and Radda, 1968), amino acids (Byrom and Turnbull, 1968; Penzer and Radda, 1968), hydroxy acids, dicarboxylic acids (Weatherby and Carr, 1970), and NADH (Radda and Calvin, 1964). Electron donors with α-carboxl groups undergo oxidative decarboxylation (Penzer and Radda, 1968; Enns and Burgess, 1965; Weatherby and Carr, 1970).

1. *Nature of the Excited State*

These photoreductions are inhibited by iodide ions (Holmström and Oster, 1961) and electron-rich compounds like indoles and phenols (Radda, 1966) under conditions where there is no quenching of flavin fluorescence. Estimates of the lifetime of the excited state, using the measured quantum yields and assuming reaction at every collision with the electron donor indicate a minimum lifetime of 10^{-5} seconds (Holmström and Oster, 1961; Radda and Calvin, 1964). The directly measured fluorescence lifetime is about 10^{-9} second (Chen *et al.*, 1967; Gordon-Walker *et al.*, 1970). These observations implicate the excited triplet as the reacting state.

2. *Reaction Mechanisms*

Most of the electron donors used are acids or bases, so it is important to know which ionic forms of the electron donors react. The variation of rate of photoreduction with pH has been measured with a variety of electron donors, and two types of behavior are found. With amines and amino acids, the rate curve follows the ionization curve of the protonated amine, showing that the positively charged form of the electron donor does not react (Penzer and Radda, 1968). A more complicated relation is found with mandelic acid (Fig. 9). The drop in rate below pH 4 indicates that the conjugate acid does not react. The rise in rate from pH 7 to pH 4

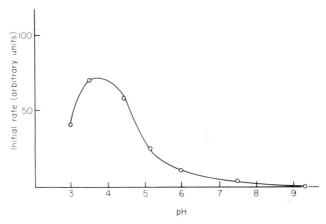

Fig. 9. The pH variation of the rate of photoreduction of 25 μM 9-(dimethylaminoethyl)isoalloxazine by 5 mM mandelic acid in phosphate buffers (ionic strength $= 0.1$).

implicates a species with a pK_a of about 5.7. A similar pH dependence has recently been reported for the reaction of dihydrophthalic acid (Weatherby and Carr, 1970). With mandelic acid, this pK_a varies among different flavins. The pK_a could be associated with the flavin triplet or with some intermediate in the reaction. Previously published values for the pK_a of the flavin triplet were obtained in glassy matrices (Lhoste *et al.*, 1966) and may not be applicable to solutions.

As in flavoprotein catalysis, it is important to distinguish between different modes of redox transfer in the photochemical reactions (electron, hydrogen atom, hydride ion, or group transfer). This problem has been approached experimentally in three ways.

1. Direct spectroscopic observation of transients using flash photolysis showed the formation of semiquinone in photobleaching and photoreduction by EDTA (Holmström, 1964) and diphenylamine (Terenin *et al.*, 1965).

2. The effect of substituents in the electron donor on the reaction rate gives information about the transition state of the rate-determining step. The relative rates of photoreduction by a series of substituted phenylglycines show a linear free energy relationship when the σ function is used for substituents. This gives a ρ value of -1.1, and shows that the flavin triplet is an electrophilic species, although the charge separation in the transition state is small (Penzer and Radda, 1968).

3. Kinetic isotope effects can be used to show whether C—H bonds are broken in rate-limiting steps, although they do not differentiate between hydrogen atom and hydride ion transfer. With α-D_1-mandelic acid as the electron donor, the kinetic isotope effect is concentration dependent. The rate of photoreduction by mandelic acid, as by phenylglycine and EDTA (Penzer and Radda, 1968), shows a hyperbolic dependence on reducing agent concentration, because quenching and reaction compete for the flavin triplet. At pH 8, the value of k_H/k_D reaches a limit of 3.5 at low concentrations and 0.62 at high concentrations. This inversion of isotope effect can be explained if the hydrogen transferred to the flavin triplet can be transferred back to the electron donor, leaving ground state flavin, or a second electron can be transferred to give reduced flavin.

$$\text{F} \xrightarrow{kI_{\text{abs}}} \text{F}_t \tag{1}$$

$$\text{F}_t \xrightarrow{kq} \text{F} \tag{2}$$

$$\text{F}_t + \text{RH}_2 \xrightarrow{k_1} \text{FH}\ldots\ldots\text{RH(I)} \tag{3}$$

$$\text{FH}\ldots\text{RH} \xrightarrow{k_2} \text{F} + \text{RH}_2 \tag{4}$$

$$\text{FH}\ldots\text{RH} \xrightarrow{k_3} \text{products} \tag{5}$$

For the isotope effect inversion to be observed, the intermediate (I) must undergo step (4) more rapidly than it exchanges the transferred hydrogen with solvent. This means that FH and RH cannot separate in solution. Penzer (1970) has suggested a similarly rapidly reversible redox transfer to account for the apparent quenching of flavin triplet by EDTA.

At pH 4, in contrast, the limiting values of k_H/k_D are 1 at high concentrations and 1.9 at low concentrations. This suggests that $k_3 \gg k_2$ at pH 4. This is supported by the limiting quantum yield at pH 4 at saturating reducing agent concentrations (0.8 ± 0.15) which is close to the maximum possible quantum yield for the triplet.

These results could be explained by the flavin triplet having a pK_a of 5.7 with different reaction and quenching rate constants for the two forms. An alternative interpretation is that it is the intermediate (I) (for which we have no direct evidence) which has a pK_a of 5.7.

B. PHOTOADDITION

In contrast to the photoreductions, excited flavins react with phenylacetic acid and α-ketoacids to give alkyl- or acyl-substituted flavins and carbon dioxide (Hemmerich et al., 1967; Brüstlein and Hemmerich, 1968).

The rate of reaction of phenylacetic acid is inhibited by 10^{-5} M iodide, phenols, and indoles, and the calculated minimum lifetime of the excited

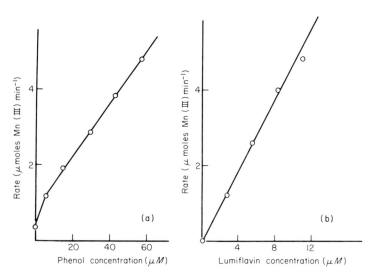

FIG. 10. Effect of (a) phenol concentration and (b) lumiflavin concentration on the rate of photosensitized oxidation of 57 μM Mn(II) in pyrophosphate buffer pH 7.6. The reaction mixtures contained (a) 11 μM lumiflavin, phenol as shown and (b) 57 μM phenol, lumiflavin as shown.

state is orders of magnitude above the measured lifetime of the singlet. The triplet is again the reactive excited state.

The phenylacetic acid reaction has a similar pH dependence to the mandelic acid reaction. The rate of reaction depends hyperbolically on reducing agent concentration and quantum yields, extrapolated to saturating phenylacetic acid concentration, are 0.01 at pH 8 and 0.028 at pH 4. No kinetic isotope effect is observed using α-D_2-phenylacetic acid at pH 4 or pH 8. Hydrogen transfer cannot be involved in the rate-determining step.

C. Photosensitization

Lumiflavin and other flavin derivatives sensitize the photooxidation of Mn(II) to Mn(III) (in the presence of pyrophosphate) or of ferrocytochrome c to ferricytochrome c. Both reactions require some other substance, one of the most efficient catalysts being phenol (cf. Andrae, 1955). The rate of photooxidation depends on light intensity (in most experiments visible light above 400 nm was used), lumiflavin and phenol con-

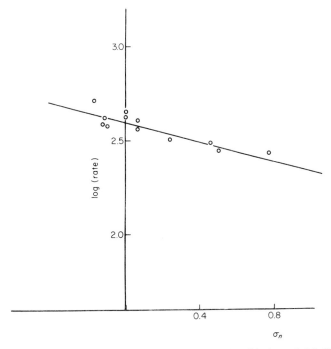

Fig. 11. Hammett plot for the rates of photosensitized oxidation of Mn(II) by substituted phenols. Reaction mixtures contained 50 μM phenol, 14 μM lumiflavin, and 49.3 μM Mn(II) in pyrophosphate buffer pH 7.6.

TABLE VII

COMPARISON OF THE INITIAL RATES OF Mn(II) PHOTOOXIDATION
SENSITIZED BY DIFFERENT ELECTRON DONORS[a]

Electron donor	Relative rate/electron donor concentration $\times 10^5$
Hydroquinone	128
Phenol	110
p-Fluorophenol	101
p-Cresol	94
p-Methoxyphenol	92
p-Chlorophenol	78
p-Hydroxymethyl benzoate	77
p-Hydroxyacetophenone	69
p-Nitrophenol	66
p-Bromophenol	20
Tyrosine	63
Tryptophan	92
N,N-Dimethylaniline	76
CMU	65
DCMU	61
Serotonin	58
Adenine	46
Adenosine	20

[a] The reaction mixtures contained approximately 0.05 mM electron donor, 0.05 mM Mn(II), and 0.014 mM lumiflavin in pyrophosphate buffer, pH 7.6.

centration, but not on the concentration of cytochrome c [or Mn(II)] or the oxygen partial pressure (Fig. 10). However, at low oxygen concentration the reaction rate is faster because the flavin triplet has a longer lifetime.

The variation in initial rate of Mn(II) photooxidation using different p-substituted phenols as accelerators can be analyzed by the Hammett equation. Using σ_n values (Wells, 1963), a ρ value of -0.24 (correlation coefficient 0.98) is obtained (Fig. 11). Electron donating substituents in the phenol ring therefore weakly accelerate the reaction. The same phenols also inhibit the photoreduction of lumiflavin by EDTA. The ρ value for the Hammett plot for this inhibition is -0.15. More generally, compounds that inhibit the photoreduction of lumiflavin which have been classified as electron donors (Radda, 1966) are also accelerators of the flavin-sensitized photooxidation of the metal ions (Table VII). The stoichiometry of the overall reaction is:

$$2H^+ + O_2 + 2\ \text{Cyt } c\ (\text{FeII}) \xrightarrow[\text{lumiflavin, phenol}]{} \text{Cyt } c\ (\text{FeIII}) + H_2O_2$$

The production of oxidized cytochrome c has been followed spectro-

photometrically (at 550 nm), that of hydrogen peroxide using cytochrome
c and cytochrome c peroxidase. Lumiflavin can be completely recovered
in the experiments, as shown spectroscopically, and phenol is also totally
unchanged (even with a large excess of Mn(II) or reduced cytochrome
c) as shown by gas–liquid chromatographic analysis.

The flavin triplet is implicated in the reaction on two grounds. The
triplet is known to be involved in hydrogen abstraction from amino acids,
EDTA, etc. The order of reactivity of different flavins toward the EDTA
reaction and as sensitizers of the Mn(II) oxidation using phenol as the
accelerator are similar (Table VIII). Because the reaction of the excited
flavin with phenol is very fast, the quenching of Mn(II) photooxidation
by iodide, oxygen, and paramagnetic ions is not as efficient as in
the EDTA reaction, but nevertheless it is still significant.

Flash photolysis experiments (Knowles and Taylor, 1970) show that
phenoxy radicals are produced when a solution of lumiflavin and phenol
are submitted to an intense flash, but Mn(II) has no significant effect
on the concentration of this radical, suggesting that the phenoxy radical
is not an intermediate in the reaction. This is also supported by the complete recovery of phenol in the steady-state illumination experiments.

TABLE VIII

COMPARISON OF Mn(II) PHOTOOXIDATION AND PHOTOREDUCTION
BY EDTA WITH DIFFERENT FLAVINS

Flavin	Relative initial rate of Mn(II) photooxidation[a]	Relative initial rate of anaerobic flavin photoreduction by EDTA[b]
6-Chloro-9-(N,N-dimethylaminopropyl) isoalloxazine	0.81	0.56
6-Methyl-9-(N,N-diethylaminoethyl) isoalloxazine	0.26	0.24
7-Chloro-9-(N,N-dimethylaminopropyl) isoalloxazine	0.56	0.26
9-(N,N-Dimethylaminoethyl)isoalloxazine	0.11	0.11
6-Chloro-7-methoxy-(ethyl-2′-N-pyrrolidino) isoalloxazine	0.56	—
Lumiflavin	1.0	1.0
Riboflavin	1.0	1.0
Isoriboflavin	0.52	—
3-Methyllumiflavin	0.89	—

[a] The reaction mixture contained 0.06 mM phenol, 0.046 mM Mn(II), and 0.014 mM
flavin in pyrophosphate buffer pH 7.6.

[b] The reaction mixture contained 4 mM EDTA and 0.07 mM flavin in phosphate
buffer pH 7.0. Taken from Radda (1966).

One scheme that accounts for the various observations is show below.

$$F_t + ArOH \rightleftarrows [F..ArOH]^*$$
$$[F...ArOH]^* \rightleftarrows [FH.ArO.]$$
$$H^+ + [FH.ArO.] + Mn(II) \rightarrow FH. + ArOH + Mn(III)$$
$$2FH. \rightleftarrows F + FH_2$$
$$FH_2 + O_2 \rightarrow F + H_2O_2$$

Here $[F..ArOH]^*$ is an excited state complex formed rapidly, and is a precursor of the oxidizing intermediate which is formed in the rate-determining step. Such a reversible electron (or hydrogen atom) transfer may be the primary mechanism of triplet quenching by phenol, and is similar to that suggested in the reaction with mandelic acid. A flavin triplet–inhibitor complex has also been implicated in earlier experiments (Radda, 1966).

This work, besides providing a model for electron transfer from oxygen

TABLE IX
Isomer Ratios for Aromatic Hydroxylations[a]

Substituted benzene	Hydroxylating system	Isomer ratio		
		o	m	p
Chlorobenzene	Lumiflavin/H_2O_2/$h\nu$	28	30	42
	2-(2'-Hydroxyethyl)iminolumiflavin/H_2O_2/$h\nu$	28	30	42
	4-Morpholinolumiflavin/H_2O_2/$h\nu$	28	29	43
	2-Morpholinolumiflavin/H_2O_2/$h\nu$	28	25	47
	Fenton's reaction[b]	42	29	29
	Fe(II)/O_2/ascorbic acid[b]	62	16	22
Fluorobenzene	Riboflavin/H_2O_2/$h\nu$	7	44	49
	Lumiflavin/H_2O_2/$h\nu$	6	43	51
	6-Chloro-9-(N,N-dimethylaminopropyl)-isoalloxazine/H_2O_2/$h\nu$	5	45	50
	7-Chloro-9-(N,N-dimethylaminopropyl)-isoalloxazine/H_2O_2/$h\nu$	6	45	49
	4-Morpholinolumiflavin/H_2O_2/$h\nu$	7	31	54
	2-(2'-Hydroxyethyl)iminolumiflavin/H_2O_2/$h\nu$	4	38	48
	Fenton's reaction[b]	37	18	45
Anisole	Riboflavin/H_2O_2/$h\nu$	47	15	38
	Fenton's reaction[b]	84	—	16
	Fe(II)/O_2/ascorbic acid[b]	61	9	30

[a] The reaction mixtures for the flavin reactions contained 5×10^{-5} M flavin, 0.02 M hydrogen peroxide, and 0.1 M substituted benzene in water, and were made anaerobic before illumination.

[b] Taken from Norman and Radda (1962).

to cytochrome c, suggests that on chemical grounds it would be reasonable to look in flavoproteins for the presence of tyrosine or tryptophan close to the flavin as functional entities. This suggestion of course assumes that in flavoproteins the flavin resembles to some extent the triplet state.

D. OTHER REACTIONS

Flavins can sensitize many other reactions (Penzer and Radda, 1967b). For instance, in the presence of hydrogen peroxide and lumiflavin, a light catalyzed aromatic hydroxylation can be brought about (Steele, 1963). Although it has been suggested that OH˙ is produced, the pattern of isomer distribution obtained in the reaction of monosubstituted benzenoid compounds differs significantly from that obtained with Fenton's reagent (Table IX). The latter is known to react via OH˙, and therefore the flavin-catalyzed reaction involves some other radical, possibly a flavin nitroxide.

IV. SOME SPECULATIONS ABOUT FLAVIN BINDING

On the basis of these models and spectroscopic observations it would be reasonable to explore two features in flavoproteins. (1) Part of the rate acceleration may be due to some distortion of the flavin nucleus to make it resemble the transition state (which might have a geometry similar to that of the triplet). (2) Aromatic groups may play more than just a passive role in catalysis, as in the cytochrome c oxidation above.

With these ideas in mind, we have initiated some studies to explore the protein binding site through the use of the fluorescent probe 1-anilino-

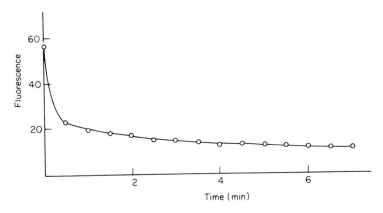

FIG. 12. Change in fluorescence of 10.7 μM ANS in the presence of D-amino acid oxidase (0.57 mg/ml) on adding 85 μM FAD. Fluorescence was excited at 385 nm and measured at 485 nm.

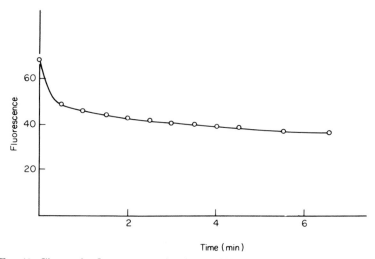

FIG. 13. Change in fluorescence of 10.7 μM ANS in the presence of D-amino acid oxidase (0.57 mg/ml) on adding 0.12 mM ADP. Fluorescence was excited at 385 nm and measured at 485 nm.

naphthalene 8-sulfonate (ANS). This binds to apo-D-amino acid oxidase with a 62-fold enhancement of its fluorescence ($K_{dis} \sim 10\ \mu M$) at approximately 3 sites per flavin binding site. Addition of FAD diminishes the fluorescence in a biphasic manner (Fig. 12), with a rate constant for the slow phase identical with that obtained by Massey and Curti (1966) by a variety of other methods. Interestingly, ADP also induces a similar change (Fig. 13). Energy transfer from tryptophan to ANS is easily observed, and from this the average ANS-tryptophan distance can be calculated. The upper limit for this distance is 19 Å.

These preliminary experiments suggest that the binding of the adenine part of FAD is partly responsible for the necessary conformational change for the "activation" of the isoalloxazine nucleus.

We have tried to show how a study of the chemistry of flavin excited states may provide some clues about flavoprotein catalysis. There is no doubt that ultimately the answers will come from studying individual enzymes in detail. We were, however, impressed by the close similarities of the reactions of flavin triplets with those of flavoproteins.

REFERENCES

Albrecht, A. C. (1961). *J. Mol. Spectrosc.* **6**, 84.
Andrae, W. A. (1955). *Arch. Biochem. Biophys.* **55**, 584.
Beinert, H. (1960). *In* "The Enzymes" (P. D. Boyer, H. Lardy, and K. Myrbäck, eds.), 2nd rev. ed., Vol. 2, Part A, p. 339. Academic Press, New York.

Bowd, A., Byrom, P., Hudson, J. B., and Turnbull, J. H. (1968). *Photochem. Photobiol.* **6**, 91.

Brocklehurst, B. (1970). *Radiat. Res. Rev.* **2**, 149.

Brüstlein, M., and Hemmerich, P. (1968). *FEBS Letters* **1**, 335.

Byrom, P., and Turnbull, J. H. (1968). *Photochem. Photobiol.* **8**, 243.

Chen, R. F., Vureck, G. G., and Alexander, N. (1967). *Science* **156**, 949.

Dhère, C., and Castelli, V. (1938). *C. R. Acad. Sci.* **206**, 2003.

Dudley, K. H., Ehrenberg, A., Hemmerich, P., and Müller, F. (1964). *Helv. Chim. Acta* **47**, 1354.

Enns, K., and Burgess, W. M. (1965). *J. Amer. Chem. Soc.* **87**, 5766.

Förster, T. (1959). *Discuss. Faraday Soc.* **27**, 1.

Fox, J. L., Laberge, S. P., Nishimoto, K., and Forster, L. S. (1967). *Biochim. Biophys. Acta* **136**, 544.

Gordon-Walker, A., Penzer, G. R., and Radda, G. K. (1970). *Eur. J. Biochem.* **13**, 313.

Harbury, H. A., LaNoue, K. F., Loach, P. A., and Amick, R. M. (1959). *Proc. Nat. Acad. Sci. U. S.* **45**, 1708.

Hemmerich, P., Massey, V., and Weber, G. (1967). *Nature (London)* **213**, 251.

Holmström, B. (1964). *Ark. Kemi* **22**, 329.

Holmström, B., and Oster, G. (1961). *J. Amer. Chem. Soc.* **83**, 1867.

Horrocks, A. R., Medinger, T., and Wilkinson, F. (1967). *Photochem. Photobiol.* **6**, 21.

Jaffé, H. H., and Orchin, M. (1962). "Theory and Applications of Ultra-violet Spectroscopy." Wiley, New York.

Jones, R. N. (1945). *J. Amer. Chem. Soc.* **67**, 2127.

Kierkegaard, P., Norrestam, R., Werner, P.-E., Ehrenberg, A., Eriksson, L. E. G., and Müller, F. (1967). *Chem. Commun.* p. 288.

Knowles, A., and Taylor, M. B. (1970). Unpublished work.

Kosower, E. M. (1958). *J. Amer. Chem. Soc.* **80**, 3253.

Koziol, J., and Knobloch, E. (1965). *Biochim. Biophys. Acta* **102**, 289.

Kurtin, W. E., and Song, P. S. (1968). *Photochem. Photobiol.* **7**, 263.

Lhoste, J. M., Haug, A., and Hemmerich, P. (1966). *Biochemistry* **5**, 3290.

Massey, V., and Curti, B. (1966). *J. Biol. Chem.* **241**, 3417.

Massey, V., and Ganther, H. (1965). *Biochemistry* **4**, 1161.

Müller, F., and Hemmerich, P. (1966). *Helv. Chim. Acta* **49**, 2352.

Müller, F., Walker, W., and Hemmerich, P. (1966). *Helv. Chim. Acta* **49**, 2365.

Nathanson, B., Brody, M., Brody, S., and Broyde, S. B. (1967). *Photochem. Photobiol.* **6**, 177.

Norman, R. O. C., and Radda, G. K. (1962). *Proc. Chem. Soc., London* p. 138.

Parker, C. A. (1968). "Photoluminescence of Solutions." Elsevier, Amsterdam.

Penzer, G. R. (1970). *Biochem. J.* **116**, 733.

Penzer, G. R., and Radda, G. K. (1967a). *Nature (London)* **213**, 251.

Penzer, G. R., and Radda, G. K. (1967b). *Quart. Rev., Chem. Soc.* **21**, 43.

Penzer, G. R., and Radda, G. K. (1968). *Biochem. J.* **109**, 259.

Radda, G. K. (1966). *Biochim. Biophys. Acta* **112**, 448.

Radda, G. K., and Calvin, M. (1964). *Biochemistry* **3**, 384.

Shiga, T., and Piette, L. H. (1964). *Photochem. Photobiol.* **3**, 213.

Steele, R. H. (1963). *Biochemistry* **2**, 529.

Sussenbach, J. S., and Berends, W. (1963). *Biochim. Biophys. Res. Commun.* **16**, 263.

Terenin, A., Tachin, V., and Shakhverdov, P. (1965). *Photochem. Photobiol.* **4,** 505.
Tollin, G. (1968). *Biochemistry* **7,** 1720.
Weatherby, G. D., and Carr, D. O. (1970). *Biochemistry* **9,** 344.
Weber, G. (1966). *In* "Flavins and Flavoproteins" (E. C. Slater, ed.), p. 15. Elsevier, Amsterdam.
Weber, G., and Teale, F. W. J. (1957). *Trans. Faraday Soc.* **53,** 646.
Wells, P. R. (1963). *Chem. Rev.* **63,** 171.

Model Studies on Flavin-Dependent Oxidoreduction

PETER HEMMERICH

Fachbereich Biologie, Universität Konstanz, Germany

I. INTRODUCTION: WHAT IS A "MODEL"?

Unfortunately, the term "model" bears a stigma for enzymologists. This is based on the fact that, up to now, no chemical "models" are (and presumably never will be) found suited to replace, substitute or even imitate, quantitatively, biocatalysts. In a way, it is the old struggle between vitalists and materialists, where the vitalists have been drawn back from whole cells to macromolecules; they stick to their last fortress, the prefix "macro," with great stubbornness—and they are, of course, right. A model in its "proper" meaning is a species of rigorously known structure, and since hardly any macromolecular structure is or can be rigorously known, a model is then taken to be an entity of low molecular weight, or, in other words, a species which exhibits nothing but a primary structure in a very limited number of possible conformations and is, in spite of this, enabled to undergo "pseudobiological" reactions.

Clearly, the term "model" as defined above, is utterly useless and even misleading except for its application to enhance the glory of macromolecules. Thus, if the need for models can be proved at all, we need another definition. Models can be taken no longer as being "enzyme models," but instead, as "active center models." Clearly, an active center cut out from a biopolymer cannot be expected to be "alive," and neither can a model. It can, however, imitate the physical properties of the center, if not the biological ones; and conclusions may be drawn from such models on chemical structures of active centers. But where to begin the search for models approximating the physical properties of active centers? The "micro class of biomolecules" consists of "bricks" for macromolecular buildup, substrates for macromolecule action, and, finally, cofactors for purposes which biopolymers alone could not fulfill. Since cofactors by definition contribute to active biopolymer centers, they seem to lend themselves most easily to model studies. Cofactors, e.g., vitamins of group B, are no "models" by themselves since they need to be activated by proteins. From this, we may gain a first definition: a "model," derived from a coenzyme or a prosthetic group, must be designed in a way to resemble the protein-bound coenzyme rather than the "free coenzyme."

Models should not be any longer conceived as "homunculi," or as "bigger elephants than nature," or as micromolecular substitutes for macromolecular catalysts, but simply as derivatives of a coenzyme or a prosthetic group or even a mere protein functional group, which help in understanding the activation of the cofactor by the protein in terms of molecular structure.

Hence, it was an important step toward *flavin* models when Harbury and co-workers (1959) showed that many flavoprotein spectra resembled the spectra of flavin in nonpolar solvents rather than in water. The protein environment of the flavin had accordingly to be accepted as lipophilic, in spite of flavins being water-soluble vitamins. At the same time, this shows that the many question marks which remain in connection with chemical structure are not confined to the range of *polymers:* flavin is a perfect example of the fact that small biomolecules may be as little rigorously known in their structure and properties as any others of bigger size.

Activation of a molecule by a change of environmental polarity seems to be a very simple phenomenon. But in fact, exactly this is rather difficult to interpret in terms of molecular structure. Fortunately, many types of coenzyme-apoenzyme interaction are known which are much more specific, in that they concern not the entire coenzyme molecule to a first approximation, but a "functional" part of it, in the most favorable case, a two-center bond, which can be defined and separated in Kekulé or valence bond terms. Two examples are given:

1. The redox-active metal cluster in iron-sulfur proteins (Palmer and Brintzinger, 1970) is nowadays known to contain atomic FeSS-arrangements of triangular type, in which the SS-distance is larger than that of a

normal organic disulfide molecule, e.g., cystine (2.04 Å). Clearly, in order to stabilize the cluster, the sulfur atoms must be kept apart by the rigid protein backbone, or else the cluster would dissociate into disulfide and free Fe^{2+}. One sees immediately the difficulties of building a micromolecular model of such a cluster which would account for the sulfur atoms being prevented from approaching each other. One may try to replace the protein clamp by a small, preferably aromatic ring structure, which induces at the same time *angular strain* and *electron delocalization* in order to prevent disulfide stability. But presumably, this would not be suited to imitate the critical *distance* of the sulfur atoms as maintained in the protein.

2. Fully reduced flavin (Fig. 1) is presently known to be a bent molecule, though the inversion time of the "butterfly wing" conformations is still far below the half time of hydrogen transfer. If, on the other hand, the flavin is fixed within a protein active site, one might guess that the flipping of the leucoflavin conformers is largely restricted, and that one conformation is stabilized. Therefore, flavin-dependent substrate dehydrogenation might exhibit a stereospecificity problem like nicotinamide-dependent dehydrogenation while free flavin is oxidoreduced unspecifically. The flavin asymmetry is removed upon detachment of the coenzyme from the protein, while that of reduced nicotinamide coenzymes is retained.

If this problem is applied to model studies, one is confined to induce rigidity into the dihydroflavin nucleus by bulky substituents, as, for ex-

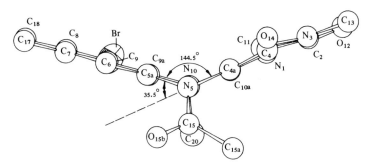

FIG. 1. Three-dimensional structure of flavohydroquinone from crystallographic measurements of Kierkegaard *et al.* (1970).

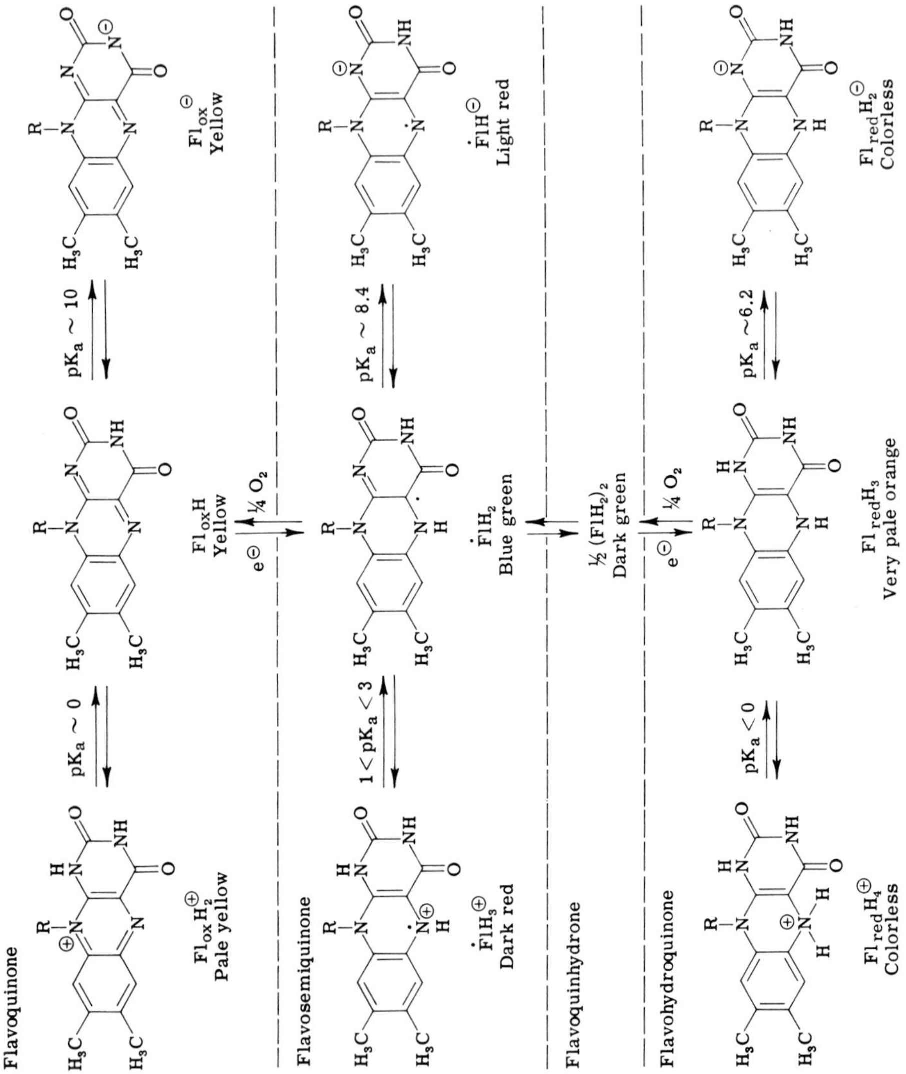

Flavoquinone

Fl_{ox} ⊖
Yellow

$Fl_{ox}H$
Yellow

$Fl_{ox}H_2$ ⊕
Pale yellow

pKa ~ 10

pKa ~ 0

Flavosemiquinone

$\dot{Fl}H$ ⊖
Light red

$\dot{Fl}H_2$
Blue green

$\dot{Fl}H_3$ ⊕
Dark red

pKa ~ 8.4

1 < pKa < 3

Flavoquinhydrone

½ $(FlH_2)_2$
Dark green

Flavohydroquinone

$Fl_{red}H_2$ ⊖
Colorless

$Fl_{red}H_3$
Very pale orange

$Fl_{red}H_4$ ⊕
Colorless

pKa ~ 6.2

pKa < 0

e⊖   ¼ O_2

e⊖   ¼ O_2

ample, in compound (A). Such a compound being a model for a bent reduced flavin may allow stereochemical studies, but it will not allow, at the
same time, the study of the behavior of reduced flavin toward molecular

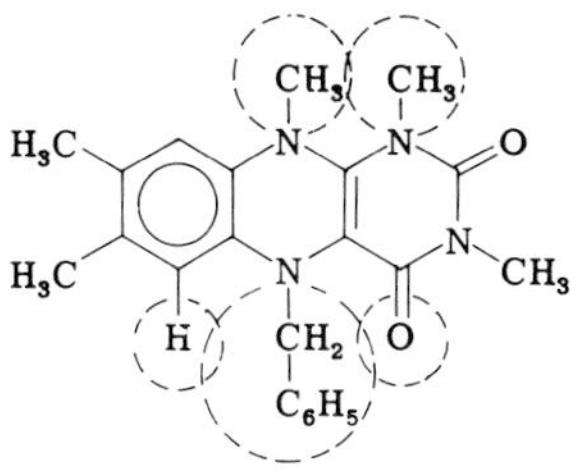

(A)

oxygen, since O_2-activation of reduced flavin must be reasonably assumed to originate from the flat state of the dihydroflavin molecule for
which compound (A) is just *no* model. Clearly, while a given protein
might stabilize the bent state of dihydroflavin, another protein might
stabilize the flat state.

Hence, a given coenzyme analog might be a model for one function of
the coenzyme, and a true "non-model" for another function of the same
coenzyme. If, like in many flavoproteins, enzyme action comprises both
functions (in our case, substrate dehydrogenation and O_2-activation by
flavin), no suitable model for both functions at the same time may be
possible at all, while there might be quite plausible models for each single
function. Free flavin is, in fact, a plausible model for O_2-activation, but
not for substrate dehydrogenation (CH-activation) by flavoproteins.

From this, a more subtle and, at the same time, more modest definition of the term "model" may be conceived. Another main feature
of models is contained in the fact that a successful model experiment
never allows safe positive conclusions as to the biological relevance of
a chemical structure or mechanism. Such a mechanism or structure can
only be *proposed* by the "modelist" to the enzymologist as a working
hypothesis which has turned out to be chemically "sound." On the other
hand, much easier and more important is the possibility of ruling out enzymological working hypotheses by model experiments which allow us to
conclude that a given hypothesis is "chemically unsound."

Again, an example from flavocoenzyme model chemistry may help to
clarify the picture.

Among the flavin species drawn in Fig. 2, only the neutral oxidized one,

FIG. 2. The flavin redox system. The pK values are given as approximations. since
the precise values depend on the nature of the substituent R.

$Fl_{ox}H$, is fluorescent *in vitro*. From this, the conclusion might be drawn that any change of fluorescence emission observed in a biological system containing flavin, e.g., mitochondria, might reflect reduction of Fl_{ox}. Model experiments may show that this working hypothesis does not hold for many possible reasons:

1. $Fl_{ox}H$ may also lose its fluorescence by protonation and deprotonation and, though the corresponding pK_a values are far from the physiological range, caution is needed. We have experimental support to propose that flavoquinone cation $Fl_{ox}H_2^+$ may be relevant in bacterial bioluminescence (Eley *et al.*, 1970).

2. These authors have also demonstrated that $Fl_{ox}H_2^+$ (Fig. 2) is non-fluorescent only in liquid, but not in solid solution. Whether the environment of flavin in a protein resembles more a liquid than a solid state cannot be decided in general. Apparently, the luciferase-bound flavin is so rigid that it behaves more like flavin in a glass than like flavin in a liquid.

3. The fluorescence of a flavin species may increase upon binding to the protein and it might as well be quenched by the protein. Hence, any change of flavin fluorescence during a biological reaction need not reflect an oxidoreduction, but maybe only a conformational change or changes connected with other oxidoreductants present in the system of the protein. Such a quenching mechanism is, e.g., exciton transfer between flavin and another aromatic donor molecule within the protein (e.g., adenine from FAD or tryptophan from the protein). Formation of a molecular complex between the exciton donor-acceptor halves is not a prerequisite. As was demonstrated by Fromherz in H. Kuhn's laboratory (Fromherz, 1969), such a radiationless transfer may penetrate a lipid layer more than 50 Å thick and does not require coplanarity between donor and acceptor.

4. While an observed change of fluorescence emission might thus not be accompanied by a change in flavin redox state, vice versa, a change in the redox state of flavin can be demonstrated by model experiments (Müller *et al.*, 1970b) which although involving only neutral flavin species, would not be indicated by a change in fluorescence. This is true for any flavoprotein shuttling between the semiquinoid and the fully reduced redox state. This shuttle has been verified to occur in flavin-dependent "low potential one-electron oxidoreduction," e.g., in flavoproteins replacing ferredoxin in iron-depleted algae (Bothe *et al.*, 1970) or bacteria (Mayhew *et al.*, 1969).

This was an example of a stringent negative conclusion from model studies: Fluorimetry is not a reliable indicator of changes in the redox state of flavoproteins.

Another example may be given in support of a "nonstringent" *positive* conclusion that lends itself as a chemically sound working hypothesis for the enzymologist. As Dr. Ehrenberg points out in this symposium, flavin metal complexes have been well characterized in the course of extensive model studies. From these, it turns out that a reasonable strength in flavin-metal chelation is found for flavin radicals as ligand species (Müller *et al.*, 1968; Hemmerich, 1964) or, conceivably, with flavoquinone and strongly back-donating metal valences like Fe(II), Mo(V) and Cu(I) (Hemmerich and Spence, 1966). Hence, it may be concluded that there is the highest probability of biological flavin-metal interaction under conditions of partial reduction of metal-flavoprotein systems and that part of the flavin may be kept under such conditions in the metal chelated state which, unfortunately, exhibits no prominent spectral characteristics, either in the optical range or—with paramagnetic metal centers—by electron spin resonance (ESR), except for the near infrared range. Therefore, Dr. Ehrenberg and I *propose* the biological relevance of flavin-iron chelates as a challenging working hypothesis for enzymologists.

II. Flavin-Substrate Complexes: Model Reactions of Flavin-Dependent Substrate Dehydrogenation

In contrast to nicotinamide coenzymes which clearly catalyze hydride transfer from alcohols and toward carbonyl compounds, the panopticum of biological activities exhibited by flavocoenzymes (Hemmerich *et al.*, 1970b) allows only one systematic conclusion concerning substrates that are dehydrogenated by flavins. With few exceptions, these substrates of the type XH do show more or less "activation" toward heterolytic dissociation $XH \rightleftharpoons X^- + H^+$. For $X = C$, carbanion formation is then followed by donation of an electron pair to the flavin and release of a carbonium ion. The most interesting recent model studies in this context come from Weatherby and Carr (1970), who demonstrated dehydrogenation of 1,2-dihydrophthalic acid or esters via carbanions by free flavocoenzymes in aqueous solution *in the dark*. These studies are parallel to older ones of Suelter and Metzler (1960), who demonstrated a similar dark reaction with free flavin and reduced nicotinamide. Though the intermediate carbanion could not be detected in this case, the transfer of electrons in pairs (and not one by one) has been documented. Those pairs, however, have been thought of in the past as being connected with hydrogen ("hydride ions") rather than with carbanions. It must be emphasized, therefore, that not the slightest evidence for a true "hydride" transfer has ever been found in flavin-dependent dehydrogenation. Experimental support has been accumulated, on the other hand, for the idea of carbanion-flavin interaction. This shall be outlined in the following:

In recent model studies, several types of *irreversible* reduction of flavo-quinone were detected:

1. Alkyl transfer, decarboxylating, was found to occur between photo-excited flavin and β,γ-unsaturated carboxylate ions (phenyl acetate, vinyl acetate, indole acetate, etc.) in the free (Walker *et al.*, 1967, 1970) as well as in the bound state (Komai and Massey, 1970), yielding a mixture of 5-(I) and 4a-alkylated (II) dihydroflavins.

2. Acyl transfer, decarboxylating, was found to occur between photo-excited flavin and α-keto acids, in the free (Brüstlein and Hemmerich, 1968) as well as in the bound state (de Kok *et al.*, 1970, amino acid oxi-dases). The acyl residue was found in position 5 of the flavin nucleus (III), where it is easily dissociated hydrolytically as well as by enforced oxidation.

3. Alkyl transfer without decarboxylation has been found recently (Knappe and Hemmerich, 1970) with organic sulfides as substrates. With tetrahydrothiophene (thiacyclopentane), for example, a product has been isolated of structure (IV).

Unlike "simple" 5-alkyl residues in dihydroflavins (e.g. I, Walker *et al.*, 1970), the tetrahydrothiophen residue is stable in the reduced state of flavin only, presumably since it is too bulky for a coplanar arrangement as required for a stable radical FlRH. Hence, autoxidation of compound (IV) is rather slow unless catalyzed by acid: Figure 3 shows the seem-ingly complex pH-dependence of this catalysis. But it is easy to see that the increase of reaction rate found upon starting from alkaline pH is interrupted by the protonation of the (IV)-anion at N(1). The "cata-lytically-active" protonation must clearly occur in the 5-substituent and is favored by deprotonation of the heteroaromatic nucleus. This proton-ation is reversible, since exposure of (IV) to acidic pH under strictly anaerobic conditions does not lead to cleavage of the 5-substituent.

(IVa)

We conclude, therefore, that (IV) is present in solution in the tauto-meric equilibrium (IV) $\rightleftarrows$ (IVa), with maximum content of (IVa) at pH 8 (Fig. 3), though not enough to be measurable directly under aqueous conditions. The mesoionic structure (IVa) should react much more easily with O_2, compared to (IV), since the $N(5)$-center is now entirely flat [cf. below (IV)]. Removal of an electron from (IVa) will, however, cause immediate hydrolysis, as also observed with (III) and unlike (I), which forms a stable radical. Investigation of the fate of the tetrahydrothiophen-residue is presently underway, as well as analogous studies in order to demonstrate a stable covalent flavin-nicotinamide complex.

For (IVa), on the other hand, a visible spectrum and possibly a long wave end absorption may be expected, like those observed in flavoprotein substrate complexes (cf. below).

4. From the above-mentioned reactions, it becomes obvious that "group transfer" might also occur in those cases where flavin substrates are dehydrogenated to yield unsubstituted dihydroflavin. Such an apparent "hydride transfer" could be simulated by alkyl transfer and subsequent fast hydrolysis.

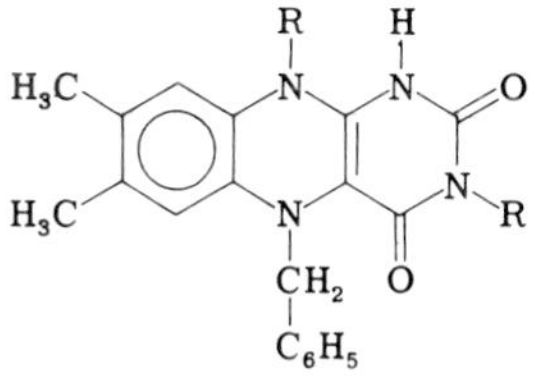

(I) 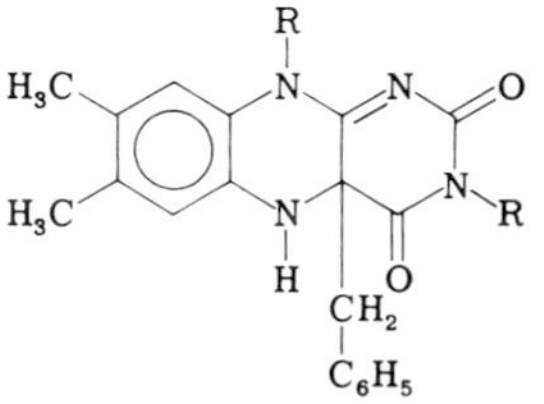   (II)

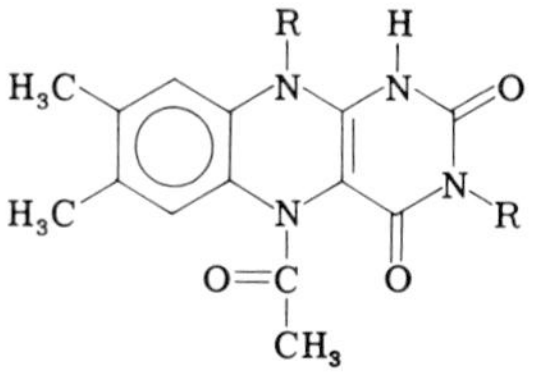

(III) 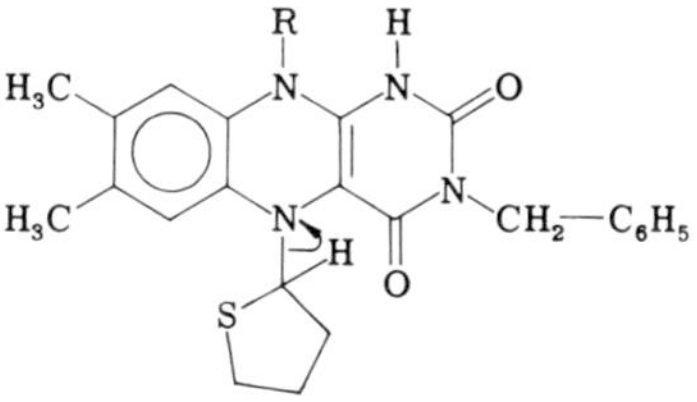   (IV)

Dr. Radda, in this symposium, has discussed in part these topics (Penzer *et al.*, this volume).

More support for the idea of "group transfer toward flavin" comes from enzymological studies, in particular by Dr. Massey's group (Massey *et al.*, 1970a), who finally succeeded in systematizing the various "flavin-substrate" or "Michaelis" complexes observed in flavoprotein-dependent substrate dehydrogenation. Let XH be the substrate, then two types of such complexes appear to be possible: HX-Fl and X-FlH. I object to these entities being conceived as "charge transfer" or π-complexes, since, accord-

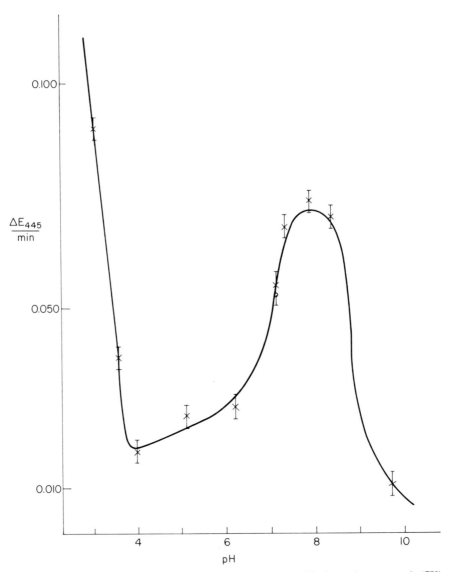

Fig. 3. Acid catalysis and pH-dependence of autoxidation of compound (IV), $7.6 \times 10^{-5}\ M$. The ordinate indicates increase in absorption at $\lambda = 445$ nm (λ_{max} of the product, 3-benzyllumiflavin) per minute. The buffer solutions were obtained by 10-fold dilution of a saturated stock solution of (IV) in methanol. The blank value for the uncatalyzed autoxidation in absolute methanol is $\Delta E_{445}/\text{min} = 0.014$. The increase at pH > 5 is due to the pK of 7.4 of compound (IV).

ing to the above-mentioned model experiences, I feel the need to postulate covalent binding. Furthermore, "π-bonding" exerted by substrates like alanine or acyl-CoA, is theoretically hard to conceive. Two main features remain to be established in order to verify this picture of the reaction sequence:

$$HX + Fl_{ox} \rightleftharpoons HX\text{-}Fl \rightleftharpoons X\text{-}FlH \rightleftharpoons HFl_{red}^- + X^+$$

a. The optical absorption of the "complexes," which is stretching out toward 500–700 nm remains to be explained. In any case, as will be outlined below, the complexes have nothing in common with flavin radicals.

b. Unclear also is the mode of rearrangement between the two "complexes," HXFl and XFlH, which might be an intramolecular hydride shift, but more probably a tautomerization accompanied by rearrangement of electron distribution within a delocalized π-system $(X\text{-}Fl)^-$.

Efforts to achieve a model demonstration of such a colored complex are presently underway in our laboratory (Brüstlein and Hemmerich, 1970). We have examined the "primary photo product" (Walker $et\ al.$, 1970) in the flavin-sensitized photodecarboxylation of phenylacetate ion. As mentioned above, the overall reaction yields 4a- and 5-benzyldihydroflavin isomers in a proportion of 1:1. At alkaline pH, both of these end products are extracted from water into chloroform, while the primary photo intermediate remains in the aqueous layer. Figure 4, curve 1, shows a spectrum of this intermediate in water at pH 11 as compared with the spectra of the two end products under the same conditions.

This behavior allows us to suggest that the primary intermediate still contains the carboxylate group. Upon acidification of the solution to pH 7.5, the intermediate changes its spectral appearance slightly (Fig. 4, curve 2) and becomes extractable by CHCl$_3$. This process is irreversible since reextraction into water at pH 11 is not possible. We conclude, therefore, that the decarboxylation step is initiated by the neutralization. The spectrum of the chloroform solution, however, shows a marked bathochromic shift which gives the solution a deep red color (Fig. 4, curve 3). This "secondary photo intermediate" is very labile and rearranges slowly but quantitatively—accelerated by acid—to yield 5-benzyldihydroflavin end product (cf. Fig. 5, curves $1–4$). In the same figure, the flavin substrate complex of L-amino acid oxidase (Massey and Curti, 1967) is shown for comparison. No structural assignment seems to be possible at present.

III. Flavin "Model" Radicals: Biologically Essential and Nonessential Flavosemiquinones

Flavin substrate complexes and flavin radicals are intimately connected, and they have been mixed up with each other since their discovery

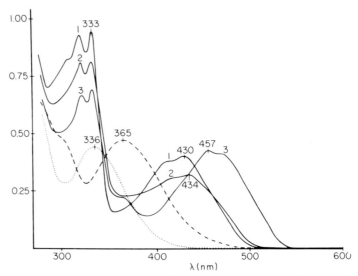

Fig. 4. Reaction of 3-methyllumiflavin with phenyl acetate, formation and decay of the "primary photoproduct"; $\lambda_{max} = 333$ nm; 4 ml $5 \times 10^{-4} M$, containing $1 M$ $C_6H_5CH_2COO^-NH_4^+$, pH 11.0 illuminated with 300 W Tungsten lamp at 0°C under argon for 1 minute. After the reaction, the end products, 4a- and 5-benzyldihydro-flavins, $\lambda_{max} = 365$ (cf. dashed curve) and 336 nm (cf. dotted curve), were removed by extraction with $CHCl_3$. Curve 1: Aqueous phase after extraction at pH 11; curve 2: aqueous phase of curve 1 acidified to pH 7.5; curve 3: $CHCl_3$-extract of aqueous phase of curve 2. Approximate molar extinctions can be obtained from the ordinate by multiplying the given values by 10^4.

by Haas (1937) and Michaelis and Schwarzenbach (1938), because radicals can obviously originate from flavin substrate complexes by homolytic dissociation

$$HX\text{-}Fl \rightarrow \overset{\cdot}{X} + \overset{\cdot}{Fl}H \leftarrow X\text{-}FlH$$

Radicals and substrate complexes absorbing in the same wavelength range could not be readily discriminated before the rise of the ESR age. In the meantime, the formation of radicals from flavin substrate complexes, which may be promoted by heat or light, has largely been acknowledged as an artificial side reaction. This has been possible only after thorough characterization of all possible species of flavin radicals in model systems: conditions have been found to keep flavins or their alkyl derivatives quantitatively in the radical anion (Ehrenberg et al., 1967) as well as the neutral radical state (Müller et al., 1970b). It has been the merit of Massey and Palmer (1966) to check most available flavoproteins with respect to the nature of the radicals they might form. From these experi-

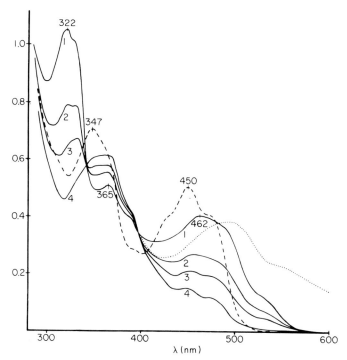

Fɪɢ. 5. Acid-catalyzed rearrangement of primary photoproduct (Fig. 4, curve *1*) after acidification to pH 5 and extraction with CHCl₃. Spectra are taken ca. 0, 20, 40, 60 minutes after acidification (curves *1–4*). Curve *4* represents mainly 5-benzyl-1,5-dihydroflavin together with some oxidized product (= starting material, 3-methyl-lumiflavin). The dashed line represents the end of autoxidation in the light, i.e., 3-methyllumiflavin (λ_{max} 449 and 346) together with some (VIa) λ_{max} 350). The dotted line gives the spectrum of ʟ-amino acid oxidase substrate complex as found by Massey and Curti (1967).

ments, two types of biologically relevant flavin radicals, i.e., the blue neutral radical (λ 570 nm) and the red anion (λ 470 nm) could be correlated with the model radicals. A thorough examination of the biological relevance of flavin radicals could take place after flavin substrate complexes, which are diamagnetic, have been rigorously discriminated from flavin radicals. From this, it has been proved that flavin radicals conform by no means to the concept of being "reactive intermediates" just by themselves. In particular, flavin radicals are not intermediates in flavin-dependent dehydrogenation reactions. This means that flavin radicals cannot be generated by substrate reduction in the case of flavoprotein dehydrogenases unless the enzyme contains secondary redox active cofactors like nonheme iron or molybdenum. If, on the other hand, a flavin radical of a dehydrogenase flavoprotein has been developed by artificial means, e.g., by photoreduction or by dithionite plus subsequent aeration, the radical is in general absolutely inert toward substrate (Massey et al., 1965). From this, it follows that for the dehydrogenase activity of flavoproteins, the radical state is not essential. Biologically essential flavin radicals, i.e., flavin radicals as true intermediates in flavin-dependent biocatalyses, appear to be found in such flavoproteins only which are concerned with true one-electron transfer. Clearly, all the known metal flavoproteins, and also others like NADP-ferredoxin oxidoreductase of chloroplasts belong to this class since physiologically they accept radical electrons from a one-electron oxidoreductant, like ferredoxin. In other words, radicals are essential intermediates only in such flavoproteins whose function consists in "splitting electron pairs" (Singer and Kearney, 1954) which are taken up by CH-activation.

It is the advantage of flavin radicals that their tendency to dimerize is, though finite, relatively small. The dimer $(FlH_2)_2$, "flavoquinhydrone," is a typical charge-transfer complex showing a diffuse absorption in the near infrared which is responsible for its greenish black appearance. Flavoquinhydrone is, however, detected only in highly polar, preferably aqueous, solution at half reduction and total flavin concentrations of more than millimolar (Gibson et al., 1962) and has not been found to occur in any flavoprotein under physiological conditions. Therefore, the flavin redox system is governed by the equation system:

$$\text{Fl}_{ox}\text{H} + \text{Fl}_{red}\text{H}_3 \overset{A}{\rightleftharpoons} 2\dot{\text{Fl}}\text{H}_2 \overset{B}{\rightleftharpoons} 2\dot{\text{Fl}}\text{H}^- + 2\text{H}^+$$
$$\updownarrow C$$
$$(\dot{\text{Fl}}\text{H}_2)_2$$

In the free chemical system, the equilibrium (A) is largely displaced toward the left, whereas practically all the known flavoproteins exhibit a strong stabilization of the radical, equilibrium (A) being shifted toward the right-hand side. The balance of equilibrium (B) depends on each single flavoapoenzyme (cf. Table I). This is a true thermodynamic stabilization of the radical state and can be explained by a specifically strong hydrogen bridge offered from the apoprotein to the flavin directed toward N-5 (Müller et al., 1970b). A similar mechanism is being established in Dr. Ehrenberg's lecture for the stabilization of flavin metal chelates.

Furthermore, there is the problem of an *additional* kinetic stabilization through restricted "interflavin contact" in the protein-bound state (Hemmerich et al., 1970b). Since most flavoproteins contain 2 flavins per active protein unit, intramolecular interflavin contact may be fast and may have biological importance.

As can be seen from the above-mentioned results, we are at the beginning of a systematization of the manifold flavin activities. The large number of known flavoproteins may be ordered and classified according to the following criteria: (1) pure flavoproteins and those containing secondary cofactors, in particular, metals; (2) flavoproteins containing one or more flavins per catalytically active unit; (3) flavoproteins exhibiting blue or red radicals; (4) flavoproteins which do react or do not react with molecular oxygen in the reduced state.

In Table I, we have tried to give a survey of flavoproteins according to these criteria. We hope that this systematization will turn out to be reasonable on the basis of molecular structure of flavoprotein active sites and their corresponding reaction mechanisms, and will be correlated to a systematization of flavin "functions" *in vivo*, i.e. XH-activation in the case of XH-bonds prepolarized in the sense $X^{\delta-} \to H^{\delta+}$, O_2-activation for $O_2 + 2e^-$ and $O_2 + e^-$ reactions, "electron pair splitting" and one more entirely open question: catalysis of the reaction

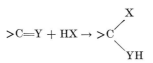

$$>C{=}Y + HX \to >C\begin{smallmatrix} \diagup X \\ \diagdown YH \end{smallmatrix}$$

by HX- (cf. above) and by $>C{=}Y$ activation (Y = O, NR, CR_2). This concerns the reversibility of flavin-dependent dehydrogenation, a still largely unexplored field. In this case, HX $= Fl_{red}H_3$. But it also concerns the "non-redox" flavoenzymes like oxynitrilase (Becker and Pfeil, 1966) and carboligase (Vennesland and Kezdy, 1969).

IV. Flavin-Dependent O_2-Activation: Discussion of Models and Nonmodels

In Table I the flavoproteins known to us are listed according to, among other properties, their ability to activate O_2. It is another question whether in any single case this given activity might be biologically essential or not. In the case of flavoprotein "oxidases," it is not known whether O_2 is a truly biological or an "incidental" acceptor. The following generalization might be proposed based upon model studies:

As mentioned above, O_2-activation is a property of the *flat* dihydroflavin. In other words, the more the dihydroflavin is bent the less easily is it attacked by O_2 (Hemmerich et al., 1970b). For the free chemical system, the flat state is a vibrationally excited state. This state might be stabilized by formation of a charge-transfer complex, e.g., a flavohydroquinone $(FlH_2)_2$, consisting of a Fl_{ox} half and a Fl_{red} half. In this arrangement, $Fl_{red}H_3$ is "flattened," and should, therefore, be expected to react

TABLE I

SURVEY OF FLAVOPROTEIN FUNCTION[a]

Enzyme (source)	Flavins per mole protein[b]	Other components	Input red/ox	Output ox/red other than O_2	Reactions $O_2 + Fl_{red}$	$SO_3^{2-} + Fl_{ox}$	1e-acceptors $+ Fl_{red}$	Type of radical
1. C—H Dehydrogenases								
Old yellow enzyme (yeast)	2(FMN)		NADPH/NADP	hFe[c]	+	−	−	Red
D-Amino acid oxidase (kidney)	2(FAD)		—CH(NH₂)COOH/ —COCOOH + NH₃		+	+	+	Red (blue with benzoate)
L-Amino acid oxidase (snake venom)	2(FAD)		—CH(NH₂)COOH/ —COCOOH + NH₃		+	+	+	Red
N(CH₃)-L-Amino acid oxidase (kidney)	?(FAD)		—CH(NH(CH₃))COOH/ —CH(NH₂)COOH + HCHO	Fl[d]	+		+	
Monoamine oxidase (kidney)	?(FAD)[e]		—CH₂NH₂/—CHO + NH₃		+			
Pyridoxamine phosphate oxidase (liver)	?(FMN)		—CH₂NH₂/—CHO + NH₃					
Pyridoxine-4-oxidase (Pseudomonas)	?(FAD)		—CH₂NH₂/—CHO + NH₃		+		+	
Pyridoxine-5-dehydrogenase (Pseudomonas)	?(FMN)		Pyridoxine/isopyridoxal				+	
Glucose oxidase (Aspergillus)	2(FAD)		β-D-Glucose/β-D-gluconolactone		+	+	−	Blue pH < 9, red pH > 9
Glycollate oxidase (spinach)	2(FMN)		HOCH₂COOH/OHCCOOH		++	+	−	Red
Pyruvate oxidase (Lactobacillus delbrueckii)	?(FAD)	TPP[g]	CH₃COCOOH + Pᵢ/ CH₃CO—P + CO₂		++		+	
Pyruvate dehydrogenase (Escherichia coli B)	4(FAD)	TPP[g]	CH₃COCOOH/ CH₃COOH + CO₂	hFe[e]			+	
Oxalate oxidase (mosses)	?(FMN or riboflavin)		HOOCCOOH/2CO₂		+			
Acyl-CoA dehydrogenase (liver)	2?(FAD)		C₆–C₁₆ Acyl-CoA/2,3 dehydro acyl-CoA	Fl[d]	−	−	−	Blue
NAD-peroxidase (Streptococcus)	?(FAD)		NADH/NAD	H₂O₂/H₂O	+	+	+	
NADH-cyt b₅ reductase (liver microsomes)	1(FAD)		NADH/NAD	hFe[e]	+	+	+	Blue

Enzyme	Flavin	Other prosthetic group	Substrate/product	Electron acceptor				Color
NADPH-cyt c reductase (liver microsomes)	2?(FAD)		NADPH/NADP	hFe[c]	+		+	Blue
NADH-dehydrogenase (heart mitochondria)	1(FMN)	SFe	NADH/NAD	hFe[e], SFe[f], CoQ			+	Red
NADPH-quinone oxido-reductase (hog liver)	?		NADPH/NADP or NADH/NAD NADPH/NADP	Quinones	-?		-?	
NADPH-vitamin K oxidoreductase (liver)	1(FAD)		NADPH/NADP	Naphthoquinones	-?		-?	
L-6-OH nicotine oxidase (*Arthrobacter*)	2(FAD)		⟩CH–N⟨ ⟩C=O + HN⟨		+		+	Red
Salicylate oxygenase (*Pseudomonas*)	1(FAD)		Salicylate/catechol NADPH/NADP		+		+	Red (blue with substrate)
p-OH-benzoate oxygenase (*Pseudomonas*)	1(FAD)		p-OH-Benzoate/3,4-di-OH-benzoate, NADPH/NADP		+	—		
Xanthine oxidase (milk)	2(FAD)	Mo, SFe	Xanthine/uric acid $-CHO/-COOH$		+		++	Blue
Aldehyde oxidase (liver)	2(FAD)	Mo, SFe	$HOOCCH_2CH_2COOH/$ $HOOCCH{=}CHCOOH$	Fl[d], CoQ	++		+	
Succinate dehydrogenase (heart mitochondria)	1(FAD)[e]	SFe	$CH_3CHOHCOOH/$ $CH_3COCOOH$	hFe[c]	—		+	
Lactate dehydrogenase (yeast)	4(FAD)		$CH_3CHOHCOOH/$ $CH_3COCOOH$	hFe[c]	+	+	+	
Lactate oxidase (*Mycobacterium*)	6(FMN)	TPP[g]	$CH_3COOH + CO_2$	SFe[f], CoQ?, Fl[d]?	+		+?	Red
Glycerol phosphate dehydrogenase (mitochondria)	1(FAD)	SFe	$CH_2OHCHOHCH_2O{-}P/$ $OHCCHOHCH_2O{-}P$	NAD/NADH	+			
Dihydroorotate dehydrogenase (*Zymobacterium*)	2(FMN) + 2(FAD)	FeS	Dihydroorotic acid/ orotic acid	NAD/NADH	+			
Choline dehydrogenase (liver mitochondria)	1(FAD)	Fe	$(CH_3)_3NCH_2CH_2OH/$ $(CH_3)_3NCH_2CHO$		+		+	
2. —S—H Dehydrogenases								
Dihydrolipoamide dehydrogenase (mitochondria)	2(FAD)	S[act][h]	Dihydrolipoamide/lipoamide	Fl[d]?	—		+	None[i]
Glutathione reductase (yeast)	2(FAD)	S[act][h]	$-S{-}S{-}{-}SH$		—	—	++	None
Thioredoxin reductase (*E. coli*)	1(FAD)	S[act][h]	$-S{-}S{-}/{-}SH$		—	—	++	Blue
3. e--Transferases								
Ferredoxin-NADP reductase (spinach)	1(FAD)		SFe(II)/SFe(III)	NADP/NADPH, hFe[c]	+		+	Blue

(Continued)

TABLE I (Continued)

Enzyme (source)	Flavins per mole protein[b]	Other components	Input red/ox	Output ox/red other than O_2	Reactions O_2 + Fl_{red}	Reactions SO_3^{2-} + Fl_{ox}	Reactions $1e^-$ acceptors + Fl_{red}	Type of radical
Electron-transferring flavoprotein	1(FAD)		Fl[d]	Fl[d]	−		+	Red
Flavodoxin (*Peptostreptococcus*)	1(FMN)			Chloroplasts	+	−	+	Blue
Azotobacter flavoprotein	?(FAD)		?	?	+	−	+	Blue
Phytoflavin (alga)	1(FMN)		NADPH/NADP	Chloroplasts	+		+	Blue
4. Other Redoxactive Flavoproteins								
Sulfite reductase (*Salmonella*)	2(FAD+FMN)	SFe	SO_3^{2-}/S^{2-}	SFe[f], hFe[e]	+?		+	Blue
Sulfate reductase (bacteria)	1(FAD)	SFe	$AMP\text{-}SO_3H/AMP + SO_4^{2-}$	SFe[f]		+	+	
Nitrate reductase (bacteria)	?(FAD)	Mo	NO_3^-/NO_2^-, NADPH/NADP	hFe[e]				
5. Redox-inactive Flavoproteins								
Glyoxylate carboligase (*E. coli*)	?(FAD)	TPP+	$2HCCOOH/OHCCHOHCOOH + CO_2$		−	−	+?	
Oxynitrilase (almonds)	1(FAD)		$C_6H_5CHOHCN/C_6H_5CHO + HCN$		+	+		Red

[a] Empty space in a given column means that no data are available. For references, see Hemmerich et al. (1970b).

[b] The numbers in this column are subject to potential error in so far as they indicate in many cases the smallest *active* subunit but in some cases it is not established whether the observed subunit is active as monomer. Therefore, the given numbers may in fact be greater by factors of 2 or 4 and in particular "one-flavin-enzymes" may act as dimers. This is supported by the fact that such proteins, e.g., phytoflavin interact rapidly with themselves, whereas "two-flavin-enzymes" in general do not.

[c] hFe = heme-iron, Fe(II)/Fe(III).

[d] Fl = flavin. It is assumed that natural electron transport runs from initial dehydrogenases in many cases through other flavoproteins, like "electron transferring flavoprotein," before it reaches ubiquinone or cytochromes.

[e] Covalently bound flavocoenzyme.

[f] SFe = iron-sulfur protein. In many cases, cf. "other components," this table. SFe is an integral part of the flavoprotein.

[g] TPP = thiamine pyrophosphate. It seems at least possible, that the immediate substrate of flavin in the TPP-flavoproteins is the "carbanion" (or enamine) of the "active acetaldehyde"

[h] S_{act} = reactive disulfide center at the enzyme active site, yielding a diamagnetic FlS-intermediate, which prevents formation of radicals in the case of the "2 FAD/Mole-Enzymes."

[i] In the presence of NAD excess the red diamagnetic intermediate can be photolysed to yield ~50% Fl presumably of the blue type.

more easily with O_2 than free $Fl_{red}H_3$. A similar flattening might be obtained at a protein active site by interaction with a flat group from the protein, e.g., tryptophan. [It might be remembered at the same time, that any other protein, having no aromatic residue in the active center, would rather stabilize the bent state of dihydroflavin.] Unfortunately, a concentration dependence of dihydroflavin autoxidation has not been measured by rapid flow techniques as yet, which could support this proposal. Also, $FADH_2$ should, in the "hairpin configuration" present at pH > 5 (Hemmerich et al., 1970a), react more rapidly with O_2 than does $FMNH_2$. The autocatalysis of $Fl_{red}H_2$-autoxidation (Gibson and Hastings, 1962) is well explained by this, rather than by FlH acting as O_2-activating intermediate.

Quite generally, there are three modes of decay for the "primary complex from dihydroflavin and O_2," HFl-OOH, which has been demonstrated by fast kinetic studies of Massey and co-workers (1970b).

$$H_2Fl\text{-}OOH \rightarrow \begin{cases} H_2\overset{\cdot}{Fl} + \overset{\cdot}{O_2^-} + H^+ & (1) \\ Fl_{ox}H + H_2O_2 & (2) \\ [H_2Fl_{ox}OH] + [O] & (3) \end{cases}$$

Path (1) has been demonstrated at alkaline pH by ESR analysis of the superoxide anion radical formed (Ballou et al., 1969). Path (2) is the "trivial" (chemical) way, but like many trivial things, it might turn out to be "unbiological." The "most biological-looking" pathway is (3), since it is the only pathway which would not produce "junk" from O_2. The term [O] is taken to be the "oxene" intermediate believed to be essential

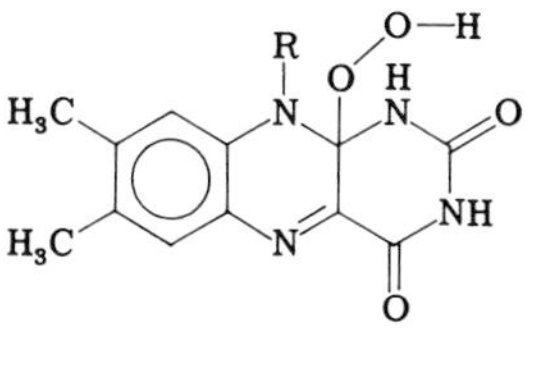

(V)

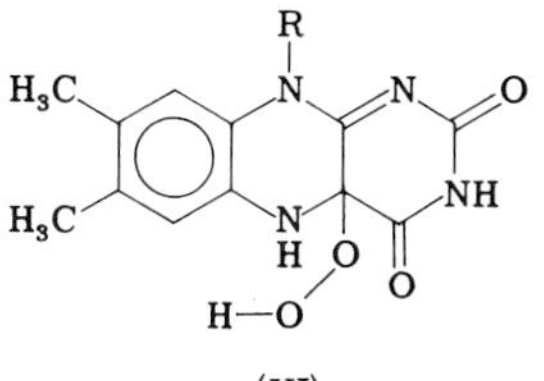

(VI)

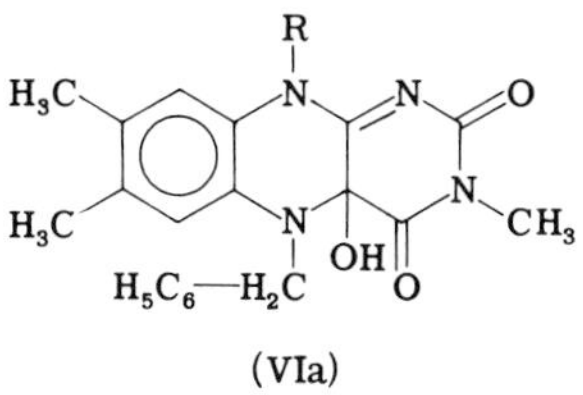

(VIa)

for biological oxygenation (Jerina *et al.*, 1970). [$H_2Fl_{ox}OH$] defines a hypothetic "flavoquinone covalent hydrate," which decays very rapidly to yield $Fl_{ox}H + H_2O$. Clearly, pathway 3 should occur "within" a ternary complex of flavin, O_2 and substrate to be oxygenated, maybe even in a quaternary complex which also includes a heavy metal ion of the enzyme. The problem to be tackled at first is the structure of H_2FlOOH. Two very nearly related structures have been proposed: (V) (Mager and Berends, 1965) and (VI) (Hemmerich, 1968).

A stable derivative of (VI) is known (VIa) (Walker *et al.*, 1967), while the proposal of Mager and Berends (1965) rests on assumptions derived from N-1-alkylated "overcrowded" models which (because of their high noncoplanarity) are, as mentioned above, "nonmodels" for flavin-dependent O_2-activation. More experiments are greatly needed.

REFERENCES

Ballou, D., Palmer, G., and Massey, V. (1969). *Biochem. Biophys. Res. Commun.* **36**, 898.

Becker, W., and Pfeil, E. (1966). *Biochem. Z.* **346**, 301.

Bothe, E., Hemmerich, P., and Sund, H. (1970). *In* "Flavins and Flavoproteins" (H. Kamin, ed.). University Park Press, Baltimore, Maryland (in press).

Brüstlein, M., and Hemmerich, P. (1968). *FEBS Letters* **1**, 335.

Brüstlein, M., and Hemmerich, P. (1970). Unpublished results.

de Kok, A., Veeger, C., and Hemmerich, P. (1970). *In* "Flavins and Flavoproteins" (H. Kamin, ed.). University Park Press, Baltimore, Maryland (in press).

Ehrenberg, A., Müller, F., and Hemmerich, P. (1967). *Eur. J. Biochem.* **2**, 286.

Eley, M., Lee, J., Cormier, M. J., Lhoste, J. M., and Hemmerich, P. (1970). *Biochemistry* (submitted for publication).

Fromherz, P. (1969). Ph.D. Thesis, University of Marburg.

Gibson, R. H., and Hastings, J. W. (1962). *Biochem. J.* **83**, 368.

Gibson, Q. H., Massey, V., and Atherton, N. (1962). *Biochem. J.* **85**, 369.

Haas, E. (1937). *Biochem. Z.* **290**, 291.

Harbury, H. A., LaNoue, K. F., Loache, P. A., and Amick, R. M. (1959). *Proc. Nat. Acad. Sci. U. S.* **45**, 1708.

Hemmerich, P., and Spence, J. (1966). *In* "Flavins and Flavoproteins" (E. C. Slater, ed.), p. 82. Elsevier, Amsterdam.

Hemmerich, P. (1964). *Helv. Chim. Acta* **47**, 464.

Hemmerich, P. (1968). *In* "Biochemie des Sauerstoffs" (B. Hess and H. Staudinger, eds.), p. 249. Springer, Berlin.

Hemmerich, P., Ghisla, S., Hartmann, U., and Müller, F. (1970a). *In* "Flavins and Flavoproteins" (H. Kamin, ed.). University Park Press, Baltimore, Maryland (in press).

Hemmerich, P., Nagelschneider, G., and Veeger, C. (1970b). *FEBS Letters* **8**, 69.

Jerina, D. M., Daly, J. W., Witkop, B., Zaltzman-Nirenberg, P., and Udenfriend, S. (1970). *Biochemistry* **9**, 147.

Kierkegaard, P., Norrestam, R., Werner, P.-E., Csöregh, I., Glehn, M. V., Karlsson, R., Leijonmarck, M., Rönnquist, O., Stensland, B., Tillberg, O., and Torbjörnsson, L. (1970). *In* "Flavins and Flavoproteins" (H. Kamin, ed.), University Park Press, Baltimore, Maryland (in press).

Knappe, W. R., and Hemmerich, P. (1970). *Angew. Chem. Int. Ed. Eng.* (in press).

Komai, H., and Massey, V. (1970). *In* "Flavins and Flavoproteins" (H. Kamin, ed.). University Park Press, Baltimore, Maryland (in press).

Mager, H. I. X., and Berends, W. (1965). *Rec. Trav. Chim. Pays-Bas* **84**, 1329.

Massey, V., and Palmer, G. (1966). *Biochemistry* **5**, 3181.

Massey, V., and Curti, B. (1967). *J. Biol. Chem.* **242**, 1259.

Massey, V., Ganther, H., Brumby, P. E., and Curti, B. (1965). *In* "Oxidases and Related Redox Systems" (T. E. King, M. Morrison, and H. S. Mason, eds.), Vol. 1, p. 335. Wiley, New York.

Massey, V., Matthews, R. G., Foust, G. P., Howell, L. G., Williams, C. H., Jr., Zanetti, G., and Ronchi, S. (1970a). *In* "Pyridine Nucleotide Dependent Dehydrogenases" (H. Sund, ed.), p. 393. Springer, Berlin.

Massey, V., Palmer, G., and Ballou, D. (1970b). *In* "Flavins and Flavoproteins" (H. Kamin, ed.). University Park Press, Baltimore, Maryland (in press).

Mayhew, S. G., Foust, G. P., and Massey, V. (1969). *J. Biol. Chem.* **244**, 803.

Michaelis, L., and Schwarzenbach, G. (1938). *J. Biol. Chem.* **123**, 538.

Müller, F., Hemmerich, P., and Ehrenberg, A. (1968). *Eur. J. Biochem.* **5**, 158.

Müller, F., Eriksson, L. E. G., and Ehrenberg, A. (1970a). *Eur. J. Biochem.* **12**, 93.

Müller, F., Hemmerich, P., Ehrenberg, A., Palmer, G., and Massey, V. (1970b). *Eur. J. Biochem.* (in press).

Palmer, G., and Brintzinger, H. (1970). *In* "A Treatise on Electron and Coupled Energy Transfer in Biological Systems" (M. Klingenberg and T. E. King, eds.) (to be published).

Singer, T. P., and Kearney, E. B. (1954). *In* "The Proteins" (H. Neurath and K. Bailey, eds.), Vol. 2, Part A, Chapter 13-IV. Academic Press, New York.

Suelter, C. H., and Metzler, D. E. (1960). *Biochim. Biophys. Acta* **44**, 23.

Vennesland, B., and Kezdy, F. J. (1969). *J. Biol. Chem.* **244**, 3991.

Walker, W. H., Hemmerich, P., and Massey, V. (1967). *Helv. Chim. Acta* **50**, 2269.

Walker, W. H., Hemmerich, P., and Massey, V. (1970). *Eur. J. Biochem.* **13**, 258.

Weatherby, G. D., and Carr, D. O. (1970). *Biochemistry* **9**, 344.

Flavin-Radical-Metal Chelates*

ANDERS EHRENBERG

*Department of Biophysics, Stockholm University, Karolinska Institutet,
Stockholm 60, Sweden*

I. Introduction

The potential chelate-forming capacity of flavin was recognized by
Albert (1950) based on the observation that flavin has a possible tauto-
meric form with a hydroxyl in peri position to a tertiary heterocyclic
nitrogen, similar to the structure of 8-hydroxyquinoline. Because of this
analogy he predicted metal ion affinity of flavin and tried to determine
stability constants for oxidized riboflavin and several divalent metal
ions (Albert, 1953). Subsequently, however, Hemmerich (1960, 1964;
Hemmerich and Fallab, 1958) made the important observation that the
oxidized and reduced states of flavin are but very poor chelating agents
with valence stable divalent metal ions, whereas the corresponding semiquinone chelates have considerable stability. The background of this
profound difference between the various redox levels of the flavin has
been reviewed extensively (Hemmerich, 1963; Hemmerich *et al.*, 1965;
Ehrenberg and Hemmerich, 1968). This difference is impressively demonstrated (Hemmerich *et al.*, 1963) by the action of added metal ions to a
half-reduced flavin solution, which shifts equilibrium (1)

$$\text{Fl}_{ox}\text{R} + \text{Fl}_{red}\text{RH}^- \underset{-H^+}{\rightleftharpoons} 2\text{FlR}^- \underset{+2\text{Me}^{2+}}{\rightleftharpoons} 2(\text{MeFl})^+ \qquad (1)$$

(R is the substituent in position 3, which is H in normal flavin) away
from radical disproportionation. These observations raised considerably
the interests of biochemists and biophysicists in the properties of those

* The works described were supported in part by the Swedish Statens Medicinska
Forskningsråd and Statens Naturvetenskapliga Forskningsråd and U. S. Public
Health Service Grant AM-05895.

chelates since they indicated possible functional modes of the chelates in the catalytic action of metalloflavoproteins.

Related to the flavin radical (flavosemiquinone) metal chelates $(Me^{n+}\dot{F}lR^-)^{(n-1)+}$ are the flavoquinone metal chelates $(Me^{n+}Fl_{ox}R)^{n+}$ which are stabilized by back-donation from the metal d-shell to the lowest empty antibonding ligand orbital, and hence are called charge-transfer chelates (Hemmerich, 1963). Only very strong (Cu^+, Ag^+) and fairly strong (Fe^{2+}, Mo^{5+}) donor ions form such charge transfer complexes of reasonable stability (Hemmerich et al., 1965; Hemmerich and Spence, 1966). The charge transfer renders the flavin ligand some properties characteristic of the flavosemiquinone and its chelates. In the following we will sum up some recent results about these chelates and discuss some important problems remaining to be solved.

II. Chelate Stability

Using electron spin resonance (ESR) for quantitative spin concentration measurements, Müller et al. (1970) determined stability constants for flavin radical chelates both in the aqueous system and in the aprotic solvent DMF (dimethyl formamide). In order to enhance solubility in these solvents flavins were used with substituents in position 3: $-CH_2COO^-$ and $-CH_2COOC_2H_5$, respectively.

The shift of equilibrium (1) upon addition of metal ions, in this case Zn^{2+}, is demonstrated in Fig. 1. From the experimental points and the equilibrium constants determined for the system in absence of metal ions (Ehrenberg et al., 1967) the stability constant

$$K_{Me\dot{F}lR}^{Me\cdot} = \frac{[(Me\dot{F}lR)^+]}{[Me^{2+}][\dot{F}lR^-]}$$

between the flavin radical anion and the metal ion could be calculated. The mean value at 20°C for the whole pH range investigated for the Zn chelate was 2.0×10^4 M^{-1}. Using this value and the earlier results from the metal-free system, the top curve of Fig. 1 could be calculated.

For the chelates in DMF, another procedure was adopted. The total spin concentration S was measured for half-reduced flavin at varied metal ion concentration. Under the assumption that $S \approx [(Me\dot{F}lR)^+] \gg \dot{F}lR_{tot}$, where the index "tot" refers to the total concentration of the species, irrespective of the protonation state, it could be deduced for the system (Müller et al., 1970) that

$$\frac{1}{S} = \frac{1}{[Me]_0 - S} \times \frac{1}{f[FlR]_0 K_{Me\dot{F}lR}^{Me\cdot}} + \frac{1}{[FlR]_0} \tag{2}$$

where $[Me]_0$ and $[FlR]_0$ are the original total concentrations of metal ion

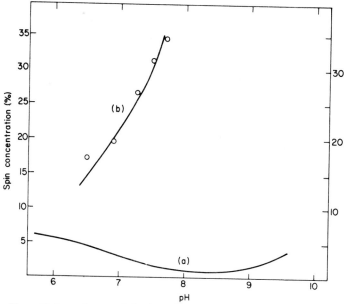

FIG. 1. The pH-dependence of flavin radical disproportionation in the presence and absence of metal ions. Radical content (% of total flavin) of half-reduced aqueous flavin solution is plotted versus pH. Curve a: 10 mM lumiflavin-3-CH$_2$COO$^-$ in the absence of metal ions (obtained as described by Ehrenberg $et\ al.$, 1967). Curve b: 1 mM lumiflavin-3-CH$_2$COO$^-$ in the presence of 10 mM Zn^{2+}. Radical concentration estimated from height and width of overmodulated electron spin resonance signal by comparison with a VOSO$_4$ standard at room temperature (0). The full-drawn curve is calculated using $\dot{K} = 4.0 \times 10^{-9} M$, $K_{red} = 5 \times 10^{-7} M$, $K_F = 2.3 \times 10^{-2}$ and $K^{Zn}_{ZnFlR} = 2.0 \times 10^4 M^{-1}$. From Müller $et\ al.$ (1970).

and flavin added to the system and $f = [\dot{F}lR^-]/([FlR]_0 - S)$. Equation (2) shows that when plotting S^{-1} versus $([Me]_0 - S)^{-1}$ a straight line should be obtained. The results for Cd^{2+} are presented in Fig. 2. The ordinate intercept is for 100% chelate formation and was, incidentally, used for quantitative calibration of the system. From the slope of the line, the value $K^{Cd}_{Cd\,FlR} = 4.0 \times 10^3 \times f^{-1} M^{-1}$ is obtained. Without metal ions added, the blank contains close to 1% of radicals. Since not all the radicals are necessarily in the form of anions $f \leq 10^{-2}$, and we found for the stability constant at room temperature in the DMF solvent system $K^{Cd}_{Cd\,FlR} \geq 4 \times 10^5\ M^{-1}$. For Zn the stability constant was about a factor of two lower.

The fact that the values obtained for K^{Zn}_{ZnFlR} from the data of Fig. 1 are practically constant over the whole pH range investigated, the standard deviation was $0.4 \times 10^4\ M^{-1}$, supports the correctness of the assump-

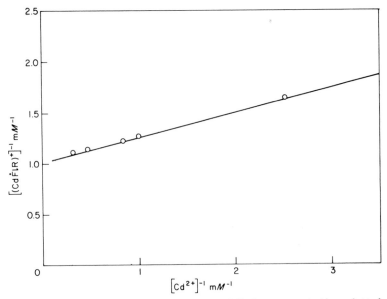

Fig. 2. Chelate concentration as function of Cd^{2+} ion concentration plotted as described in text [Eq. (2)]: 1 mM half-reduced 3-$CH_2COOC_2H_5$-10-methylisoalloxazine in the presence of 4 mM Et_3N. Solvent system: 80% dimethyl formamide, 16% CH_3CN, and 4% $CHCl_3$. From Müller et al. (1970).

tion about a 1:1 chelate formation. Because of the assumptions involved in deducing Eq. (2), the straight line obtained in Fig. 2 provides further support for the existence of this kind of chelate.

The stability constant of the lumiflavin radical Zn chelate determined as described, with the ESR technique in aqueous solution at 20° is $2 \times 10^4 M^{-1}$ (Müller et al., 1970), which is in fair agreement with the value $5 \times 10^4 M^{-1}$ derived from acidimetric measurements on tetra-O-acetyl-riboflavin-3-methyl in ethanol–water (1:1, v/v) at 50° (Hemmerich, 1964). The Cd and Zn chelates have about equal stability: in DMF the Cd chelates are somewhat more stable (Müller et al., 1970); in ethanol, the Zn chelates (Hemmerich, 1964). There is about a 10-fold increase in stability constant when going from water to DMF. The latter solvent is aprotic, has a larger dipole moment than water but a lower dielectric constant, and is amphiphilic, i.e., it is both hydro- and lipophilic (hydrophobic). In flavoproteins there could well be situations with such properties of the protein region at the flavin, including steric arrangements, and a high local metal-ion activity, which could give the flavin–radical–metal chelates considerable stability and possibly make them important for stabilizing the intermediate redox state of the flavin. There are in fact flavoproteins for which Zn has been claimed as cofactor (see, e.g., Dixon and Webb, 1964). The stability of Fe, Mo, and Cu chelates could be enhanced similarly.

III. Electron Spin Resonance

The hyperfine interactions within the flavin radical ligand and with the chelated Zn and Cd ions have been studied in great detail (Ehrenberg et al., 1966; Müller et al., 1967, 1970). The natural abundance of non-magnetic ^{64}Zn is 95.9%, and the influence of the 4.1% of magnetic ^{67}Zn could be neglected for practical purposes when studying the radical ligand.

In order to resolve the hyperfine interactions in the radical ligand the technique of specific isotopic and chemical substitution was applied (Müller et al., 1970). In Fig. 3 this technique is illustrated by some of the spectra recorded. The second spectrum of the top row shows that there is only a small spin density in position 7 (for position numbering see Fig. 4). Substitution of ^{15}N in positions 1 and 3 did not markedly change the top left spectrum, proving that there is only negligible spin density on those nitrogens. The spectra of the second and third rows demonstrate the strong couplings of the nitrogens in positions 5 and 10 and of the methyl groups in positions 8 and 10, and consequently the high spin density in those positions. All substitutions tested with the radical chelates affected the number of hyperfine lines in the same way as for the radical anion (Eriksson and Ehrenberg, 1964, 1965; Ehrenberg et al., 1967). The main differences between the two sets of spectra (Müller et al., 1970) is that in case of the chelate there is a slightly larger total width and a somewhat poorer coincidence of the hyperfine lines in the central region, decreasing the amplitudes and increasing the resolution in that part of the spectrum.

With high spectrometer gain the positions of the outermost lines of the spectra, those of Fig. 3 and others, could be determined and the total widths of the spectra could be measured. The change in total width upon specific isotopic or chemical substitutions could be determined and the corresponding hyperfine couplings computed (Müller et al., 1970). In Table I these coupling constants are compared with those of the radical anion. The close correspondence is apparent and demonstrates that the flavin radical ligand is a slightly perturbed anion radical. This is in agreement with the light absorption (Müller et al., 1968), see below, and with the observed release of one proton equivalent from half-reduced flavin when metal ion is added (Hemmerich, 1964) [cf. equilibrium (1)].

It has been discovered that the electronic spin of the radical ligand is also delocalized to the metal ion (Ehrenberg et al., 1966). With highly enriched isotopes of Cd and Zn the coupling constants of the metal ions

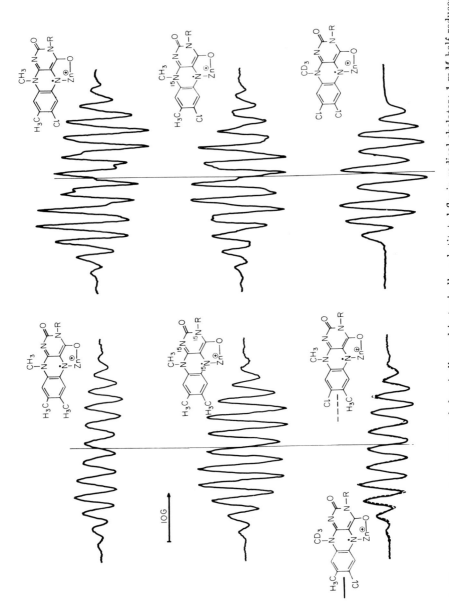

Fig. 3. Electron spin resonance spectra of chemically and isotopically substituted flavin radical chelates; 1 mM half-reduced flavin in dimethyl formamide with 4 mM Et₃N and 4 mM Zn²⁺. G = gauss. From Müller et al. (1970).

TABLE I

Isotropic Hyperfine Coupling Constants in Gauss for 3-Alkylated
Lumiflavin Radical Chelates Compared with Coupling Constants
for the Nonchelated Anionic Radical
both in Dimethyl Formamide

Coupling constant	Radical chelate		Anionic radical	
	ESR[a]	ENDOR[b]	ESR[c]	ENDOR[b]
a_5^N	7.7 ± 0.3	—	7.3 ± 0.3	—
a_6^H	3.5 ± 0.5	—	3.5 ± 0.5	—
$a_8^H(CCH_3)$	3.9 ± 0.2	3.72 ± 0.04	4.0 ± 0.5	4.08 ± 0.04
a_9^H	Small	—	0.9 ± 0.1	—
a_{10}^N	3.1 ± 0.5	—	3.2 ± 0.3	—
$a_{10}^H(NCH_3)$	3.1 ± 0.2	3.51 ± 0.04	3.0 ± 0.2	3.19 ± 0.04
a^{111Cd}	16.65 ± 0.10	—	—	—
a^{113Cd}	17.55 ± 0.10	—	—	—
a^{67Zn}	2.59 ± 0.05	—	—	—

[a] Electron spin resonance (Müller *et al.*, 1970).
[b] Electron nuclear double resonance (Eriksson *et al.*, 1969).
[c] Ehrenberg *et al.* (1967).

could be determined with high precision (Müller *et al.*, 1967, 1970) (see Table I). Some relevant recordings are shown in Fig. 4. From these data it was estimated that the spin density or spin polarization transferred to the nucleus of Cd is about double that in case of Zn.

Various mechanisms for spin transfer to the metal nucleus and factors causing a difference between Cd and Zn have been discussed (Müller *et al.*, 1970). The main conclusion is that the metal ion must be coordinated by a partly double bond to a site of the ligand with nonvanishing spin density, probably $N(5)$ where the ligand has its highest spin density, see Table I. The partly double bond reflects back donation from metal hybrid orbitals to the ligand π-orbital. This mechanism of electron transfer between flavin and a redox-active metal ion, e.g., Fe^{2+}, could be of importance in the action of metalloflavopriteins.

IV. Electron Nuclear Double Resonance (ENDOR)

The lumiflavin-radical Zn chelates were selected for our first work with ENDOR on flavin radicals, because of their comparative ease of preparation, the possibility to obtain high spin concentration in both organic and aqueous media, and the stability of the samples (Hyde, 1967; Eriksson *et al.*, 1969). The ENDOR spectrum of the radical chelate in liquid DMF is shown in Fig. 5. In a proton ENDOR display there should be a peak for each proton or group of equivalent protons. Three peaks from strongly

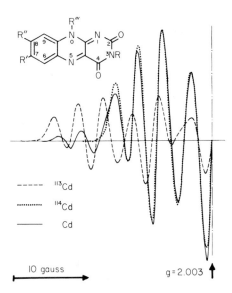

Fig. 4. Low-field part of electron spin resonance recordings of cadmium flavin radical chelates. The spectra are normalized to the same radical concentration. 1 mM flavin (R = CH$_2$COOC$_2$H$_5$; R' = R'' = Cl; R''' = CD$_3$); 3 mM Cd(NO$_3$)$_2$; 3 mM triethylamine. Solvent system: dimethyl formamide (1 ml), chloroform (1 ml) acetonitrile (0.4 ml) and triethylamine (0.1 ml). Reduction to about 50% with hydrogen in palladium. From Ehrenberg *et al.* (1966).

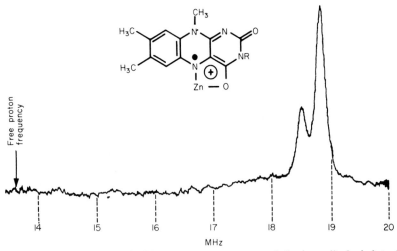

Fig. 5. Electron nuclear double resonance spectrum of flavin radical chelate in dimethyl formamide at −70°. Total flavin concentration 8 mM, triethylamine and Zn(ClO$_4$)$_2$ 32 mM. Reduced to 50% with H$_2$/Pd. Spectrum of cadmium chelate is identical. From Eriksson *et al.* (1969).

coupling protons, H(6), CH$_3$(8), and CH$_3$(10), would be expected from the ESR data on the radical chelate, but only two peaks are seen in the recording of Fig. 5. These peaks were assigned to the two strongly coupling methyl groups by measurements on the 8-Cl derivative and a sample with the 10-methyl group deuterated, as is shown in Fig. 6 (Eriksson *et al.*, 1969). The methyl protons have low anisotropy and are especially favorable for ENDOR detection. The α-proton in position 6, on the other hand, is very anisotropic, and its ENDOR signal is broadened beyond detection under the experimental conditions applied. Similar experiments were also made on the lumiflavin anionic radical (Eriksson *et al.*, 1969). From the frequencies of the ENDOR signals, very accurate coupling constants were obtained. These constants are included in Table I and are in very good agreement with the ESR results.

The ENDOR studies were also extended to frozen solutions (Eriksson *et al.*, 1969) as a model for planned experiments on flavoprotein radicals. Under these conditions so-called powder ENDOR spectra are obtained (Hyde *et al.*, 1968) as illustrated in Fig. 7. Here each methyl-ENDOR signal is broadened and often obtains an asymmetric double peaked shape, characteristic of a group with axial symmetry. Resolution and assignment of the two overlapping signals could be accomplished with chemical and isotopic substitution as in case of the liquid samples. Each methyl powder-ENDOR signal has its absorption centered closely at the same frequency as the corresponding signal from the liquid sample. At

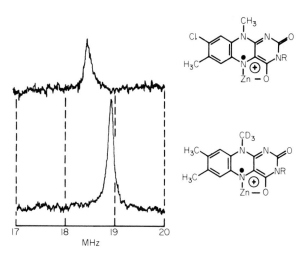

FIG. 6. Electron nuclear double resonance recordings of radical chelates in dimethyl formamide at −74°. Concentration of isoalloxazine derivative 4 m*M*, triethylamine and metal salt 16 m*M*. Spectra recorded under identical conditions. From Eriksson *et al.* (1969).

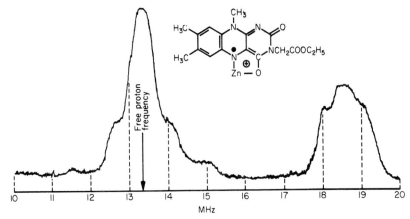

FIG. 7. Electron nuclear double resonance spectrum of lumiflavin radical chelate in dimethyl formamide at about −160°. Total flavin concentration 4 mM, triethylamine and metal salt 16 mM. From Eriksson et al. (1969).

the free proton frequency an intense signal is obtained. This is called the matrix-ENDOR signal (Hyde et al., 1968) and is due to weakly interacting protons in the immediate surroundings of the radical. On the slopes of the matrix signal, bumps are observed that have been assigned to the weakly coupling protons in positions 7 and 9.

Based on this experience from the model compounds the ENDOR studies have been extended to flavoproteins (Ehrenberg et al., 1968, 1970; Eriksson et al., 1969). The results demonstrate that with the ENDOR technique useful information is obtained from the 8-methyl coupling concerning the state of protonation of the flavin radical, and from the matrix signal concerning the interaction between the radical and the protein and possibly also nearby water molecules. ENDOR measurements have further provided very crucial evidence concerning the covalent attachment of the peptide to position 8 of the flavin in the flavinpeptide prepared from succinic dehydrogenase (Walker et al., 1969).

V. LIGHT ABSORPTION

The light absorption of the radical chelates have recently been studied in detail by Müller et al. (1968). Typical spectra are shown by the Cd chelates of tetraacetylriboflavin, which are presented in Fig. 8. There is an intense double peak in the region 370–405 nm, a weaker and broader band, often with a double peak, in the region 450–600 nm, and a still weaker band in the far-red and near-infrared region 600–900 nm.

Below about 550 nm the spectrum of the chelate is very similar to that of the flavin radical anion (Ehrenberg et al., 1967). This part of the spec-

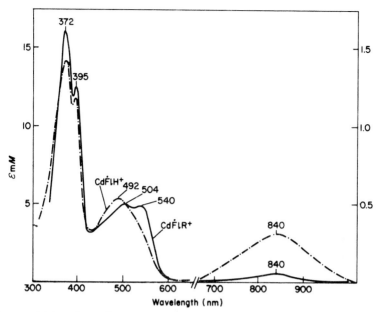

Fig. 8. Light absorption spectra in the visible and near-infrared regions of (CdFlH)$^+$, $-\cdot-\cdot-$, and (CdFlR)$^+$ —, in dimethyl formamide using tetraacetylriboflavin and tetraacetalriboflavin-3-C$_2$H$_5$, respectively. Sample preparation: 6 ml 1.25 mM half-reduced flavin in DMF $+$ 1.2 ml 25 mM Cd(NO$_3$) in CH$_3$CN $+$ 0.3 ml 100 mM Et$_3$N in CHCl$_3$. From Müller et al. (1968).

trum may therefore be used for identification of the radical chelate only under conditions when no radical anion can be formed, or vice versa. Also the charge-transfer chelates have in this wavelength region spectra of somewhat similar appearance (Bamberg and Hemmerich, 1961; Hemmerich, 1963). In the case of ions with instable valence, e.g., the iron ions, this is particularly troublesome. In a reaction mixture containing the radical chelate, as in the case illustrated in Fig. 10, it is not possible to decide whether some charge-transfer chelate is also formed (Müller et al., 1968).

The near-infrared band is easily distinguished from the broader bands of the dimolecular flavin complexes (Gibson et al., 1962; Ehrenberg et al., 1965). Linear relationships between the light absorptions and the ESR intensities were obtained in experiments where the diamagnetic metal ion (Cd^{2+} or Zn^{2+}) or the half-reduced flavin concentration was varied (see Fig. 9) (Ehrenberg and Hemmerich, 1964; Müller et al., 1968). This provides strong evidence that all the bands are due to the monomeric chelate species, not to more compounded aggregates. At the rather high

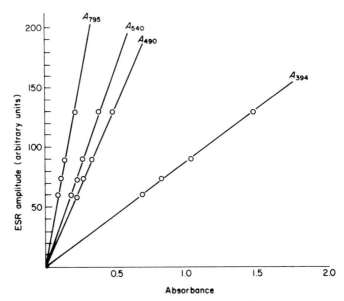

Fig. 9. Comparison of electron spin resonance (ESR) amplitude (which is proportional to spin concentration) with light absorption in the visible and near-infrared regions for (ZnFlR)$^+$ in pyridine. Flavin concentration was varied from about 0.5 to about 1.5 mM. The flavin species was 7,8-dichloro-10-methylisoalloxazine with R(3) = CH$_2$COOC$_2$H$_5$. The magnetic field was overmodulated so that the hyperfine structure was unresolved, but the overall electron spin resonance sensitivity was greatly increased. Light path was 0.1 cm. From Müller et al. (1968).

total flavin concentration of 10 mM needed for the measurements of paramagnetic susceptibility (see below) the near-infrared band was found to develope gradually (Eriksson, 1970). The final maximum extinction coefficient was more than 10-fold enhanced in comparison with the value at 1 mM flavin. Alkylation in position 3 affects the light absorption in a rather irregular way (Müller et al., 1968). In case of the Cd chelate in DMF (see Fig. 8), the band in the region 450–600 nm is altered to show a more pronounced splitting and the near-infrared band is greatly decreased by 3-alkylation. These large effects of 3-substitution have led to the hypothesis (Müller et al., 1968) that in the unsubstituted radical ligand the proton should be located at N(1), not at N(3), since in the latter case mere substitution of alkyl for H would not be expected to provoke very marked spectral changes (Dudley et al., 1964).

The near infrared absorption has been observed for flavin radical chelates with various metal centers (Zn^{2+}, Cd^{2+}, Mn^{2+}, Fe^{2+}, Co^{2+}, Ni^{2+}, Cu$^+$, and Mo^{5+}) in aprotic polar solvents (Müller et al., 1968). The important case of the radical chelate with Fe^{2+} is illustrated in Fig. 10,

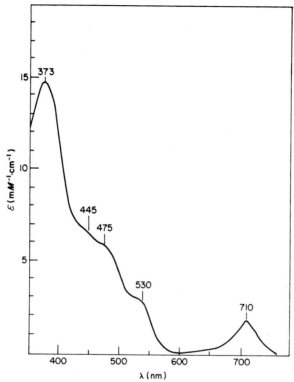

Fig. 10. Light absorption spectrum of $(Fe^{2+}\dot{F}lH^-)^+$ obtained from half-reduced 1 mM tetraacetylriboflavin in pyridine in the presence of 2 mM $(C_6H_5CH_2N(CH_3)_3)_2$ Fe(II)Cl$_4$ and 4 mM Et$_3$N. The shoulders at 445 and 475 nm indicate the presence of some free Fl$_{ox}$H. From Müller et $al.$ (1968).

under conditions when it was formed nearly completely. The extinction of the near-infrared band is (except in case of chelates with Ni^{2+} and Mo^{5+}) enhanced by solvents that may bind as quaternary ligands, e.g., pyridine and acetonitrile. It was therefore proposed (Müller et $al.$, 1968) that the near-infrared absorption reflects the symmetry of the flavosemi-quinone–H$_2$O–solvent complex. The real nature of this transition is, how-ever, still obscure. The extinction coefficient, falling in the range between 10 and 2 $\times$ 10^3 M^{-1} cm^{-1}, varies between the different metal ions, but no regular relationship is discerned.

Nevertheless, as we have pointed out (Müller et $al.$, 1968) the light absorption in the near infrared region as well as in the region 370–405 nm should be indicative of the formation of flavin radical chelates, in partic-ular possible Fe and Mo chelates in metalloflavoproteins. In the model system with Fe^{2+} the near infrared, absorption is not detected or remains very diffuse in the absence of pyridine. Hence, in case of a metalloflavo-protein it might be worthwhile to look for a possible enhancement of the near-infrared absorption by addition of agents, such as pyridine or aceto-nitrile, to the protein at a suitable stage of oxidoreduction.

VI. Paramagnetic Susceptibility

No ESR signals have been detected from flavin radical chelates with paramagnetic metal ions or from charge-transfer chelates. In these cases any statement about magnetic states and multiplicity must await suscep-tibility measurements. Some experiments bearing on this point have re-cently been performed in our laboratory (Eriksson, 1970).

The radical chelates of diamagnetic Cd^{2+} and Zn^{2+} were found to be paramagnetic as expected from previous ESR data. At the high concentra-tion of 10 mM flavin necessary for the susceptibility measurement only about 60% of the expected paramagnetism was however obtained. The same yield of paramagnetic species could be determined by a quantitative ESR measurement. This indicates that at the concentration used some diamagnetic complexes of unknown structure are formed, or part of the flavin radicals could be disproportionated by stabilization of the oxidized (or the reduced) form in some kind of complex.

The flavin radical chelate of one paramagnetic ion, Ni^{2+}, was carefully investigated. The flavin radical has the spin $S = \frac{1}{2}$ and the Ni^{2+} is in a triplet state with $S = 1$. The measured paramagnetism for the chelate revealed that the spins are coupled in a state with $S = \frac{3}{2}$. This explains the absence of any ESR signal from the radical ligand in the chelate. A spin coupling of this type might exist in other chelates where no ESR signal is obtained.

As an example of a charge-transfer chelate, the Ag^+-flavin complex was studied. Within the sensitivity limits of the method no paramagnetism could be detected. This proves that the ground state is a singlet and that there is not significant population of any excited paramagnetic triplet state.

VII. Some Concluding Remarks

The existence of flavin-radical-metal chelates and of flavoquinone-metal charge-transfer chelates has been well established in the model sys-tems and their properties have been determined in some details. So far, however, there is no single case where any such chelate has been demon-strated in a flavin-metal containing protein. With metalloflavoproteins containing Mo and/or Fe, it has been observed in the native enzyme that only part of the flavin and the metal can under the conditions explored be recovered as species that give ESR signals. The possibility has been discussed that the missing portions of both species could be present as radical-metal chelates (Müller *et al.*, 1968; Hemmerich and Spence, 1966), which would become indetectable by ESR. This could possibly be demonstrated by the characteristic paramagnetic susceptibility of such a chelate. Such measurements would require great sensitivity and accuracy since several centers in the metalloflavoprotein must change their paramagnetism and each individual change depends critically on the redox state of the protein.

A very promising approach to the elucidation of the interaction between paramagnetic metal centers and flavin radicals in metalloflavoproteins is the enhancement of the radical relaxation discovered and explored by Beinert and co-workers (Beinert and Hemmerich, 1965; Beinert and Orme-Johnson, 1967). A deeper knowledge of the underlaying processes might be crucial for an understanding of the interplay between metal and flavin in the catalysis of these enzymes. In general it can be said that more refined and sophisticated work will be needed until we know whether the radical chelates really play a role in the enzyme systems and how electrons are transferred between metal ions and flavin in metalloflavoproteins.

REFERENCES

Albert, A. (1950). *Biochem. J.* **47**, xvii.
Albert, A. (1953). *Biochem. J.* **54**, 646.
Bamberg, P., and Hemmerich, P. (1961). *Helv. Chim. Acta* **44**, 1001.
Beinert, H., and Hemmerich, P. (1965). *Biochem. Biophys. Res. Commun.* **18**, 212.
Beinert, H., and Orme-Johnson, W. H. (1967). *In* "Magnetic Resonance in Biological Systems" (A. Ehrenberg, B. G. Malmström, and T. Vänngård, eds.), p. 221. Pergamon Press, Oxford.
Dixon, M., and Webb, E. C. (1964). "Enzymes," 2nd ed. Academic Press, New York.
Dudley, K. H., Ehrenberg, A., Hemmerich, P., and Müller, F. (1964). *Helv. Chim. Acta* **47**, 1354.
Ehrenberg, A., and Hemmerich, P. (1964). *Acta Chem. Scand.* **18**, 1320.
Ehrenberg, A., and Hemmerich, P. (1968). *In* "Biological Oxidations" (T. P. Singer, ed.), p. 239. Wiley (Interscience), New York.
Ehrenberg, A., Eriksson, L. E. G., and Hemmerich, P. (1965). *In* "Oxidases and Related Redox Systems" (T. E. King, H. S. Mason, and M. Morrison, eds.), p. 179. Wiley, New York.
Ehrenberg, A., Eriksson, L. E. G., and Müller, F. (1966). *Nature (London)* **212**, 503.
Ehrenberg, A., Müller, F., and Hemmerich, P. (1967). *Eur. J. Biochem.* **2**, 286.
Ehrenberg, A., Eriksson, L. E. G., and Hyde, J. S. (1968). *Biochim. Biophys. Acta* **167**, 482.
Ehrenberg, A., Hyde, J. S., Eriksson, L. E. G., and Walker, W. (1970). In preparation.
Eriksson, L. E. G. (1970). *Biochim. Biophys. Acta* **208**, 528.
Eriksson, L. E. G., and Ehrenberg, A. (1964). *Acta Chem. Scand.* **18**, 1437.
Eriksson, L. E. G., and Ehrenberg, A. (1965). *Arch. Biochem. Biophys.* **110**, 628.

Eriksson, L. E. G., Hyde, J. S., and Ehrenberg, A. (1969). *Biochim. Biophys. Acta* **192**, 211.

Gibson, Q. H., Massey, V., and Atherton, N. M. (1962). *Biochem. J.* **85**, 369.

Hemmerich, P. (1960). *Experientia* **16**, 534.

Hemmerich, P. (1963). *In* "Wirkungsmechanismen von Enzymen," Vol. 14, p. 183. Springer, Berlin.

Hemmerich, P. (1964). *Helv. Chim. Acta* **47**, 464.

Hemmerich, P., and Fallab, S. (1958). *Helv. Chim. Acta* **41**, 498.

Hemmerich, P., and Spence, J. (1966). *In* "Flavins and Flavoproteins" (E. C. Slater, ed.), B. B. A. Library, Vol. 8, p. 82. Elsevier, Amsterdam.

Hemmerich, P., Dervartanian, D. V., Veeger, C., and Van Voorst, J. D. W. (1963). *Biochim. Biophys. Acta* **77**, 504.

Hemmerich, P., Müller, F., and Ehrenberg, A. (1965). *In* "Oxidases and Related Redox Systems" (T. E. King, H. S. Mason, and M. Morrison, eds.), p. 19. Wiley, New York.

Hyde, J. S. (1967). *In* "Magnetic Resonance in Biological Systems" (A. Ehrenberg, B. G. Malmström, and T. Vänngård, eds.), p. 63. Pergamon Press, Oxford.

Hyde, J. S., Rist, G. H., and Eriksson, L. E. G. (1968). *J. Phys. Chem.* **72**, 4269.

Müller, F., Ehrenberg, A., and Eriksson, L. E. G. (1967). *In* "Magnetic Resonance in Biological Systems" (A. Ehrenberg, B. G. Malmström, and T. Vänngård, eds.), p. 281. Pergamon Press, Oxford.

Müller, F., Hemmerich, P., and Ehrenberg. A. (1968). *Eur. J. Biochem.* **5**, 158.

Müller, F., Eriksson, L. E. G., and Ehrenberg, A. (1970). *Eur. J. Biochem.* **12**, 93.

Walker, W., Salach, J., Gutman, M., Singer, T. P., Hyde, J. S., and Ehrenberg, A. (1969). *FEBS Letters* **5**, 237.

The Existence of Nonfunctional Active Sites in Milk Xanthine Oxidase; Reaction with Functional Active Site Inhibitors*

VINCENT MASSEY, HIROCHIKA KOMAI, GRAHAM PALMER, AND GERTRUDE B. ELION

Department of Biological Chemistry and Biophysics Research Division, The University of Michigan, Ann Arbor, Michigan and The Wellcome Laboratories, Research Triangle Park, North Carolina

I. INTRODUCTION

Previous studies on xanthine oxidase have been complicated by the existence of a biphasic bleaching of the enzyme by xanthine and all other substrates tested. This phenomenon was first observed by Morell (1952) and ascribed to the presence of inactive species which were slowly reduced by the reduced active form of the enzyme. Bray and his associates (1961, 1966; Avis *et al.*, 1955; Hart *et al.*, 1970) had also obtained considerable evidence for the existence of inactive forms of xanthine oxidase. Their evidence was indirect, and based on varying contents of the iron, flavin,

* This work was supported by grants from the U. S. Public Health Service, GM 11106 and GM 12176, and by a Career Development Award to G. P. (GM-K3-31,213).

505

and molybdenum components found in different preparations, and on correlation of these components with the xanthine-oxygen reductase activity. They concluded that two inactive species of xanthine oxidase, i_1 and i_2 existed in their preparations; i_1 having a Mo:flavin:Fe ratio of 1:1:4 and i_2 having the ratio 0:1:4. Enzyme prepared in our laboratory (Massey et al., 1969) routinely contained its full complement of molybdenum, flavin, and iron, and possessed catalytic activity at least as high as any previously reported preparation. Such enzyme still retained the biphasic reduction pattern first observed by Morell. However, it was noted (Massey et al., 1969) that the rate of reduction in the slow phase varied considerably with the substrate used; hence it was concluded that Morell's interpretation was unlikely and that the biphasic reduction pattern was a property intrinsic to the enzyme. Recent results, however, have made it clear that Morell's interpretation was indeed correct, and that the best preparations of xanthine oxidase so far reported in the literature are at most 75–80% functional, and sometimes 50% functional or even less. The lack of recognition of this phenomenon has lead to considerable confusion, especially in recent years. For example, Bray and Watts (1966) showed that reaction of xanthine oxidase with iodoacetamide is greatly accelerated in the presence of xanthine and reaction of 1 mole of the reagent per mole of enzyme (i.e., per two molcules of FAD) resulted in complete loss of xanthine-oxygen reductase activity. They concluded (McGartoll and Bray, 1969) that iodoacetamide reacted with a single protein sulfhydryl and therefore that the active site of xanthine oxidase must comprise in some way its two FAD molecules, 2 molybdenum atoms, and 8 atoms of iron (with its associated labile sulfide). In fact, it has been shown recently (Komai and Massey, 1970) that the findings of Bray and colleagues were a consequence of nonfunctional enzyme. We have shown that it is the reduced flavin which reacts with iodoacetamide rather than a protein sulfhydryl group; the alkylation of reduced flavin by iodoacetamide requires the prior reduction of the flavin by xanthine. Evidently Bray and co-workers used enzyme containing approximately 50% functional sites; in our experiments, where enzyme containing approximately 70% functional sites were present, we required reaction of 0.7 mole of iodoacetamide for inactivation. Furthermore, inactivation, stoichiometric with extent of alkylation of total flavin, was obtained when the nonspecific reductant dithionite was used instead of the substrate, xanthine, or when the enzyme was reduced to varying total extents by prolonged contact with xanthine before reaction with iodoacetamide. In this work it was also shown that photoalkylation of the enzyme flavin with phenylacetate ions, a nonspecific method not relying on prior reduction of the flavin (Hemmerich et al., 1967; Walker et al.,

1967), also results in inactivation stoichiometric with the extent of alkylation.

Definitive evidence for the existence of nonfunctional active sites in xanthine oxidase has come from studies with allopurinol and a series of related pyrazolo[3,4-d]pyrimidines. This work has been reported in part in another publication (Massey *et al.*, 1970) and also at the 3rd International Flavin Conference at Durham, 1969. From previous studies (Elion *et al.*, 1966) it was known that allopurinol (4-hydroxypyrazolo-[3,4-d]pyrimidine) is a potent inhibitor of the xanthine-oxygen reductase activity of xanthine oxidase, and that alloxanthine (4,6-dihydroxy-pyrazolo[3,4-d]pyrimidine) is the product of xanthine oxidase reaction with allopurinol.

Allopurinol   Alloxanthine

It has also been observed (Elion, 1966) that low concentrations of allopurinol inactivated xanthine oxidase when preincubated with the enzyme for several minutes before addition of xanthine. With low concentrations of alloxanthine, on the other hand, preincubation with enzyme caused no decrease in activity, but there was progressive inactivation after the substrate, xanthine, was added. These findings suggested that inactivation was due to reaction of the inhibitor with a modified form of the enzyme produced during the catalytic reaction.

In a recent communication, Spector and Johns (1968) reported that allopurinol was an effective substrate for xanthine oxidase when phenazine methosulfate was used as electron acceptor, but not when molecular oxygen was the acceptor. They claimed that this phenomenon was due to the inability of allopurinol to reduce the flavin (and presumably nonheme iron) constituent of the enzyme, and that the observed catalysis was probably due to electron transfer involving only the molybdenum component of the enzyme. In the present paper we have investigated the effect on xanthine oxidase of a number of pyrazolo[3,4-d]pyrimidine derivatives. In contrast to the results of Spector and Johns (1968) we find that, provided there is no substituent at position 6 of the substrate, rapid reduction of all the chromophores of xanthine oxidase is obtained. However, on air reoxidation, a modified spectrum of the enzyme is obtained; this form of the enzyme is completely inactive in the xanthine-oxygen reductase reaction. Evidence is presented that the inactive modified

enzyme is a complex of alloxanthine (or other 6-hydroxypyrazolo[3,4-d]
pyrimidine derivatives) with a lower valence state of molybdenum than
that present in the unmodified enzyme. Such complex formation prevents
further electron uptake from xanthine and is presumably the basis of the
strong inhibitory action of this class of compounds and of their therapeutic action. Recently, Spector and Johns (1970) have obtained results
contrary to their originally reported ones, in agreement with our findings.

II. Materials and Methods

Milk xanthine oxidase was prepared as described previously (Massey
et al., 1969). Xanthine-oxygen reductase activity was measured spectrophotometrically at 295 nm and at a temperature of 25°. Following the
original work of Avis et al. (1955), such catalytic activity is also expressed as $AFR^{25°}$ values. This value is obtained by dividing the change
in absorbancy per minute at 295 nm by the absorbancy at 450 nm of the
xanthine oxidase employed in the assay. Avis et al. (1955) made their
determination at 23.5°; the activity at 25° is 1.12 greater than at 23.5°
(Massey et al., 1969).

The pyrazolo[3,4-d]pyrimidines were prepared by methods described
in the literature (Falco and Hitchings, 1956; Robins, 1956; Taylor et al.,
1967). The synthesis of the alloxanthine-6-^{14}C used in this work has been
reported previously (Elion et al., 1966); it had a specific activity of 0.69
μCi per μmole. The pyrazolo[4,3-d]pyrimidines used were generously
provided by Dr. Sidney Hecht. The triazolopyrimidines and 4-hydroxy-
pyrrolopyrimidines were prepared as described previously (Roblin et al.,
1945; West, 1961).

Electron paramagnetic resonance spectra were determined with Varian
equipment as described previously (Palmer and Massey, 1969).

III. Results and Discussion

A. Reduction of Xanthine Oxidase by Allopurinol

Under anaerobic conditions, xanthine oxidase was found to be readily
reduced by allopurinol. Figure 1 illustrates several of the properties of this
system. On the addition of allopurinol anaerobically, there was an immediate reduction of the enzyme to the same level as that found in the
rapid phase of reduction with xanthine (Massey et al., 1969). However,
with xanthine further reduction occurred over several hours to a level
close to that given by dithionite (Massey et al., 1969), whereas with allopurinol there was only a small secondary decrease in absorbance which
was complete in 2–3 minutes (Fig. 1 inset). No further changes occurred
even on incubation for as long as 24 hours. When air was admitted a

rapid return of color was obtained, with an absorption spectrum slightly modified from that of the original enzyme (Fig. 1). An aliquot of this modified enzyme tested in the xanthine-oxygen reductase assay showed less than 0.1% of the original activity. When the system was made anaerobic again and a second aliquot of allopurinol (or xanthine) was added, no reduction was obtained, even after several hours of incubation. The failure of Spector and Johns (1968) to obtain reduction in their experiments was probably due to incomplete removal of oxygen in their anaerobic experiments; this would result in the production of inhibited enzyme incapable of reduction. In contrast, added NADH slowly produced maximal bleaching of the enzyme as it does with untreated enzyme (Massey *et al.*, 1969). The NADH-ferricyanide reductase activity of the modified enzyme is the same as that of untreated enzyme. This finding

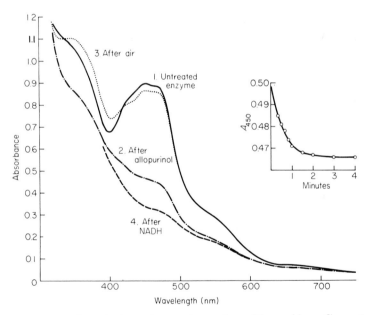

Fig. 1. Effect of allopurinol on the spectrum of xanthine oxidase. Curve *1*, untreated enzyme, $2.38 \times 10^{-5} M$ with respect to FAD, in $0.1 M$ pyrophosphate pH 8.5, 25°C. Curve *2*, spectrum recorded 5 minutes after the addition of $1.67 \times 10^{-4} M$ allopurinol anaerobically. The spectrum remained unchanged over a period of 2 hours. Curve *3*, immediately after mixing with air. Further addition of allopurinol or xanthine anaerobically resulted in no spectral changes over a period of 2 hours. Curve *4*, 4 hours after the further anaerobic addition of $3 \times 10^{-4} M$ NADH. The inset shows on an expanded scale the absorbance changes occurring in the first few minutes after the addition of allopurinol to untreated enzyme. In this curve the rapid phase of bleaching is not shown.

is consistent with the concept (Komai *et al.*, 1969) that electron transfer in this catalytic activity requires only the flavin and iron-sulfur chromophores of the enzyme.

B. Inactivation of Xanthine Oxidase by Alloxanthine

The results on the inactivation of the xanthine oxygen reductase activity with allopurinol show that, under anaerobic conditions, this compound is a very effective reductant of xanthine oxidase; however, after reoxidation, a modified form of the enzyme is obtained which is incapable of reduction by either xanthine or allopurinol. These results and the previous demonstration (Elion, 1966) that alloxanthine inactivated the enzyme, even under aerobic conditions, when xanthine was present as substrate, suggested that the product of allopurinol oxidation, alloxanthine, might be the reactive agent responsible. That alloxanthine is indeed responsible for inactivation, but only under conditions where the enzyme is reduced, was shown in several ways. When added to oxidized enzyme, even in considerable excess, alloxanthine failed to produce any significant spectral perturbation. On adding xanthine anaerobically to enzyme previously mixed with alloxanthine, results identical with these shown in Fig. 1 were

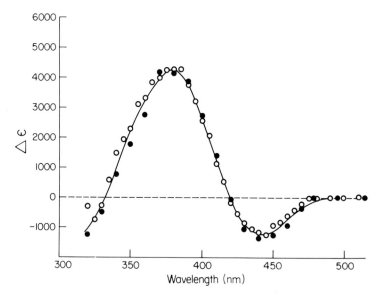

FIG. 2. Difference spectrum between alloxanthine-inhibited and native xanthine oxidase. ○, The difference between curves *3* and *1* of Fig. 1; ●, results from a similar experiment where the enzyme was reduced with xanthine in the presence of alloxanthine, and air was admitted. The results are expressed as Δ extinction coefficient per molecule of enzyme flavin.

obtained; i.e., there was an initial fast reduction of the enzyme, followed by a further slight decrease in absorbancy for 2 minutes, after which no further reaction was obtained. When air was admitted, the same modified reoxidized absorption spectrum was found as when allopurinol used as the reductant, and the xanthine-oxygen reductase activity was completely abolished. Figure 2 shows the difference spectrum between untreated enzyme and the modified enzyme obtained after reduction either with allopurinol or with xanthine plus alloxanthine, followed by air reoxidation. Similar results were obtained when enzyme was first reduced anaerobically with xanthine followed by addition of alloxanthine and finally reoxidized with air. Furthermore, as shown in a later section, the enzyme inactivated anaerobically with allopurinol was found to contain 1.0 mole of tightly bound alloxanthine per functional active site.

C. REACTIVATION OF ALLOXANTHINE-INHIBITED ENZYME

Complete reversal of alloxanthine inhibition could be obtained by incubation anaerobically with excess phenazine methosulfate or $K_3Fe(CN)_6$. After dialysis of enzyme treated in this way, the absorption spectrum of the product had returned quantitatively to that of native enzyme. Similar recovery of catalytic activity and absorption spectrum was found on prolonged incubation in the presence of air; such reactivation was found to be markedly dependent on temperature. In $0.1\,M$ pyrophosphate, pH 8.5, the half-time of reactivation at 25° was approximately 300 minutes; at 0° less than 10% reactivation was obtained in 24 hours. In all cases the extent of reactivation correlated well with the extent of return of the absorption spectrum of native enzyme. These data indicate that the inhibited enzyme is a complex of alloxanthine and partially reduced enzyme, since reactivation is obtained only under oxidizing conditions. The fact that on rapid air reoxidation (cf. Fig. 1, curve 3), the absorption spectrum of the inhibited enzyme is identical with that of native enzyme at wavelengths greater than 500 nm (the region of nonheme iron absorption) shows that the iron–sulfur chromophores are reoxidized in the inhibited enzyme. Similarly, from the changes in absorbancy at 450 nm occurring immediately after the admission of air, it is clear that flavin reoxidation occurs rapidly. It therefore follows that the reduced forms of these chromophores are not involved in the binding of alloxanthine, thereby implicating the molybdenum component as the reactive moiety.

The valency state of the molybdenum involved can be determined by titration with ferricyanide (under anaerobic conditions) of the inhibited enzyme (Fig. 3). As shown in curve A, almost 1 equivalent of $Fe(CN)_6^{3-}$ per atom of enzyme-bound molybdenum resulted in very little reacti-

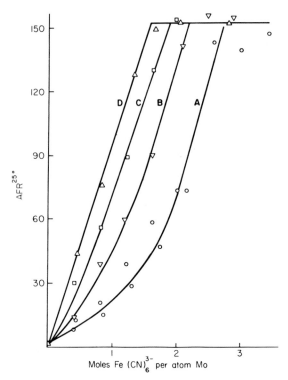

FIG. 3. Reactivation of alloxanthine-inhibited enzyme by ferricyanide. Xanthine oxidase ($6.91 \times 10^{-5} M$ with respect to bound FAD) was inactivated by incubation anaerobically for 20 minutes with $2.5 \times 10^{-4} M$ alloxanthine and $4 \times 10^{-4} M$ xanthine (experiments A, B, and C) or with $3 \times 10^{-4} M$ allopurinol (experiment D). The inhibited enzyme was separated from reaction products on a column of Sephadex G-25 (1.2×30 cm) equilibrated at $4°$ with $0.1 M$ pyrophosphate pH 8.3. Typically enzyme emerged in the effluent after 12–17 ml, allopurinol in an approximately 10-ml fraction centered at 55 ml and alloxanthine in a 15-ml fraction centered at 79 ml. Aliquots of enzyme of 1-ml volume were diluted to a known concentration (approximately $1.8 \times 10^{-5} M$) and incubated anaerobically with the appropriate concentrations of $K_3Fe(CN)_6$ and phenylmercuric acetate for 2 days at $0°$. Air was then admitted, and the xanthine-oxygen reductase activity was measured. Curves A, B, C, and D contained, respectively, 0, 3, 6, 9 moles phenylmercuric acetate per atom of enzyme bound molybdenum. When the phenylmercuric acetate concentration was increased to 15 moles/atom Mo the activated enzyme had a specific activity only 20% that of native enzyme; however, the same end point of ferricyanide titration was found as for curve D.

vation. (This was accompanied by only a small extent of return of the spectrum of native enzyme.) Approximately 2.7 equivalents of $Fe(CN)_6^{3-}$ were required for complete reactivation. These results suggested that $Fe(CN)_6^{3-}$ was being consumed in a competing reaction. From unpublished results of titration of native enzyme with 5,5′-dithiobis-2-nitrobenzoic acid) it was known that unmodified enzyme contained one reactive sulfhydryl group per molecule of enzyme-bound FAD; the possibility therefore existed that reaction of this sulfhydryl group with $Fe(CN)_6^{3-}$ was the competing reaction. Titrations were therefore carried out in the presence of phenylmercuric acetate. Results in the presence of 3, 6, and 9 molecules of phenylmercuric acetate per molecule of enzyme flavin are shown in curves B, C, and D. In the presence of 9 moles phenylmercuric acetate a linear titration plot was obtained, with 1.6 equivalents $Fe(CN)_6^{3-}$ required for full reactivation of the alloxanthine-inhibited enzyme. In light of the data indicating that the enzyme used in these experiments contained only 73% of its active sites in a functional form capable of binding alloxanthine (see later section), the value of 1.6 equivalents of $Fe(CN)_6^{3-}$ required for full reactivation corresponds to 2.2 equivalents per functional active site. Thus, these data indicate that in the alloxanthine-inhibited enzyme the molybdenum had been trapped at the MoIV level.

D. ELECTRON PARAMAGNETIC RESONANCE EVIDENCE

Rapid reaction studies of Bray et al. (1964) have demonstrated that anaerobic mixing of xanthine oxidase and xanthine results in the rapid appearance and disappearance of electron paramagnetic resonance (EPR) signals attributable to MoV and flavin radical and to the rapid appearance of the characteristic EPR spectrum of reduced nonheme iron chromophores. Recent work has also revealed the rapid appearance of a newly recognized EPR signal with a g value of 2.11 (Palmer and Massey, 1969). These time-dependent changes in EPR signals are well correlated with rapid reaction spectrophotometric studies (Massey et al., 1969; Palmer and Massey, 1969). Such changes are complete within approximately 1 second at pH 8.5, 25°. If the reaction with excess substrate is allowed to proceed for somewhat longer times (~1–2 minutes) virtually the only EPR species present in significant amount are the reduced iron–sulfur chromophores. Anaerobic incubation for still longer times (hours to days) results in the production and subsequent decay of flavin radicals, the reappearance of reduced species of molybdenum, and further intensification of the signals of the iron–sulfur chromophores (Bray et al., 1961; Palmer and Massey, 1969). These changes appear to be correlated with the secondary slow phase of bleaching of the enzyme first reported by Morell (1952) and by all subsequent workers. As described in a previous section, the presence of alloxanthine abolishes the slow phase of bleaching of the enzyme by xanthine. It was, therefore, of considerable interest to determine the effect of alloxanthine in companion EPR studies. Figure 4 shows the effect of anaerobic incubation of xanthine oxidase with

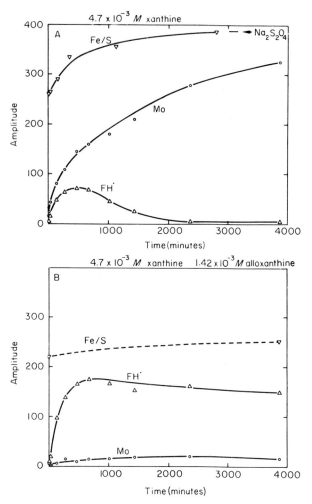

Fig. 4. Comparison of amplitudes of EPR signals of $3.2 \times 10^{-4}\,M$ xanthine oxidase (AFR[25°], 150), incubated with $4.7 \times 10^{-3}\,M$ xanthine in the absence (A) and the presence (B) of $1.4 \times 10^{-3}\,M$ alloxanthine at room temperature in $0.1\,M$ pyrophosphate, pH 8.5. Molybdenum and flavin signals were recorded at 124°K; iron–sulfur signal at 24°K. The amplitudes of the molybdenum and flavin signals were measured at magnetic fields were there is no contribution from other species. The amplitude of the iron-sulfur signal was measured at high field (g_x) and may have contributions from the $g = 2.11$ as well as the $g = 1.94$ species.

xanthine in the absence and presence of alloxanthine. It can be seen that alloxanthine virtually abolishes the slow reappearance of molybdenum signals; in contrast, however, its presence leads to greater reappearance of flavin radical signals. As expected, the $g = 1.94$ and $g = 2.11$ signals of the reduced iron-sulfur chromophores appear rapidly on mixing with xanthine, even in the presence of alloxanthine. Preliminary experiments indicate approximately the same level of reduction as found rapidly with xanthine as substrate in the absence of alloxanthine. While more definitive experiments need to be done, the results shown in Fig. 4, coupled with the evidence presented in later sections, can be explained as follows. Within 2 minutes of anaerobic addition of xanthine, the functional xanthine oxidase molecules have accepted a total of 6–7 reducing equivalents, $(FAD \rightarrow FADH_2; \ 2(Fe/S)_{ox} \rightarrow 2(Fe/S)_{red}; \ MoVI \rightarrow MoIV \ or \ MoIII)$. Such enzyme shows essentially no EPR absorption except for that due to the reduced Fe/S chromophores. Subsequently, with a time course roughly paralleling that of the slow phase of substrate bleaching of the optical spectrum (Massey et al., 1969), the reduced functional enzyme slowly reduces the nonfunctional enzyme, accounting for the appearance and disappearance of flavin radical signals, the appearance of molybdenum signals and the intensification of the Fe/S signals to the same level as that given with dithionite. When the reaction is carried out in the presence of alloxanthine, the alloxanthine complexes with reduced active enzyme and the subsequent slow reduction of nonfunctional enzyme is prevented, thus accounting for the failure of appearance of molybdenum signals and the insignificant changes in the intensity of the signals due to the reduced iron–sulfur chromophores. The slow appearance of flavin radical signals (greater in quantity than with uninhibited enzyme) and their long-term stability is readily explained by a dismutation reaction between reduced functional enzyme and oxidized nonfunctional enzyme:

$$FADH_2\text{-enz}_{(active)} + FAD\text{-enz}_{(inactive)} \rightleftharpoons FADH\cdot\text{enz}_{(active)} + FADH\cdot\text{enz}_{(inactive)}$$

Such slow dismutation reactions of oxidized and reduced flavin to yield semiquinone are common with flavoproteins (Massey and Curti, 1967).

E. Stoichiometry of Alloxanthine Binding: Evidence for Alloxanthine as a Functional Active Site Label

The extreme avidity of alloxanthine in binding to reduced xanthine oxidase is shown in Fig. 5. In these experiments enzyme of $AFR^{25°}$ of 153 was incubated anaerobically at 25° with different concentrations of alloxanthine in the presence of xanthine and then assayed for residual xanthine-oxygen reductase activity. A decrease in activity, linear with increasing alloxanthine concentration, was found, with complete inactivation corresponding to the reaction of 0.73 mole alloxanthine per atom of enzyme bound molybdenum. This puzzling finding was confirmed by studies with alloxanthine-^{14}C, which are summarized in Table I. In the initial experiments enzyme with an $AFR^{25°}$ value of 140 was used. After

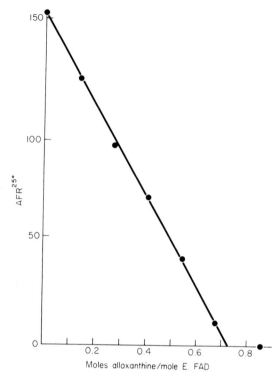

Fɪɢ. 5. Stoichiometry of alloxanthine-inactivation of xanthine oxidase. Enzyme, $6.91 \times 10^{-6} M$ with respect to flavin content was incubated anaerobically in $0.1 M$ pyrophosphate pH of 8.5, at 25° for 60 minutes with $3.33 \times 10^{-4} M$ xanthine and the molar ratios of alloxanthine shown. Air was then admitted and xanthine-oxygen reductase activity was determined.

incubation anaerobically with xanthine and alloxanthine-^{14}C the reaction mixture was chromatographed on a Sephadex G-25 column at 4°. Complete separation of labeled enzyme and excess alloxanthine-^{14}C was obtained and the AFR$^{25°}$ values of the labeled enzyme fractions were found to be less than 1% the initial value. By radioisotope analysis the amount of alloxanthine bound was found to be 0.73 mole per atom of enzyme bound molybdenum. Treatment of the inactivated enzyme with ferricyanide before the gel filtration step led to quantitative return of catalytic activity and loss of bound radioactivity.

The explanation for complete loss of catalytic activity by binding of less than a stoichiometric amount of alloxanthine came from studies with enzyme of lower specific activity. The amount of ^{14}C-alloxanthine bound was found to be proportional to the AFR value (Table I).

TABLE I

ALLOXANTHINE-^{14}C BINDING TO XANTHINE OXIDASE[a]

	Experiment	AFR$^{25°}$ initial	AFR$^{25°}$ inhibited	Alloxanthine-^{14}C per atom of enzyme-bound Mo	AFR initial/ bound alloxanthine
I	Standard	140	1.5	0.73	192
	After reoxidation with ferricyanide	140	135	0.007	—
II	Standard	150	0.9	0.76	197
III	Standard	150	1.0	0.73	205
IV	Standard	45	0.8	0.24	188
V	Standard	145	1.2	0.67	216
	Reacted 20 hours with xanthine before alloxanthine	145	1.1	0.65	223
VI	Standard	67	0.6	0.33	203
	Reacted 20 hours with xanthine before alloxanthine	67	0.7	0.33	203

[a] Standard conditions: xanthine oxidase reacted anaerobically at 25°C with xanthine and an excess of alloxanthine-^{14}C for 15–30 minutes before admitting air and chromatography at 4° on a column of Sephadex G-25 (1.3 × 18 cm). Fractions of 1–2 ml volume were collected; complete separation of the protein from unreacted alloxanthine was obtained (cf. legend to Fig. 9). Radioactivity measurements were carried out with 0.3 ml samples from the fractions containing the enzyme. The AFR value, spectrum and radioactivity were determined for each fraction to yield the AFR$^{25°}$ of the inhibited enzyme and the alloxanthine-^{14}C content per atom of enzyme-bound molybdenum. The background count on either side of the labeled enzyme fraction was of the order of 20–30 cpm compared to values of 1000–5000 cpm for the enzyme fractions.

In experiment I an aliquot of the inhibited enzyme was incubated anaerobically at 25° for 2 hours with excess Fe(CN)$_6^{3-}$ before Sephadex chromatography at 4°.

In experiments V and VI, in addition to the standard conditions, enzyme was allowed to be reduced fully by reaction anaerobically with xanthine for 20 hours before addition of alloxanthine-^{14}C.

In all experiments the buffer used was 0.1 M pyrophosphate, pH 8.5. The enzyme concentration was 3–4 × 10^{-5} M with respect to bound molybdenum. Xanthine concentration, 3.33 × 10^{-4} M; alloxanthine-^{14}C concentration; 1.67 × 10^{-4} M (0.69 μCi/μmole).

These results, and those of Fig. 5, indicate that alloxanthine is an active site label of xanthine oxidase, binding only to complete, functional active sites. If this hypothesis is correct, it is evident that the most active preparations of xanthine oxidase so far obtained, even though they contain molybdenum, flavin and the iron–sulfur chromophores in ratios of 1:1:4 (Massey et al., 1969), still contain active sites which are non-functional. The data of Fig. 5 obtained with enzyme of an AFR$^{25°}$ value of 153 and binding 0.73 mole alloxanthine, indicate that completely functional xanthine oxidase would have an $AFR^{25°}$ value of 208. The allo-xanthine-^{14}C binding experiments of Table I indicate completely functional enzyme to have $AFR^{25°}$ values in the range 188–223, with an average value of 203. This conclusion is confirmed by studies of inactivation by iodoacetamide, which also shows complete inactivation with less than stoichiometric reaction (Komai and Massey, 1970). Furthermore, this conclusion is strongly supported by a study of the extent of rapid bleaching of the absorption of the enzyme by xanthine. As shown by Morell (1952), xanthine oxidase when reacted anaerobically with xanthine is bleached in a distinctly biphasic fashion, an "immediate" bleaching followed by a further reaction extending over several hours. Morell interpreted these results as being due, respectively, to active and inactive species of the enzyme, the latter being reduced via reaction with the active enzyme. In a recent publication (Massey et al., 1969), we reported on the rates of reaction in both fast and slow phases with a variety of substrates, and concluded that the interpretation of Morell was probably not correct because quite different reaction rates were found in the slow phase depending on the substrate used. However, the present finding that alloxanthine can bind with great avidity to partially reduced xanthine oxidase, and prevent further reduction, i.e., eliminating the slow phase, suggests that other substrates or their products may do the same thing to lesser extents, and hence influence the rate of reduction in the slow phase. Thus if the extent of the fast phase of reduction is a measure of the content of catalytically functional enzyme, one should expect different extents of reduction in this phase depending on the catalytic activity of the enzyme. Indeed such a correlation was shown by Morell (1952) and confirmed in the present study (Fig. 6). It is seen that the extent of rapid bleaching of the enzyme is directly proportional to the AFR value, whereas, the total bleaching (fast plus slow phases) is the same no matter what the AFR value. If it is assumed that no slow phase of reduction would exist in fully functional enzyme, then one can predict by extrapolation that the $AFR^{25°}$ value of such enzyme would be 207. This value is within experimental error the same as that predicted above from the alloxanthine binding studies, and adds considerable weight to the conclusion that hitherto we (and all other previous workers) have been working with enzyme of at most 75–80% maximal activity, even though the analytical data give no evidence for the presence of proteins other than xanthine oxidase. This conclusion has considerable implications concerning the interpretation of data previously obtained with this enzyme. In particular, it should be noted that Bray and his colleagues (Bray et al., 1966; Bray and Watts, 1966; McGartoll and Bray, 1969)

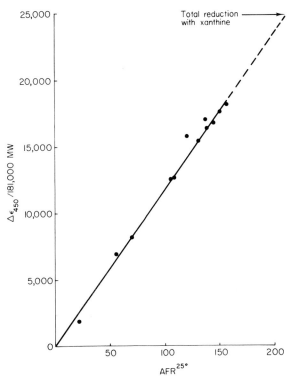

FIG. 6. Correlation of the extinction changes at 450 nm during the rapid phase of reduction of xanthine oxidase with xanthine and the $AFR^{25°}$ value. Experiments were carried out anaerobically in 0.1 M pyrophosphate, pH 8.5, 25°. In all cases the total extinction change after 24 hours was the same, even though the changes occurring in the first 30 sec after addition of xanthine ($3.33 \times 10^{-4} M$) varied widely as shown.

have concluded that xanthine oxidase must possess a single active site comprising 2 atoms of molybdenum, 2 molecules of FAD, 8 atoms of nonheme iron and 8 labile sulfur residues. This conclusion was based on the finding that reaction of less than one molecule of iodoacetamide per molecule of enzyme bound flavin is required for complete loss of xanthine-oxygen reductase activity. As discussed in a separate communication (Komai and Massey, 1970) this result is due to the presence of non-functional active sites; indeed the inactivation is due to alkylation of reduced flavin (Komai and Massey, 1970) rather than reaction with protein sulfhydryl groups (Bray et al., 1966; Bray and Watts, 1966) or loss of flavin (McGartoll and Bray, 1969) as previously claimed. It should be noted from Table I that, in distinction to the results obtained with iodoacetamide inactivation (Komai and Massey, 1970), the amount of alloxanthine fixed to the enzyme is not changed by allowing complete reduction of the enzyme to occur (by long-term incubation with substrate or by addition of dithionite) before reaction with alloxanthine. Thus the binding of alloxanthine appears to be simply a measure of the content of functional active sites, independent of the method of reduction of the enzyme. It is hoped that a thorough study of this phenomenon will throw light on the nature of the lesion responsible for loss of functionality and perhaps in so doing provide more information on the reaction mechanism of this enzyme.

F. STOICHIOMETRY OF ALLOPURINOL REDUCTION

In the experiments reported in Fig. 3, where xanthine oxidase inactivated by anaerobic reaction with allopurinol was separated from unreacted substrate by gel filtration with Sephadex G-25, it was found that in addition to that bound to the inactivated enzyme, alloxanthine was also present in the free form. With a column of Sephadex G-25 (1.2×30 cm) equilibrated with $0.1\,M$ pyrophosphate, pH 8.3, inactivated enzyme was found to emerge in the void volume (15 ml), unreacted allopurinol at 55 ml and alloxanthine at 81 ml. The separation of allopurinol and alloxanthine was quantitative, and from the measured extinction coefficient of alloxanthine at 242 nm of $8.25 \times 10^3\,M^{-1}\,cm^{-1}$ (in $0.1\,M$ pyrophosphate pH 8.3) the yield could be estimated.

Figure 7 shows the spectra of the compounds used in the experiments described in this and the next section. The xanthine oxidase is routinely stored in the presence of approximately $10^{-3}\,M$ salicylate as stabilizer; hence this component is present in all column effluents. It is readily distinguished from other compounds of interest because of its characteristic absorption spectrum. The results of a typical experiment to determine the stoichiometry of alloxanthine production by anaerobic reaction of xanthine oxidase with allopurinol are summarized in Table II and Fig. 8. Figure 8 shows the separation of inactivated enzyme, unreacted allopurinol, salicylate and alloxanthine produced in excess of that bound to the inactive enzyme. From Table II it can be seen that nearly quantitative recovery of allopurinol as unreacted material and alloxanthine product is obtained, with a total of 3.28 moles alloxanthine produced per mole functional E.FAD.

That the product firmly bound to the enzyme is indeed alloxanthine was demonstrated as follows. In the above experiment the inactive enzyme (obtained by allopurinol reduction and separated from alloxanthine and unreacted allopurinol) was denatured by heating at 100° for 2 minutes. The supernatant solution was subjected to gel filtration

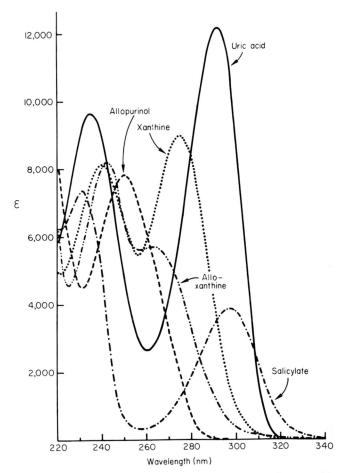

FIG. 7. Absorption spectra of salicylate, allopurinol, alloxanthine, xanthine and uric acid under the conditions used to analyze the fractions collected in the experiments reported in Figs. 8 and 9. The spectra were determined at a concentration of $10^{-4} M$, in $0.1 M$ pyrophosphate, pH 8.3, 20°, and are expressed as extinction coefficients $(cm^{-1}M^{-1})$.

on the same Sephadex column, and 1.0 mole alloxanthine per mole functional enzyme was found to emerge at a volume of 81 ml. The alloxanthine was identified and estimated quantitatively by its absorption spectrum and by its ability to inhibit xanthine oxidase in experiments similar to those shown in Fig. 5.

From the spectrophotometric and EPR results already discussed it is evident that allopurinol reduces both the flavin and iron–sulfur

TABLE II

STOICHIOMETRY OF ANAEROBIC REACTION OF ALLOPURINOL
WITH XANTHINE OXIDASE[a]

1. Enzyme reacted	0.2075 μmole E.FAD (total)
2. —	≡0.152 μmole E.FAD (73% functional)
3. Allopurinol taken	0.80 μmole
4. Unreacted allopurinol	0.294 μmole
5. Free alloxanthine	0.346 μmole
6. Bound alloxanthine	0.152 μmole (assumed)
7. Sum of 4 to 6	0.792 μmole
8. Sum of 5 + 6	0.498 μmole (3.28 moles alloxanthine per mole functional E.FAD)
9. Alloxanthine-inactivated enzyme used for heat denaturation	0.1935 μmole E.FAD total
	≡0.141 μmole E.FAD functional
10. Alloxanthine recovered	
Estimated by spectrophotometry	0.141 μmole
Estimated by inhibition as in Fig. 5.	0.140 μmole

[a] Milk xanthine oxidase (AFR$^{25°}$, 153) was reacted anaerobically with allopurinol in the presence of 0.1 M pyrophosphate pH 8.5 for 25 minutes at 25°. The reaction mixture was then cooled in ice, air was admitted, and the inactive enzyme (2.0 ml) was passed through a Sephadex G-25 column, as shown in Fig. 7.

chromophores of the enzyme. There are two different pairs of iron–sulfur chromophores in xanthine oxidase, each of which can accept one electron (Palmer and Massey, 1969). Hence the iron–sulfur chromophores plus the flavin prosthetic group account for the production of 2 moles of alloxanthine. Reduction of MoVI to MoIV would then account nicely for the formation of the third mole of product; the observed stoichiometry of 3.28 moles of alloxanthine per mole of functional E.FAD perhaps indicating still further reduction to MoIII.

G. STOICHIOMETRY OF URIC ACID PRODUCTION ON ANAEROBIC REDUCTION OF
  XANTHINE OXIDASE BY XANTHINE, USING ALLOXANTHINE TO PREVENT
  FURTHER TURNOVER

It is a matter of some interest to determine the total number of reducing equivalents that can be accepted by the enzyme from xanthine and other substrates. In previous studies, where both the fast and slow phases of reduction were taken into account, it was estimated that, per molecule of enzyme-bound flavin, 7 electron equivalents can be accepted from a variety of substrates and 8 from dithionite (Massey et al., 1969). These results were corroborated by EPR titration studies with dithionite (Palmer and Massey, 1969), and the suggestion was made that, in order

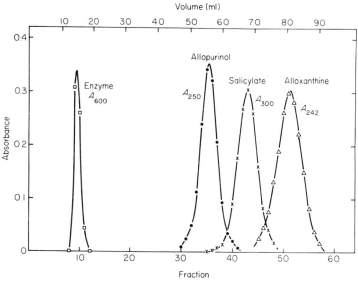

Fig. 8. Separation of allopurinol-inactivated enzyme from unreacted allopurinol, salicylate, and alloxanthine. Enzyme, in a volume of 2.0 ml, was reacted anaerobically with allopurinol as described in Table II, and chromatographed on a column of Sephadex G-25. Fractions of 1.58 ml volume were collected and spectra were recorded for all fractions. The spectra obtained for most fractions showed the existence of only one compound, except in the overlap fractions. The absorbance values shown above are corrected in these fractions for the contribution of the contaminating compound by use of the data of Fig. 7.

to account for such results, molybdenum must be reduced finally to the level of MoIII with substrates and to the level of MoII with dithionite. These results and conclusions have not been readily accepted (Hart *et al.*, 1970), although for no compelling experimental reasons. The finding of very potent binding of alloxanthine to reduced enzyme, preventing reaction of the enzyme with oxygen, offered the possibility of another sensitive method of determining the electron uptake of the enzyme by estimation of the uric acid produced. This method would be free of the objection raised by Pick and Bray (1969) that our previous estimations might be in error due to *binding* of xanthine rather than utilization of it. The results of such experiments are summarized in Fig. 9 and Table III. In the first experiment, alloxanthine was mixed with enzyme before the anaerobic addition of xanthine. As shown in Fig. 1, no bleaching of the enzyme occurred beyond the level equivalent to the phase of rapid bleaching. Thus the yield of uric acid produced in this experiment should be related to the level of *functional* active sites. As detailed in Table III,

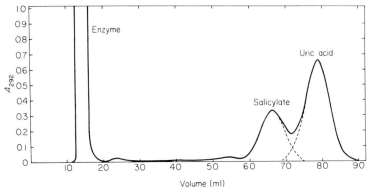

FIG. 9. Separation of alloxanthine-inactivated enzyme from salicylate and the uric acid produced by anaerobic reaction of xanthine oxidase with xanthine. The figure shows the analysis of the column effluents from Sephadex G-25 of the second experiment of Table III. Unreacted xanthine elutes at the same position as salicylate; the small excess of alloxanthine employed elutes at approximately the same position as uric acid but makes an insignificant contribution to the total absorbance at 292 nm (cf. Fig. 7) (the same stoichiometry of uric acid production was estimated from the observed absorbance at 300 nm).

this is equivalent to 3.49 moles of uric acid produced per functional active center. In the second experiment, complete substrate-bleaching of the enzyme was obtained by prolonged incubation with xanthine before the addition of alloxanthine. In this case the total yield of uric acid was appreciably more than in the first experiment, and equivalent to 3.44 moles per mole of total E.FAD (functional + nonfunctional active sites).

Not only are these results in striking quantitative agreement with our previous titration data, but they also permit more incisive interpretation. Previously, it was thought that the slow electron uptake occurring after the rapid phase of substrate bleaching was of no catalytic significance, merely reflecting slow kinetic events that could occur with the enzyme under anaerobic conditions. However, the results obtained above make it clear that these changes also occur rapidly with *functional* enzyme, and that serious consideration of their possible catalytic significance should be made. Thus within the 1–2-minute period possibly required for inactivation by alloxanthine, 7 electron equivalents per functional active site are accepted by the enzyme from xanthine. In the absence of evidence for other electron accepting groups in the enzyme than flavin (which could accept 2 electrons), the two iron–sulfur chromophores (which together could account for a further 2 electron uptake) and molybdenum, it becomes compelling to consider that the molybdenum must be reducible by substrate to the Mo(III) state. From the previous studies it must

TABLE III

STOICHIOMETRY OF URIC ACID PRODUCTION ON REDUCTION OF XANTHINE OXIDASE
BY XANTHINE, USING ALLOXANTHINE TO PREVENT FURTHER TURNOVER[a]

Experiment	Enzyme applied to column	Uric acid produced	Uric acid
1. Alloxanthine before xanthine	0.136 μmole E.FAD (total)	0.349	2.56 moles per mole total E.FAD
	0.100 μmole (functional)		3.49 moles per mole functional E.FAD
2. Extended reaction with xanthine before alloxanthine	0.130 μmole E.FAD (total)	0.440	3.44 moles per mole total E.FAD

[a] Two anaerobic reaction cuvettes containing identical reaction mixtures, but differing in the order of additions, were incubated at 25° as shown below, then cooled in ice; air was admitted, and the contents were chromatographed on Sephadex G-25, as shown in Fig. 9. Each cuvette contained in a total volume of 2.06 ml: 170 μmoles pyrophosphate, pH 8.5; 0.138 μmole xanthine oxidase (as total FAD content); 0.667 μmole xanthine; 0.2 μmole alloxanthine. To maintain strict anaerobiosis, 100 μmoles glucose and 7.74 nmoles of glucose oxidase (as E.FAD) were also present. In the first experiment, alloxanthine was present with the enzyme before the xanthine was mixed from a side arm; incubation was continued for 3 hours, during which time no further bleaching of the enzyme occurred beyond that shown in Fig. 1. In the second experiment, alloxanthine and xanthine were in separate side arms. The enzyme was reacted with xanthine for 18 hours before the alloxanthine was added; reaction was then continued for a further 2 hours. The level of bleaching obtained was close to that shown in Fig. 1, curve *3* of Massey *et al.* (1969).

therefore be concluded that with dithionite as reductant, the Mo(II) state is reached.

H. REACTION OF OTHER PYRAZOLO[3,4-*d*]PYRIMIDINES WITH XANTHINE OXIDASE

In addition to allopurinol and alloxanthine, the effects of other pyrazolo[3,4-*d*]pyrimidines on xanthine oxidase were tested. As expected, those compounds which were unsubstituted in the C-6 position were able to reduce xanthine oxidase rapidly, and on reoxidation yield inactivated enzyme incapable of further reduction. Compounds substituted at the C-6 position were unable to reduce xanthine oxidase anaerobically, and like alloxanthine failed to produce any spectral perturbation of the enzyme. However, like alloxanthine, they did not prevent anaerobic reduction by xanthine, and on reoxidation marked spectral changes from that of the original enzyme were obtained with complete loss of xanthine-oxygen reductase activity. The spectral perturbations obtained varied markedly with the different compounds. To emphasize these effects, Fig.

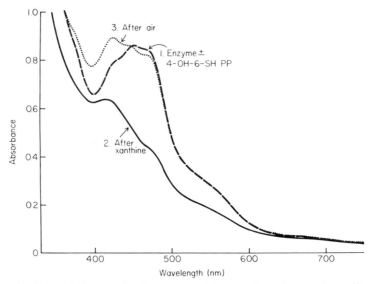

Fig. 10. Spectral changes in the course of inactivation of xanthine oxidase by 4-hydroxy-6-mercaptopyrazolo[3,4-d]pyrimidine. Curve 1, enzyme in 0.1 M pyrophosphate pH 8.5, before and after the addition of 4-hydroxy-6-mercaptopyrazolo[3,4-d]-pyrimidine ($1.33 \times 10^{-4} M$). Curve 2, 5 minutes after the anaerobic addition of $1.1 \times 10^{-4} M$ xanthine. Curve 3, immediately after admitting air.

10 shows the result of reaction of xanthine oxidase anaerobically with xanthine in the presence of 4-hydroxy-6-mercaptopyrazolo[3,4-d] pyrimidine, and the spectrum obtained immediately after admitting air. The spectra should be compared with those obtained with alloxanthine (Fig. 1). It is readily seen that the spectrum of the reduced enzyme is quite different from that obtained in the presence of alloxanthine. Furthermore, the spectrum obtained directly after air reoxidation is markedly different from that of the initial enzyme or that obtained by reduction and reoxidation in the presence of alloxanthine. From the results of Fig. 3, it appears highly probable that the changed spectrum of the alloxanthine-inactivated enzyme is due to a complex between alloxanthine and a reduced form of molybdenum, probably Mo(IV). The results of Fig. 9 indicate that this same complex exists in the reduced enzyme since similar spectral perturbations exist between this spectrum and that obtained on reduction of xanthine oxidase by xanthine in the absence of any inhibitor. Indeed this has been found to apply to all the pyrazolo[3,4-d]pyrimidines tested, as shown in Fig. 11. In this figure are recorded the difference spectra between enzyme reduced by xanthine

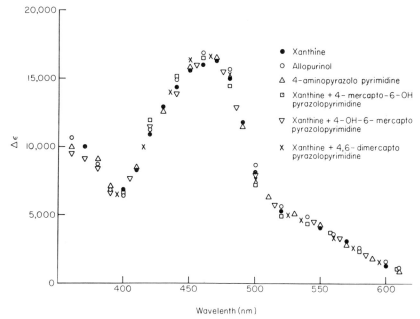

Wavelength (nm)

FIG. 11. Difference spectra (expressed as Δε based on concentration of enzyme-bound flavin) between air-reoxidized enzyme and enzyme reduced as indicated. With xanthine as reductant the difference calculated was between oxidized enzyme and the spectrum produced immediately after addition of xanthine (Massey *et al.*, 1969). The difference spectra obtained with the pyrazolo[3,4-*d*]pyrimidines was, for example, that between curves *3* and *2* of Figs. 1 and 10.

and that immediately after air reoxidation, *in the absence or in the presence of the inhibitors.* It can be seen that there is no significant or systematic difference in such difference spectra, indicating that the only effect of the immediate air reoxidation is the reoxidation of the reduced flavin and iron–sulfur chromophores, leaving the complexed Mo(IV) still intact. From these data it can also be concluded that in the uninhibited enzyme the conversion of Mo(VI) to Mo(IV) results in no significant spectral change. On the other hand, it is evident that the complexed Mo(IV) has considerably altered spectral characteristics compared to uncomplexed Mo(VI) or Mo(IV). The change in absorption spectrum on complexing can be obtained from the difference spectrum of the untreated enzyme and that obtained immediately after air reoxidation of the inhibited enzyme. Such difference spectra are shown in Fig. 12, illustrating the pronounced effect of changing substituents in the pyrazolo[3,4-*d*] pyrimidine nucleus.

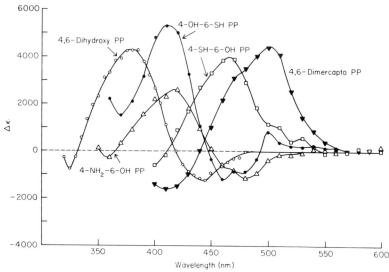

Fig. 12. Difference spectra between xanthine oxidase inactivated with various pyrazolo[3,4-*d*]pyrimidines and native enzymes. The spectra represent, for example, the difference between curves *3* and *1* of Figs. 1 and 10. ○, 4,6-Dihydroxypyrazolo-[3,4-*d*]pyrimidine; ●, 4-hydroxy-6-mercaptopyrazolo[3,4-*d*]pyrimidine; △, 4-amino-6-hydroxypyrazolo[3,4-*d*]pyrimidine; □, 4-mercapto-6-hydroxypyrazolo[3,4-*d*]pyrimidine; ▼, 4,6-dimercaptopyrazolo[3,4-*d*]pyrimidine.

TABLE IV

Stability of Pyrazolo[3,4-*d*]pyrimidine Complexes of Xanthine Oxidase[a]

Complex with	Time for half reactivation (min)
4-Mercapto-6-hydroxypyrazolo[3,4-*d*]pyrimidine	70
4,6-Dimercaptopyrazolo[3,4-*d*]pyrimidine	270
4-Amino-6-hydroxypyrazolo[3,4-*d*]pyrimidine	160
4,6-Dihydroxypyrazolo[3,4-*d*]pyrimidine (alloxanthine)	300
4-Hydroxy-6-mercaptopyrazolo[3,4-*d*]pyrimidine	1220
4-(3-Hydroxypropylamino)pyrazolo[3,4-*d*]pyrimidine[b]	50
4-Hydroxy-5-*N*-propylpyrazolo[3,4-*d*]pyrimidine[b]	1100

[a] Inhibited enzyme obtained as described in text was incubated aerobically in 0.1 *M* pyrophosphate pH 8.5 at 25° and activity determined at intervals. Excellent agreement between return of activity and return of native enzyme spectrum was observed in each case.

[b] Used as substrates; by analogy with the other compounds the inhibitory complex is probably with the 6-hydroxypyrazolo[3,4-*d*]pyrimidine products.

I. Stability of Pyrazolo[3,4-d]pyrimidine Complexes of Xanthine Oxidase

As was found with alloxanthine-inactivated enzyme, all the other complexes investigated were slowly destroyed in the presence of air, with full return of catalytic activity and the absorption spectrum of uncomplexed enzyme. The rate of such reoxidation of the Mo(IV), and hence the

TABLE V

Effect of Allopurinol-Analogues on Xanthine Oxidase

Compound	Structure	Effect
Allopurinol (4-Hydroxypyrazolo-(3,4-d)pyrimidine)	(4-hydroxypyrazolo[3,4-d]pyrimidine structure, OH)	Rapid reduction of enzyme, resulting in spectral perturbations and complete inactivation
7-Hydroxypyrazolo(4,3-d) pyramidine	(structure, OH)	Rapid reduction of enzyme, no spectral perturbations, no activation
7-Hydroxy-3-methylpyrazolo-(4,3-d)pyrimidine	(structure, OH, CH₃)	Slow reduction of enzyme, no spectral perturbations, no inactivation
4-Hydroxypyrrolopyrimidine	(structure, OH)	Rapid reduction of enzyme, no spectral perturbations, no inactivation
7-Hydrovy-ν-triazolo[d]-pyrimidine	(structure, OH)	Rapid reduction of enzyme, no spectral perturbations, no inactivation
7-Amino-ν-triazolo[d]-pyrimidine	(structure, NH₂)	Rapid reduction of enzyme, no spectral perturbations, no inactivation

All compounds were tested anaerobically at 25° in 0.1 M pyrophosphate pH 8.5 under conditions similar to those shown in Fig. 1.

stability of the complex, varies considerably with the nature of the pyrazolo[3,4-d]pyrimidine used. Results are shown in Table IV. An interesting difference in stability is evident between the complex with 4-mercapto-6-hydroxypyrazolo[3,4-d]pyrimidine (half-life, **70** minutes) and that with 4-hydroxy-6-mercaptopyrazolo[3,4-d]pyrimidine (half-life, **1220** minutes). It should be noted that bulky substituents can be accommodated in the pyrimidine ring without affecting adversely the strong binding of the pyrazolo[3,4-d]pyrimidines to the reduced enzyme. This offers the possibility of attaching such compounds to an inert carrier and making use of the extremely tight binding to *functional* xanthine oxidase as a chromatographic method for obtaining fully functional xanthine oxidase preparations.

J. STRUCTURAL REQUIREMENTS FOR INACTIVATION

The location of the N atoms in the five-membered ring of the pyrazolo-[3,4-d]pyrimidine series has been found to be quite critical for tight binding to reduced enzyme and concomitant inactivation. Two pyrazolo-[4,3-d]pyrimidines, two triazolopyrimidines and 4-hydroxypyrrolopyrimidine were tested and found to be substrates of xanthine oxidase. However, in no case did these compounds prevent the secondary slow phase of bleaching of the enzyme, cause spectral perturbations after reoxidation, or cause any inactivation. The compounds tested are listed in Table V. An exciting area of research is thus opened up to determine what features of the structure of the pyrazolo[3,4-d]pyrimidines makes them unique in their ability to bind so tightly to the reduced molybdenum component of xanthine oxidase.

REFERENCES

Avis, P. G., Bergel, F., and Bray, R. C. (1955). *J. Chem. Soc.* p. 1100.
Bray, R. C., and Watts, D. C. (1966). *Biochem. J.* **98**, 142.
Bray, R. C., Pettersson, R., and Ehrenberg, A. (1961). *Biochem. J.* **81**, 178.
Bray, R. C., Palmer, G., and Beinert, H. (1964). *J. Biol. Chem.* **239**, 2667.
Bray, R. C., Chisholm, A. J., Hart, L. I., Meriwether, L. S., and Watts, D. C. (1966).
    In "Flavins and Flavoproteins" (E. C. Slater, ed.), p. 117. Elsevier, Amsterdam.
Elion, G. B. (1966). *Ann. Rheum. Dis.* **25**, 608.
Elion, G. B., Kovensky, A., Hitchings, G. H., Metz, E., and Rundles, R. W. (1966).
    Biochem. Pharmacol. **15**, 863.
Falco, E. A., and Hitchings, G. H. (1956). *J. Amer. Chem. Soc.* **78**, 3143.
Hart, L. I., McGartoll, M. A., Chapman, H. R., and Bray, R. C. (1970). *Biochem. J.*
    (in press).
Hemmerich, P., Massey, V., and Weber, G. (1967). *Nature* (*London*) **213**, 728.
Komai, H., and Massey, V. (1970). *Proc. 3rd Int. Symp. Flavins Flavoproteins, 1969*
    (in press).
Komai, H., Massey, V., and Palmer, G., (1969). *J. Biol. Chem.* **244**, 1692.

McGartoll, M. A., and Bray, R. C. (1969). *Biochem. J.* **114**, 443.

Massey, V., and Curti, B. (1967). *J. Biol. Chem.* **242**, 1259.

Massey, V., Brumby, P. E., Komai, H., and Palmer, G. (1969). *J. Biol. Chem.* **244**, 1682.

Massey, V., Komai, H., Palmer, G., and Elion, G. B. (1970). *J. Biol. Chem.* **245**, 2837.

Morell, D. B. (1952). *Biochem. J.* **51**, 657.

Palmer, G., and Massey, V. (1969). *J. Biol. Chem.* **244**, 2614.

Pick, F. M., and Bray, R. C. (1969). *Biochem. J.* **114**, 735.

Robins, R. K. (1956). *J. Amer. Chem. Soc.* **78**, 784.

Roblin, R. O., Lampen, J. O., English, J. P., Cole, Q. P., and Vaughan, J. R. (1945). *J. Amer. Chem. Soc.* **67**, 290.

Spector, T., and Johns, D. G. (1968). *Biochem. Biophys. Res. Commun.* **32**, 1039.

Spector, T., and Johns, D. G. (1970). *Biochem. Biophys. Res. Commun.* **38**, 583.

Taylor, E. C., McKillop, A., and Warrener, R. N. (1967). *Tetrahedron* **23**, 891.

Walker, N. H., Hemmerich, P., and Massey, V. (1967). *Helv. Chim. Acta* **50**, 2269.

West, R. A. (1961). *J. Org. Chem.* **26**, 4959.

Quinones and Nicotinamide Nucleotides Associated with Electron Transfer*

A. KRÖGER AND M. KLINGENBERG

*Institut für Physiologische Chemie und
Physikalische Biochemie, University of Munich,
Munich, Germany*

This paper concentrates on the principles of function of nicotinamide nucleotides† and of menaquinone and ubiquinone in terminal substrate oxidation. In mitochondria, NAN and quinones have been considered as members of the respiratory chain. In particular for the NAN, this association is too limited since by the pool function the NAN is linked to

* This work was supported by grants from the Deutsche Forschungsgemeinschaft and the Fonds der Chemischen Industrie.

† Abbreviations: NAN, nicotinamide nucleotides; UQ, ubiquinone; MQ, menaquinone; FCCP, *p*-trifluoromethoxycarbonylcyanidephenylhydrazone; HQNO, 2-*n*-heptylhydroxyquinoline-*N*-oxide; TMPD, N,N,N′,N′-tetramethyl-1,4-phenylene-diamine; TRA, triethanolamine.

the majority of cellular redox reactions. In animal cells one may concentrate on the mitochondrial NAN system, whereas in protists and plants the extramitochondrial NAD also is directly linked to the respiratory chain. In prekaryotic cells this compartmentation of NAN does not exist. Here, particularly interesting principles of function for the quinones are revealed. In view of these various associations, the function of the coenzymes will be considered both in terminal oxidation and in the substrate-substrate hydrogen transfer. A number of relevant review articles have been published (Klingenberg, 1961, 1964b, 1968; Klingenberg and Kröger, 1966; Kröger and Klingenberg, 1967).

I. GENERAL ASPECTS

A. REDOX POTENTIAL AND COENZYME LINKAGE

A major factor for associating a substrate with a specific coenzyme is its redox potential. In Scheme 1 a number of important substrate redox couples associated with the terminal oxidation are assembled according to the redox potentials together with their coenzymes. A range from about $+80$ down to -500 mV is covered by the combined functions of quinones

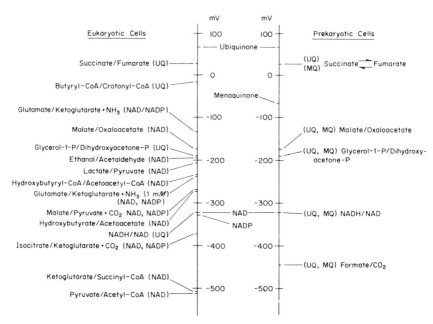

SCHEME 1. Redox potentials and coenzyme linkage of various (mitochondrial) substrate-redox systems. The redox potentials refer to midpotentials (pH 7.0) at standard conditions (Krebs and Veech, 1970; Mathews and Vennesland, 1950; Young and Pace, 1958; Borsook, 1935; Bäcklin, 1958; Johnson, 1960; Rodkey, 1959).

and NAN. It is clear that the actual redox potential of the substrate couples may deviate greatly from the midpotentials. This explains why there is a rather poor correlation of the substrate redox potential and the associated coenzymes. The difference of the redox potentials in the steady state, $\Delta E = E_{substrate} - E_{coenzyme}$, can be expected to be negative if the substrate is feeding hydrogen into the coenzyme pool, and positive if it accepts hydrogen. Both effects are inseparably linked, and therefore the function of the coenzymes in substrate reduction will be appropriately considered. Substrate reduction appears to be responsible for the occurrence of menaquinone as well as ubiquinone and of NADP in addition to NAD. Whereas the quinones have a midpotential difference of 120 mV, those of NAD and NADP are equal. However, the actual redox potentials of NAD and NADP in the cell appear to differ widely because of the association of NADP with substate couples of more negative redox potential, as shown in Scheme 1. The difference in redox potential between both NANs is not an inherent property of the coenzyme and therefore is subject to regulation by energy transfer, as discussed below.

The redox potential of UQ has been measured directly in submitochondrial particles by coupling to succinate/fumarate. The midpotential measured, $E' = 65$ mV (Urban and Klingenberg, 1969) is about 50 mV more negative than estimated for isolated UQ in ethanol (Schnorf, 1966; Morton, 1965). This difference has been interpreted as being caused by the particular binding of UQ in the lipid phase of the membrane with the quinone reaching into the hydrophilic phase. Also for membrane-bound MQ a similar decrease of E_0 compared to that in ethanol solution can be expected.

B. The Molar Relations between Coenzymes, Respiratory Carriers, and Dehydrogenases in Mitochondria

In Table I a survey of the content of NAD, NADP, and UQ in mitochondria from various sources is given (cf. Klingenberg, 1962; Kröger and Klingenberg, 1967). In animal mitochondria, the content of NAD ranges between 3 and 6 μmoles per gram of protein. The UQ content is closely parallel to that of NAD. In contrast, the content of NADP varies from 5 to 0.3 μmoles/gm protein. NAD and UQ are directly linked to the terminal oxidation and therefore to the main function, and thus they are relatively constant, whereas NADP is linked to special functions and therefore varies strongly according to the source of mitochondria. In mitochondria from various protists and from plants a relatively high content of NAD and little or no NADP are found.

The enzyme activity of various NAN-linked dehydrogenases has been measured in a variety of animal mitochondria and related to the NAN content. When referred to the content of the key enzyme of respiration,

TABLE I

CONTENT OF NICOTINAMIDE NUCLEOTIDES (NAN) AND UBIQUINONE (UQ) IN
MITOCHONDRIA FROM VARIOUS SOURCES[a,b]

Mitochondrial source	NAD	NADP	UQ
Liver, rat	3.2	4.8	1.8
Adrenal, calf	5.5	2.8	—
Breast muscle, pigeon	4.8	1.2	3.9
Heart muscle, rat	4.5	1.1	4.0
Kidney, rat	4.5	0.9	1.6
Skeletal muscle, rat	5.1	0.8	3.0
Brain, rat	2.0	0.4	—
Flight muscle, locust	4.2	0.3	3.5
Saccharomyces carlsbergensis	4–6	0.3	5.4
Neurospora crassa: wild	7	0	0.5
mi-1	6.2	0	7
Plants (mung bean)	4.1	—	1.6

[a] Data from Klingenberg (1962), Kröger and Klingenberg (1967), Ohnishi et al.
(1967), Weiss et al. (1970), Chance et al. (1968).

[b] Values are expressed as micromoles per gram of protein.

cytochrome a, the NAD-linked dehydrogenases, i.e., the main dehydrogenases of the oxidative pathway, are found to be contained in various
mitochondria in constant proportion to the cytochromes and the NAD
content. The NADP-linked dehydrogenases follow the larger variations
of the NADP content (Klingenberg, 1964b; Klingenberg and Pette, 1962;
Goebell and Klingenberg, 1963).

TABLE II

MOLAR COMPOSITION OF RESPIRATORY CHAIN: APPROXIMATE VALUES FOR RAT
HEART MITOCHONDRIA[a]

Cytochrome a_3	≡1
Cytochrome a	1
Cytochrome c	1
Cytochrome c_1	0.5
Cytochrome b	1
Ubiquinone	11
Succinate-DH	0.16
NADH-DH	0.1
NAD	11
NADP	3
MDH	0.4
GluDH	0.01
IDH$_{NAD}$	0.03
IDH$_{NADP}$	0.25

[a] Data from Klingenberg (1964b, 1968).

Of particular interest are the molar ratios of the coenzymes vs. the associated enzymes. The approximate molar contents are summarized for rat heart mitochondria in Table II, calculated from the enzyme activities and turnover numbers (Klingenberg, 1964b, 1968). Three groups may be differentiated: the cytochromes with an approximate molar ratio of 1:1, the coenzymes NAN and UQ with approximate molar contents one order of magnitude greater than those of the cytochromes, and the dehydrogenases with ratios approximately 1 to 2 orders of magnitude lower than the cytochromes. This illustrates that the dehydrogenases are not related to the cytochromes in a fixed stoichiometric manner, building up "chains" or "complexes" (contrast, Chance, 1965; Green, 1963), but rather form a more statistical relation to the cytochromes. This results not only from the stoichiometric discrepancy, but also from the wide variation of molar ratios of special dehydrogenases to cytochromes.

C. Topochemical Organization of the Hydrogen-Transferring Coenzymes and Enzymes in the Mitochondrial Membrane

On the basis of the molar content of the various components and on estimation of the available inner membrane surface, the occupation of the inner membrane with these components is schematically described in Fig. 1 (cf. Klingenberg, 1968). The components are projected on the membrane, assuming globular structure and molecular weights from the literature. The scheme is based on the estimate that one molecule of cytochrome a is found on a membrane surface of approximately 6×10^4 Å^2. As a result, the average distance between cytochrome a and the two major membrane-bound dehydrogenases, succinate-DH and NADH-DH, is about 150–250 Å. This distance has to be bridged by UQ, which diffuses two-dimensionally on the lipid layer between the components. The diffusion time is much below the time resolution of hydrogen transfer to be measured. In the hydrophilic layer above this membrane are the NADH-linked dehydrogenases in a "dilute" distribution similar to that of the cytochromes. The NAD has to diffuse between these dehydrogenases and the NADH-DH on the membrane for the terminal oxidation.

The transverse cut through the membrane demonstrates the sidedness of the components (Klingenberg and von Jagow, 1970). This is of particular interest for the function of UQ. Most of the membrane-bound dehydrogenases are located on the inner surface. An exception in animal mitochondria is glycerolphosphate dehydrogenase (Klingenberg and Buchholz, 1970) and, in mitochondria from protists and plants, also NADH-dehydrogenase (von Jagow and Klingenberg, 1970), which are located on the outer surface. Apparently these outer dehydrogenases feed to the same UQ pool as the inner dehydrogenases. This indicates that UQ

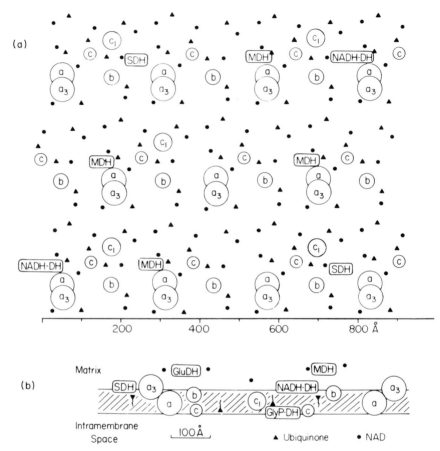

FIG. 1. (A) Projection of respiratory components, dehydrogenases, and coenzymes on the inner mitochondrial membrane. Carrier distribution is based on data in Table II. The dimensions of carriers are estimated from molecular weights, assuming globular structure. (B) Cut through the inner mitochondrial membrane.

diffuses not only "horizontally," but also vertically through the membrane. Such a transmembrane hydrogen transfer may be of great importance for the concept of the H^+ pump associated with the energy coupling of electron transport to oxidative phosphorylation (Mitchell, 1966; Mitchell and Moyle, 1967).

D. The Pool Function of NAD and Ubiquinone

It is clear that the stoichiometric discrepancy and variability require a linkage between the dehydrogenases and the cytochromes by a mobile hydrogen carrier system, such as provided by the low molecular weight coenzymes. While this has never been disputed for the dehydrogenases linked to the NAN system, the corresponding role for UQ has been contested frequently (cf. Chance, 1965). This is due to the membrane fixation of UQ and the associated dehydrogenases which has led to a misunderstanding of the function of the membrane in binding enzymatically active components. Most of the UQ-linked dehydrogenases are membrane-bound, as are the cytochromes. The membrane was considered to form a structural matrix which provides proximal localization of the components for ensuring their interaction in an ordered sequence. This concept is wrong in explaining both the association of the cytochromes to the membrane and their linkage to the dehydrogenases.

This aspect may be illustrated in two important examples, succinate-DH and NADH-DH. Both are present in a ratio of only 0.1 or 0.15 to cytochromes. The distance from a cytochrome, such as cytochrome b, to the nearest dehydrogenase may exceed 300 Å (cf. Fig. 1). Nevertheless, from one type dehydrogenase all cytochromes are rapidly reduced by either succinate or NADH. It is clear that only a diffusible metabolite can bridge these distances and therefore such a mobile hydrogen carrier should have been postulated even before the rather late detection of UQ. In particular a H-transfer between dehydrogenases requires also a H-carrier. Such a H-transfer has been demonstrated early for the reversibility of oxidative phosphorylation, e.g., H-transfer from succinate to NADH (Klingenberg et al., 1959; Chance and Hollunger, 1960).

In some bacteria the function of H-transfer to a substrate appears to be a main function of menaquinone, as discussed below. Furthermore, only with a mobile coenzyme linkage to the cytochromes can the great variation in the dehydrogenase content, associated with particular cell function and adaptation, be accommodated. This is clearly accepted for the NAN-linked dehydrogenases; however, variability is required also on the level of the membrane-bound flavoproteins. As a striking example, the glycerol-phosphate dehydrogenase might be mentioned. In liver mitochondria the content of this enzyme can be increased 20-fold in a hyperthyroid state, without corresponding changes of the cytochromes, UQ or other dehydrogenases (Kadenbach, 1966; Y. P. Lee et al., 1959). There are numerous examples of wide variation in bacteria, depending on the growth conditions.

The principles of function of the coenzymes linked to terminal oxidation may be summarized as follows:

1. Both types of coenzymes, the quinones (UQ and MQ) and nicotinamide-nucleotides (NAD and NADP) are low molecular weight compounds accepting or donating hydrogen equivalents.

2. Both coenzymes are in most cases easily dissociable from the de-

hydrogenases and do not form (with exceptions) tightly bound prosthetic groups with the enzymes.

3. The NAN as hydrophilic molecules localized in the hydrophilic space (matrix space of mitochondria) and correspondingly associated mainly with "soluble" enzymes. The lipophilic quinones are bound to the inner mitochondrial membrane associated with the membrane-bound quinone-specific dehydrogenases, mainly flavoproteins.

4. The great molar excess of the coenzymes to dehydrogenases and cytochromes corresponds to the function of the coenzymes as hydrogen carrier pool in which the coenzymes diffuse between the various acceptor and donor sites of the dehydrogenases.

5. The separation of the dehydrogenases from the cytochrome chain by a hydrogen transferring carrier pool permits great variability in the composition of the dehydrogenases.

6. The diffusible hydrogen carrier pool permits that from one dehydrogenase electrons can be transferred to a number of cytochrome chains orders of magnitude higher.

E. COMPARTMENTATION OF COENZYMES IN THE MITOCHONDRIAL MEMBRANE

The NAN are unable to penetrate the inner mitochondrial membrane, in all mitochondria tested (Purvis and Lowenstein, 1961; Klingenberg and Pfaff, 1965; von Jagow and Klingenberg, 1970). The major share of hydrogen for the respiratory chain is generated inside the mitochondrion. The linkage of the extramitochondrial NAN system to the terminal oxidation is therefore bridged by auxiliary substrate shuttle systems which reach the respiratory chain, as summarized in Scheme 2.

The most simple system is the direct oxidation of cytosolic NADH by an external NADH dehydrogenase located on the outer surface of the inner membrane, in addition to an inner NADH dehydrogenase available to the endogenous NAD (T. Ohnishi et al., 1966a; von Jagow and Klingenberg, 1970). This arrangement is found in eukaryotic protists and plants (Storey and Bahr, 1969; Weiss et al., 1970). In animal mitochondria, auxiliary systems of hydrogen transfer operate in the absence of an external NADH dehydrogenase. In particular in insect muscle, but also in nerve cells, hydrogen from NADH is first transferred to glycerol phosphate, which is then dehydrogenated by an externally located dehydrogenase linked to the membrane-bound UQ (Bücher and Klingenberg, 1958; Klingenberg and Buchholz, 1970). The substrate shuttle is thus a result of the cooperation of cytosolic and membrane-bound dehydrogenase. In other hydrogen shuttles, the substrate permeates the membrane and reacts with two analogous dehydrogenases in both com-

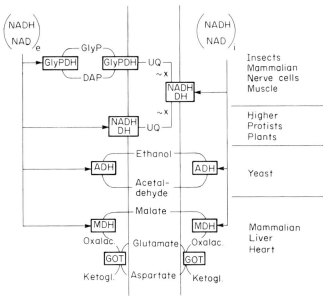

SCHEME 2. Hydrogen transfer systems between intra- and extramitochondrial NAD at the inner membrane from various mitochondria. Oxalac. = oxaloacetate; Ketogl. = ketoglutarate.

partments. One example is the ethanol-acetaldehyde shuttle in yeast mitochondria (von Jagow and Klingenberg, 1970). Of great importance in animal mitochondria is the H-transfer via the malate system catalyzed by a specific membrane carrier (Borst, 1963; Chappell, 1968). The oxidized partner, oxaloacetate, can itself permeate only indirectly via membrane carrier for two coupled amino acids, glutamate and aspartate.

The impermeability of the inner membrane for NAD and NADH is related to the fact that the extramitochondrial NADH is maintained in the animal cell at a considerably higher redox potential ($E' = -230$ mV) as compared to the intramitochondrial NAD system ($E' = -280$ mV) (Bücher and Klingenberg, 1958; Williamson et $al.$, 1967). This fact has been elucidated and discussed in great detail in metabolic studies, particularly in liver (Williamson et $al.$, 1967; Bücher, 1970). One main factor in maintaining this difference is the opposite dependence of the redox potential of NADH on the phosphorylation potential of ATP in both compartments (Klingenberg, 1965). This is based on the difference in the mechanisms of the substrate level phosphorylation in glycolysis and the electron transport phosphorylation in mitochondria. The substrate shuttles must be constructed in such a way as to maintain this difference between the two NAD-systems. It is conceivable that this difference is maintained via the substrate permeation shuttle by the membrane potential or pH difference at the inner membrane (Klingenberg *et al.*, 1969; Chappell, 1969).

II. The Redox State of Nicotinamide
Nucleotides in Mitochondria

The redox state of the NAD and NADP in mitochondria in various states has early been investigated by the application of highly sensitive enzymatic analysis on mitochondrial extracts (Klingenberg and Slenczka, 1959; Klingenberg *et al.*, 1959). More qualitative results, in particular on the kinetics, are obtained by recording of absorption or of fluorescence changes (Chance and Williams, 1956; Chance and Baltscheffsky, 1958). The factors which control these changes are considered to be strictly a function of donor and acceptor activities. No postulated intermediate of oxidative phosphorylation of NAD could be confirmed experimentally. The strong influence of the activity of oxidative phosphorylation on the mitochondrial NAD system is mainly explained by a control of the acceptor activity for NADH of the NADH dehydrogenase.

An example for this control is illustrated in Fig. 2 for the fatty acid oxidation in heart mitochondria (Klingenberg, 1963). In the controlled state, in the absence of added ADP, the intramitochondrial NAD is largely reduced and becomes oxidized on stimulation of respiration by the addition of ADP or on uncoupling. The redox state of NAD as well as of other respiratory components is considered to be close to equilibrium which is sustained by the coupling to the high potential of the energy-rich intermediate and ATP. The energy-linked redox equilibrium of NAD incorporates the energy-linked reduction of NAD from flavin-linked substrates such as succinate or glycerol phosphate as one of its consequences (Klingenberg and Bücher, 1959; Klingenberg, 1961, 1964a). As a result, redox equivalents at the level of UQ and flavoproteins are in equilibrium with those of the NADH, in dependence on the energy level.

In this state the redox state of NAN should be a function of both the reducing power and phosphorylation potential. Since the phosphorylation potential is also a function of the reducing power, an increase of the redox state of NAN alone with the reducing power can be expected. This is illustrated in Fig. 3, where the redox state of NAN increases with the respiratory activity of a variety of substrates over a wide range (Klingenberg and Kröger, 1967; Kröger and Klingenberg, 1967). A high level of reduction of NAD is observed only with a sufficiently active substrate. In the equilibrium state the entrance point of reducing equivalents,

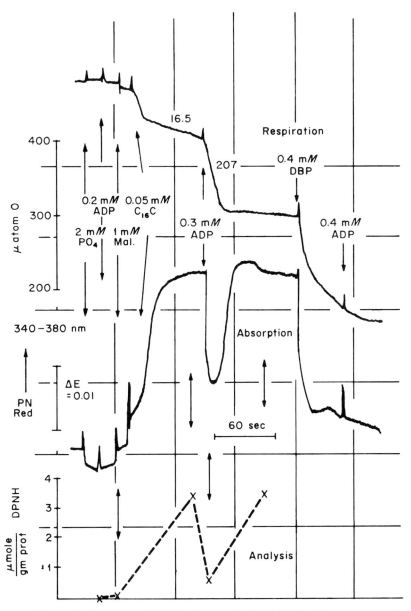

FIG. 2. The redox behavior of NAD in heart mitochondria. Simultaneous recording of respiration, NADH absorption, and enzymatic NADH analysis in a suspension of heart mitochondria, incubated in 0.25 M sucrose, 1 mM EDTA medium at 25°, pH 7.2. From Klingenberg and Bode, 1965.

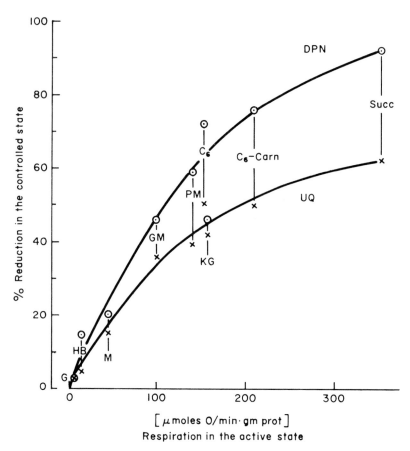

FIG. 3. Correlation of redox state of NAD and UQ in mitochondria and the hydrogen donor activity of various substrates, as measured by the respiratory rate in the active state. G = glutamate, HB = β-hydroxybutyrate, GM = glutamate + malate, PM = pyruvate + malate, C₆-Carn. = hexanoylcarnitine, KG = α-ketoglutarate, Succ = succinate, M = malate. From Klingenberg and Kröger (1966).

whether at cytochrome c (TMPD + ascorbate), UQ or NAD, is irrelevant for the redox state of NAD. The equivalence of the NAD-linked and flavoprotein-linked substrates in the reduction of NAD is clearly demonstrated by the homogeneity of the increase of NAD only as a function of the dehydrogenase activity. Earlier concepts of special pathways for hydrogen from succinate and compartmentation of NAD for succinate have thus been disproved (Chance and Hollunger, 1960, 1961).

Further support for this concept comes from the redox state of NAD in mitochondria from *Saccharomyces carlsbergensis*, where the first phos-

TABLE III

The Relation of Internal and External NAD-Systems to Energy Transfer[a]

Source	Maximal P/O		Reduction of endogenous NAD in controlled state (%)
	Endogenous NADH	Exogenous NADH	
Animals	3	2.3	70–80
Eukaryotic protists			
Saccharomyces carlsbergensis	2	2	5
Torulopsis utilis	3	2	—
Neurospora crassa: wild	3	2	20
mi-1	3	2	—
Plants (skunk cabbage)	3	2	25

[a] Data from von Jagow and Klingenberg (1970) and Storey and Bahr (1969).

phorylation site is missing and therefore the NAD is not included in the energy-linked redox equilibration at the respiratory chain (T. Ohnishi *et al.*, 1967). Therefore the NAD stays oxidized both with NAD-linked and quinone-linked substrates in the controlled state. A survey on the linkage of the NAD system to oxidative phosphorylation is given in Table III, where data on the presence and absence of the first phosphorylation site are summarized for various mitochondria and for the oxidation of both exogenous and endogenous NADH. In contrast to animal mitochon-

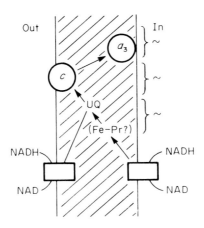

Scheme 3. Sidedness at the inner membrane of two different dehydrogenases for oxidation of endogenous and exogenous NADH, and the occurrence of the first coupling site, in mitochondria from higher protists and plants (cf. von Jagow and Klingenberg, 1970).

dria, the first phosphorylation site is missing in mitochondria from *S. carlsbergensis* (T. Ohnishi *et al.*, 1966a), iron-deficient *Torulopsis utilis* (Light *et al.*, 1968), and for the oxidation of exogenous NADH in all higher protists studied (Weiss *et al.*, 1970) (cf. Scheme 3). The consequences for the intra- and extramitochondrial redox potential of the NAD were discussed above.

RELATION BETWEEN MITOCHONDRIAL NAD AND NADP SYSTEMS

The NAD and NADP systems are linked by at least two substrate couples with a dual specificity both for NAD and NADP, and by the transhydrogenase. Only the NAD is directly linked to the respiratory

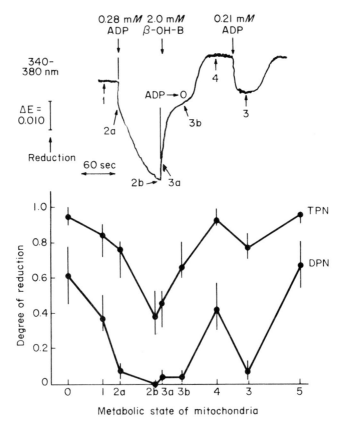

FIG. 4. Comparison of recordings of NAD (DPN) and NADP (TPN) in liver mitochondria in various metabolic states. Simultaneous recording of absorption changes and enzymatic analysis of NAD and NADP in a suspension of liver mitochondria in isotonic sucrose medium, pH 7.2, 25°. Substrate: β-hydroxybutyrate (β-OH-B). From Klingenberg and Slenczka (1959).

chain by the NAD specificity of the NADH dehydrogenase in animal mitochondria. In some higher protists and plants, NADPH can apparently also be oxidized without a transhydrogenase by the respiratory chain (Ikuma and Bonner, 1967; Weiss *et al.*, 1970). Although both coenzymes have equal midpotentials, the actual redox potential of the NAD appears to be more positive than that of the NADP, both in the cytosol and intramitochondrial space.

For the mitochondria this was early demonstrated by following the redox changes of the NADP parallel to those of NAD, as shown in Fig. 4 for liver mitochondria (Klingenberg and Slenczka, 1959). NADP is always more reduced than NAD. Making the simplifying assumption that the activity coefficients for both systems are equal in the mitochondria, the redox ratios have been taken to estimate the redox potential difference under various conditions. As shown in Fig. 5, NADP is always about 30 mV more negative in coupled mitochondria than the NAD system, whereas both are equal in the uncoupled state. This has been considered as a first indication for an energy-linked transhydrogenation from the NAD to the NADP system. The existence of this transhydrogenation could later be confirmed on sonic particles of mitochondria and has been

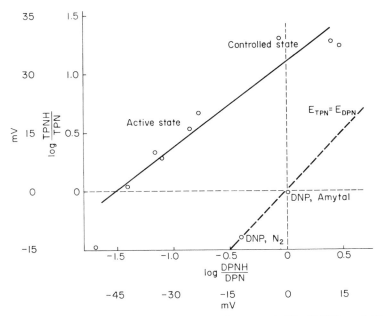

Fig. 5. Energy-dependent redox equilibrium between NAD (DPN) and NADP (TPN) systems in liver mitochondria. The values are measured by enzymatic analysis, as shown in Fig. 4. From Klingenberg and Slenczka (1959).

widely applied in elucidating energy transfer mechanisms (cf. C. P. Lee and Ernster, 1966).

The linkage of intramitochondrial dehydrogenases either to the NAD or NADP systems can be most appropriately demonstrated by eliminating the influence of the respiratory chain with respiratory inhibitors and following only substrate-substrate hydrogen transfer through the NAD and NADP systems. Malate, hydroxybutyrate, and isocitrate are used as donors; and ketoglutarate + NH_3 or +CO_2, and acetoacetate as acceptors (Klingenberg and von Häfen, 1963; Tager and Slater, 1963; Klingenberg *et al.*, 1965) (Fig. 6). As shown in Fig. 7, mainly NADPH is oxidized with ketoglutarate + NH_3 and therefore the linkage of glutamate dehydrogenase to mitochondrial NADPH can be deduced. NADPH is again reduced more in the combined action of malate and ATP, indicating the transhydrogenation of the NADPH and demonstrating the effect of an energy-dependent transhydrogenation which brings hydrogen from NAD-linked malate to NADPH.

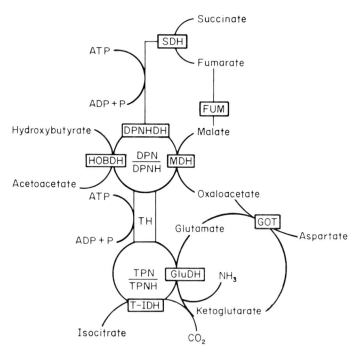

Fig. 6. Pathways of inter-substrate H-transfer mediated by the intramitochondrial NAD and NADP. HOBDH = β-hydroxybutyrate dehydrogenase; SDH = succinate dehydrogenase; IDH = isocitrate dehydrogenase; GOT = glutamic-oxaloacetic transaminase; GluDH = glutamate dehydrogenase. From Klingenberg *et al.* (1965).

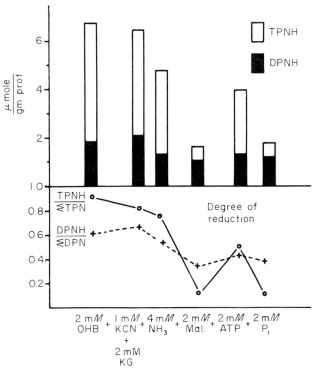

F<small>IG</small>. 7. Redox changes of intramitochondrial NAD and NADP systems during the intersubstrate H-transfer. The experiment demonstrates H-transfer from β-hydroxy-butyrate (HOB) as H-donor for NAD and ketoglutarate + NH₃ as acceptors for hydrogen from NADPH. Energy-linked H-transfer from NADH to NADP is demonstrated by the ATP-driven reduction of NADPH. From Klingenberg et al. (1965).

III. U<small>BIQUINONE</small> <small>IN</small> M<small>ITOCHONDRIAL</small> E<small>LECTRON</small> T<small>RANSPORT</small>

The experimental evidence until about 1966 of the functions of the quinones in electron transport has been reviewed in several articles (Chance, 1965; Redfearn, 1966; Crane and Löw, 1966; Kröger and Kling-enberg, 1967; Crane, 1968). This section is concerned with recent developments in the field of respiration and not with the function of quinones in photosynthetic systems. It is well established that UQ undergoes redox reactions dependent on the respiratory process and that it interacts only in the quinone and quinol form. Only 0.2–1.5% of UQ is found in the radical form in the anaerobic state (Bäckström et al., 1970; Weber et al., 1965). Its position in the mitochondrial respiratory chain is still under discussion. On the basis of kinetic arguments, Chance and Pring (1968) and Chance et al. (1969) concluded that UQ is in a blind alley of the electron pathway, whereas UQ and cytochrome b form branches in the respiratory system according to Storey and Chance (1967) and Storey (1968). Similar schemes were put forward by Redfearn (1966) and Crane (1968; Crane and Löw, 1966) on the basis of extraction-reactivation experiments. On the other hand, Klingenberg and Kröger (1967) proposed that UQ is the only component transporting reducing equivalents from the flavo-dehydrogenases to the cytochromes. This concept was recently confirmed by Ernster *et al.* (1969) by means of a convincing extraction-reactivation method.

A. KINETICS OF THE REDOX REACTIONS OF UBIQUINONE

1. *Reduction of Ubiquinone*

The position of UQ in the respiratory chain was judged from its rate of reduction on the addition of the substrate in the presence of an inhibitor (Chance, 1965; Redfearn, 1966; Kröger and Klingenberg, 1967; Chance *et al.*, 1969; Klingenberg & Kröger, 1966; Storey, 1967). This rate cannot be regarded as maximum rate since it is largely controlled by the activity of the dehydrogenases. Accordingly, Klingenberg and Kröger (1966) found the rates of reduction of UQ by succinate and NADH to be about equal to the respiratory rates. Those of the cytochromes were 2–4 times slower.

The activity of the dehydrogenase at the moment of the addition of the substrate is not necessarily equal to that calculated, e.g., from the respiratory rate (Minikami *et al.*, 1964). This may explain the data of Storey (1967), who found equal reduction rates of UQ and cytochromes b and c with succinate, which are 20 times lower than the respiratory rate.

In contrast to Klingenberg and Kröger (1966), Storey and Chance (1967) found extremely low rates of the reduction of UQ by NADH. The rates of reduction of the cytochromes were 2–4 times slower than the respiratory rate, in agreement with Klingenberg and Kröger (1966). The discrepancy resides probably in the experimental conditions. Klingenberg and Kröger used sulfide in concentrations sufficient for complete inhibition of respiration, whereas Storey and Chance applied the inhibitors (antimycin or KCN) and the NADH in low amounts so that the reduction of UQ could be expected not to continue after the flow period. Under these conditions, however, the absorption change due to the reduction of UQ can be obscured by the interference of the NADH (Szarkowska and Klingenberg, 1963). The difficulties in measuring the rate of reduction of UQ with NADH are overcome if the quench-flow method is used instead of the direct optical method. With this technique Redfearn and Kröger (1967) found the rate of reduction of UQ to be faster than that of cytochromes b and c.

2. *Oxidation of Ubiquinone*

It is now generally agreed that the rate of oxidation of UQ in submito-chondrial particles is faster than the maximum respiratory rate (Kröger and Klingenberg, 1967; Chance and Pring, 1968; Storey, 1968; Klingenberg and Kröger, 1966). Hence UQ can shift its redox state at rates compatible with its interaction in a linear sequence of the respiratory components. Although Storey (1968) measured an extremely fast rate in ETP, he proposed a scheme with a parallel interaction of UQ and cytochrome *b* in a branched system (Storey and Chance, 1967; Storey, 1968). This scheme is based on the oxidation rate of UQ in the presence of small levels of inhibitors. UQ is more rapidly oxidized with antimycin present than with KCN, whereas the opposite holds for cytochrome *b* (Storey, 1967). The conclusion is unjustified, however, considering that the differences were observed at less than 1% of the uninhibited oxidation rates.

Table IV summarizes the results on the oxidation rates of UQ as obtained by the different authors with various preparations. The kinetics of the oxidation of UQ in ETP is characterized by a halftime of 3–5 msec according to Storey (1968). In contrast, Chance and Pring (1968) observed a lag phase of about 25 msec in uncoupled pigeon heart mitochondria and a subsequent oxidation of UQ with a halftime of about 0.2 second. In uncoupled E-SMP the oxidation proceeded without a lag phase and a similar halftime (Chance and Pring, 1968). According to these authors (Chance and Pring, 1968; Chance *et al.*, 1969), UQ responds too slowly to interact in the main path of the electron pathway. Its position is thought to be on a blind alley of the respiratory system, and the fast oxidation rate measured in the ETP was explained as an artifact of the preparation. A similar explanation (Chance and Pring, 1968) was applied to the earlier results of Klingenberg and Kröger (1966), who measured an oxidation rate of UQ in sonic particles, which is compatible with an interaction in a linear sequence of the carriers. The interpretation of the kinetics of the redox reactions of UQ depends greatly on the molecular organization of the respiratory system. On the basis of the assumption of respiratory units (Chance, 1965) composed of carriers in a mole to mole stoichiometry, Chance and Storey (Chance and Pring, 1968; Chance *et al.*, 1969; Storey, 1968) judge the kinetics from the halftimes. They expect that each respiratory unit responds as an entity with the halftime of the components only dependent on the position in the chain. The conclusion of these authors is based on the discrepancy between the halftimes of UQ and those of the cytochromes, which is about two orders of magnitude.

TABLE IV

COMPARISON OF THE KINETIC DATA ON THE OXIDATION REACTION OF UBIQUINONE OCCURRING ON ADDITION OF OXYGEN TO THE ANAEROBIC PREPARATIONS[a]

Authors	Preparation and temperature (°C)	Component	Reactive pool size (C_0) (μmoles e^-/gm protein)	Lag phase (msec)	Rate measured (μmoles e^-/sec/gm protein)	$t_{1/2}$ (msec)	TN = $0.69/t_{1/2}$ (sec^{-1})	Rate = TN × C_0 (μmoles e^-/sec/gm protein)
Storey (1968)	ETP, 24°	UQ	1	—	—	4.5	150	150
Chance and Pring (1968)	E-SMP, 25°	UQ	≡8	—	—	180	3.8	30
Kröger and Klingenberg (1970)	SP, 23°	UQ	7.6	—	42	250	—	—
Chance and Pring (1968)	Mitochondria (pigeon heart), 25°	UQ	≡9	25	—	220	3.1	28
Kröger (1969)	Mitochondria (rat heart), 23°	UQ	9.2	—	35	210	—	—
Storey (1968)	ETP 24°	Cyt c	0.4	—	—	2.8	250	100
Chance and Pring (1968)	Mitochondria (pigeon heart), 25°	Cyt c	≡0.5	—	—	3	230	115

[a] TN = turnover number; ETP = electron transport particles; E-SMP = sonic particles + EDTA from beef heart mitochondria; SP = sonic particles from beef heart mitochondria.

The fact, however, that UQ is in a big molar excess over the cyto-chromes led Klingenberg and Kröger (1966) to the assumption of a pool, in which each molecule of UQ can react with each acceptor cytochrome chain. Thus in the steady state each cytochrome has to transport the same amount of reducing equivalents as the total pool of UQ, although the capacities for redox equivalents differ by almost 20. If equal and first-order rates of the oxidation reactions are assumed for the two components, the ratio of $t_{1/2}$ of the oxidation reaction of UQ is expected to be about 20 times greater than that of cytochrome c. Therefore the kinetics should be judged by the molar rate (μmoles/min/gm protein) at which the UQ pool can conduct redox equivalents, rather than by $t_{1/2}$. This rate was ac-curately measured by the quench-flow method (Fig. 8). For comparison,

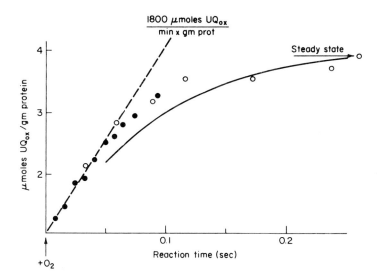

Fig. 8. Comparison of the direct optical to the quench-flow method applied for measuring the oxidation rate of ubiquinone (UQ). Freshly prepared rat heart mito-chondria in 0.25 M sucrose, 20 mM TRA, pH 7.2, 5 μM rotenone, 5 μM p-trifluoro-methoxycarbonylcyanidephenylhydrazone, 10 mM succinate, 23°. The respiratory rate (120 μatoms of oxygen per minute per gram of protein) was adjusted by malonate. The solid line was replotted from direct absorption measurements at 280–289 nm with the moving mixing apparatus (Klingenberg, 1964c); 2.5 mg protein per milliliter; optical path length, 0.2 cm. The points were obtained with the quench-flow apparatus: 1 ml of the anaerobic mitochondrial suspension was mixed with 1 ml of sucrose-TRA-medium and quenched with 10 ml of a mixture of 70% (v/v) methanol and petroleum ether (b.p. 40°–60°) at the reaction times indicated. The redox state of UQ was de-termined according to Kröger and Klingenberg (1966). Contents of the reaction chambers: ● 17 μl, ○ 120 μl. Total amount of UQ:4.5 μmoles per gram of protein (Kröger and Klingenberg, 1970).

the $t_{1/2}$ given by Storey and Chance are converted to rates on the basis of the pool sizes, assuming first-order reactions (Table IV). As seen when comparing columns 6 and 9, the computed rates are very close to those measured by Kröger and Klingenberg and Kröger. There are two exceptions: the lag phase observed in pigeon heart mitochondria and the extremely high rate computed for ETP. As seen from Fig. 8 this lag phase does not occur in rat heart mitochondria. The oxidation rate of cytochrome c is only about 3 times higher than that of UQ. This may reflect the position of cytochrome c on the oxygen side of UQ.

The rate of UQ oxidation is consistent with the function of UQ as the only electron donor of the cytochrome chain. This was supported by comparison to the maximum flux of reducing equivalents through the cytochrome chain (Kröger, 1969). Complete reduction of cytochrome a was observed at a rate of respiration with ascorbate $+$ TMPD which is equal to the oxidation rate of UQ.

The direct optical method applied by Klingenberg and Kröger (1966) and the quench-flow method are compared in the experiment of Fig. 8. There is close agreement on the course of the oxidation of UQ, although the optical trace could not be evaluated until 50 msec after oxygen was added. This confirms the validity of both methods.

In summary, the discrepancies on the position of UQ derived from kinetic studies by the various authors reside mainly in the different concepts of the respiratory system, rather than in different experimental results.

B. Requirement for Ubiquinone in Electron Transport, as Shown by Extraction-Reactivation Experiments

In principle, measurements of the kinetics of oxidation and reduction cannot prove that UQ is a component necessary for respiration, whereas extraction-reactivation experiments are especially suited to answer this question. Earlier attempts failed to solve the problem either because of incomplete extraction or the lack of specificity or irreversible damage of the enzymes. The extraction with acetone caused the irreversible breakdown of the NADH dehydrogenase, and a reactivation of the succinate oxidase was observed in the absence of UQ on the addition of cytochrome c. This led Redfearn (1966) and Crane (1968) to accept the concept of a branched system. Pentane extraction of UQ after lyophilization preserves the NADH dehydrogenase. The respiratory activities with both succinate and NADH are fully inhibited and can be restored specifically by UQ (Szarkowska, 1966). As UQ was added in excess to aqueous solutions, the short-chain homologs are more active than the natural ones, and it was questionable whether the added UQ interacts at the natural site.

This problem was recently overcome by application of the natural long-chain homologs of UQ in pentane solution to lyophilized preparations which were depleted from UQ by pentane (Ernster *et al.*, 1969). Thus UQ is reincorporated by a procedure complementary to that of the depletion and leads very probably to the insertion of the UQ into the original place, the lipid phase of the membrane. This is supported by the finding that only amounts of UQ equal to the original content are required for full restoration.

By this method, it was demonstrated that the electron transport from the flavodehydrogenases to the cytochromes as well as the respiratory activity and the reduction of fumarate by NADH depend specifically on the presence of UQ. These experiments strongly favor the concept that UQ collects the hydrogen provided by the various dehydrogenases and feeds it into the cytochrome chain. They contradict the concept that UQ is bypassed or on a blind alley.

C. Demonstration of Ubiquinone Pool

1. *Titration with Succinate Dehydrogenase*

The variability of the molar ratios of the dehydrogenase to the cytochrome chain and the order of magnitude lower content of the dehydrogenase compared to the cytochromes have been a strong argument in favor of the existence of a diffusible quinone pool, as discussed above. The problem can be examined making use of the reconstitution of succinate oxidase by additions of succinate dehydrogenase (SDH) to an SDH-depleted oxidase preparation containing the cytochromes. For this purpose, a reconstitutively active succinate dehydrogenase and SDH-depleted Keilin-Hartree preparation were prepared (King, 1967) by incubation at high pH. For reconstitution, SDH was added in amounts varying over a range of two orders of magnitude relative to the SDH-depleted cytochrome oxidase. In each reconstituted incubation, the activity of succinate oxidation and the redox levels (percent reduction) of UQ and of cytochrome b were measured, both in the aerobic steady state and in the cyanide-inhibited state. In order to obtain the molar ratios of SDH to cytochromes, the FAD-content in the SDH-preparation and the cytochrome aa_3 content in the oxidase were determined.

The result of a reconstitution study is shown in Fig. 9, where percent reduction and respiration are plotted dependent on the log of the molar ratio SDH/cytochrome aa_3. In the aerobic steady state the reduction and respiration rise continuously with the amounts of SDH. The steady-state reduction reaches saturation at a ratio SDH/cytochrome $aa_3 = 0.1$, respiration is not yet at maximum. In the anaerobic state the reduction both

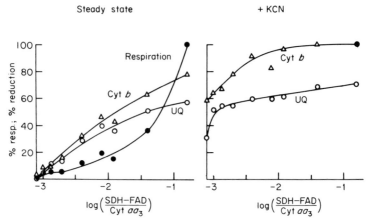

FIG. 9. Titration of cytochrome particles with succinate dehydrogenase (SDH). Simultaneous measurement of the respiration and the redox states of ubiquinone (UQ) and cytochrome b. SDH and cytochrome particles were prepared according to King (1967). The reconstituted respiratory activity (100% = 155 μatoms of oxygen per minute per gram of particle protein) was measured at 25°. The redox state of cytochrome b was recorded at 562–575 nm, that of UQ was measured by extraction (Kröger and Klingenberg, 1966). The maximum amount of cytochrome b reducible by succinate in the presence of KCN was 0.37 μmole per gram of protein ($\equiv$100% reduction). The total amounts of UQ and cytochrome aa_3 were 3.6 and 0.4 μmole per gram of protein. The active amount of FAD in the SDH was calculated from the difference spectrum (plus succinate versus untreated) (Hülsmann et al., 1969).

of UQ and cytochrome b reaches a high maximum level already at ratios SDH/cytochrome $a < 0.01$. This demonstrates that even at a ratio SDH/cytochrome $aa_3 = 1:300$ and at SDH/UQ $= 1:1200$, all the maximal reducible UQ can be reduced by succinate, i.e., reached by reducing equivalents that originate from the SDH. Previously in similar reconstitution studies of C. P. Lee et al. (1965), the reduction of the cytochromes was followed in dependence on the amount of SDH added. The results were interpreted by a branching of electron transfer at the cytochromes. However, the molar discrepancies between SDH and the cytochromes were not taken into account, and the function of UQ ignored.

2. Titration with Antimycin

The nonlinear dependence of the respiration on the concentration of antimycin has been explained by assuming that antimycin is an allosteric inhibitor (Bryla et al., 1969; Ernster et al., 1970). This interpretation is based on the concept of the existence of respiratory units. As it is generally accepted that antimycin binds stoichiometrically to a respiratory component (Rieske *et al.*, 1967), a linear dependence is expected. The nonlinear dependence without the additional assumption of an allosteric interaction of antimycin can be derived from the function of UQ as a freely diffusible carrier between the statistically distributed flavodehydrogenases (E_1) and cytochrome chains (E_2) (I. Y. Lee *et al.*, 1970; Klingenberg and Kröger, 1969). The inhibitor attacks the second nonrate-limiting step:

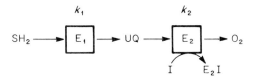

k_1 and k_2 are the specific rates of the steps catalyzed by E_1 and E_2. The overall rates without (v_0) and with the inhibitor (v) are:

$$v_0 = \frac{k_1 \cdot k_2}{k_1 + k_2} \tag{1a}$$

$$v = \frac{k_1 \cdot k'_2}{k_1 + k'_2} \tag{1b}$$

The inhibitor decreases k_2 in a linear dependence by stoichiometric binding to E_2.

$$k'_2 = \frac{n}{n_0} k_2 \tag{2}$$

where $k'_2 =$ the activity of E_2 under the influence of the inhibitor, $n_0 =$ total amount of E_2; and $n =$ free E_2, i.e., not bound as E_2I.

Assuming that all the added I is bound as E_2I, it follows that $n_0 - n =$ I. The overall rate in dependence on the inhibition follows from Eqs. (1b) and (2):

$$v = \frac{k_1 \cdot \dfrac{n}{n_0} k_2}{k_1 + \dfrac{n}{n_0} k_2} \tag{3}$$

v/v_0 is obtained by division of Eq. (3) by Eq. (1a):

$$\frac{v}{v_0} = \frac{\dfrac{n}{n_0}\left(1 + \dfrac{k_1}{k_2}\right)}{\dfrac{n}{n_0} + \dfrac{k_1}{k_2}} \tag{4}$$

The model is illustrated in Scheme 4, in analogy to a flow system. Re-

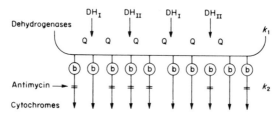

SCHEME 4. Quinone function and its influence on the titration curve with anti-mycin. Electron transfer from the flavodehydrogenases to the cytochrome chains, which are statistically distributed over the membrane surface, is achieved by the diffusion of ubiquinone.

dox equivalents are fed into a vessel representing the pool of UQ. Here they are redistributed to a number of outlets representing the cytochrome chains. As the concentration of antimycin is increased, an increasing number of cytochrome chains are blocked, with a corresponding linear de-crease of k_2. As long as not all the cytochrome chains are blocked, UQ can channel the redox equivalents from all the dehydrogenases through the uninhibited chains by virtue of its pool function. As a consequence the titration of respiration with antimycin A (overall rate) should follow the nonlinear kinetics of the two-enzyme sequence.

The shapes of the curves derived from Eq. (4) depend on the ratios k_1/k_2. Nonlinear curves are obtained only with small values for k_1/k_2, whereas linear curves result from larger values (Fig. 10A).

The redox state of UQ in the simplified steady-state condition is:

$$\frac{Q_{red}}{Q_{ox}} = \frac{k_1}{k'_2} \tag{5}$$

The degree of reduction in dependence on the inhibition is obtained by substitution of k'_2 by Eq. (2):

$$\frac{Q_{red}}{Q} = \frac{\dfrac{k_1}{k_2}}{\dfrac{n}{n_0} + \dfrac{k_1}{k_2}} \tag{6}$$

Equation (6) is plotted in Fig. 10B. With increasing k_1/k_2, the curves become more linear in a manner similar to the respiratory curves.

The response of cytochrome b to the titration with antimycin should differ from that of UQ, if its position is assumed to be between UQ and the point of action of the inhibitor. Whereas the total amount of UQ participates in the steady state electron flow during the titration, the part of cytochrome b in the blocked chains should be in redox equilibrium with UQ. With this assumption, as shown in Fig. 10C, a distinctly different re-

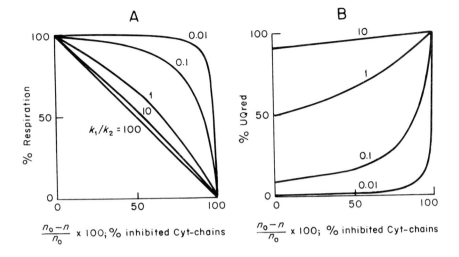

FIG. 10. Theoretical antimycin titration curves for the respiration activity and the redox states of ubiquinone (UQ) and cytochrome b dependent on k_1/k_2. A, evaluated from Eq. (4); B, from Eq. (6); C, from the equation:

$$\frac{b_{red}}{b} = \frac{1 - (n/n_0)}{1 + \sqrt{\dfrac{n \cdot k_2}{n_0 \cdot k_1}} \cdot \exp \dfrac{\Delta E \cdot F}{R \cdot T}} + \frac{1}{\dfrac{n_0}{n} + \dfrac{k_2}{k_1}}$$

where b_{red} is the concentration of reduced cytochrome b, b the total reducible amount, and ΔE ($\equiv -30$ mV in Fig. 10C) the difference in the redox potentials between UQ and cytochrome b.

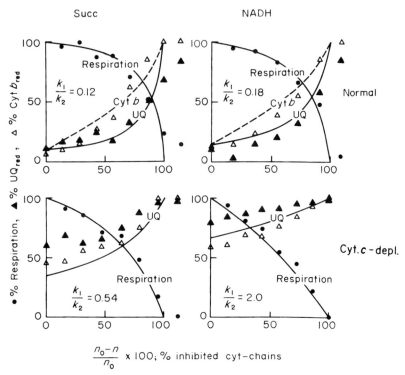

Fɪɢ. 11. Titration with antimycin of the respiration and the redox states of UQ and cytochrome b (points) in comparison to the theoretical curves. The respiratory activities (25°) and the absorption at 562–575 nm were recorded and extracts for the determination of the redox state of UQ (Kröger and Klingenberg, 1966) were sampled simultaneously during the titration with antimycin. Submitochondrial particles were prepared from beef heart mitochondria by sonication either in 0.25 M sucrose (normal) or 0.15 M phosphate pH 7.2 (cytochrome c depleted). In the normal preparation k_2 was measured as the saturating respiratory activity with TMPD + ascorbate. From k_2 and v_0, k_1 was calculated according to Eq. (1a). In the preparation depleted of cytochrome c, k_1 was measured as the respiratory activity with PMS, and k_2 was calculated from Eq. (1a) and v_0. n_0 is obtained from the end point of the titration by extrapolation. The curves were plotted from the Eq. (4) and (6) and from the equation given in the legend of Fig. 10. (Kröger and Klingenberg, 1970).

sponse of UQ and cytochrome b is expected for low values of k_1/k_2, as cytochrome b responds more linearly.

From the rates of oxidation and reduction of UQ it can be deduced that $k_1/k_2 < 1$ in normal preparations. This results in nonlinear titration curves according to the model. In preparations depleted of cytochrome c, it should be $k_1/k_2 > 1$ and almost linear curves are expected.

The comparison between the model and the experiments is given in Fig. 11. The respiration with succinate and NADH of the two types of preparations is titrated with antimycin. Simultaneously with the respiratory activities the redox states of UQ and cytochrome b are measured. The theoretical curves are evaluated from Eqs. (4) and (6) for the corresponding ratios k_1/k_2. The experimental points fit the theoretical tritration curves of the respiration with both substrates, k_1/k_2 varying by a factor of almost 20. The strongly bent curves at low ratios k_1/k_2 as well as the almost straight curves for higher ratios which are predicted by the model are confirmed by the experimental data. Consistency is in principle also observed for the response of UQ, although the steady state equation (Eq. 5) fails to predict the absolute redox state of UQ at higher ratios of k_1/k_2. The experimental points for cytochrome b also fit the theoretical curves fairly well. A measurable difference in the response of cytochrome b and UQ is expected only at smaller k_1/k_2. Accordingly, the response of cytochrome b is more linear than that of UQ at smaller k_1/k_2, and a similar response of both components is measured at higher ratios.

In conclusion, the response of the respiration to antimycin titration can be explained in a simple manner on the basis of the concept of the pool function of UQ. There is no need for the assumption of an allosteric interaction of antimycin. The shapes of the titration curves can vary from the bent to the straight form by mere variation of the activity of cytochrome chains relative to that of the dehydrogenase.

A similar change in the titration curves with antimycin of the respiration with menadiole has been reported to occur on pentane extraction of the UQ (Ernster et al., 1970). Menadiole is assumed to react with the respiratory chain at the level of cytochrome b. This change in the titration curves is expected from the model (Scheme 4) and even confirms it. On the removal of UQ the distribution of the reducing equivalents among the cytochrome chains is abolished and straight titration curves are expected at any donor and acceptor activities.

IV. The Function of Ubiquinone and Menaquinone in Bacteria

Most of the aerobic gram-negative bacteria contain UQ as the sole quinone components, whereas the aerobic gram-positive bacteria contain MQ (Bishop et al., 1962). Only some enterobacteria contain both UQ and MQ. It is widely accepted that the respiratory system is localized in the cytoplasmic membrane (Mitchell and Moyle, 1956; Weibull and Bergström, 1958). This view is substantiated by the observation that the quinones are found in the membrane fraction together with the membrane-bound cytochromes on fractionation of the cells (Bishop and King, 1962;

TABLE V

CONTENTS OF RESPIRATORY COMPONENTS IN MEMBRANES

Source	UQ	MQ (μmoles/gm protein)	Cyt b	NADH-oxidase ($\frac{\mu atoms\ 0}{min/gm\ protein}$)
Mitochondria[a] (beef heart)	6	0	0.9[d]	850
Micrococcus[a] denitrificans (NCIB 8944)	1.5	0	0.18[d]	570
Bacillus megaterium[b] (ATCC 14581)	0	5.4	0.87[e]	985
Proteus rettgeri[c]	5.4	3.4	0.46[e]	657

[a] Sonic particles.

[b] Lysed protoplasts.

[c] Lysed spheroplasts.

[d] From $\Delta A_{562-575nm}$ on the addition of $Na_2S_2O_4$ using the extinction coefficient $20\ mM^{-1} \times cm^{-1}$ (K. Ohnishi, 1966).

[e] From $\Delta A_{557.5-575nm}$ on addition of $Na_2S_2O_4$ using the extinction coefficient $17.5\ mM^{-1} \times cm^{-1}$ (Deeb and Hager, 1964).

Smith, 1968; Daniel and Redfearn, 1968; Kröger and Dadak, 1969). The equipment with respiratory components of the membranes of the three different types of bacteria mentioned above is compared to that of the mitochondrial membrane in Table V. On a protein basis, the contents of the quinones and of the b-type cytochromes as well as the respiratory activities with NADH are of the same order of magnitude. This indicates the functional similarity with respect to the respiration of the cytoplasmic and the mitochondrial membranes. The approximately 10-fold molar excess of the quinones over the individual cytochromes suggests a similar function for the quinones in bacteria and mitochondria.

A. UBIQUINONE IN BACTERIA

Redox reactions of the UQ in fragments prepared from *Acetobacter vinelandii* have been observed by Knowles and Redfearn (1966; Redfearn, 1966), UQ was found to be partially reduced in the steady state of respiration and highly reduced in the presence of KCN. The oxidation of NADH by this organism was demonstrated to depend on the presence of UQ by Swank and Burris (1969). A similar situation was described for *Acetobacter xylinum* by Benziman and Goldhamer (1968). In agreement with the observations in mitochondria (Kröger and Klingenberg, 1967) the redox state of UQ in the steady state of respiration was found to vary

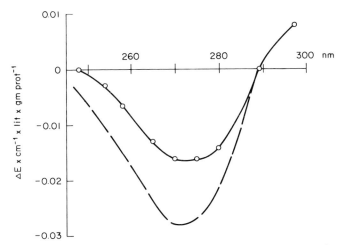

Fig. 12. Difference spectrum of sonic particles from *Micrococcus denitrificans* (NCIB8944) compared to that of ubiquinone. Absorbance differences at various wavelengths on the transition from the steady state of respiration with lactate to the anaerobic state recorded with the dual wavelength spectrophotometer (reference wavelength 289 nm). Dashed line, difference spectrum calculated for the reduction of the total content of UQ (2.5 μmoles per gram of protein) (Kröger and Dadak, 1968).

with the substrate, whereas on inhibition by KCN almost complete reduction is found with each substrate. These authors propose a position of UQ between the flavodehydrogenases and the cytochromes, similar to the situation in mitochondria.

An example for redox reactions of UQ in bacteria is given in Fig. 12. The reduction of UQ on the transition from the steady state of respiration to the anaerobic state is demonstrated by direct spectrophotometry. The absorption changes observed on the exhaustion of oxygen in a suspension of sonic particles from *Micrococcus denitrificans* are similar to the spectrum of the totally extracted UQ. Thus the absorption changes of the bacterial particles indicate the partial reduction of UQ and confirm that UQ undergoes redox reactions linked to the electron transport in bacteria.

B. MENAQUINONE IN BACTERIA

The role of MQ in the electron transport systems of the aerobic gram-positive bacteria is similar in several respects to that of UQ in mitochondria and gram-negative bacteria. The earliest studies were done on *Mycobacterium phlei* (Asano and Brodie, 1964), which contains vitamin K_9H (Gale *et al.*, 1963). From irradiation-reactivation studies it was concluded that MQ interacts between the dehydrogenases for NADH, and malate, and the cytochromes, and that the succinic dehydrogenase is linked to cytochrome *b*. The irradiation as well as the reactivation, as applied to *M. phlei* by Brodie and co-workers, is rather unspecific (Asano and Brodie, 1963). The lack of specificity was observed for the irradiation method also with sonic fragments from *Micrococcus lysodeikticus* (Fujita *et al.*, 1966) and for several extraction-reactivation methods (Downey *et al.*, 1962; Weber and Rosso, 1963). Therefore, the necessity of MQ for respiration has not been demonstrated unequivocally in these cases.

Experiments with added derivatives of quinones led Brodie to the suggestion that MQ may be involved also in the phosphorylation reaction (Brodie, 1965). White (1965) studied the redox state of demethyl-MQ in *Hemophilus parainfluenzae* in the anaerobic state. He found demethyl-MQ to occur only in its quinone and quinol forms and concluded that the total content of the quinone is functionally divided into parts, each of which is specifically linked to a dehydrogenase. However, the validity of the extraction procedure used is doubtful and has not been proved by a direct optical method.

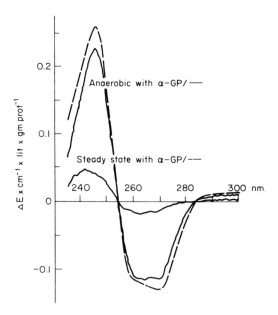

Fig. 13. Difference spectra of the membrane fraction from *Bacillus megaterium* (ATCC14581) compared to that of menaquinone (MQ). The membrane fraction was prepared by lysozyme treatment and osmotic shock. The dashed spectrum represents the total content of MQ (9.1 μmoles per gram protein) (Kröger, 1970).

The role of the normal MQ of the typical gram-positive organism *Bacillus megaterium* has been shown to be that of a redox pool between the various flavodehydrogenases and the cytochromes (Kröger and Dadak, 1969). MQ was found to interact in the electron transport from NADH, malate, and glycerol 1-phosphate to oxygen and fumarate as the acceptors. The interaction is restricted to the transfer of redox equivalents, since the constituent MQ undergoes only two reactions, the reduction of the quinone to the quinol and the reverse reaction. This is demonstrated in Fig. 13 by difference spectra of the membrane fraction. The difference spectra both in the steady and anaerobic state are identical to that of authentic MQ. Of the constituent menaquinone, 85% is reduced in the anaerobic state with glycerol 1-phosphate, and 10–15% in the steady state with oxygen.

The position of the respiratory components relative to each other is illustrated in Scheme 5. The scheme is based on the redox response of MQ, the mode of action of the inhibitor HQNO, and extraction-reincorporation experiments. The whole pool of the constituent MQ is equally accessible to each flavodehydrogenase since the same extent of reduction is observed in the anaerobic state with NADH, malate, and glycerol-1-phosphate. This result, obtained both by direct spectrophotometry and the extraction method, is in contrast to the results reported for *H. parainfluenzae* (White, 1965). In the steady state the degree of reduction is controlled by the activity of the individual dehydrogenase. It was shown by the extraction-reincorporation technique with pentane that MQ is obligatory for the electron flow from each substrate to oxygen and fumarate. The

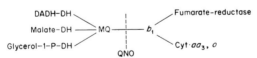

SCHEME 5. Electron transport system of *Bacillus megaterium* (Kröger and Dadak, 1969).

activities could be reactivated by reincorporation of about the original amount of MQ but not with UQ. In the reconstituted particles MQ is again reducible and the electron transfer sensitive to HQNO. The pathways from MQ to both acceptors share a common step which is located between MQ and cytochrome b_1 and is sensitive to HQNO.

C. BACTERIA CONTAINING UBIQUINONE AND MENAQUINONE

The individual roles of the quinones in some enterobacteria which contain both MQ and UQ at about equal amounts is still under discussion. Since there is no indication that the quinones are associated with two morphologically separate membranes, it has to be assumed that both quinones are located in the cytoplasmic membrane (Smith, 1968).

Snoswell and Cox (1968; Cox *et al.*, 1968) report that mutants of *Escherichia coli* which are unable to synthesize UQ, oxidize all the substrates which are also oxidized by the wild type. This may be interpreted to indicate that both quinones have the same role and can replace each other. On the other hand, the quinones might differ in their specificity for the redox acceptor rather than for the dehydrogenases, since enterobacteria can use nitrate and fumarate in addition to oxygen. This is supported by the observation that *E. coli* can shift the quinone contents according to the oxygen supply during the growth (Polglase *et al.*, 1966). On vigorous aeration MQ disappears whereas anaerobic cultures do not contain UQ. This would suggest that UQ is specific for the aerobic and MQ for the anaerobic pathway.

The role of the quinones in the formate-nitrate reductase pathway was studied by an extraction-reactivation technique (Itagaki, 1964). On acetone-extraction the activity was fully inhibited and could be partially restored by either MQ or UQ, the latter being more efficient. This result argues against the specific interaction of MQ in the pathway for nitrate reduction and favors the view that the quinones may functionally replace each other. It is feasible, however, that the unspecificity for the quinones is caused by the procedure applied (Asano and Brodie, 1963; Downey *et al.*, 1962; Fujita *et al.*, 1966; Weber and Rosso, 1963).

On the other hand, Kashkett and Brodie (1963a,b) proposed, for *E. coli*, that UQ interacts in the succinate- and MQ in the NADH pathway. Both pathways are thought to converge at the level of cytochrome *b*. This scheme is based on an assay employing cytochrome *c* reductase with NADH or succinate in irradiation-reactivation experiments. However, since the system used by Kashkett and Brodie contains MQ only at the amount of 5% of that of UQ, it is unlikely that MQ interacts in either pathway. A similar system has been studied by Bragg and Hou (1967).

The membrane fraction of *Proteus rettgeri* grown aerobically on complex media catalyzes the oxidation of succinate, NADH, and formate by oxygen and the oxidation of formate and NADH by fumarate (Kröger *et al.*, 1970). The fumarate reductase activities were more pronounced in bacteria grown anaerobically. Concomitantly, the content of UQ is decreased 10-fold as compared to MQ. This suggests that UQ is involved in the electron transport with oxygen as the acceptor, whereas MQ serves as a carrier in the anaerobic pathways of electron transport.

Both quinones were found to undergo redox reactions. UQ is reducible by all the substrates respired, whereas MQ is reduced only by formate

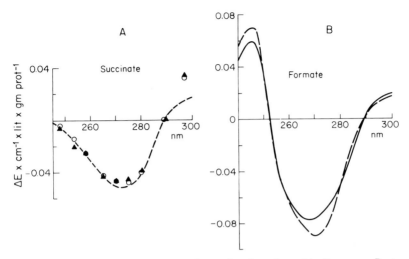

Fɪɢ. 14. Difference spectra of the membrane fraction of aerobically grown *Proteus rettgeri* (167-3 Hygiene Institute, Marburg) compared to those of the quinones. The membrane fraction was prepared by osmotic shock of ampicillin spheroplasts grown in a complex medium at 37°C and 15 liters of air per minute in 10-liter batches. (A) Absorbance differences recorded on the transition from the steady state of respiration to the anaerobic state with the dual wavelength spectrophotometer (reference wavelength 289 nm). Dashed line, difference spectrum calculated for the reduction of the total content of ubiquinone (UQ) (4.55 μmoles per gram of protein). (B) Solid line, suspension of the membrane fraction anaerobic with formate (sample) recorded against the untreated suspension (reference). Dashed line, difference spectrum calculated for the reduction of the contents of both quinones (UQ 4.55 and MQ 2.6 μmoles/g protein) (Kröger *et al.*, 1970).

and NADH. This is shown in Fig. 14, where difference spectra of the membrane and extracts are compared. The difference spectrum with succinate (Fig. 14A) corresponds to the total content of UQ as reduced on the transition to the anaerobic state. The difference spectrum with formate (Fig. 14B) corresponds to almost the total amounts of both UQ and MQ. It is concluded that the total pool of UQ is accessible to each substrate, whereas MQ is linked specifically to the formate and NADH dehydrogenase.

The respiratory activities with the three substrates exhibit equal sensitivities to HQNO (Fig. 15A), indicating identical pathways to oxygen. HQNO interacts on the oxygen side of UQ, since the reduction of UQ increases with the inhibition (Fig. 15B). The individual roles of UQ and MQ are also studied by the extraction-reincorporation method, as shown

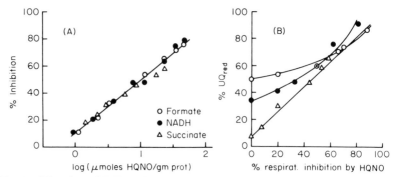

Fig. 15. Titration with HQNO of the respiratory activity (A) and the redox state (B) of ubiquinone (UQ) of the membrane fraction of *Proteus rettgeri* (167-3, Hygiene Institute, Marburg). For preparation of the membrane fraction, see legend to Fig. 14. (A) Respiratory activities without inhibitor in 0.1 M P_i, pH 7.0, 25°C (μatoms of oxygen per minute per gram of protein): formate, 2370; NADH, 955; succinate, 540. (B) Titration of the respiratory activity and simultaneous determination of the redox state of UQ by extraction, 0.1 M TRA, pH 7.4, 15°. Respiratory rates without inhibitor (μatoms of oxygen per minute per gram of protein): formate, 1160; NADH, 205; succinate, 87. Total content of UQ:4.55 μmoles per gram of protein. From Kröger *et al.* (1970).

in Table VI, for *P. rettgeri* grown under limited oxygen supply. Ninety-five percent of the quinones were extracted by pentane, resulting in an inhibition of the electron transport from all the substrates to both acceptors. The reincorporation of UQ restores the electron transport to oxygen, but not to fumarate. Reincorporation of MQ restores only the electron transport to fumarate.

The results of these experiments are summarized in Scheme 6. UQ interacts in the pathway to oxygen, and MQ mediates the electron transport to fumarate. The activities of succinate oxidation and fumarate reduction belong to two different enzymes. This is shown by the specificity for the quinones (Table VI). The same conclusion was drawn for *E. coli* from genetic experiments (Hirsch *et al.*, 1963).

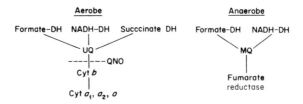

Scheme 6. Electron transport system of *Proteus rettgeri* (Kröger *et al.*, 1970).

TABLE VI

DEPENDENCE OF VARIOUS ELECTRON TRANSPORT ACTIVITIES OF *Proteus rettgeri*
ON UQ AND MQ[a,b]

Acceptor:	Oxygen			Fumarate	
Substrate: Preparation	Succinate	NADH	Formate (% of lyophilized preparation)	NADH	Formate
Depleted	30	4	3	30	9
Depleted + MQ	24	13	17	245	113
Depleted + UQ	131	95	68	18	11
Depleted + MQ + UQ	101	95	88	222	99

[a] From Kröger *et al.* (1970).

[b] The membrane fraction of *P. rettgeri* (167-3, Hygiene Institute, Marburg) prepared as indicated in the legend of Fig. 14 from bacteria grown at 1 liter of air per minute was subjected to the procedure of Ernster *et al.* (1969). The activities of the lyophilized preparation measured at 25° with oxygen as the acceptor were (µatoms of oxygen per minute per gram of protein): succinate, 136; NADH, 760; formate, 1280; and with fumarate (µmoles of fumarate per minute per gram of protein): NADH, 56; formate, 85.

D. PRINCIPLES OF DIFFERENCE IN THE FUNCTION OF UBIQUINONE AND MENAQUINONE AND THEIR RELATION TO THE DEVELOPMENT OF ELECTRON TRANSPORT PHOSPHORYLATION

As discussed in the introductory chapter, the redox potential of the coenzymes are a major guideline for the substrate linkage. After description of the role of MQ and UQ in bacterial electron transport, the general rules for the difference in the function of MQ and UQ might again be considered.

The great difference of redox potential between MQ and UQ clearly separates the substrate interaction of MQ from that of UQ. As an acceptor MQ should be linked to substrates of relatively low potential, as a donor it should be effective for substrates of higher redox potential. With the same substrates UQ could only function as an acceptor, unless participating in energy-dependent "reversed" electron transfer. These principles are exemplified for succinate-fumarate. The oxidation of succinate involves UQ in bacteria containing UQ but not MQ. In bacteria which contain only MQ, succinate oxidation is quinone-independent. The reduction of fumarate is a main function of MQ and therefore important in bacteria containing this quinone.

With this background a broader understanding of the quinone function may be reached in an attempt to visualize the occurrence of MQ and UQ in the development of bacterial electron transport (Scheme 7). Three stages are differentiated according to the type of phosphorylation: (1) Stage with exclusive reliance on substrate level phosphorylation (Decker *et al.*, 1970). Here the redox reactions are performed in the hydrophilic cell matrix preferentially with NAD, which transfers hydride. (2) Stage with phosphorylation from electron transport with substrate acceptors such as SO_4^{2-}. Here the redox reactions are linked to the membrane, which enables the separation of electron from proton transfer. (3) Stage with phosphorylation from membrane-bound electron transport to oxygen. These three stages coincide with the sequential appearance of first MQ and then UQ. Stage 1 is represented by obligate anaerobes such as *Clostridium*, which do not have electron transport phosphorylation and do not contain quinones. Then the electron transport with substrate acceptors is developed. This is linked to the appearance of MQ, still in obligate anaerobes before the advent of oxygen. An example is *Desulfovibrio* which contains only MQ (Maroc *et al.*, 1970). Consequently the advent of higher potential acceptors for electron transport such as nitrate and oxygen is accompanied by the occurrence of the higher redox potential quinone, UQ. Before the transition to the classical aerobes both high and low potential electron acceptors were used, and therefore some of these bacteria retained MQ besides UQ. Examples for this stage are *Escherichia*

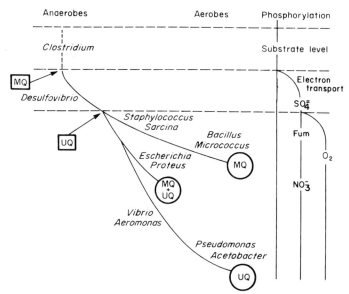

SCHEME 7. Relative positions of menaquinone (MQ) and ubiquinone (UQ) in the evolution of membrane-bound electron transfer phosphorylation.

and *Proteus*. From these descend the obligate aerobes with an exclusive content of UQ, such as *Pseudomonas* and *Acetobacter*. In a parallel branch no UQ was incorporated despite the transition to obligate aerobes. These organisms contain only MQ. Examples are the obligate aerobe bacilli and micrococci.

REFERENCES

Asano, A., and Brodie, A. F. (1963). *Biochem. Biophys. Res. Commun.* **13**, 423.
Asano, A., and Brodie, A. F. (1964). *J. Biol. Chem.* **239**, 4280.
Bäcklin, K. J. (1958). *Acta Chem. Scand.* **12**, 1279.
Bäckström, D., Norling, B., Ehrenberg, A., and Ernster, L. (1970). *Biochim. Biophys. Acta* **197**, 108.
Benziman, M., and Goldhamer, H. (1968). *Biochem. J.* **108**, 311.
Bishop, D. H. L., and King, H. K. (1962). *Biochem. J.* **85**, 550.
Bishop, D. H. L., Pandya, K. P., and King, H. K. (1962). *Biochem. J.* **83**, 606.
Borsook, H. (1935). *Ergeb. Enzymforsch.* **4**, 1.
Borst, P. (1963). *In* "Funktionelle und morphologische Organisation der Zelle" (P. Karlson, ed.), p. 137. Springer, Berlin.
Bragg, P. D., and Hou, C. (1967). *Arch. Biochem. Biophys.* **119**, 194.
Brodie, A. F. (1965). *In* "Biochemistry of Quinones" (R. A. Morton, ed.), p. 356. Academic Press, New York.
Bryla, J., Kaniuga, Z., and Slater, E. C. (1969). *Biochim. Biophys. Acta* **189**, 317.
Bücher, T. (1970). *In* "Pyridine Nucleotide Dependent Dehydrogenases" (H. Sund. ed.), p. 439. Springer, Berlin.
Bücher, T., and Klingenberg, M. (1958). *Angew. Chem.* **70**, 552.
Chance, B. (1965). *In* "Biochemistry of Quinones" (R. A. Morton, ed.), p. 460. Academic Press, New York.
Chance, B., and Baltscheffsky, H. (1958). *J. Biol. Chem.* **233**, 736.
Chance, B., and Hollunger, G. (1960). *Nature (London)* **185**, 666.
Chance, B., and Hollunger, G. (1961). *J. Biol. Chem.* **236**, 1534.
Chance, B., and Pring, M. (1968). *In* "Biochemie des Sauerstoffs" (B. Hess and Hj. Staudinger, eds.), p. 102. Springer, Berlin.
Chance, B., and Williams, G. P. (1956). *Advan. Enzymol.* **14**, 65.
Chance, B., Bonner, W. D., and Storey, B. T. (1968). *Annu. Rev. Plant Physiol.* **19**, 295.
Chance, B., Azzi, A., Lee, I. Y., Lee, C. P., and Mela, L. (1969). *In* "Mitochondria—Structure and Function" (L. Ernster, ed.), p. 233. Academic Press, New York.
Chappell, J. B. (1968). *Brit. Med. Bull.* **24**, 150.
Chappell, J. B. (1969). *In* "Inhibitors—Tools in Cell Research" (T. Bücher and H. Sies, eds.), p. 335. Springer, Berlin.
Cox, G. B., Snoswell, A. M., and Gibson, F. (1968). *Biochim. Biophys. Acta* **153**, 1.
Crane, F. L. (1968). *In* "Biological Oxidations" (T. P. Singer, ed.), p. 533. Wiley (Interscience), New York.
Crane, F. L., and Löw, H. (1966). *Physiol. Rev.* **46**, 662.
Daniel, R. M., and Redfearn, E. R. (1968). *Biochem. J.* **106**, 49P.
Decker, K., Jungermann, K., and Thauer, R. K. (1970). *Angew. Chem.* **82**, 153.
Deeb, S. S., and Hager, L. P. (1964). *J. Biol. Chem.* **239**, 1024.
Downey, R. J., Georgi, C. E. and Militzer, W. E. (1962). *J. Bacteriol.* **83**, 1140.
Ernster, L., Lee, I. Y., Norling, B., and Persson, B. (1969). *Eur. J. Biochem.* **9**, 299.

Ernster, L., Lee, I. Y., Norling, B., and Persson, B. (1970). *In* "Electron Transport and Energy Conservation" (J. M. Tager *et al.*, eds.). Adriatica Editrice, Bari (in press).

Fujita, M., Ishikawa, S., and Shimazono, N. (1966). *J. Biochem.* (*Tokyo*) **59**, 104.

Gale, P. H., Arison, B. H., Trenner, N. R., Page, A. C., Folkers, K., and Brodie, A. F. (1963). *Biochemistry* **2**, 200.

Goebell, H., and Klingenberg, M. (1963). *Biochem. Biophys. Res. Commun.* **13**, 209.

Green, D. E. (1963). *Proc. 5th Int. Congr. Biochem., 1961,* Plen. Lect.

Hirsch, D., Rasminsky, M., Davis, B. D., and Lin, E. C. (1963). *J. Biol. Chem.* **238**, 3370.

Hülsmann, S., Kröger, A., and Klingenberg, M. (1969). Unpublished results.

Ikuma, H., and Bonner, W. D. (1967). *Plant Physiol.* **42**, 67.

Itagaki, E. (1964). *J. Biochem.* **55**, 432.

Johnson, M. J. (1960). *In* "The Enzymes" (P. D. Boyer, H. Lardy, and K. Myrbäck, eds.), 2nd rev. ed., Vol. 2, p. 407. Academic Press, New York.

Kadenbach, B. (1966). *Biochem. Z.* **344**, 49.

Kashkett, E. R., and Brodie, A. F. (1963a). *Biochim. Biophys. Acta* **78**, 52.

Kashkett, E. R., and Brodie, A. F. (1963b). *J. Biol. Chem.* **238**, 2564.

King, T. E. (1967). *Methods Enzymol.* **10**, 322.

Klingenberg, M. (1961). *In* "Zur Bedeutung der freien Nukleotide," 11. Mosbach Coll. p. 82. Springer, Berlin.

Klingenberg, M. (1962). *In* "Funktionelle und morphologische Organisation der Zelle" (P. Karlson, ed.), p. 69. Springer, Berlin.

Klingenberg, M. (1963). *In* "Energy-Linked Functions of Mitochondria" (B. Chance, ed.), Discussion comment, p. 270. Academic Press, New York.

Klingenberg, M. (1964a). *Angew. Chem., Int. Ed. Engl.* **3**, 54.

Klingenberg, M. (1964b). *Ergeb. Physiol., Biol. Chem. Exp. Pharmakol.* **55**, 129.

Klingenberg, M. (1964c). *In* "Rapid Mixing and Sampling Techniques in Biochemistry" (B. Chance *et al.*, eds.), p. 61. Academic Press, New York.

Klingenberg, M. (1965). *In* "Control of Energy Metabolism" (B. Chance *et al.*, eds.), p. 149. Academic Press, New York.

Klingenberg, M. (1968). *In* "Biological Oxidations" (T. P. Singer, ed.), p. 3. Wiley (Interscience), New York.

Klingenberg, M., and Bode, C. (1965). *In* "Recent Research in Carnitine" (G. Wolf, ed.), p. 87. M. I. T. Press, Cambridge, Massachusetts.

Klingenberg, M., and Bücher, T. (1959). *Biochem. Z.* **331**, 312.

Klingenberg, M., and Buchholz, M. (1970). *Eur. J. Biochem.* **13**, 247.

Klingenberg, M., and Kröger, A. (1966). *In* "Biochemistry of Mitochondria" (E. C. Slater *et al.*, eds.), p. 11. Academic Press, New York.

Klingenberg, M., and Kröger, A. (1969). *In* "Electron Transport and Energy Conservation" (J. M. Tager *et al.*, eds.), p. 135. Adriatica Editrice, Bari.

Klingenberg, M., and Pette, D. (1962). *Biochem. Biophys. Res. Commun.* **7**, 430.

Klingenberg, M., and Pfaff, E. (1965). *In* "Regulation of Metabolic Processes in Mitochondria" (J. M. Tager *et al.*, eds.), p. 180. Elsevier, Amsterdam.

Klingenberg, M., and Slenczka, W. (1959). *Biochem. Z.* **331**, 486.

Klingenberg, M., and von Häfen, H. (1963). *Biochem. Z.* **337**, 120.

Klingenberg, M., and von Jagow, G. (1970). *In* "Electron Transport and Energy Conservation" (J. M. Tager *et al.*, eds.), p. 281. Adriatica Editrice, Bari.

Klingenberg, M., Slenczka, W., and Ritt, E. (1959). *Biochem. Z.* **332**, 47.

Klingenberg, M., von Häfen, H., and Wenske, G. (1965). *Biochem. Z.* **343**, 452.

Klingenberg, M., Heldt, H. W., and Pfaff, E. (1969). *In* "The Energy Level and Metabolic Control in Mitochondria" (S. Papa *et al.*, eds.), p. 237. Adriatica Editrice, Bari.

Knowles, C. J., and Redfearn, E. R. (1966). *Biochem. J.* **99**, 33P.

Krebs, H. A., and Veech, R. L. (1970). *In* "Pyridine Nucleotide Dependent Dehydrogenases" (H. Sund, ed.), p. 416. Springer, Berlin.

Kröger, A. (1969). *In* "Electron Transport and Energy Conservation" (J. M. Tager *et al.*, eds.), p. 145. Adriatica Editrice, Bari.

Kröger, A. (1970). *In* "Electron Transport and Energy Conservation" (J. M. Tager *et al.*, eds.). Adriatica Editrice, Bari.

Kröger, A., and Dadak, V. (1968). *Z. Physiol. Chem.* **349**, 9.

Kröger, A., and Dadak, V. (1969). *Eur. J. Biochem.* **11**, 328.

Kröger, A., and Klingenberg, M. (1966). *Biochem. Z.* **344**, 317.

Kröger, A., and Klingenberg, M. (1967). *In* "Current Topics in Bioenergetics" (D. R. Sanadi, ed.), Vol. 2, p. 176. Academic Press, New York.

Kröger, A., and Klingenberg, M. (1970). To be published.

Kröger, A., Dadak, V., Klingenberg, M., and Diemer, F. (1970). To be published.

Kröger, A., and Klingenberg, M. (1970). Unpublished results.

Lee, C. P., and Ernster, L. (1966). *In* "Regulation of Metabolic Processes in Mitochondria" (J. M. Tager *et al.*, eds.), p. 218. Elsevier, Amsterdam.

Lee, C. P., Estabrook, R. W., and Chance, B. (1965). *Biochim. Biophys. Acta* **99**, 32.

Lee, I. Y., Kröger, A., and Klingenberg, M. (1970). *Fed. Proc., Fed. Amer. Soc. Exp. Biol.* **29**, 899.

Lee, Y. P., Takemori, A. E., and Lardy, H. A. (1959). *J. Biol. Chem.* **234**, 3051.

Light, A., Ragan, C., and Garland, P. (1968). *FEBS Letters* **1**, 4.

Maroc, J. R., Azerad, R. Kamen, M. D., and Le Gall, J. (1970). *Biochim. Biophys. Acta* **197**, 87.

Mathews, M. B., and Vennesland, B. (1950). *J. Biol. Chem.* **186**, 667.

Minikami, S., Schindler, F. J., and Estabrook, R. W. (1964). *J. Biol. Chem.* **239**, 2049.

Mitchell, P. (1966). *Biol. Rev.* **41**, 445.

Mitchell, P., and Moyle, J. (1956). *Biochem. J.* **64**, 19P.

Mitchell, P., and Moyle, J. (1967). *Biochem. J.* **105**, 1147.

Morton, R. A. (1965). *In* "Biochemistry of Quinenes." p. 4, Academic Press.

Ohnishi, K. (1966). *J. Biochem.* **59**, 1.

Ohnishi, T., Kawaguchi, L., and Hagihara, B. (1966a). *J. Biol. Chem.* **241**, 1797.

Ohnishi, T., Sottocasa, G. L., and Ernster, L. (1966b). *Bull. Soc. Chim. Biol.* **48**, 1189.

Ohnishi, T., Kröger, A., Heldt, H. W., Pfaff, E., and Klingenberg, M. (1967). *Eur. J. Biochem.* **1**, 301.

Polglase, W. J., Pun, W. T., and Withaar, J. (1966). *Biochim. Biophys. Acta* **118**, 425.

Purvis, J. L., and Lowenstein, J. M. (1961). *J. Biol. Chem.* **236**, 2794.

Redfearn, E. R. (1966). *Vitam. Horm. (New York)* **24**, 465.

Redfearn, E. R., and Kröger, A. (1967). Unpublished results.

Rieske, J. H., Baum, H., Stoner, C. D., and Lipton, S. H. (1967). *J. Biol. Chem.* **242**, 4854.

Rodkey, F. L. (1959). *J. Biol. Chem.* **234**, 188.

Schnorf, U. (1966). Dissertation, No. 3871. Eidgenössische Technische Hochschule, Zürich.

Smith, L. (1968). *In* "Biological Oxidations" (T. P. Singer, ed.), p. 55. Wiley (Interscience), New York.

Snoswell, A. M., and Cox, G. B. (1968). *Biochem. Biophys. Acta* **162**, 455.

Storey, B. T. (1967). *Arch. Biochem. Biophys.* **121**, 261.

Storey, B. T. (1968). *Arch. Biochem. Biophys.* **126**, 585.

Storey, B. T., and Bahr, J. T. (1969). *Plant Physiol.* **44**, 115.

Storey, B. T., and Chance, B. (1967). *Arch. Biochem. Biophys.* **121**, 279.

Swank, R. T., and Burris, R. H. (1969). *J. Bacteriol.* **98**, 311.

Szarkowska, L. (1966). *Arch. Biochem. Biophys.* **113**, 519.

Szarkowska, L., and Klingenberg, M. (1963). *Biochem. Z.* **338**, 674.

Tager, J. M., and Slater, E. C. (1963). *Biochim. Biophys. Acta* **77**, 227.

Urban, P. F., and Klingenberg, M. (1969). *Eur. J. Biochem.* **9**, 519.

von Jagow, G., and Klingenberg, M. (1970). *Eur. J. Biochem.* **12**, 583.

Weber, M. M., and Rosso, G. (1963). *Proc. Nat. Acad. Sci. U. S.* **50**, 710.

Weber, M. M., Hollocher, T. C., and Rosso, G. (1965). *J. Biol. Chem.* **240**, 1776.

Weibull, C., and Bergström, C. (1958). *Biochem. Biophys. Acta* **30**, 340.

Weiss, H., von Jagow, G., Klingenberg, M., and Bücher, T. (1970). *Eur. J. Biochem.* **14**, 75.

White, D. C. (1965). *J. Biol. Chem.* **240**, 1387.

Williamson, D. H., Lund, P., and Krebs, H. A. (1967). *Biochem. J.* **103**, 514.

Young, H. L., and Pace, N. (1958). *Arch. Biochem. Biophys.* **75**, 125.

Au Revoir

HUGO THEORELL

Ladies and Gentlemen: Dr. Harris has invited me to say a few words of "farewell." After all that has happened to us during these two days, I am sure you all agree with me that the more optimistic French expression "au revoir" would be more appropriate, since we all would like to meet again somewhere at some time.

This has been a fantastic meeting. Let me, on behalf of the participants, convey our heartfelt thanks to Professor Harris, Professor Wiss, Dr. Weber, and the remainder of the organizing committee for organizing this excellent symposium, to Hoffmann-Le Roche Company for its generosity in supporting it, and for the overwhelming friendliness which has surrounded these meetings.

I myself have a very special reason to thank you. It is a great honor you have bestowed on me in dedicating this symposium to my name. I don't think I have deserved it. You have given me too many flowers. On the other hand, have you ever heard of anyone who refused to accept flowers because there were too many? So please, receive my heartfelt thanks!

I feel that organizing an excellent scientific meeting is like presenting a marvelous concert. May I ask you to join me in expressing gratitude to our hosts and to all participants in the same way as in a concert hall or theater, by giving them a "standing ovation"?

Author Index

Numbers in italics indicate the page on which the complete reference is listed.

A

Aarskog, D., 13, 16, 22, 26, *30*
Abaturov, L. V., 168, *190*
Abbott, J. C., 436, *440*
Abeles, R. H., 401, *414*
Abraham, S., 227, *242*
Abramovich, D. R., 12, 15, 19, 20, *30*
Achiwa, K., 400, *414*
Acs, Z., 14, *35*
Actis, A. S., 381, 391, *397*
Adam, P. A. J., 39, 40, 85, *87*
Adams, D. H., 117, *134*
Adams, E., 400, *414*
Adams, M. J., *87*, 199, 201, *209*
Adamsons, K., 28, *34*
Adesman, J., 84, *99*
Aebi, H., 206, *210*
Aguilar-Parada, E., 65, 80, *97*
Ahn, C. S., 74, *97*
Aho, I., 105, 116, *137, 138*
Ailhaud, G. P., 330, *343*
Akagami, H., 234, 237, *242*
Akerblom, H. K., 79, *96*
Akeson, A., 206, 207, *209, 210*
Akhtar, M., 400, *414*
Akre, P. R., 38, 43, *87*
Albert, A., 489, *503*
Albert, J. D., 269, *290*
Alberts, A. W., 215, 228, 229, *241, 242*, 330, 340, *343*, 351, *363*
Albrecht, A. C., 446, *464*
Albright, F., 105, *134*
Aleman, V., 305, *314*
Alexander, N., 456, *465*
Allen, W. M., 6, *34*
Allison, S. P., 81, *87*
Allison, W. S., 201, *209*, 325, *326*
Allmann, D. W., 218, 227, *241*
Alric, R., 75, *95*
Amick, R. M., 304, *314*, 442, *465*, 468, *486*

Ammon, J., 81, *97*
Anast, C., 106, 110, *134, 138*
Anderson, A. B. M., 28, *30*
Anderson, E., 79, *87*
Anderson, G. E., 65, *87*
Anderson, J., 76, *99*
Anderson, K. J. I., 43, *96*
Andrae, W. A., 459, *464*
Anfinsen, C. B., 50, 59, *100*
Angers, M., 5, *32*
Angevine, D. M., 10, 21, 22, *30*
Anker, H. S., 215, 238, *242*
Antonini, E., 178, 183, *191*
Aoji, O., 84, *101*
Apella, E., 195, *209*
Aprile, M. A., 42, *96*
Arata, H., 366, 376, *396*
Archer, D. F., 8, 9, 24, *35*
Arens, A., 44, 45, *99*
Arias, I. M., 225, *241*, 292, *300*
Arigoni, D., 407, 411, *413*
Arison, B. H., 563, *572*
Arnaud, C. D., Jr., 104, 106, 110, 114, *134, 138*
Arnott, J. H., 42, *94*
Arquilla, E. R., 41, 42, 43, *87, 91*
Arrio-Dupont, M., 167, *191*
Asano, A., 563, 564, 566, *571*
Asano, T., 69, *92*
Aschheim, S., 2, *30*
Ashcroft, S. J. H., 55, 56, 57, 67, 75, *87*, *97*
Ashmore, J., 37, 72, *95, 96*
Ask-Upmark, M. E., 6, *30*
Asplund, K., 85, *87*
Aten, B., 39, 44, 59, 60, *99*
Atherton, N. M., 499, *504*
Athos, W., 20, *32*
Au, W. Y. W., 113, *138*
August, J. T., 47, *87*
Auhagen, E., 365, *394*

577

Subject Index